Acute Nursing Care

Delays in recognising deterioration, or inappropriate management of people in acute care settings can result in late treatment, avoidable admissions to intensive care units and, in some instances, unnecessary deaths. As the role of the nurse in healthcare settings continues to change and evolve, today's nursing and other healthcare students need to be equipped with the fundamental skills to recognise and manage deterioration in the patient in a competent and confident manner, appreciating the complexities of caring for those who are acutely unwell as you learn to become practitioners of the future.

Using a body systems approach, and fully updated in light of new NEWS2 and NMC future nurse standards, as well as acknowledging the challenges faced by people with delirium in acute care settings, the second edition of this book provides a comprehensive overview of the essential issues in this important subject. Topics covered include recognition and identification of physiological and mental deterioration in adults; identification of disordered physiology that may lead to a medical emergency linked to deterioration of normal function; relevant anatomy and physiology; pathophysiological changes and actions that need to be taken; immediate recognition and response; investigations, diagnosis and management issues; and teaching and preventative strategies.

Including case studies and test yourself questions, this book is an essential tool for student nurses who are required to undertake acute care experiences and are assessed in theory and practice.

Ian Peate, OBE FRCN; Visiting Professor of Nursing, St George's University of London and Kingston University, London; Visiting Professor Northumbria University; Visiting Senior Clinical Fellow University of Hertfordshire; Head of School, School of Health Studies, Gibraltar; Editor in Chief, *British Journal of Nursing*.

Ian began his nursing career at Central Middlesex Hospital, becoming an Enrolled Nurse practicing in an intensive care unit. He later undertook three years of student nurse training, becoming a Staff Nurse, then a Charge Nurse. He has worked in nurse education since 1989. His key areas of interest are nursing practice and theory. Ian has published widely. He was awarded an OBE in the Queen's 90th Birthday Honours List for his services to Nursing and Nurse Education and was bestowed a Fellowship from the Royal College of Nursing in 2017.

Helen Dutton, RGN; ENB100; RNT; BA Nursing Education (Manchester); MSc (London); Senior Fellow of the Higher Education Academy; Senior Lecturer Critical Care, College of Nursing Midwifery and Healthcare, University of West London.

Helen completed her RGN at Addenbrooke's Hospital, Cambridge. After gaining experience in medical and surgical nursing, she moved to St Thomas' Hospital, London to work in intensive care, then moved to become a Sister in Cardiothoracic Intensive Care at the Royal Brompton and Harefield NHS Trust. Her education career started at the Royal Brompton, then moved on to higher education. She is currently employed as a Senior Lecturer in Critical Care at the University of West London. Helen is course leader for BSc (Hons) Clinical Practice. Intensive and critical care nursing have been her main focus, leading the development of post qualifying critical care courses at the Univerity of West London. She has published in her areas of interest: acute/enhanced/high dependency care, physical examinations skill for health care professionals and the early recognition and treatment of those who are at risk of deterioration.

Acute Nursing Care

Recognising and Responding to Medical Emergencies

Second Edition

Ian Peate and Helen Dutton

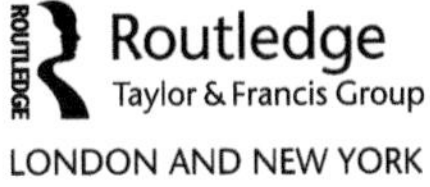
LONDON AND NEW YORK

Second edition published 2021
by Routledge
2 Park Square, Milton Park, Abingdon, Oxon, OX14 4RN

and by Routledge
52 Vanderbilt Avenue, New York, NY 10017

Routledge is an imprint of the Taylor & Francis Group, an informa business

First edition published by Pearson 2012

British Library Cataloguing-in-Publication Data
A catalogue record for this book is available from the British Library

Library of Congress Cataloguing-in-Publication Data
Names: Peate, Ian, author. | Dutton, Helen, author.
Title: Acute nursing care: recognising and responding to medical emergencies/ Ian Peate and Helen Dutton.
Description: Second edition. | Milton Park, Abingdon, Oxon; New York, NY: Routledge, 2020. | Includes bibliographical references and index. |
Identifiers: LCCN 2020012414 (print) | LCCN 2020012415 (ebook) |
ISBN 9781138352001 (hardback) | ISBN 9781138352018 (paperback) |
ISBN 9780429434938 (ebook)
Subjects: LCSH: Intensive care nursing. | Emergency nursing.
Classification: LCC RT120.I5 P33 2020 (print) | LCC RT120.I5 (ebook) |
DDC 616.02/8–dc23
LC record available at https://lccn.loc.gov/2020012414
LC ebook record available at https://lccn.loc.gov/2020012415

ISBN: 978-1-138-35200-1 (hbk)
ISBN: 978-1-138-35201-8 (pbk)
ISBN: 978-0-429-43493-8 (ebk)

Typeset in Bembo
By Deanta Global Publishing Services, Chennai, India

This text is dedicated to the health and social work workforce who lost their lives to COVID-19

Contents

Figures

Tables

Contributors

Luke Cox, BSc (Hons), RN, PGDip (Clin Ed), FHEA
Lecturer in Simulated Learning, University of West London
Luke has worked as a senior nurse in a variety of acute clinical settings, including Coronary Care at St. Bartholomew's Hospital, and St. Thomas' Hospital Emergency Department. Alongside contributions to nursing education, he has an interest in how human factors contribute to safety in clinical settings. Luke is now a lecturer in pre-registration and post-graduate nursing courses at the University of West London.

Sharon Elliott, MSc, BA(Hons), RCNT RN
Head of Pre-Registration Nursing, University of West London
Sharon began her nursing a career in 1983 at The Royal London Hospital as a registered nurse working in Head and Neck Surgery and Trauma. Her key areas of interest are nursing practice, simulated learning and curriculum design and development.

Adrian Jugdoyal, Pg Dip, PgCAP, BSc (Hons), BSc (Hons), Dip HE, Dip HE, Cert HE, RGN, RMN, NMP, TCH, FHEA
Senior Lecturer, Middlesex University, London
Adrian is currently a Director of Programmes/Senior Lecturer at Middlesex University. He teaches across the nursing curriculum and is interested in simulated learning and augmented realty in clinical assessments. He is a committee member of the the British Association of the study of the Liver (BASL), British Liver Nurses Association (BLNA) British Society of Gastroenterology, (BSG) International Nurses Society in Addictions (IntNSA) as well as the Chapter President of IntNSA. He is a member of Drug and Alcohol Nurses of Australia (DANA) and The society of Acute Medicine (SAM) as well as on the Editorial Panel for Gastrointestinal Nursing Journal. Adrian is heavily involved in projects in the UK and around the world working towards widening awareness of SUD and liver disease in non specialist practitioners.

Muili Lawal, BSc (Hons), PGDE, MA, PhD
Senior Lecturer, University of West London, London
Muili is a Senior Lecturer at the University of West London, and his education and teaching experience span through three different continents: from Europe to North America and Africa. Muili is currently an external examiner for two UK universities, and he promotes the ethos of self-management in long-term conditions through teaching, conference presentations and published work.

Rebecca Maindonald, RN, MSN
Senior Lecturer, Adult Nursing, University of West London
Rebecca has worked as a nurse for 15 years in both the United States and the United Kingdom. Her experience in acute care includes Staff Nurse and Charge Nurse in Cardiology, Orthopaedics, Neurology, and Gastrointestinal care. Rebecca's education experience ranges from lecturing to bedside clinical instruction and simulation, and she has been lucky enough to teach nursing students at Texas Tech University, University of Texas at Austin, Austin Community College, and most recently University of West London.

John Mears, BSc (Comb Hons), MSc, Dip N (Lond), Cert Ed (Post 16), RNT, SRN
John trained at St George's hospital London, 1976 to 1978. This was followed by a Staff Nurse post on a mixed cardiology/cardiac surgery ward. During this time, he was seconded to the School of Nursing for periods of time to assist. From 1981 onwards, he held a number of educational posts within the changing and evolving nursing education system in West London, eventually taking a senior lecturer post in the University of West London.

He is now retired, but continues to lecture in anatomy, physiology and pathophysiology underpinning clinical practice.

Ian Naldrett, RN, RNT FHEA, Advanced DipHE (Acute care nursing), BSc Hons (Intensive care nursing), MSc Professional practice
Ian Naldrett qualified as a nurse in 2008 working in a variety of acute inpatient areas and has worked in intensive care since 2010. Currently, he holds the position of Lecturer Practitioner in intensive care nursing across the Royal Brompton Hospital and University of West London. He is currently on the British association of critical care national board as a regional advisor, is the representative from British Association of Critical Care Nurses (BACCN) for European federation of Critical Care Nurse associations (EfCCNa) and is on the BACCN board.

Caroline Smales, MSc, BSc, RGN, Cert Ed
Senior Lecturer, College of Nursing, Midwifery and Health Care, University of West London (UWL)
Caroline began her nursing career as a student at the Middlesex Hospital, London, before moving to Northwick Park Hospital as a staff nurse in infectious diseases, then moving into intensive care nursing before becoming a ward Sister in acute medical care and infectious diseases. She currently delivers infection control link nurse courses and is part of the team delivering an MSc Infection Prevention and Control course at UWL.

Kit Tong, BSc in Healthcare (Nursing), PGCE, MSc in Advancing Practice, FHEA,
Senior Lecturer in Adult Nursing, University of West London
Kit completed her nursing training in 1992 and became a Staff Nurse in a High Dependency and surgical ward in Singapore General Hospital. After two years, she transferred to the Intensive Care Unit and further trained as a Critical Care Nurse. Currently, she is working in the University of West London as a Senior Lecturer, teaching in the Pre-Registration Nursing Programme and supporting the postgraduate teaching and learning as well. She has a special interest in Critical Care Nursing, in particular neurology, preceptorship and learning in the workplace.

Michelle Treacy, RGN, RNT, FHEA, BSc (Nursing), MSc, PhD student
Senior Lecturer, College of Nursing, Midwifery and Healthcare, University of West London

Michelle qualified as an adult nurse at St. Angela's College, Sligo, Ireland. Following a period as a staff nurse at Sligo General Hospital, she then moved to the Royal Berkshire NHS Trust. Here, she specialised in intensive care nursing alongside developing a passion for education. Michelle leads on the intensive care course and is course leader for the advanced clinical practitioner degree. She is committed to evolving the NHS workforce through education. Her key areas of interests are: patient deterioration, sepsis recognition and delirium in the ICU. Concurrently, she is undertaking a PhD focused on the implementation of early warning scores in acute care.

Anthony Wheeldon, MSc (Lond), PGDE, BSc(Hons), DipHE, RN
Department of Nursing, Health and Wellbeing, School of Health and Social Work, University of Hertfordshire

Anthony began his nursing career at Barnet College of Nursing and Midwifery in 1992. After qualification, he worked as a staff nurse and senior staff nurse in the Respiratory Directorate at the Royal Brompton and Harefield NHS Trust in London. Since 2006, Anthony has worked at the University of Hertfordshire, where he teaches on pre and post registration nursing courses. He is currently an Associate Subject Group Lead for Adult Nursing.

Preface

Ian Peate and Helen Dutton

We were delighted to have been asked to edit a second edition of the very popular *Acute Nursing Care. Recognising and Responding to Medical Emergencies*. The feedback from readers of the first edition were very generous and complementary, and we are pleased to provide you with a fully updated and revised copy of the first edition. The aims of this new edition are similar to the previous edition; this text sets out to meet the needs of a range of health care workers, including student nurses who are working towards graduate status and professional registration, the trainee nursing associate who has become an integral part of the health and social care multidisciplinary team, those practitioners returning to practice as well as the newly qualified practitioner who has chosen to begin their professional career in the acute care setting.

There are, and there will continue to be changes in how health and social care is delivered, demonstrating that a larger proportion of care will take place outside of traditional care settings. This strategic shift for nursing, from hospital to community, for example, will focus on prevention, with patients and the public as the drivers of their care. Nurses have to be aware of changes in health care settings and the needs of the communities they offer services to, responding to both current and future need. The need to care for and respond appropriately to people who are experiencing medical emergencies is also changing and is ongoing as the technological support provided to people continues to advance. Medical advances and major developments in technology mean that the nurse of the future must be prepared to work safely and confidently in a number of care environments, providing care that is compassionate and effective. The knowledge base provided here is one that is rooted in applied physiology and some of the disorders that may give rise to a medical emergency.

The Nursing and Midwifery Council (NMC) have issued standards that must be achieved prior to registration with the NMC to practise as a nurse. These include a standards framework for nursing and midwifery education (NMC 2019) and proficiencies for the registered nurse (NMC 2018a) and the nursing associate (NMC 2018b). The proficiencies lay out what must be achieved when the student is at the point of registration. This text was written with those standards and proficiencies in mind, helping you to achieve the skills required within the sphere of medical emergencies. The practice of delivering nursing care involves a capacity not only to participate actively in care provision, but also to accept accountability and responsibility for the effective and efficient management of that care, practised within a safe environment. This involves:

- The capacity to understand and accept accountability.
- Taking responsibility for the delegation of aspects of care to others.

- Effectively supervising and facilitating the work of such carers.
- The capacity to work effectively within the nursing and wider multidisciplinary health and social care team.
- Accepting leadership roles, where appropriate, within such teams, and demonstrating overall competency in care and case management.

As well as being proficient practitioners, nurses must also be concerned with the environment of care and the interest and safety of people in their care. The nurse must make concerns about failing standards of public protection known to the NMC, and do this through the *Code of Conduct* (NMC 2018c). Nurses have a duty to protect the vulnerable in our society. The *Code* makes clear what is expected of the nurse and is a key tool in delivering effective public protection. While the student nurse is not subjected to the *Code of Conduct*, they should strive to meet those standards under the auspices of a registered nurse; the content in this book aims to advance this. This text will help you become a proficient nurse as well as encourage you to uphold the reputation of our profession.

It is the student nurse who will become the dynamic, responsive nurse of tomorrow, with the ability to adapt to meet the dynamic and changing needs of the public in a number of situations and settings. This text provides you with the principles on which to offer effective, safe, acute medical care to adults in a hospital setting. The nurse works with other highly skilled health and social care professionals, and this interdisciplinary role will be emphasised throughout. The registered nurse is required to demonstrate that they have the skills associated with higher level decision-making, become an autonomous practitioner and have at the heart of all you do the safety of the people you have the privilege to care for.

The coming years will see a change in the way health and social care is delivered, with a focus upon the need to continue to maximise the contribution that nurses make to the demands placed upon health and social services by society, government and technological changes.

You will be required to respond effectively to medical emergencies, and this text will enable you to learn the fundamentals in order to do this as you learn to become a practitioner of the future – the future nurse. There is a clear need for change to enable nurses to meet the demands arising from a contemporary health service; being aware of this, and honing the skills required to make that change and to be an effective member of health and social services are absolute prerequisites.

Future career frameworks will take into account nurses from all fields providing broad categories of service delivery. One category particularly pertinent to this text (but not exclusively) is acute and critical care. Other categories, for example, the first contact, access and urgent care and managing long-term conditions, are also worthy of consideration.

Care provision is becoming more complex. An ageing population, technological developments, shorter length of stay and higher consumer expectations will result in the provision of a higher level of care than has been previously offered. You will therefore need to be equipped with the skills to recognise and manage deterioration in the patient in a competent and confident manner.

Delays in recognising deterioration in a patient's condition and treating and managing that condition appropriately can and does result in avoidable admission to intensive care units and, in some cases, unnecessary deaths. This text will help you improve and develop competence and confidence when caring for the acutely ill patient.

The level at which the information contained in this book is presented makes this a unique text. A fundamental approach is used to enable and encourage you to apply the content to contexts that you may find yourself in. It adopts a user-friendly approach. There are a number of features in the book that help this process happen.

In order to apply theory to practice, each chapter provides a range of teaching features, for example, the inclusion of case studies that can make the understanding and application of some complex concepts easier to come to terms with and assimilate. The case studies will 'set the scene' for the application of chapter content to (as near as possible) clinical practice. There are aims and objectives that provide you with structured, guided learning. A glossary of terms at the end of each chapter is provided to help you to develop your nursing and medical vocabulary even further.

The chapters within the text provide you with links to relevant and related websites to help guide and support learning, links to professional and statutory websites such as the Nursing and Midwifery Council (NMC), the Department of Health and Social Care (DHSC), National Institute for Health and Care Excellence (NICE) and the Scottish Intercollegiate Guidelines Network (SIGN). A bank of multiple-choice test questions is provided with the aim of reinforcing your learning.

The use of illustrations is key to this text, providing you with visual stimulation which promotes learning and aids retention. Line drawings are used, and outlines of diagnostic and investigatory tests and procedures provided. Where appropriate, the provision of diagnostic test outcomes will be supplied to demonstrate the 'normal' and 'abnormal', for example, a 'normal' electrocardiograph (ECG) and an 'abnormal' ECG depicting a cardiac arrhythmia.

A word or two on normal values is important. There are a variety of techniques that those who analyse blood, for example, use in the laboratory to identify the various components. These techniques may differ from laboratory to laboratory, and it is essential that when assessment of blood results is carried out, referral to the local laboratory's normal values is made. The values provided here are related to a full blood count and are offered only as a guide, rather than a fixed indicator of limits. Variation occurs across the UK, Europe and globally. These variations will also occur with a person's age, gender and co-morbidity. Any variation has the potential to artificially alter a situation, triggering a response that may not be appropriate when the person is stable and not in danger.

The overarching aim of the text is to help you better understand the fundamental aspects associated with a number of acute medical conditions in order to provide skilled and effective care to patients in various situations. The use of a contemporary evidence base will encourage safe and effective practice.

It is hoped that you will develop your caring skills with a sound knowledge base underpinning the delivery of care – preparing you for registration with the NMC. This book is based upon the principles of care and is a foundation text that will encourage you to grow and develop.

The structure promotes the concept of lifelong learning, supporting you and encouraging you to delve deeper and discover further, to become even more curious. Referral to the *Code* (NMC 2018c) encourages you to practise ethically and morally, with the patient's best interests at the heart of all that is done.

The book is designed to be used as a reference text in either the clinical setting, the classroom or at home, and is not intended to be read from cover to cover in one sitting. It will provide you with the help you need to respond in a confident and competent manner to a variety of medical emergencies you may come across.

We have enjoyed revising and reviewing this second edition, and we very much hope that you will find it useful and enjoyable. It is our wish that by using this book and applying the principles within it to the care that you offer to the people you nurse, you will be able minimise their distress and the anxieties that are associated with acute illness and critical care.

References

Nursing and Midwifery Council. (2018a). *Future Nurse. Standards of Proficiency for Registered Nurses.* Available from https://www.nmc.org.uk/globalassets/sitedocuments/education-standards/future-nurse-proficiencies.pdf. Accessed October 2019

Nursing and Midwifery Council. (2018b). *Standards of Proficiency for Nursing Associates.* Available from https://www.nmc.org.uk/globalassets/sitedocuments/education-standards/nursing-associates-proficiency-standards.pdf. Accessed October 2019

Nursing and Midwifery Council. (2018c). *The Code. Professional Standards of Practice and Behaviour for Nurses, Midwives and Nursing Associates.* Available from https://www.nmc.org.uk/globalassets/sitedocuments/education-standards/nursing-associates-proficiency-standards.pdf. Accessed October 2019

Nursing and Midwifery Council. (2019). *Standards Framework for Nursing and Midwifery Education.* Available from https://www.nmc.org.uk/globalassets/sitedocuments/education-standards/education-framework.pdf. Accessed October 2019

Acknowledgements

Ian would like to thank his partner, Jussi Lahtinen, for his continued support and Helen Dutton, who has been an absolute joy to work with.

Helen would like to thank her academic and clinical colleagues for their support and enthusiasm with the preparation of this book. All comments and suggestions have been constructive and gratefully received. She would also like to thank Geoff, Emma and Mike for their love, patience and encouragement during this project.

We would like to acknowledge the contributions that previous contributors have made to the first edition. We are appreciative to them for their support and for setting the foundation for this second edition.

Chapter 4: Liz Allibone
Chapter 5: Carl Margereson and Sarah Withey
Chapter 6: Andrew Sargent
Chapter 8: Jacqui Finch
Chapter 9: Katie Scales
Chapter 10: Julian Howard and Angela Morgan
Chapter 11: Julian Howard, Angela Morgan and Margaret Kirkby
Chapter 12: Andrea Blay and Jacqui Finch
Chapter 13: Jacqui Finch

Our appreciation also goes to those who were kind enough to give of their time to review the chapters.

1 Assessment and recognition of emergencies in acute care

Helen Dutton

AIM

This chapter aims to give the reader an insight into the assessment and early identification of risk of clinical deterioration, and the skills required to escalate care in an appropriate and timely manner.

OBJECTIVES

After reading this chapter you will be able to:

- Give an overview of developments to date aimed at supporting the adult who has the potential to become acutely unwell.
- Understand that there are usually clinical signs of deterioration many hours before most life-threatening events.
- Use the National Early Warning Score (NEWS) 2 as a tool to calculate risk, escalate care and become familiar with interdisciplinary communication tools, such as SBAR.
- Perform, analyse and interpret a rapid clinical assessment of a patient who is at risk of deterioration/medical emergency.
- Understand how a 'chain of prevention' can be used to structure processes to detect patient deterioration.
- Have a context on which to base future chapters in recognising and responding to medical emergencies.

Introduction

The ultimate medical emergency, cardiopulmonary arrest, has long been the focus of education and training of health care professions. Resuscitation teams were formed as early as the 1930s, although it was not until 1966 that the first **cardiopulmonary resuscitation (CPR)** guidelines were published. Guidance on CPR continues to be updated every five years and is available at https://www.resus.org.uk. Techniques in addressing cardiopulmonary arrest are improving but results remain disappointing, with survival rates to discharge for in-hospital arrests at 20.4% (National Cardiac Arrest Audit 2017). Previously, much attention was placed on after-arrest care; more recently, however, the emphasis has shifted towards recognising those patients who are at risk of deterioration, with the aim of preventing medical emergencies, such as cardiac arrest, occurring. Expert advice, in the form of **medical emergency teams (MET)** and/or **outreach services,** is now a key feature in acute trusts, alongside tools that identify those at greatest risk of deterioration. The aim is to recognise those at increased risk and to provide timely interventions to prevent deterioration.

Recognition of the problem

Patients who deteriorate and present as a **medical emergency** require critical care. Whatever the cause or precipitating factor of a medical emergency, the physiological consequences for the patient are similar. Medical emergencies affect oxygen delivery to cells, tissues and organs. Oxygen is essential for glucose metabolism and ATP production as, without oxygen cellular and organ dysfunction, failure and death will inevitably ensue. Prompt responses are required to support failing organs until recovery or death, and this often requires the support of critical care services.

The problem is not a new one, with a number of studies in the 1990s highlighting problems with the recognition and management of the acutely unwell patient on adult wards (Goldhill et al. 1999; Schein et al. 1990; McQuillan et al. 1998) The evidence indicated that patients who deteriorate do not normally do so 'out of the blue' but have abnormal clinical parameters often some hours before the presentation of a medical emergency. Findings, such as abnormal respiratory rate, heart rate, adequacy of oxygenation or deteriorating mental status, were strong indicators that a patient was at risk of clinical deterioration. The conclusion drawn from these and other studies was that, if the patient had been identified and treated appropriately earlier, it was likely that the emergency may have been prevented.

Early identification

Although most people in hospital are unlikely to become seriously unwell, a significant number will require interventions in order to prevent or treat acute illness. Individuals move from experiencing minor physiological derangements through a period of deterioration and more serious illness, which, if left undetected and untreated, may progress to a life-threatening medical emergency, culminating in cardiopulmonary arrest. As people move along this continuum of wellness to the stage where death is imminent, they will be experiencing major physiological changes. The body will be attempting to restore homoeostasis by the activation of compensatory mechanisms, such as increased breathing rate or heart rate. These compensatory mechanisms in themselves require additional energy, placing extra physiological demands on the individual. In the early stages of acute illness, these mechanisms may be sufficient to meet the extra demands, healing may occur and the problem resolve. However, if the underlying problem remains untreated, or is unresponsive to treatments, deterioration will continue. There may be a rapid progression of severity of illness resulting in cardiac arrest. Clinical assessment will detect these physiological changes, but the information gained needs to be understood and acted upon to prevent the progression of illness. Examples of acute illnesses that may or may not deteriorate to a medical emergency are included in Table 1.1.

Understanding that signs of compensation may be indicative of acute illness, with the risk of rapid deterioration, helps the nurse interpret the vital signs recorded, so problems

Table 1.1 Examples of acute illnesses that may lead to a medical emergency. Note how compensatory mechanisms of increased RR, HR and decreased adequacy of oxygenation are a feature of most examples

Example of acute illness	*Physiological derangementsand clinical consequences*	*Signs of compensation that may be evident*
Airway swelling	Airway obstruction Failure to ventilate causing hypoxaemia and hypercarbia	Raised HR and blood pressure Intercostal retraction
Acute asthma	Bronchoconstriction reducing airflow through bronchioles and alveoli. Work of breathing increased. SpO_2 falls, hypercarbia may follow	Raised respiratory rate, HR, BP Use of accessory muscles
Pneumothorax	Presence of air in the pleural space, leading to lung collapse Pain Hypoxaemia	Sensation of breathlessness, Use of accessory muscles increasing RR, HR and BP
Myocardial infarction	Death of myocardium due to blockage of a branch of a coronary artery Pain	Raised RR, HR, BP, peripheral vasoconstriction.
Acute left ventricular failure	Failure of the left ventricle to pump blood effectively into the aorta and round the body. Pulmonary venous pressures rise, causing the development of pulmonary oedema, hypoxaemia, frothy sputum	Profound respiratory difficulty and distress Raised RR & HR Use of accessory muscles, peripheral vasoconstriction.
Hypovolaemic shock	Reduction of amount of blood/fluid in the circulation Hypoxaemia	Raised respiratory rate, lowered HR, lowered BP, peripheral vasoconstriction
Sepsis	A dysregulated response to infection causing organ damage Inflammatory mediators cause vasodilation and increased capillary permeability	'New confusion' Raised HR, RR Warm and dilated peripheries Lowered BP

can be addressed early in the continuum of deterioration, averting the medical emergency. Unfortunately, this is not always the case; when problems are recognised, the appropriate treatment and management is not always followed, adversely affecting patient outcome.

The changing nature of acute health care delivery

Over the past few decades, the emphasis has moved from hospital care towards managing health care in the primary sector. The number of overnight and acute beds has fallen, with a reduction of 43.4% between 1987/8 and 2016/17 (King's Fund 2017). The UK currently has fewer acute beds per population than in equivalent health care systems in other, comparable countries.

Changing patterns, in both the population requiring hospital admission and the environment in which acute care is delivered, are evident. The population of the UK has seen a rise of 6.1 years in median age from 1974 to 2014 (ONS 2016). The increasingly aging population, combined with advances in management of many chronic illnesses, has increased the number of older people with several co-morbidities and complex health care needs (DH 2015; Lacobucci 2017). This increases the pressure on hospital admissions and A&E services, with a record number (almost 23.7 million) attendees to A&E recorded in the UK in 2016/17. The seasonal variations in admissions, noted in the winter bed crisis of 1998/9 (Lipley 2000), continue, with the greatest proportion of admissions occurring in the winter months, stretching health care services at this time (NHS Digital 2017). Those admitted require more resources, with greater input from multi-disciplinary teams, as they are much sicker. Advances in health care technology mean that some treatments, previously considered to be high risk, are now considered as a standard of care, placing an increased demand on a stretched acute care delivery service.

The upward trend in number of hospital admissions, mean age and proportion of emergency admissions continues, but with a decreasing mean length of stay. Even though the overall number of patients in hospital is reduced, the number of patients treated is continuing to increase. The growth in critical care provision has continued, with numbers of critical care beds almost doubling from 2,200 in 1999, to 4,018 in June 2018 (Government Statistical Service 2018). However, the high critical care occupancy still causes a significance number of urgent operations to be cancelled due to lack of available critical care beds (Government Statistical Service 2018).

National initiatives in acute and critical care

A major change in configuration of critical care services was recommended by a national expert group report *Comprehensive Critical Care – A Review of Adult Critical Care Services* (DH 2000). Patients were classified according to their level of need, with the appropriate care and necessary resources brought to them, regardless of location. The now familiar four levels of care (level 0–level 3) were identified, and have been clarified with more detailed examples by the Intensive Care Society (2009) (see Table 1.2).

The emphasis on delivering competent care according to clinical need, regardless of patient location, opening access to staff with critical care skills, outside of the pressurised intensive care units, expanded the ability to deliver critical care. The development of **critical care outreach** services was encouraged, and seen to be key to supporting patients who were acutely ill in the ward environment.

The problems of recognising and responding appropriately to prevent clinical deterioration remains an issue for acute care, identified in reports by the National Confidential Enquiry into Patient Outcome and Death (NCEPOD) over the past 15 years (NCEPOD 2017, 2012, 2005). The 2005 report considered the management of acutely unwell medical patients, including a review of 1677 patient over 226 hospitals. Pre-ITU medical review was deemed not acceptable in 10% of ITU admissions, with only 58% of patients receiving prompt and appropriate interventions. Respiratory rate monitoring was poor, and written requests, regarding the type and frequency of observations, rare (NCEPOD 2005). The National Patient Safety Agency (NPSA 2007) found further evidence that sub-optimal care was continuing to contribute to preventable deaths. The most recent report (NCEPOD 2017) focused on patients requiring **non-invasive ventilation** (NIV). They identified that vital signs were not assessed or monitored sufficiently to prevent patient deterioration.

The National Institute for Health and Clinical Excellence (NICE) considered the evidence for physiological **track and trigger systems** and care escalation strategies

Table 1.2 Classification of severity of illness: Level 1 patients are usually cared for in acute wards, Level 2 in acute wards or HDU, Level 3 equivalent to ITU or some HDUs. ICS (2009) Levels of Critical Care for Adult Patients [DOH (2000)]

	DH 2000	*ICS 2009 A selection of specific examples*
Level 0	Those patients whose needs are met through general ward care in an acute hospital.	Intravenous therapy. Observations needed less often than 4-hourly.
Level 1	Those at risk of their condition deteriorating, or patients recently relocated from higher levels of care where their needs can be met on an acute ward with extra advice and support from the critical care team.	Minimum of 4-hourly observations. Observations aligned to clinical need. Patients requiring ongoing oxygen therapy. Those receiving epidural analgesia or patient-controlled analgesia. Post-operative patients still requiring 4-hourly observations. Patients with diabetes receiving a continuous infusion of insulin. Abnormal vital signs but not requiring a higher level of critical care.
Level 2	Patients requiring more detailed observation or intervention which includes support for a single failing organ system or post-operative care, and patients stepping down from higher levels of care.	Basic respiratory support such as requiring 50% oxygen or supported ventilation by face mask (e.g., CPAP, NIV). Basic cardiovascular support. Treatment of a circulatory uncertainty. Use of a CVP line for basic monitoring or central venous access to provide therapeutic agents. Use of an arterial line for basic monitoring of arterial pressure and/or arterial blood sampling. Single intravenous vaso-active drug, supporting or controlling arterial pressure, cardiac output or organ perfusion.
Level 3	Patients requiring advanced respiratory support alone or basic respiratory support along with support of at least two organ systems. This level includes all complex patients needing support for multi-organ failure.	As per DH 2000.

(NICE 2007). They published guidelines for the frequency and type of clinical observations recorded. A pathway describing assessment, recognition of and response to acute illness in adults supported the use of Track and Trigger tools and referral to a team of personnel with core competences in the care of the acutely unwell. A more detailed 'chain of response' (DH 2009) suggested roles for health care teams at each stage of the recognition and care escalation process (see Figure 1.1).

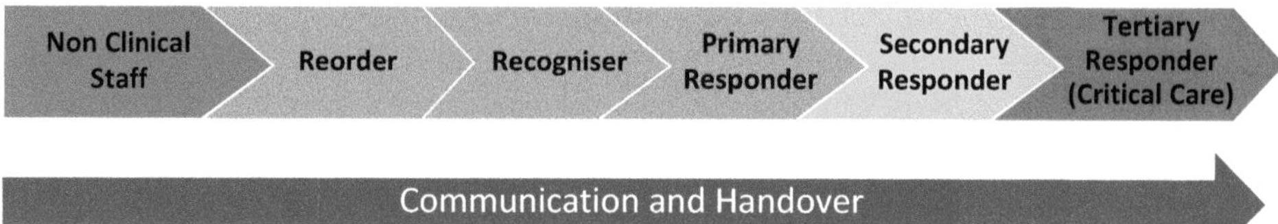

Non- Clinical staff	May also be the 'alerter' may include the patient or visitor.
The recorder	Takes designated measurements, records observations and information.
The recogniser	Monitors the patient's condition, interprets designated measurements, observations and information and adjusts the frequency of observations and level of monitoring.
The primary responder	Goes beyond recording and further observation by interpreting the measurements and initiating a clinical management plan e.g., commencing oxygen therapy, insertion of airway adjuncts, selection of Intravenous fluids and administration of a bolus of fluid.
The secondary responder	Likely to be called to attend when the patient fails to responds to the primary intervention, or continues to 'trigger' or 're-trigger' a response. This individual will assess the clinical effect of the primary intervention, formulate a diagnosis, refine the management plan, initiate a secondary response and will have the knowledge to recognise when referral to Critical Care is indicated.
Tertiary responder (Critical Care)	This role will be undertaken by staff possessing appropriate Critical Care competences such as advanced airway management, resuscitation, and clinical examination and interpretation of critically ill patients.

Figure 1.1 Chain of response (Adapted from DH 2009). Reproduced under terms of the Click-Use Licence available from http://www.dh.gov.uk/prod_consum_dh/groups/dh_digitalassets/documents/digitalasset/dh_096988.pdf.

Nurses as **recognisers** need excellent assessment skills and the ability to interpret signs within the clinical context, in order to fulfil this role.

Additional skills for the **nurses** in the **primary responder** role may include: airway manoeuvres, giving supplemental oxygen, initiating CPAP or NIV, IV cannulation, considering/initiating IV fluids, initiating additional investigations such as ABG and CXR, and escalating to secondary responder as appropriate.

The **recorder** component of the chain is often performed by Health Care Assistants (HCA), who are delegated the task of taking vital signs as part of their role. Formal training of HCAs in assessment skills has been lacking, despite its pivotal role in the chain of response. The responsibility for delegating this role resided with the registered nurse, who ultimately remained accountable (NMC 2018a). Recent developments in clinical roles, such as that of the nursing associate, should, to some extent, fill the gap between heath assistants and registered nurses (HEE 2017). This new nursing associate role is regulated by the NMC, with the nursing associate registering with the NMC on the new nursing associate part of the register (NMC 2018b). The ability to recognise (**recogniser**), traditionally part of the registered nurses' role, may now be supported by these newer members of the health care team. The response (**primary responder**) to signs of deterioration is key to the chain. The individuals performing these roles may vary, but aspects of responder roles are likely to fall within the registered nurses' domain of care (DH 2009), supported by outreach and medical staff. Foundations for physical assessment and prescribing skills are now incorporated into the Registered Nurse curriculum (NMC 2018c), giving opportunities for more skills to be developed in this area for the future workforce. Additional training and responsibilities may be necessary for aspects of the primary responder role, with assessment and interpretative skills being essential for competent execution. The **secondary responder** assesses and evaluates initial interventions, refines the management plan and refers to the tertiary responder if no improvement is seen. The **tertiary responder** requires core competencies in critical care, such as advanced airway management, and will normally be part of the critical care team.

Roles of critical care outreach service

- To identify, initiate and support treatment of patients who are deteriorating in ward areas
- To avert admission to ITU, or, if necessary, to support a timely transfer to critical care
- To educate and support ward staff in caring for acutely unwell patients
- To enable discharge from critical care, by monitoring recovery of discharged patients on wards

The Critical Care Outreach team supports the chain of response from recogniser through to the tertiary responder. Several factors have influenced a reduction in the core skills of ward nurses in caring for acutely unwell patients and the need for education and training to support a competent workforce has been recognised. Safe staffing levels were highlighted as an issue in the Francis report (2013), with lower levels of nursing staff associated with poorer patient outcome. The Faculty of Intensive Care Medicine (FICM) (2019) recommended a nursing staff ratio of one nurse to two patients for Level 2 dependency, but with no recommended level for Level 1 dependency. NICE (2018) considered safe staffing across all acute and critical care provision, suggesting an increased staff: patient ratio for Level 1 patients. The proportion of qualified nurses on acute wards, however, has been reduced, along with expanding demands on their time. This increased dependence on unqualified staff to undertake patient observations should be ameliorated with new roles within health care, such as the **nursing associate**.

Critical care outreach services have expanded and developed to educate and support nurses working in acute wards, and to enable a smooth transfer to a higher level of care, when necessary. They have evolved locally, with no standard levels of personnel or hours of cover, but, in the UK, are normally nurse led, supported by the medical team focussing on pre-critical care admission. They may provide a 7-days-a-week service or hand over cover after hours to a 'hospital at night' team. Rapid response teams, such as outreach, are more costly, but benefits may be seen in terms of reduced numbers of avoidable adverse events, such as cardiac arrest. An increase in **DNAR** orders and an overall increase in length of stay, but a small decrease in ICU stay (NICE 2018), have been observed. Outreach teams are an accepted part of good practice in the UK.

Where are we now?

Critical and acute care organisation

The Faculty of Intensive Care Medicine (FICM) (2019) has published its second Guideline for the Provision of Intensive Care Units, which encompasses both Level 2 and Level 3 care. The standards apply to Intensive Care, Critical Care Units and High-Dependency Units (HDU). The standards require that care is led by a consultant in Intensive Care Medicine, with a dedicated Lead Nurse for each critical care unit. The ITU consultant is able to support and advise management of those who are at risk of deterioration, to avert or support admission to a higher level of care. Increasingly, Level 2 beds are being located within intensive care units, but ward-based Level 2 beds care and separate HDUs currently remain a part of acute care delivery. A new category of **'Enhanced Care'** is being considered for those who do not require admission to a high-dependency unit but require a higher level of care than can normally be provided on a general ward. Examples include post-operative or post-anaesthetic care, or maybe patients receiving acute medical care in a 'Level 1^{+}' environment (FICM 2019). A national strategy for education and competence development for nurses working in higher levels of care has been developed by the Critical Care National Network leads (CC3n), with a range of competencies for qualified nurses working in Enhanced Care areas (CC3n 2018a), with STEP 1–4 competencies to support qualified nurses staff working in Level 2 and Level 3 dependency areas (CC3n 2018b). A co-ordinated approach to competency attainment across acute and critical care areas, supported by both local training and post-qualifying education for the health care workforce, is instrumental in developing the required skills to meet the increasing needs of the in-patient population.

Track and Trigger tools to aid identification of deterioration

NICE (2007) *CG 50*, embraced the use of a physiological 'track and trigger system' to monitor all patients in acute care, with every patient being monitored at least every 12 hours. Many different early warning scores (EWS) are available and recognised as contributing to assessment of clinical risk (Donahue and Endacott 2010). EWS establish a score based on physiological variables. Commonly, they are **weighted, aggregated scoring tools,** completed as part of the routine observations process. A score is obtained by adding together points that are assigned to deviations from normal observation values. The score identifies patients in low-, medium- and high-risk groups and forms part of a graded response strategy. NICE (2007) described **six essential physiological parameters** for inclusion and these have continued to form the basis of the National Early Warning Score (RCP 2012, 2017). Trigger thresholds alert staff to the deterioration risk and a protocol is followed, to enable a clear response for escalation. Evidence suggests that implementation of early warning tools have improved patient outcomes, detection rates and timely appropriate actions. An increase has been noted in the accuracy of recording observations, in particular the respiratory rate (Kyriacos et al. 2015; Mackintosh et al. 2012).

Initially, there was a lack of standardisation of EWS across the NHS that prevented it from becoming part of routine training for all health care professionals. Variation led to lack of familiarity with different tools and trigger levels, as staff moved between clinical areas and hospital trusts. The development and publication of a validated National Early Warning Score (NEWS) in 2012 (RCP 2012) provided benefits of clarity and consistency. Whilst widely embraced by acute care trusts, NEWS continued to be developed in response to feedback from users and professional bodies. In 2017, a revised edition, NEWS 2, was released, with full adoption in March 2019 (NHS England 2018).

National Early Warning Score (NEWS) 2

Key features of NEWS 2

- Use of the ABCDE structure
- A choice of two scales on which to record SpO_2
- Improved documentation for oxygen flow and delivery device
- Parameter ranges for each clinical variable
- ACVPU ('new confusion' added as a trigger)
- A revised colour scheme

NEWS 2 is now in use for adult patients in UK acute hospitals and ambulance trusts as the standard, to record clinical observations and assess risk of deterioration (see Figure 1.2). Please note that, in this chapter, NEWS 2 will be used, but, for future chapters, NEWS 2 will simply be referred to as NEWS. The Royal College of Physicians gives detailed rationale for and guidance on using NEWS 2, available at https://www.rcplondon.ac.uk/projects/outputs/national-early-warning-score-news-2. NEWS 2 is used in the case studies in each of the book chapters, to inform assessment of deterioration risk and care escalation strategy. Modifications from NEWS (RCP 2012) are aimed to:

- Improve sepsis identification.
- Risk identification for those with hypercapnic respiratory failure.
- Highlight the important of 'new confusion' as an indicator of clinical deterioration.
- Change the chart's colour scheme for ease of use for HCPs who may be colour blind, by removing the red/green banding.

NEWS 2 score allocation

White: Score 0
Yellow: Score 1
Orange: Score 2
Red: Score 3

NEWS key 0 1 2 3	FULL NAME	
	DATE OF BIRTH	DATE OF ADMISSION

Parameter	Range	Score	Range
	DATE / TIME		DATE / TIME
A+B Respirations Breaths/min	≥25	3	≥25
	21–24	2	21–24
	18–20		18–20
	15–17		15–17
	12–14		12–14
	9–11	1	9–11
	≤8	3	≤8
A+B SpO_2 Scale 1 Oxygen saturation (%)	≥96		≥96
	94–95	1	94–95
	92–93	2	92–93
	≤91	3	≤91
SpO_2 Scale 2† Oxygen saturation (%) Use Scale 2 if target range is 88–92%, eg in hypercapnic respiratory failure	≥97 on O_2	3	≥97 on O_2
	95–96 on O_2	2	95–96 on O_2
	93–94 on O_2	1	93–94 on O_2
	≥93 on air		≥93 on air
	88–92		88–92
†ONLY use Scale 2 under the direction of a qualified clinician	86–87	1	86–87
	84–85	2	84–85
	≤83%	3	≤83%
Air or oxygen?	A=Air		A=Air
	O_2 L/min	2	O_2 L/min
	Device		Device
C Blood pressure mmHg Score uses systolic BP only	≥220	3	≥220
	201–219		201–219
	181–200		181–200
	161–180		161–180
	141–160		141–160
	121–140		121–140
	111–120		111–120
	101–110	1	101–110
	91–100	2	91–100
	81–90		81–90
	71–80		71–80
	61–70	3	61–70
	51–60		51–60
	≤50		≤50
C Pulse Beats/min	≥131	3	≥131
	121–130	2	121–130
	111–120		111–120
	101–110	1	101–110
	91–100		91–100
	81–90		81–90
	71–80		71–80
	61–70		61–70
	51–60		51–60
	41–50	1	41–50
	31–40	3	31–40
	≤30		≤30
D Consciousness Score for NEW onset of confusion (no score if chronic)	Alert		Alert
	Confusion		Confusion
	V	3	V
	P		P
	U		U
E Temperature °C	≥39.1°	2	≥39.1°
	38.1–39.0°	1	38.1–39.0°
	37.1–38.0°		37.1–38.0°
	36.1–37.0°		36.1–37.0°
	35.1–36.0°	1	35.1–36.0°
	≤35.0°	3	≤35.0°
NEWS TOTAL			TOTAL
	Monitoring frequency		Monitoring
	Escalation of care Y/N		Escalation
	Initials		Initials

Figure 1.2 National Early Warning Score (NEWS) 2. Chart Reproduced with kind permission form the Royal College of Physicians National Early Warning Score (NEWS) 2 Standardising the assessment of acute-illness severity in the NHS. Report of a working party London (RCP 2017) https://www.rcplondon.ac.uk/projects/outputs/national-early-warning-score-news-2.

The ABCDE structure to assessment is well recognised for its benefits in assessing the acutely unwell (Resuscitation Council UK 2015), so presenting the observation chart to be consistent with this is welcomed by many. Recording of temperature has been located under Exposure (moved to the bottom of the chart). Parameters for each clinical variable are clear on the chart, reducing confusion around borderline measurements. For example, a temperature of 38°C can been clearly seen as scoring 0, without reference to an additional chart clarifying trigger parameters.

NEWS2 SpO_2 Scale 1 is used for **most patients** who have a target saturation range of 94–98%.

NEWS2 SpO_2 Scale 2 is used for those with a target saturation range of 88–92%, with confirmed hypercapnic respiratory failure, either currently or on a previous admission, **only** after assessment by a competent decision maker. This is recorded in the notes.

The scale not in use must be crossed out on the observation chart.

In Section A+B, the recording of oxygen saturations has two scales: Scale 1 is use for those with no chronic disordered respiratory physiology, and Scale 2 for those with a previous record of **type 2 respiratory** failure (T2RF). Scale 2 is designed to reflect the impact of chronic altered physiology associated with hypercapnic respiratory failure or type 2 respiratory failure (T2RF). This is most commonly, but not exclusively, seen in patients with Chronic Obstructive Pulmonary Disease (COPD). Patients are assessed by the medical team, the risk of/evidence for hypercapnia is assessed, the appropriate scale (Scale 1 or Scale 2) identified and recorded along with the target oxygen saturations. Interestingly, a recent study (Pimental et al. 2019) found that NEWS2 was not superior to NEWS in identifying in-hospital mortality risks, for patients with T2RF. The two scales, though, may be less confusing for nursing staff, reducing ambiguity regarding the trigger point for this client group.

For both scales the use (in litres) of supplemental oxygen is recorded and scored, to reflect the disordered physiology associated with the inability to maintain oxygen saturations within the normal range on room air. The device/method of oxygen delivery is also recorded for clarity, as the patient may change from nasal specs at 2L of flow, to high-flow oxygen delivery *via* a non-rebreathe face mask. This change in oxygen requirements reflects deteriorating respiratory status, so recording this information is important as part of a recorded assessment.

In Section C, the recording of observations of circulation are unchanged, including heart rate and blood pressure. The systolic blood pressure is the variable to be scored.

ACVPU classification

A = alert
C = new confusion
V = responds to voice
P= responds only to painful stimuli
U = unresponsive to all stimuli

RCP (2017)

Section D includes 'new confusion', as an additional trigger. If confusion is evident, this should be assumed to be new, unless previous confusion is documented or confirmed by relatives.

Section E includes recording of temperature. This can be a reminder to the nurse to assess the patient carefully for any signs which might indicate injury or infection, that could lead to sepsis.

The scores from each section are added to give an overall NEWS 2, with a low, medium or high score being obtained as part of an aggregated weighted scoring system. This score should be interpreted, actioned and communicated in conjunction with comprehensive clinical assessment, using the ABCDE (Airway, Breathing Circulation Disability, Exposure) approach.

Assessment priorities – the ABCDE approach

The use of ABCDE is a recurring theme in each of the chapters of this book. This simple mnemonic was first used in cardiopulmonary resuscitation, but is now also recommended for acute care patients as it supports a rapid assessment of the patient at risk of deterioration (NICE 2007; Resuscitation Council UK 2015; RCP 2017).

A: assess **airway** and treat if needed
B: assess **breathing** and treat if needed
C: assess **circulation** and treat if needed
D: assess **disability** and treat if needed
E: expose and **examine** patient fully, once ABCD are stable

(Cooper et al 2006, Resuscitation Council UK 2015)

In order to prevent medical emergencies, nurses must understand the clinical priorities of potentially life-threatening problems, to enable them to respond to and treat problems in a prioritised order. Used in combination with track and trigger tools, such as NEWS 2, good communication and care escalation, early intervention to treat clinical problems is aided. A systematic assessment is an expansion of what may be seen as the 'task' of filling in observation charts and calculating NEWS 2. Using information from what is seen (look), felt (feel), heard (listen), what can be measured (measure) with additional information from investigations (investigate), ensures that all the senses are used to gather information that informs the interpretation of vital signs. The approach to a rapid ABCDE assessment will be discussed (see Table 1.3 for a summary), but please note that later chapters contain detailed discussion of assessment, focusing on each of the main systems.

A comprehensive approach to assessment should include:

Look **(inspect)**
Listen **(auscultate)**
Feel **(palpate/percuss)**
Measure
Investigate

Table 1.3 Checklist for a rapid ABCDE assessment

ABCDE assessment checklist

Professional behaviour
Be respectful and non-discriminatory at all times (NMC 2018).
Ensure comfort and dignity of patient.
Demonstrate professional behaviour throughout (NMC 2018).

Preparation
Wash hands/apply hand gel/universal precautions as appropriate.

Communication skills
Introduce self to patient, make clear requests, communicate effectively with patient, and seek consent.
Note appropriateness of response: orientated, vague or confused.

Perform a quick systematic (ABCDE) assessment, accurately recording assessment findings, taking action as appropriate at each stage.

AIRWAY

Assess patency

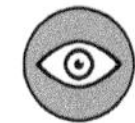

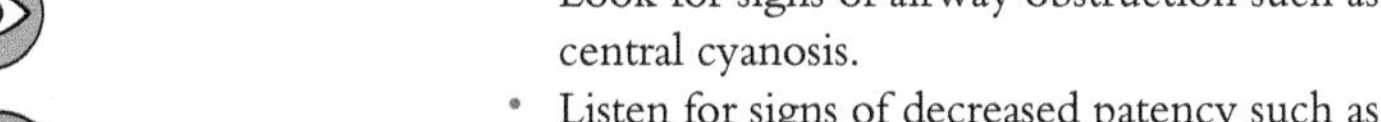
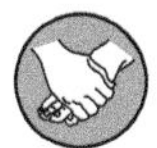

- Look for signs of airway obstruction such as paradoxical breathing, central cyanosis.
- Listen for signs of decreased patency such as stridor, snoring, crowing, wheezing or gurgling.
- Note ability to cough and clear airway secretions.
- Feel for moving air as necessary.

ACTION appropriately
Positioning, simple suction, nasopharyngeal/guedel airway insertion.
Call for help if required.

BREATHING

Observe patient's colour and position

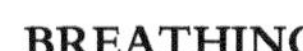
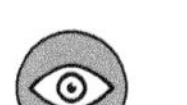
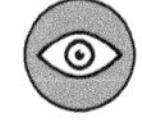
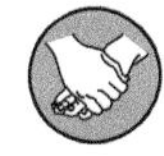
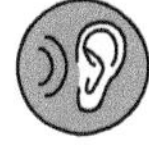
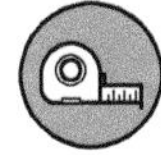

- Centrally – lips and oral mucosa for cyanosis.
- Peripherally – fingers for cyanosis/clubbing.
- Use of accessory muscles.
- Check the trachea is in the midline position.
- Look and feel for bilateral chest expansion, note depth and rhythm of breathing.
- Listen to what patient is saying and the ease with which they are talking.
- Listen and observe patient's breathing for one full minute, noting rate.
- Listen to breath sounds using a stethoscope.
- Assess oxygen saturations, check that acceptable target ranges for patient have been recorded by medical staff. Use correct scale for recording on NEWS 2.
- Note that oxygen percentage and delivery method is prescribed and given.
- Listen and observe patient's breathing for one full minute, noting rate and rhythm.

ACTION appropriately
Reposition in upright position as necessary.
Titrate oxygen requirements to meet specified range, if competent to do so as per BTS 2017 guidance to maintain target saturations.
Call for help if required.

(*Continued*)

Table 1.3 Continued

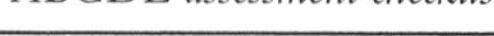

	ABCDE assessment checklist
CIRCULATION 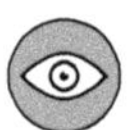 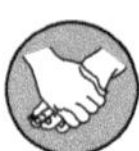 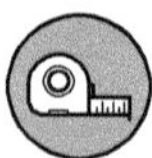	• Look at colour/pallor. • Look for obvious signs of blood loss. • Feel limbs, noting warmth and perfusion. • Note temperature change along all limbs. • Palpate pulse (radial) for 30 seconds if regular (60 seconds, if irregular) noting rate, rhythm and characteristics. • Assess capillary refill in finger (apply pressure for 5 seconds with finger above heart level). • Palpate with thumb for five seconds for signs of pitting oedema. • Record blood pressure (calculate pulse pressure and mean arterial pressure (MAP) as appropriate). • Measure urine output at > 0.5mL/kg/hour. • Assess fluid balance. **ACTION appropriately** **Call for help if required.** Insert a large-bore cannula (12–14fg) if you think shock is present or likely.
DISABILITY 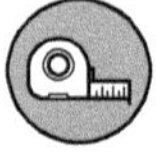 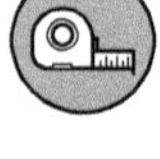	• Use ACVPU to correctly assess level of wakefulness. • Check blood glucose level. **ACTION appropriately** **Call for help if required.**
EXPOSURE	• Record temperature. • Inspect wounds/drains. • Check skin for rashes/erythema. • Check invasive lines for phlebitis.
Investigations	Identify and interpret relevant information gained from simple initial investigations such as: • Hb, urea, creatinine electrolytes (K^+ and Na^+, Mg^{2+}). • 12-lead ECG. • White blood cell count (WBC), C-reactive protein (CRP). • Chest X-ray (CXR). • Simple arterial blood gas analysis: acid-base status hypoxaemia, hypercarbia, BE, lactate.
Care escalation	• Complete observations on chart. • Calculate NEWS 2, adjust frequency of observations accordingly. • Escalate care using NEWS 2 trigger levels, relay to the appropriate clinician, using SBAR as communication tool.

Assessment approach

When initially approaching the patient, take note of their appearance, whether they are collapsed, in obvious respiratory distress, or unable to talk coherently. This immediate observation will give you an indication of the urgency of the assessment.

> Patient collapsed, with no response and showing no signs of life, necessitates a call for help and commencement of CPR (see Chapter 7)

Airway

Airway patency and adequacy of cerebral perfusion can be assumed if a patient is engaging in a conversation and demonstrating understanding and awareness. However, partial airway obstruction is not always immediately obvious, so should always be specifically excluded by ensuring that any increased respiratory effort, abnormal sounds, such as stridor, grunting, gurgling or wheezing, are observed and noted (Smith and Bowden 2017). Any of these signs require immediate management and are covered fully in Chapter 7. These should be treated prior to moving onto assessment of breathing. Asking a patient to demonstrate an effective cough can give insight into risks of aspiration, and forms part of airway assessment.

Breathing

Changes in respiratory status can occur due to respiratory, metabolic, neurological or cardiovascular compromise, and is therefore a sensitive indicator of deterioration. Respiratory assessment is covered in detail in Chapter 5. Respiratory pattern should be determined, looking for patient indicators of distress, such as the use of accessory muscles, paradoxical breathing, position and difficulty in talking in complete sentences. Central cyanosis seen as a bluish hue on the lips/oral mucosa, is a late sign of hypoxaemia and should be excluded. Palpation to assess equal chest expansion can exclude medical emergencies, such as a large or tension pneumothorax, and auscultation can identify adventitious sounds indicative of respiratory deterioration. The importance of measuring respiratory rate (RR) cannot be overemphasised, with 20 breaths per minute a cause for concern, and 30 breaths per minute or more indicating significant risk, necessitating immediate action. When RR >25, it may be helpful to record it as a number on the NEWS 2 chart. This enables even small changes to be monitored to track patient progress that will not affect the NEWS 2 but will reflect further clinical deterioration. Respiratory rate is one of the most sensitive markers of a patient's condition but is often poorly documented (Philip et al. 2015; Flenady et al. 2017).

When using pulse oximetry, always record the flow device and the amount of oxygen the patient is receiving
Use the correct scale on NEWS 2 to record SpO_2
Always check target SpO_2 range set by medical staff

(O'Driscoll *et al.*, 2017, RCP 2017)

Pulse oximeters give valuable information regarding oxygen saturations, enabling hypoxaemia to be detected. O'Driscoll et al. (2017) refer to SpO_2 as the 'fifth vital sign'. However, care must be taken when interpreting SpO_2 levels within the normal range, when other factors, such as inspired oxygen percentage, underlying chronic disordered physiology, respiratory rate and work of breathing, must be taken into account. The British Thoracic Society has published guidelines on oxygen therapy (O'Driscoll et al. 2017) and recommends that target ranges for oxygen saturation should be recorded for each patient. NEWS 2 includes two scales for oxygen saturation recording and trigger levels. Scale 1 is used for most patients who have no evidence of chronic disordered respiratory physiology, with a target SpO_2 range of 94–98%. Scale 2 is used if the patient is at risk of hypercapnic respiratory failure, and a target SpO_2 range of 88–92% will be selected. Scale 2 is used only on the specific direction of a qualified clinician (RCP 2017). The flow rate of oxygen and delivery device is noted, as this is an important factor to note on patient assessments and for interpretation of SpO_2. Supplemental oxygen therapy attracts an additional score of 2 on NEWS2.

Remember

Pulse oximetry does not detect hypercapnia

In patients whose SpO_2 falls below 94%, ABG analysis should be considered, to check for hypercapnia or metabolic problems

SpO_2 monitoring will not detect hypercapnia, which can be reliably ascertained only from arterial blood gas (ABG) analysis. Patients with SpO_2 falling below 94% may need ABG's to be assessed for acid-base balance and hypercapnia. In clinical practice, venous blood gas (VBG) analyses are easier to obtain if no arterial line is *in situ*. VBGs can give valuable information regarding trends or confirming near-normal values, but do not reliably reflect altered values in the critically unwell, so should be interpreted with caution.

Recording measurements on the observation chart and noting any triggers on the NEWS 2 alerts the nurse to deterioration risk. If urgent issues such respiratory distress, marked wheezing or reduced SpO_2 are present, these should be addressed promptly. If assessment suggests a possible tension pneumothorax or acute severe asthma, help is urgently required to get these treated and should be sought before completing a detailed cardiovascular assessment.

Circulation

The circulatory system is the transport mechanism by which the oxygenated blood is distributed to the tissues. A detailed cardiovascular assessment is discussed in Chapter 6. Looking at the patient should reveal any obvious massive blood loss, though internal bleeding is not readily apparent. Patient pallor, as a result of sympathetic nervous system-mediated vasoconstriction, is an indicator of poor cardiac output. A grey sweaty patient is extremely unwell, and expert help should be sought immediately.

Has your patient got an irregular pulse?

- Is this a new event?
- Perform a 12-lead ECG
- Check that serum electrolytes, K^+ and Mg^{2+} are within the normal range

Palpation of pulses aids assessment of the circulation. A weak and thready pulse, or one with a low pulse volume, is associated with low cardiac output, most likely due to hypovolaemia, though cardiac failure needs to be considered. A strong and bounding pulse is associated with the vasodilation of sepsis or anaphylaxis. Peripheral temperature tends to be cooler (feel hands and feet to see if they are cool or warm) and capillary refill time is prolonged if cardiac output is reduced. Pitting oedema can alert the nurse to possible cardiac, renal or fluid balance problems. A normal heart rate varies in the range 60–100 beats per minute; values outside the range will score on NEWS 2. Normally, the HR will be a lower value than the systolic blood pressure, if the pulse rate is rising, or is greater than the systolic BP; this is a cause for concern and should be reported. An irregular pulse requires investigation with a 12-lead ECG, to identify and enable treatment of arrhythmias, such as atrial fibrillation. A new finding of an irregular pulse should be treated with a degree of urgency and communicated to the medical team. Guidelines for immediate treatments of tachyarrhythmia or bradyarrhythmia have been formulated by the RCUK (2015) and should form the basis of clinical decision making (see Chapter 7). Rates above 150 or below 40 are unlikely to be consistent with adequate cardiac output, so expert help is required immediately.

If the *heart rate* is higher than the *systolic blood pressure*, this is a cause for concern

Heart rate •
SBP ∨
DBP ∧

Blood pressure measurements vary with age, but normal systolic values are in the range 90–140mmHg. A drop of more than 40mmHg in the systolic pressure is a cause for concern, even if the value remains above 100mmHg. Changes in blood pressure are often a late sign of deterioration as the sympathetic response of vasoconstriction and increased force of myocardial contraction tend to compensate in the earlier stages of shock. The diastolic pressure reflects the degree of vasoconstriction and is usually greater than 60mmHg. Vasoconstriction (as in hypovolaemia or cardiogenic shock) will raise the diastolic pressure and narrow the pulse pressure. Vasodilation will reduce the diastolic pressure (as in sepsis or anaphylaxis) and raise the pulse pressure.

What is pulse pressure?

The difference between systolic and diastolic blood pressure
Normal range is 35–45mmHg

The average pressure throughout the cardiac cycle (mean arterial pressure) needs to be adequate to maintain organ perfusion. Indicators of good organ perfusion would be a urine output of more than 0.5–1mL/kg/h and an alert, orientated patient. Fluid balance is integral to the circulatory assessment and would normally be about 500mL positive over a 24-hour period.

Mean arterial pressure (MAP)

MAP=1/3 pulse pressure + diastolic pressure
MAP reflects organ perfusion, and should be above 70mmHg

After completing the assessment of circulation, record the observations and note the parameters that trigger on the observation chart. Consider whether expert help is needed immediately, and/or if concern is sufficient to require that the patient is cannulated with a large-bore cannula (12–14fg) to enable rapid fluid resuscitation, as necessary. If the patient is sufficiently stable, move on to assessment of disability.

Disability

In your initial approach, you will have noted whether your patient is talking to you. Further probing helps clarify whether the patient is confused, which can be used as part of the assessment of level of consciousness, using the ACVPU method of assessment. New confusion (C) has been identified as a marker of deterioration, and should be noted, scoring 3 on NEWS 2. Relatives are helpful in helping determine whether the confusion is worse than normal for those patients with short-term memory problems. If the level of consciousness is reduced, then the Glasgow Coma Scale (GCS) is a useful tool with which to assess neurological status. For a detailed neurological assessment, please see Chapter 9. A GSC of eight or less is a particular cause for concern; the patient needs positioning to protect the airway and an expert is required for airway maintenance/protection. Blood glucose level needs to be assessed as either hyper- and hypoglycaemia can present as a medical emergency, requiring urgent treatment. Hypotension, hypoxia or sepsis, as causes of altered neurological status, must be considered and treated, as a matter of priority.

Exposure

The central temperature must be recorded and noted that a temperature above 38 degrees centigrade (i.e. 38.1°C) is consistent with, but not necessarily present in, infection and sepsis. The trust policy for performing a septic screen to help identify possible pathogens should be checked. A head-to-toe examination is necessary to ensure that every detail is considered. Signs such as urticaria may signify an allergic reaction, an inflamed area on the buttock may indicate a source of infection and/or sepsis, and rashes indicative of meningitis are examples of clinical signs that can aid diagnosis and treatment. In addition to considering initial interventions, a full review of the patient's charts, looking for trends, requests and reviews of relevant investigations, and decisions regarding the level of care required, should be considered.

NEWS 2 to identify deterioration risk and clinical response

As part of the ABCDE assessment, vital signs are recorded on NEWS 2 and an aggregate score obtained. Figure 1.3 summarises the score given to each clinical parameter as it moves away from the normal physiological ranges. The total NEWS 2 needs to be checked for accuracy and compared with previous scores to evaluate changes in clinical status.

The total score defines the graded response. Levels of response are described, with directions for frequency of observations (see Figure 1.4). Individual trusts may vary in the way the escalation strategy is structured, but RCP (2017) recommends that the trigger levels remain unchanged and, at each level, the speed/ urgency of response, and the clinician with the appropriate skills match the grades of acute illness severity. The increased frequency of monitoring The increased frequency of monitoring to a minimum of hourly for those that score three in a single parameter, or five or more (**urgent**

National Early Warning Score (NEWS2)

Physiological parameter	Score 3	2	1	0	1	2	3
Respiration rate (per minute)	≤8		9–11	12–20		21–24	≥25
SpO_2 Scale 1(%)	≤91	92–93	94–95	≥96			
SpO_2 Scale 2(%)	≤83	84–85	86–87	88–92 ≥93 on air	93–94 on oxygen	95–96 on oxygen	≥97 on oxygen
Air or oxygen?		Oxygen		Air			
Systolic blood pressure (mmHg)	≤90	91–100	101–110	111–219			≥220
Pulse (per minute)	≤40		41–50	51–90	91–110	111–130	≥131
Consciousness				Alert			CVPU
Temperature (°C)	≤35.0		35.1–36.0	36.1–38.0	38.1–39.0	≥39.1	

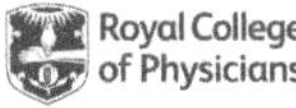

Figure 1.3 The NEWS scoring system. Reproduced with kind permission from the Royal College of Physicians National Early Warning Score (NEWS) 2 Standardising the assessment of acute-illness severity in the NHS. Report of a working party London RCP 2017) https://www.rcplondon.ac.uk/projects/outputs/national-early-warning-score-news-2.

response threshold) and for those that score seven or more recorded continuously (**emergency response threshold**), provides a challenge to nurses working in acute care. It is, though, an important part of the clinical response, ensuring that those most at risk are monitored closely, re-enforcing the escalation strategy if NEWS 2 continues to rise, or requires a different response.

The urgent response threshold (five or more) is set lower than in the first version of NEWS and is the trigger for urgent review. The RCP urges that a score of five triggers the suspicion of sepsis in those with known/suspected infection or who are at significant risk of infection. The emergency threshold of seven requires not only that the medical team be informed, but for this to be, at least, at specialist registrar level. Review is required by a team with critical care competencies in airway management. A score of seven should prompt the team to consider whether the patient need to be transferred to a higher level of care, or whether the needs of the patient can be met in the current environment. Many patients may respond quickly to timely appropriate interventions, with NEWS 2 falling to a lower trigger level. Those who remain in the emergency threshold after initial treatment, however, are sicker and are likely to require a higher level of care (Level 2 or 3). This may be delivered on the ward, if Level 2 beds and appropriately trained staff are available but will often require transfer to a critical care unit, under the supervision of the critical care team.

NEW score	Frequency of monitoring	Clinical response
0	Minimum 12 hourly	• Continue routine NEWS monitoring
Total 1–4	Minimum 4–6 hourly	• Inform registered nurse, who must assess the patient • Registered nurse decides whether increased frequency of monitoring and/or escalation of care is required
3 in single parameter	Minimum 1 hourly	• Registered nurse to inform medical team caring for the patient, who will review and decide whether escalation of care is necessary
Total 5 or more Urgent response threshold	Minimum 1 hourly	• Registered nurse to immediately inform the medical team caring for the patient • Registered nurse to request urgent assessment by a clinician or team with core competencies in the care of acutely ill patients • Provide clinical care in an environment with monitoring facilities
Total 7 or more Emergency response threshold	Continuous monitoring of vital signs	• Registered nurse to immediately inform the medical team caring for the patient – this should be at least at specialist registrar level • Emergency assessment by a team with critical care competencies, including practitioner(s) with advanced airway management skills • Consider transfer of care to a level 2 or 3 clinical care facility, ie higher-dependency unit or ICU • Clinical care in an environment with monitoring facilities

Figure 1.4 Clinical response to the NEWS trigger thresholds. Reproduced with kind permission from the Royal College of Physicians National Early Warning Score (NEWS) 2 Standardising the assessment of acute-illness severity in the NHS. Report of a working party London RCP 2017) https://www.rcplondon.ac.uk/projects/outputs/national-early-warning-score-news-2.

CASE STUDY 1.1 JÓZEF BREZEZINSKI PART 1

It's 14.30h and you are caring for Józef Brezezinski, aged 63, who has been admitted earlier this morning with a 3-4 day history of a productive cough, expectorating green sputum. He was previously fit and healthy and has initially been treated by his GP with a course of antibiotics. He has failed to improve and is now extremely breathless.

On approaching Józef, you notice that he is sitting upright and looks in some respiratory difficulty. You introduce yourself to him, as you wash your hands and apply hand gel. The screens are pulled round and you ask Józef if he is happy for you to perform an assessment. Józef replies that he is fine for you to examine him, but not to ask too many questions as he is very tired. You note that he appears orientated but has some difficulty in continuing the conversation.

Airway: You assess his airway as clear but listen carefully for stridor or gurgling that may indicate partial airway obstruction. You ask him to cough, which he is able to do effectively and so you surmise that he is at low risk of aspiration. As he is in no immediate danger, you continue with your assessment.

Breathing: Józef's lips and oral mucosa show no evidence of central cyanosis, but Józef's use of accessory muscles indicates respiratory distress. Peripherally, his fingers look a little pale. You attach the oxygen saturation probe to obtain a reading of 91% on 2L of oxygen, which he is receiving *via* nasal specs. You check his admission status and note that the reading has fallen from 96%. This is outside the target saturation of 94–98% which has been set by your medical colleagues. Scale 1 is being used to record SpO_2 on NEWS 2.

You are aware of the BTS guidance (O'Driscoll et al. 2017), so increase the oxygen flow to 4L, making a mental note to recheck the saturations in a few minutes. You are concerned that he is mouth breathing and think that a face mask may be more appropriate for him. After counting his respiratory rate at 24 breaths per minute (a rise of four from his previous observations), you record this number on the observation chart and note that it is in the orange area, scoring 2 on NEWS 2. His reduced SpO_2 and the fact that he is receiving oxygen therapy, score 4 (Scale 1 SpO_2 2 + supplemental oxygen 2).

After seeking Józef's consent, you auscultate his lungs. You think you hear some crackles on inspiration, but, as this is a skill that you are just developing, you will ask the medical staff to confirm your findings. On palpation, you note equal lung expansion, that the trachea is midline, but his breathing is shallow and laboured.

You recheck the oxygen saturations and note they have increased to 94%, (which scores 1 on NEWS 2), despite his mouth breathing, with no change in respiratory rate. You are reassured that there has been some response to this initial intervention but decide to suggest an arterial blood gas sample is taken to evaluate acid-base status. You feel that he is stable enough for you to continue your assessment.

Breathing NEWS 2 (2+3+2) =7 (on 2L of oxygen)
Breathing NEWS 2 (2+1+2) = 5 (on 4L of oxygen)

Circulation: Józef looks a little pale, but there is no obvious blood loss, and his radial pulse is easy to palpate, with a good pulse pressure. His wrist feels warm, and the pulse is regular, but tachycardic at 108 beats per minute (increased from 98 from the previous observation). Capillary refill is at 2 seconds, and his blood pressure is 125/85mmHg. You note the normal pulse pressure, but do not calculate the mean arterial pressure at this point. The HR falls in the yellow band, generating an additional score of 1.

Józef explains that he passed urine before being admitted 2 hours ago and has no desire to go again. He has no signs of ankle oedema, skin turgor is poor and his mouth appears dry. You are concerned about his fluid status, knowing that his raised respiratory rate can lead to increased insensible losses, and he feels too breathless to drink. You decide to commence a record of his intake and output on a fluid balance chart.

Circulation NEWS 2 (2+0) = 2

Disability: Józef is able to respond appropriately, aware of time and place, with no sign of confusion. Neurological status is important as this can be affected by hypoxaemia, hypercapnia or sepsis. The blood glucose level is checked, but it is within normal limits at 5mmols/L.

Disability NEWS 2 = 0

Exposure: His temperature is raised, at 38.0 °C, scoring 0 on NEWS 2. You complete a quick head-to-toe examination looking for additional sign of infection, detecting no abnormalities.

Exposure NEWS 2 =0

You calculate the **total NEWS 2 as 7**, which places him in the emergency response threshold. A brief scan of his observation chart indicates an upward trend in respiratory rate and heart rate, borderline pyrexia and a downwards trend in oxygen saturations, with increasing oxygen therapy requirements.

NEWS 2 requires that you call the patient's primary medical team, at specialist registrar level. You also plan to call outreach. You ask a member of your team to stay with Józef and recheck his observations in 10 minutes, while you escalate care.

Escalating care

The recording of assessment findings, i.e., calculation of NEWS 2, and using this to determine the appropriate response, is key to the recognition of the patient at risk of deterioration, or a medical emergency. The next step of care escalation requires that the nurse's concerns are communicated to the health care team in a clear and coherent manner. NPSA (2007) identified failure of communication as the biggest problem area with the deteriorating patient. Nurses do not always use the same language as their medical colleagues when discussing patients at risk of deterioration, which may cause confusion and misunderstandings. Nurses are often alerted to the acutely unwell patient by the feeling that 'something is wrong'. This 'feeling of concern' is incorporated into NEWS 2 as an additional trigger factor. However, a nursing observation that 'the patient just does not look well' may not enable doctors to appreciate the urgency of a situation as clearly as 'the patient is peripherally vasoconstricted, cold, clammy, with a capillary refill time of greater than three seconds'. Nurses who pick up early signs of deterioration may have difficulty in convincing the doctor to take timely action due to problems in articulating concerns in a manner that is clearly understood. NEWS 2 can help overcome these barriers by providing objective 'calling criteria'. On the other hand, more information than just NEWS 2 is needed. Medical staff/outreach cover large numbers of patients in differing geographical locations, so they have to prioritise their workload, and the information given to them needs to enable this process. In order to improve communication, a couple of moments organising one's thoughts can be beneficial. The patient at risk of deterioration needs that information to be communicated with total clarity, so that the person being called is immediately aware of the impending emergency, and can instantly start helping with the clinical decision-making process. Systems such SBAR (Situation, Background, Assessment, Recommendation) (NHS Improvement 2018) ensures that both the caller and the recipient are familiar with the structure of information giving (see Table 1.4). There is evidence that SBAR improves patient safety, especially when used to structure phone handovers (Muller et al. 2018). For senior students, newly qualified nurses/nursing associates and health care professionals, the stress and urgency of a patient who is deteriorating can cause minds to go completely 'blank'; the security of a simple, structured system can help allay anxiety and ensure that a full and comprehensive request for help is responded to.

Tips when escalating care

- Ensure you are making contact with the appropriate health care professional
- Stand by the phone, if possible, to receive response to the bleep
- Have the patient's chart and notes to hand
- Use SBAR to guide the conversation

Additional considerations when using NEWS 2

Whereas NEWS 2 generates an objective score supporting decision making with regard to care escalation, it is wise to consider this in conjunction with a comprehensive patient assessment. The alignment of the NEWS 2 chart with the ABCDE approach (see Figure 1.3) may aid the nurse to consider the importance of the assessment, alongside the recording of vital signs. Grant (2018) argues that an ABCDE assessment should be performed routinely on all patients, with physiological findings interpreted, in addition to generating the score. After a full review, additional information could be noted. For example, a patient may be displaying trends over a period of time on one or a number of variables, moving towards a

Table 1.4 Examples of systems for communication of deterioration in hospitals

SBAR	
Situation	Identity yourself and from where you are calling Identify patient by name, consultant, location resuscitation status and reason for concern **State NEWS 2**
Background	Brief overview of reason for admission, date, PMH, medications allergies, pertinent results
Assessment	**ABCDE** assessment Give a **succinct** overview of findings Use the ABCDE approach to structure your handover, including vital clinical signs as appropriate *Avoid just giving lists of observations* Identify what you think the problem may be, and state what actions have been taken already
Recommendation	Be specific about what you need, make suggestions, clarify expectations Ask if there is anything else you should do Repeat instructions to ensure accuracy

SBAR adapted from IHI (2018) https://improvement.nhs.uk/resources/sbar-communication-tool/

trigger point. A patient with a normal heart rate of 60 beats per minute, whose rate increases by 5 beats per minute progressively over the day, is demonstrating a trend of deterioration. It may be wise to seek advice before the trigger point is reached, as this could be a sign of a developing acute illness. Whereas cluttering a chart with numbers is generally discouraged, small changes and trends can be significant and so recording exact clinical values of HR, BP, SpO_2 and temperature will be appropriate in some circumstances, to aid assessment of deterioration risk and patient response to urgent therapeutic interventions. It should also be remembered that the patient's normal medication may influence the physiological response to illness. For example, a patient taking beta-blocker medication will have a blunted sympathetic response and signs, such as increased heart rate, may not be readily apparent.

Nurses require a sound understanding of potentially worrying observations that do not trigger on NEWS 2. O'Driscoll et al. (2017) and RCUK (2015) emphasise that a normal target range for SpO_2 should be 94–98%. Patients with an SpO_2 > 98%, who are receiving oxygen, may be at risk from increased levels of oxygen free radicals, resulting in alveolar swelling, reperfusion injury post-myocardial infarction and/or coronary artery/cerebral vasoconstriction (Grant 2018). Nurses, therefore, should aim to keep within the target range of SpO_2 for those requiring supplemental oxygen, keeping below 99%, unless different specific requirements have been indicated.

The high value for systolic blood pressure on NEWS 2 for a trigger is 219mmHg. This extremely high pressure is associated with poor outcome, yet is significantly higher than the physiologically normal higher values of 130–140mmHg (NICE 2019). Nurses need to recognise raised systolic or diastolic pressures, so that appropriate assessment of organ damage/management of hypertension can be considered (Grant 2018), regardless of the lack of a NEWS 2 trigger. A new irregular pulse is not recorded as such on NEWS 2, only the rate, but this is part of an ABCDE assessment and is an important clinical observation. New cardiac arrhythmias, such as atrial fibrillation, require further investigation and treatment.

While acknowledging some of these constraints, the association between high NEWS scores and serious adverse events is evident (Smith et al. 2016). Its validity has also been demonstrated in emergency departments (Bilben et al. 2016). The implementation of NEWS was shown to speed up the clinical response to patients at risk of deterioration, with Spiers et al. (2015) recording an increase in attendance by clinicians within 1 hour, increasing from 33% to 85% within 6 months of implementation. NEWS 2 is a valuable tool, to be used by nurses in conjunction with good clinical assessment skills, good clinical reasoning skills and the ability to clearly articulate concerns.

Moving care forward

The chain of response (DH 2009) does not stop with the arrival of outreach or the patient's primary medical team. Suboptimal care is still possible, and teamwork is required to move care forward. It is important that nurses have a clear understanding of the physiological basis of deterioration, in order to monitor the response to the interventions prescribed. Interventions need to be appropriate and timely, and should result in improvements in clinical status, reflected in a reduction of NEWS 2 Newly qualified doctors and nurses may feel unsure in the management of the deteriorating patient, and education, advice and support from outreach services, supervising consultant and ICU should be utilised (NCEPOD 2005; RCP 2017). The chain of response will involve a secondary and maybe a tertiary responder, who will have competencies in critical care (DH 2009). Early advice should be sought if the patient does not respond to initial therapies, or requires continuing therapy to retain stability, as admission to a higher level of care may be appropriate.

Track and Trigger

- Check that you have correctly calculated NEWS 2
- Recheck score after each intervention, and use it to track progress
- If the score stays the same or increases after interventions, your patient is deteriorating: continue to seek appropriate help

CASE STUDY 1.2 JÓZEF BREZEZINSKI PART 2

Józef has been admitted with Community-Acquired Pneumonia (CAP) and, after an assessment at 14.35, you are concerned that he is deteriorating as he has triggered on NEWS 2. His heart rate and respiratory rate have a rising trend, indicating an increased level of compensation, and deteriorating status. Mr. Brezezinski is at risk of becoming a medical emergency, with the NEWS 2 of 7 requiring an emergency response.

You check that you know which team Józef is under the care of, and that you have the charts and notes with you. You make sure that Józef is comfortable and hand him the call bell, while you bleep the specialist registrar. Your ward uses the SBAR system as a communication tool and when the doctor responds to his bleep, you give the following information.

SITUATION: Hello Dr Jones, thanks for calling back so promptly. This is S/N Wills from 2 South and I am calling because I am concerned about Józef Brezezinski, a 63-year-old gentleman your team admitted earlier today. Józef has a NEWS of 7.

BACKGROUND: Józef Brezezinski was admitted at 10.30 this morning with community-acquired pneumonia. He had a history of a cough which was productive, with green sputum, and he has become increasingly breathless. His chest X-ray showed some consolidation and he was started on antibiotics and 2L of oxygen *via* nasal specs, with a target saturation of 94–98%. His past medical history includes hypertension for which he is taking Candasartan 16mg and Bisoprolol 5mg.

ASSESSMENT: His airway is clear. His oxygen saturations had dropped to 92% but are now 94% after increasing oxygen from 2 to 4L. His respiratory rate has gone up to 24 and he looks distressed. I think I heard some new crackles on auscultation, but I am not confident, so I would like you to check. His blood pressure is 135/95, and his capillary refill is 2 seconds. His heart rate has increased from 92 to 109 over the past couple of hours. He has not passed urine for a few hours. I am worried that his respiratory failure is worsening and that he may deteriorate quickly, and, as NEWS 2 >5, sepsis needs to be considered.

RECOMMENDATIONS:

Please come and assess him urgently. He may need an arterial blood gas sample taken, some intravenous antibiotics and IV fluids as he is not drinking. Would you like me to organise a repeat chest X-ray and chase up the blood results? I was also thinking of cannulating him for IV access.

When will you be able to get here?
Is there anything else you would like me to do.?
So, can I just confirm that you would like me to cannulate him and arrange a chest X-ray? Thanks, see you in 15 minutes.

You go back to Józef to explain that his doctor is coming to review him, and notice that his oxygen saturations have slipped back down to 92%. You repeat his observations and note that his respiratory rate has increased to 30, and his heart rate to 112. He cannot complete sentences in one breath and is still finding it hard work to breath. You decide to place him on a non-rebreathe mask at 15L oxygen; while you are waiting for the doctor/Outreach to attend, his oxygen saturations increase back to 94%, and you are pleased that they arrive promptly. You note that the NEWS 2 has now increased from 7 to 9; he is deteriorating.

Dr Jones arrives, reviews Józef, noting his deteriorating clinical status. His oxygen saturations have increased to 94% on 15L of oxygen, and an arterial blood gas reveals a pH of 7.35, PaO_2 8.2kPa, and a $PaCO_2$ of 3.6kPa. BE, HCO_3^- and lactate are within the normal range; type one respiratory failure is confirmed. His repeat CXR reveals a worsening of consolidation. Dr Jones asks you to call Outreach with a view to commencing CPAP or NHFLOT as his response to oxygen therapy is limited. You discuss moving Józef to a higher level of care. He is cannulated and, after blood cultures and a sputum specimen have been obtained, commenced on IV Augmentin 1.2g and Clarithromycin 500mg. 1L of IV normal saline is started, to run over 8 hours.

Outreach arrive and commence CPAP on 50% oxygen with a PEEP of 5cm H_2O. The critical care team is consulted, and it is agreed that the response to CPAP will be assessed. Within 30 minutes, there are signs of clinical improvement. Józef appears more comfortable, with less evidence of accessory muscle use. His respiratory rate reduces to 21 breaths /minute and his oxygen saturations rise to 96%. Heart rate is reduced to 98 beats /minute as his effort to breathe decreases. NEWS 2 has reduced into the urgent category and Outreach stay with Józef until he is stable enough for transfer to a Level 2 bed, where he will be with nurses who are able to monitor arterial blood gases, have competence in caring for a patient requiring CPAP and have sufficient staff to increase the frequency of observations as required.

After 48 hours, Józef returns back to your ward and he is discharged home, two days later.

Chain of prevention

Recognising and responding appropriately to patient deterioration and medical emergencies requires complex skills and effective multidisciplinary education and teamwork. The 'chain of prevention' (Smith 2010) is an illustration of the components necessary to promote safe and effective care in the acute hospital setting (see Figure 1.5). Many rings of the chain have been considered in this chapter, and the themes of assessment (monitoring) recognition, asking for help and appropriate response, are evident in subsequent chapters in this book. Every link in the chain need to be strong, as the chain is only as strong as the weakest link.

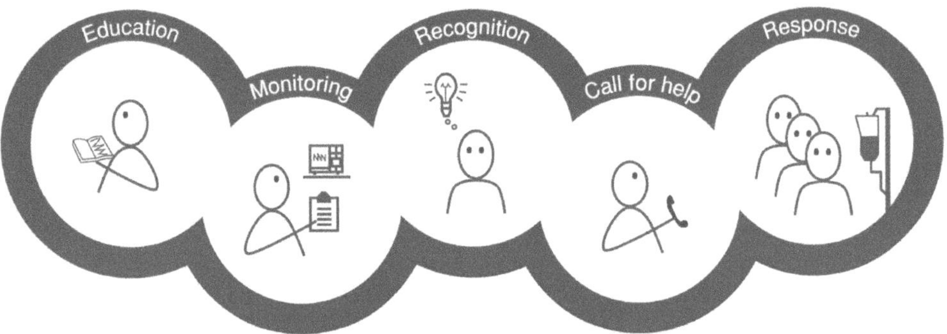

Figure 1.5 Chain of Prevention (Smith 2010). *Source*: Smith (2010) In-hospital cardiac arrest: is it time for an in-hospital 'chain of prevention'? *Resuscitation*, 81(a), 1209–1211.

'Education', the first link of the chain, is essential to ensure competence of the health care professional in patient assessment, recording and interpreting vital signs, calculating NEWS and escalating care appropriately. The NMC (2018c) Standards for Pre-registration Nursing Education reflect this need, recognising that all nurses (in each of the four fields) must be able to recognise and interpret signs of normal and deteriorating mental and physical health, and to respond promptly. The early signs of illness must be detected by making accurate assessments, starting appropriate and carrying out timely management of those who are acutely ill and at risk of clinical deterioration, or requiring emergency care (NMC 2018c). Nurses do not care for patients in isolation, so that education needs to address the multi-professional team, using effective methods such as clinical simulation training. Importantly, not all patients benefit from or want invasive curative therapy. The health care team, alongside patients and relatives, needs to consider whether a 'do not attempt to resuscitate' (DNAR) order would be beneficial. Active treatment may be chosen, but decisions regarding 'ceilings of treatment' to avoid futile aggressive therapies, with inappropriate arrest calls for patients in the terminal stage of their illness, are an important contribution to providing individualised patient-centred care.

The quality of 'monitoring', namely the frequency, completeness and the recording of observations forms the second link. Qualified nurses are accountable for their practice and must ensure that they are competently performed and regularly reviewed. The third ring of the chain, 'recognition', is supported by the use of NEWS 2 and has potential to standardise calling criteria, to assist health care professionals in the early recognition of deterioration. The 'call for help' is the fourth ring of the chain. The use of tools, such as SBAR, may improve the quality of communication tools, both within and between disciplines. The final ring in the chain 'response' considers the functioning of teams such as Critical Care Outreach Services (CCOS), a dedicated team with specific skills in managing the acutely ill patient, namely the medical and critical care team. The speed of response and level of support provided by these teams are crucial to moving patient care forward. Kolic et al. (2015) concluded from their study that clinical response to NEWS was significantly worse at weekends, highlighting possible patient safety concerns. Factors such as ward culture, workload and staffing issues can negatively influence the successful introduction of Rapid Response Systems (McGaughey et al. 2017). Organisational culture needs to be supportive, not criticising staff for calling for help, while ensuring that an adequate clinical response is not impeded by lack of staff, or the time of the call.

Conclusion

The problem of early recognition of acute illness, with appropriate and timely response to prevent medical emergencies occurring, is not a new one. Early recognition of deterioration, with timely and appropriate interventions, is beneficial in improving patient outcomes in a number of acute conditions, such as sepsis and acute kidney injury. National strategies have been implemented to support the organisation of acute care services, opening up critical care expertise outside the ITU environment. Education of the multidisciplinary team in terms of the identification and management of the acutely unwell patient is ongoing. NEWS 2 is instrumental in identifying deterioration risk, and systems such as SBAR enhance multi- and intra-disciplinary communications. However, the early detection of an impending medical emergency is largely reliant on nurses performing a comprehensive patient assessment and accurately recording abnormal vital signs. Nurses need to understand the physiological basis of deterioration and have the competence and confidence to use NEWS 2 appropriately to escalate care. Critical care outreach teams and medical staff are dependent on nurses assessing their patients and adhering to NEWS 2 criteria. Caring for patients at risk of becoming acutely unwell can be challenging, but, ultimately, rewarding. Expanding knowledge and expertise in recognition of and organising response to medical emergencies is a good step forward in improving the quality of care for those at risk of becoming acutely unwell.

Glossary

Care escalation Care moved forward in order that a set of timely appropriate interventions prescribed by clinicians with competence in critical care, aimed at treating/preventing acute deterioration, are commenced. May involve advice from Critical Care Outreach, ITU, and transfer to a higher level of care.

Ceiling of Care Ceiling of care decisions are made by the patient and their family in conjunction with the health care team, when their baselines problems limit the ability to recover from their present illnessDecisions after a 'ceiling of care' discussion may result in: full treatment, treatment that can be delivered out of a critical care environment, or palliative care, treatment that enhances comfort rather than focusing on recovery.

CPAP (Continuous Positive Airways Pressure) A respiratory support therapy in which continuous positive pressure is delivered *via* a face mask, nasal mask or mouthpiece. Positive end-expiratory pressure (PEEP) is achieved through a PEEP valve. This increases the lung functional residual capacity, and aids oxygenation.

CPR Cardiopulmonary resuscitation (CPR) is an emergency procedure used to manually support the circulation, thereby preserving blood flow to the brain.

Critical Care Outreach A team, often multi-professional, that provides clinical and educational support in the recognition and treatment at the onset of deteriorating health of adult patients on general wards. They also provide for patients after a period of critical illness when they are discharged back to a lower level of care on the general wards.

DNAR (Do not actively resuscitate) or DNACPR (Do not actively perform cardiopulmonary resuscitation) A DNAR/DNACPR decision is made to provide guidance to heath care professionals on the best course of action to be taken in the event of a cardiac arrest or sudden death. It does not preclude other active treatment of an unwell patient.

Enhanced care Care that involves enhanced observation and support. In the context of the unwell patient; this may be seen as Level 1+ care, not yet requiring critical care.

EWS (Early Warning Score/System) System: a process by which objective criteria are used to generate a score, which is used as an indicator for 'calling for help'. Score: Each of six physiological variables generates a number as it deviates from acceptable ranges. The EWS is the sum of those numbers.

Hypoxaemia Low level of oxygen in the blood.

Medical emergency An acute life-threatening event, usually preceded by a period of physiological deterioration and changes in vital signs.

Medical Emergency Teams (MET) A team of health care professionals who have advanced life support skills, who are able to respond to patients who have abnormal physiological signs indicative of clinical deterioration. MET were first used in Australia.

Multi-Parameter Early Warning System Multi-parameter systems trigger on two or more physiological variables that fall outside a predetermined range.

High-Flow Nasal Oxygen Therapy High-flow oxygen therapy is for those not responding to conventional oxygen therapy. It delivers *via* nasal cannula up to 60L/min of oxygen/air mixture, thereby assisting breathing during inspiration, and providing a low level of positive end-expiratory pressure to enhance oxygenation during expiration. It is generally well tolerated by patients.

National Early Warning Score NEWS 2 The 2017 update of the National Early Warning Score published by the Royal College of Physicians in 2017.

Non-Invasive Ventilation (NIV) A process which enables different pressures to be delivered during inspiration and expiration and providing ventilatory support. NIV is delivered *via* face or nasal mask, does not require intubation, and is most commonly used for patients with type 2 respiratory failure.

Nursing Associate This a role new within the nursing team. A registered nursing associate supports the registered nurse to deliver patient care.

Physiological Variable A clinical measurement such as heart rate, respiratory rate, that varies over time.

SBAR Situation. Background, Assessment. Recommendation. An easy-to-use mechanism used to structure communication, to accurately communicate the clinical situations that require a clinician's attention.

Six essential physiological parameters Described by NICE 2007 and RCP 2017, as those physiological parameters that should be measured, recorded, and scored (using NEWS 2) at least every 12 hours in the acute care setting. These six variables are: respiratory rate, SpO_2, heart rate, blood pressure, ACVPU, temperature.

Track and Trigger tool A set of predetermined objective criteria used as indicators for 'calling for help' in the management of a patient at risk of clinical deterioration.

Type 1 respiratory failure (T1RF) Also known as hypoxaemic respiratory failure, present when PaO_2 falls below 8.0kPa, and $PaCO_2$ remains at or below 6.0kPa.

Type 2 respiratory failure (T2RF) Also known as hypercapnic respiratory failure, present when $PaCO_2$ rises to 6.1kPa or above, and the pH falls below 7.35.

Weighted Aggregated Early Warning tools Allocate points in a weighted manner (e.g., the more the parameter has deviated from normal, the higher the score generated) and these points are added to generate the early warning score. This allows the generation of low-, medium- and high-risk categories as recommended by NICE (2007).

TEST YOURSELF

1 Patients who have a cardiopulmonary arrest:
  a. Can often do so when there are no signs of anything being wrong with them.
  b. Usually collapse within an hour of developing a temperature.
  c. Often have abnormal vital signs in the 24 hours before arrest.
  d. Always have low oxygen saturations 6 hours before the arrest.
2 The six physiological parameters that should be included in a track and trigger system are:
  a. Heart rate, respiratory rate, central venous pressure, urine output, temperature and peak expiratory flow rate.
  b. Heart rate, respiratory rate, blood pressure, urine output, temperature and level of consciousness.
  c. Heart rate, oxygen saturations, level of consciousness, temperature, systolic blood pressure and respiratory rate.
  d. Heart rate, oxygen saturations, respiratory rate, systolic blood pressure and urine output.
3 Which of the following do not form part of a compensatory mechanism to acute illness?
  a. Respiratory rate.
  b. Blood pressure.
  c. Heart rate.
  d. Hypoxaemia.
4 When using NEWS 2, patients who do not trigger on the observation chart:
  a. Need to have the 6 physiological parameters measured at least every 12 hours, with NEWS 2 calculated.
  b. Need to have the 6 physiological parameters measured only if the patient says they do not feel well.
  c. Can be taught how to measure their own respiratory rate, heart rate, temperature, blood pressure and oxygen saturations.
  d. Need only to have temperature, heart rate, respiratory rate and blood pressure measured every 4 hours.
5 You are with a qualified nurse and you assess a young man admitted with abdominal pain. He has a respiratory rate of 24, oxygen saturations of 92% on room air and appears distressed. His target saturations are 94–98%, with oxygen prescribed. Which of the following is the best course of action?
  a. Carry on with an ABCDE assessment and calculate NEWS 2.
  b. Reposition him in as upright a position as tolerated, draw round the screens and pull the emergency bell.
  c. Tell the doctor the next time they are on the ward.
  d. Reposition the patient in as upright a position as tolerated, commence oxygen at 2L/min *via* nasal specs, continue to complete an ABCDE assessment, calculate NEWS 2 and action accordingly.
6 **SBAR** is a communication tool that does which of the following?:
  a. Gives a simple structured well-understood system for conveying information regarding a deteriorating patient to health care professionals.
  b. Tells the doctor that they have to come and see your patient immediately.

c. Enables communication across the healthcare team, using the mnemonic for situation, background, qssessment and response.
d. Summons the cardiac arrest team when a patient collapses.

7 Qualified nurses may fulfil which roles in the 'chain of response' (DH 2009)?
a. Recorder and recogniser only.
b. Recorder, and secondary responder, if they have been qualified for 2 years.
c. Recorder, recogniser and primary responder in the areas they have received training and have appropriate competencies.
d. Can perform the role of primary and secondary responder if the Matron says that is now part of their role.

8 The problem of early recognition of acute illness, with appropriate and timely response to prevent medical emergencies occurring:
a. Is not a new problem, has been recognised since the 1990s.
b. Has only been a problem since everybody started using NEWS.
c. Is only a problem in the United Kingdom.
d. Is a product of an increasing number of patients in hospital at any one time.

9 The accurate measurement and recording of respiratory rate is:
a. Best done while talking to the patient so they relax and RR is not falsely elevated.
b. Quickly and accurately calculated by counting the breaths over 15 seconds and multiplying by 4.
c. Not an important part of the ABCDE assessment if the patient is monitored for SpO_2.
d. Counted over 1 full minute, as even small deviations can be clinically significant.

10 Many acute trusts have developed a Critical Care Outreach Service. The primary role of outreach is:
a. To use their specific skills in managing the acutely ill patient to support and advise nurses and medical staff in the immediate management of the deteriorating patient.
b. To look after patients who are not well and transfer them to the intensive care unit as necessary.
c. To teach doctors the skills of advanced life support.
d. To support relatives whose loved ones have died while receiving critical care.

Answers

1 c
2 c
3 d
4 a
5 d
6 c
7 c
8 a
9 d
10 a

References

Bilben B, Grandal L and Søvik S. (2016). National Early Warning Score (NEWS) as an emergency department predictor of disease severity and 90-day survival in the acutely dyspneic patient—a prospective observational study. *Scandinavian Journal of Trauma, Resuscitation and Emergency Medicine*, 24, 80.

Critical Care Network-National Nurse Leads (CC3n a). (2018a). *National Competency Framework for Registered Practitioners: Level 1 Patients and Enhanced Care Areas*. Available from https://www.cc3n.org.uk/uploads/9/8/4/2/98425184/level_1_competencies_final_7.7.18.pdf. Accessed on 8 February 2019.

CC3n. (2018b). *Step Competency Framework*. Accessible from https://www.cc3n.org.uk/step-competency-framework.html.

Cooper N, Forrest K and Cramp P. (2006). *Essential Guide to Acute Care*. London: BMJ Books, Blackwell Publishing.

DH. (2000). *Comprehensive Critical Care: A Review of Adult Critical Care Services*. London: Department of Health, The Stationary Office.

DH. (2009). *Competencies for Recognising and Responding to Acutely Ill Patients in Hospital*. London: DH.

DH. (2015). *Comorbidities a Framework of Principles for System-Wide Action*. Available from https://assets.publishing.service.gov.uk/government/uploads/system/uploads/attachment_data/file/307143/Comorbidities_framework.pdf. Accessed on 2 February 2019.

Donohue LA and Endacott R. (2010). Track, trigger and teamwork: communication of deterioration in acute medical and surgical wards. *Intensive and Critical Care Nursing*, 26, 10–17.

Faculty of Intensive Care Medicine. (2019). *Guidelines for the Provision of Intensive Care Services*. Available from https://www.ics.ac.uk/ICS/ICS/GuidelinesAndStandards/GPICS_2nd_Edition.aspx. Accessed on 27 September 2019.

Flenady T, Dwyer T and Applegarth J. (2017). Accurate respiratory rates count: so should you! *Australasian Emergency Nursing Journal*, 20, 45.

Francis R. (2013). *Report of the Mid Staffordshire NHS Foundation Trust Public Inquiry*. London: The Stationery Office. Available from https://webarchive.nationalarchives.gov.uk/20150407084231/http://www.midstaffspublicinquiry.com/report. Accessed on 8 February 2018.

Goldhill D, White A and Summer A. (1999). Physiological values and procedures in the 24-h before ICU admission from the ward. *Anaesthesia*, 54, 529–534.

Government Statistical Service. (2018). *Statistical Press Notice Monthly Critical Care Beds and Cancelled Urgent Operations Data, England June 2018*. Available from https://www.england.nhs.uk/statistics/wp-content/uploads/sites/2/2018/08/June-18-Monthly-SitRep-SPN-IIDo3-V2.pdf. Accessed on 11 January 2019.

Grant S. (2018). Limitations of track and trigger systems and the National Early Warning Score. Part 1: areas of contention. *British Journal of Nursing*, 27(11), 24–31.

Health Education England. (2017). Nursing Associate Curriculum Framework. Available from https://www.hee.nhs.uk/sites/default/files/documents/Nursing%20Associate%20Curriculum%20Framework%20Feb2017_0.pdf. Accessed on 2 February 2019.

King's Fund. (2017). *NHS Hospital Bed Numbers: Past, Present, Future*. Available from https://www.kingsfund.org.uk/publications/nhs-hospital-bed-numbers. Accessed on 11 January 2019.

Kolic I, Crane S, McCartney S, Perkins Z, Taylor A (2015). Factors affecting response to National Early Warning Score (NEWS). *Resuscitation*, 90, 85–90.

Kyriacos U, Jelsma J, James M and Jordan S. (2015). Early warning score system versus standard observation charts for wards in South Africa: a cluster randomized controlled trial. *Trials*, 16(1), 103. doi:10.1186/s13063-015-0624-2. Available from https://www.ncbi.nlm.nih.gov/pmc/articles/PMC4374204/pdf/13063_2015_Article_624.pdf. Accessed on August 2019.

Lacobucci G. (2017). NHS in 2017: 'keeping pace with society'. *BMJ*, 356, i6738. Available from https://www.bmj.com/content/356/bmj.i6738. Accessed on 10 January 2019.

Lipley N. (2000). Government takes early action to avert another NHS winter of chaos. *Nursing Standard*, 14(37), 4–5.

Mackintosh N, Rainey H and Sandal J. (2012). Understanding how rapid response systems may improve safety for the acutely ill patient: learning from the front line. *BMJ Quality & Safety*, 21, 135–144.

McGaughey J, O'Halloran P, Porter S and Blackwood B. (2017). Early warning systems and rapid response to the deteriorating patient in hospital: a systematic realist review. *Journal of Advanced Nursing*, 73, 2977–2891. doi:10.1111/jan.13398.

McQuillan P, Pilkington S, Allan A, Taylor B, Short A, Morgan G, Nielson M, Barret D and Smith G. (1998). Confidential enquiry into quality of care before admission to intensive care. *British Medical Journal*, 316, 1853–1858.

Muller M, Jurgens J, Redaelli M, Klinberg K, Haust W and Stock S. (2018). Impact of the communication and patient hand-off tool SBAR on patient safety: a systematic review. *BMJ Open*, 8, e022202. doi:10.1136/bmjopen-2018-022202. Accessed from https://bmjopen.bmj.com/content/8/8/e022202. Accessed on 1 February 2019.

National Cardiac Arrest Audit. (2017). *Key Statistics from the National Cardiac Arrest Audit.* Available from https://www.icnarc.org/DataServices/.../39d06a50-74e7-e811-80ef-1402ec3fcd79. Accessed on 1 February 2019.

National Patient Safety Agency. (2007). *Recognising and Responding Appropriately to Early Signs of Deterioration in Hospitalised Patients.* London: NPSA.

NCEPOD. (2005). An acute problem? In *National Confidential Enquiry into Patient Outcome and Death.* London: NCEPOD.

NCEPOD. (2012). *Time to Intervene.* Available from https://www.ncepod.org.uk/2012report1/downloads/CAP_summary.pdf. Accessed on January 2019.

NCEPOD. (2017). *Inspiring Change A Review of the Quality of Care Provided to Patients Receiving Acute Non-Invasive Ventilation.* Available from https://www.ncepod.org.uk/2017report2/downloads/InspiringChange_ExecutiveSummary.pdf. Accessed on February 2019.

NHS Digital. (2017). *Hospital Accident and Emergency Activity.* Available from https://digital.nhs.uk/data-and-information/publications/statistical/hospital-accident--emergency-activity. Accessed on 11 January 2019.

NHS Digital. (2019). *Hospital Episode Statistics (HES).* Available from https://digital.nhs.uk/data-and-information/data-tools-and-services/data-services/hospital-episode-statistics. Accessed on 11 January 2019.

NHS England. (2018). *National Early Warning Score (NEWS).* Available from https://www.england.nhs.uk/ourwork/clinical-policy/sepsis/nationalearlywarningscore/. Accessed on 10 February 2019.

NHS Improvement. (2018). *SBAR Communication Tool-Situation, Background, Assessment Recommendation.* Available from https://improvement.nhs.uk/resources/sbar-communication-tool/. Accessed on February 2019.

NICE. (2007). *Acutely Ill Patients in Hospital GC50.* London: NICE.

NICE. (2018). *Critical Care Outreach Teams Emergency and Acute Medical Cover in the Over 16's: Service Delivery and Organisation NG94.* Available from https://www.nice.org.uk/guidance/ng94/evidence/27.critical-care-outreach-teams-pdf-172397464640. Accessed February 2019.

NICE. (2019). *Hypertension in Adults: Diagnosis and Management NG10054.* Available from https://www.nice.org.uk/guidance/indevelopment/gid-ng10054. Accessed August 2019.

NMC. (2018a). *The Code: Professional Standards of Practice and Behaviour for Nurses, Midwives and Nursing Associates.* Available from https://www.nmc.org.uk/globalassets/sitedocuments/nmc-publications/nmc-code.pdf. Accessed on 2 February 2019a.

NMC. (2018b). *Becoming a Nursing Associate.* Available from https://www.nmc.org.uk/education/becoming-a-nurse-midwife-nursing-associate/becoming-a-nursing-associate/. Accessed on 2 February 2019.

NMC. (2018c). *Standards Framework for Nursing and Midwifery Education.* Available form https://www.nmc.org.uk/standards-for-education-and-training/standards-framework-for-nursing-and-midwifery-education/. Accessed on 2 February 2019.

NPSA. (2007). *Safer Care for the Acutely Ill Patient: Learning from Serious Incidents.* London: NPSA.

O'Driscoll R, Howard L, Earis J, Mak V, Bajwah S, Beasley R, Curtis K, Davison A, Dorward A, Dyer C, Evans A, Falconer L, Fitzpatrick C, Gibbs S, Hinshaw K, Howard R, Kane B, Keep J, Kelly C, Khachi H, Asad M, Khan I, Kishen R, Mansfield L, Martin B, Moore F, Powrie D, Restrick L, Roffe C, Singer M, Soar J, Small I, Ward L, Whitmore D, Wedzicha W, Wijesinghe M and BTS

Emergency Oxygen Guideline Development Group On behalf of the British Thoracic Society. (2017). BTS guideline for oxygen use in adults in healthcare an emergency settings. *Thorax*, 72(S1), i1–i20.

Office for National Statistics. (2016). *Overview of the UK Population*: February 2016. Available from https://www.ons.gov.uk/peoplepopulationandcommunity/populationandmigration/populationestimates/articles/overviewoftheukpopulation/february2016. Accessed on 10 January 2019.

Philip K, Pack E, Cambiana V, Rollmann H, Weil S and O'Beirne J. (2015). The accuracy of respiratory rate assessment by doctors in a London Teaching Hospital: a cross sectional study. *Journal of Clinical Monitoring and Computing*, 29, 455–460.

Pimental M, Redfern O, Gerry S, Collins G, Malycha J, Prytherch D, Schmidt P, Smith G and Watkinsin P. (2019 in press). A comparison of the ability of the National Early Warning Score and the National Early Warning Score 2 to identify patients at risk of in-hospital mortality: a multi-centre database study. *Resuscitation*, 134, 147–156.

Resuscitation Council UK. (2015). *Advanced Life Support* (3rd Edition). UK: Resuscitation Council (UK).

Royal College of Physicians. (2012). *National Early Warning Score (NEWS) Standardising the Assessment of Acute-Illness Severity in the NHS*. Available from https://www.rcplondon.ac.uk/file/32/download?token=5NwjEyTq. Accessed January 2019.

Royal College of Physicians. (2017). *National Early Warning Score (NEWS) 2 Standardising the Assessment of Acute-Illness Severity in the NHS*. Available from http://www.rcplondon.ac.uk/resources/national-early-warning-score-news. Accessed on 14 January 2019.

Schein R, Hazday N, Pena N and Ruben B. (1990). Clinical antecedents to in-hospital cardiopulmonary arrest. *Chest*, 98, 1388–1392.

Smith G. (2010). In-hospital cardiac arrest: is it time for an in-hospital 'chain of prevention?' *Resuscitation*, 81, 1209–1211.

Smith GB, Prytherch DR, Jarvis S, et al. (2016). Comparison of the ability of the physiologic components of medical emergency team criteria and the U.K. National Early Warning Score to discriminate patients at risk of a range of adverse clinical outcomes. *Critical Care Medicine*, 44(12), 2171–2181. doi:10.1097/CCM.0000000000002000. Accessed on 9 February 2019.

Smith D and Bowden T. (2017). Using the ABCDE approach to assess the deteriorating patient. *Nursing Standard*, 29(32), 51–63.

Spiers L, Singh Mohal J, Pearson-Stuttard J, Greenlee H, Carmichael J and Busher R. (2015). Recognition of the deteriorating patient. *BMJ Quality Improvement Reports*, 4, 1. doi:10.1136/bmjquality.u206777.w2734. Accessed on 9 February 2019.

2 Vulnerability in the acutely ill patient

Ian Peate

> **AIM**
>
> This chapter aims to provide the reader with insight and understanding concerning the vulnerable adult in the acute care setting and those whose health and wellbeing is at risk of deterioration.

> **OBJECTIVES**
>
> After reading this chapter you will be able to:
>
> - Describe key terms.
> - Understand the rights of vulnerable adults in acute care situations.
> - Examine the health and social policy provisions for vulnerable adults.
> - Ensure that the voice of the vulnerable adult is heard and action taken.
> - Outline some of the ethical considerations relevant to the care and treatment of vulnerable people in the acute care setting.
> - Discuss the key issues concerning delirium in the acute care setting.

Introduction

Regardless of the setting in which the nurse works, safeguarding is a part of every nurse's practice, every single day; it is everyone's business. Michaels and Moffett (2012) suggest that nurses encounter vulnerability at all levels: cellular, physiological systems, mind–body, individuals, communities and societies. It is not always the case that adults can protect and care for themselves ('Adults' in this chapter refers to people aged 18 years or over). Providing care for vulnerable adults is an essential aspect of the role of the nurse. There are many reasons people may be thought of as vulnerable.

This chapter discusses the issue of vulnerability, reminding the reader that they are patient's advocates and as a result of this privilege they must always act with the patient's, best interests in mind, ensuring that the patient is at the heart of all that is done. One of the many aspects of professional practice is to ensure that those for whom you care come to no harm (Peate 2016).

Vulnerability

A number of high-level adverse incidents have occurred over the years in hospital and social care settings putting people at risk or actually causing harm. Not everyone is receiving good care (Care Quality Commission [CQC] 2018). Often in large and complex organisations such as the National Health Service (NHS) things can go wrong, and it is essential that organisations report and learn from such incidents so that changes can be implemented and then become embedded in practice. Those with long-term conditions, those who present with co-morbidities and those with medical emergencies are more vulnerable and are placed at higher risk by the increasingly complex nature of acute care.

Vulnerability is a multifaceted state that is not easy to quantify. A vulnerable person can be defined as a person who has or may have a care need (broadly defined) arising from a mental or other disability, age or illness (Disclosure and Baring Service [DBS] 2012). Having 'a care need' means that the person needs someone to assist in caring for them. The nurse is centrally placed, often as a member of a multi-disciplinary team working in partnership, to assist people.

Each one of us is potentially at risk of abuse and ill-treatment. Any of the following conditions have the possibility to increase vulnerability, for example:

- having a learning disability;
- experiencing mental health problems;
- having physical/sensory impairment;
- being frail or an older person;
- being acutely ill;
- having a long-term condition;
- being incarcerated;
- being homeless.

This chapter discusses the complex issue of vulnerability and how nurses can help others with their care needs, with an emphasis on the vulnerable person who may be experiencing an acute medical emergency and their significant others. Nurses must work in partnership with others to ensure that they safeguard and protect the most vulnerable and to promote high-quality care (Mencap 2007; RCN 2014b). In order to protect the public and those who are deemed vulnerable it is essential to have an understanding of the moral theories and ethical frameworks that will impact on patient outcomes. This chapter will provide a very brief introduction to some of the ethical frameworks that can have an important influence on health care practice.

There had been an absence of adult safeguarding systems within the NHS that enabled healthcare incidents that cause concern to be raised and addressed (Michael and the Independent Inquiry into Access to Healthcare for People with Learning Disabilities 2008; DH 2010). In 2011, The Parliamentary and Health Service Ombudsman had reported on the care and treatment of 10 older people who had received care in the NHS. The report considered 10 complaints made to the Ombudsman about the standard of care those older people had received. The accounts of care discussed provided a picture of an NHS that was failing to respond to the needs of older people with care and compassion.

There is an ongoing need to ensure that nurses and other health and social care professionals have a key role in the identification of abuse, harm and neglect and in response to this putting together appropriate strategies. This will also mean that health and social care professionals work in a collaborative manner with local authorities if needs be when adult safeguarding concerns arise during the delivery of health care (see Case study 2.1). Working in a collaborative manner is termed an integrated approach. In some areas of care posts have been created, for example, designated nurse posts for the safeguarding of adults. These nurses have responsibility for strengthening safeguarding processes across health and social services.

Potential and actual abuse of vulnerable adults can take many forms. Allegations can be made about physical abuse; the highest number of allegations concerning abuse is related to physical abuse, however, it is incorrect to assume that only those people who are battered people are abused, but emotional scars are just as serious as physical injuries. There are some vulnerable groups and communities that have a significantly poorer life expectancy than the general population, often as a result of their vulnerable status.

CASE STUDY 2.1 STUDENT NURSE JAVELLE

A third-year student nurse Javelle is on placement on an arterial high-dependency unit. She is on this clinical placement for 12 weeks and this is her second week. She has been allocated a mentor/supervisor but, unfortunately, her mentor/supervisor has been off sick for most of the two weeks she has been there.

For the last three days Javelle has been working with Sister Isharm. They are caring for a patient with learning disabilities who is recovering from major arterial surgery but he is still too unwell to return to the general ward and he needs one-to-one nursing care.

Javelle is concerned about some aspects of Sister Isharm's work style. Sister Isharm has been making derogatory, patronising and sarcastic comments about the patient, his physical appearance and also about some of his family members. She has been using offensive terms such as 'fatty' and 'slowcoach'. Her comments are being made in an insensitive manner. Sister Isharm's actions are making Javelle feel increasingly uncomfortable.

Javelle has confided in another staff nurse. The staff nurse tells Javelle that Sister Isharm is the most senior nurse on the unit and is highly respected by other nurses and other health care professionals. The staff nurse told Javelle to keep her head down and she also reminds her that Sister has a lot of sway when it comes to assessing clinical practice and the completion of her practice assessment documentation.

Vulnerability and safeguarding is everyone's concern and all staff have a duty to raise and report any concerns about any aspect of care that they consider to be unacceptable. Javelle is aware of the various routes that can be taken to raise concerns and she contacts her link lecturer to discuss the issues further.

The Law

The principles of protection are enshrined in various legislative and policy directives. The Human Rights Act 1998 is made up of articles, which state that no person should be subjected to any form of torture or cruel or inhumane or degrading treatment or punishment, that each person has a right to life, liberty and security. There is also a prohibition against discrimination.

Implemented in April 2015, the Care Act 2014 gave safeguarding adults a legal framework for the first time. Fundamental standards of safety and quality were introduced that apply to all providers of regulated health and social care. The standards set the benchmark for care provision. One of the standards relates to safeguarding. The nurse must remember that since devolution, the laws within the four UK countries may differ and it is essential that they work within the laws of the country in which they are practicing (Nursing and Midwifery Council (NMC) 2018a).

The Equality Act 2010

This Act came into force on 1 October 2010 bringing together over 116 separate pieces of legislation into one single Act. Combined, they provide a legal framework to protect the rights of individuals and advance equality of opportunity for all. The Act simplifies, strengthens and harmonises legislation to provide Britain with a new discrimination law which protects individuals from unfair treatment and promotes a fair and more equal society.

From the Equality Act comes the Equality and Human Rights Commission, taking over the functions of the Commission for Racial Equality, the Disability Rights Commission and the Equality Opportunities Commission, and bringing them all under one umbrella in 2007.

There are many more laws that can be cited when considering safeguarding and vulnerability. It is not the intention of this chapter to provide a discussion of the law, but you must be aware of the legal and professional issues that arise when you are caring for a person who is acutely ill.

No secrets

Guidance (No Secrets) was produced in 2000 (in England) relating to how to develop policies and procedures to safeguard vulnerable adults from abuse, it brought about major changes in adult protection procedures. The equivalent was also produced in Wales in 2000 (National Assembly for Wales 2000). In Scotland, this is the Adult Support and Protection (Scotland) Act 2007 providing legislation that aims to protect vulnerable people from harm. The aim of these publications is to provide protection for those adults who are believed vulnerable in our society, those who are at risk of abuse and those who may need protection. Local authorities through the social services they provide are obliged to act and conform to the general guidance issued in the *No Secrets* publication (DH and Home Office 2000). Policy and procedures have to be in place to safeguard those who are considered at risk. *No Secrets* states that there can be no secrets and no hiding places when it comes to exposing the abuse of adults (DH and Home Office 2000).

Safeguarding Adults (DH 2009) is a review of *No Secrets*, and also provides guidance on devising and implementing multi-agency policies and procedures to protect vulnerable adults from harm. The aim of the review was to determine whether and how the *No Secrets* guidance needed to change in order to assist society in keeping adults safe from harm or abuse.

No secrets and other similar guidance brought together a large number of key stakeholders, including the police, various organisations within the NHS, the social services and independent and voluntary organisations as they worked together to reach a consensus regarding the protection of vulnerable adults. For the first time, it laid down a framework for responding to the abuse of vulnerable adults in all settings.

The government has revised its 2000 guidance (DH 2009) as there have been many changes in the field of adult protection, including a reconsideration of 'safeguarding'. No Secrets operates within the context of current legislation and case law and the legal landscape has developed significantly since it was published.

The Government's policy objective is to prevent and reduce risk of significant harm to vulnerable adults from abuse or other types of exploitation, whilst at the same time supporting individuals in keeping control over their lives and in making informed choices without coercion (DH 2011a).

No Secrets and subsequent reviews are needed so as to focus on how people are protected as well as how abuse is prevented. Present systems need to be continually reviewed and revised to ensure that people are protected and early interventions put in place to address actual or potential harm. Legislation around safeguarding needs to be monitored to determine if it is fit for purpose and that policies and practices that emerge from legislation are contemporary.

Key terms

Guidance has been provided to help health and social care professionals to work in partnership, produce policies and ensure that appropriate procedures and practices are in place and carried out (DH and Home Office 2000; DH 2009, 2010). This guidance is very often derived from statute. It is not law, but the government expects that the guidance is adhered to and should only be deviated from in exceptional circumstances. The guidance covers issues of definition concerning the various and often complex terms associated with vulnerability. Other terms synonymous with vulnerability include liability, exposure and susceptibility.

It must be reiterated that regardless of the care setting (and the acute care setting is no exception) the important issue of safeguarding and vulnerability must be paramount for all of those who are recipients of care. The key aim is to make sure that there are robust processes in place that ensure adult safeguarding arrangements become fully integrated into healthcare systems.

There are several terms that are used when considering adult protection issues and it is imperative that these key terms are defined. Understanding these terms can assist you when helping the people you care for. Northway and Jenkins (2018) note that definitions vary over time and also with regards to geographical variation, which may present difficulties in interpretation and practice.

Safeguarding

This term is associated with the need to feel safe and free from exploitation and is often seen as one of our most basic needs. Any threat to a person's safety will directly threaten their health and well-being, therefore identifying what the threat to the person's safety is and addressing it is one way of providing high-quality holistic care (De Chesnay 2012).

Safeguarding is associated with various legal frameworks and policies that aim to protect an adult's fundamental right to be safe. This is of particular importance for those who are, as a result of their situation or circumstances, unable to keep themselves safe; this also applies to those people who are acutely ill.

Safeguarding vulnerable adults from abuse and harm is everyone's concern and this is now a significant aspect of everyday healthcare provision. In 1954 Maslow (a psychologist) postulated that humans have a hierarchy of needs, and this remains a popular theory (see Figure 2.1).

The theory suggests that each person has a hierarchy of needs and the individual must satisfy each level before they are able to move onto the next level. Five hierarchical levels are identified:

1 *Physiological needs*: the need for food, water, sexual satisfaction. These needs are required in order to survive.
2 *Safety needs*: we all need to feel safe within our environment. These needs also refer to emotional and physical safety.
3 *Social needs*: the need for love, friendship and a sense of belonging.
4 *Esteem needs*: the need for self-respect and recognition from others.
5 *Self-actualisation*: this is the point of reaching your full potential.

It is suggested that prior to moving onto another level an individual must satisfy their most basic needs, hence physiological needs must be met before being able to meet safety needs and safety needs have to be met prior to being able to meet social needs and so forth.

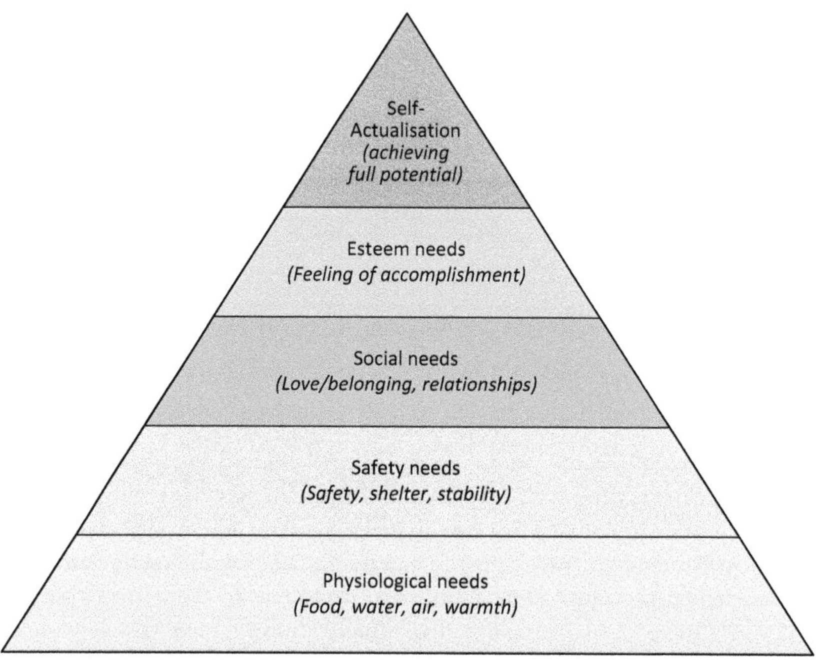

Figure 2.1 Maslow's hierarchy of needs. Source: Maslow, A. (1987) Motivation and Personality, 3rd ed. Upper Saddle River, NJ: Pearson.

Feeling safe and being safe, physically and emotionally, are therefore essential. If a person feels vulnerable or feels their health and well-being are at risk this may prevent them from making a full recovery. Sometimes, the health of a patient in hospital may deteriorate suddenly and the person becomes acutely ill. There are times when this is more likely to happen, for example, if the patient is an emergency admission to hospital, after surgery and after discharge from a critical care area such as a high-dependency unit. Becoming acutely ill can happen at any time during an illness and this increases a person's risk of needing to stay longer in hospital, not making a full recovery or dying. At all stages Maslow's hierarchy will need to be given consideration. Think of patients who are acutely ill and apply Maslow's model to those patients. All of those who are acutely ill are vulnerable and this may be from a physiological, emotional or psychological perspective.

Vulnerable adults

Every one of us is vulnerable at some point in our lives, we can all be considered as adults at risk. Penhale and Parker (2008) note that labelling a person as vulnerable can automatically assign them to a category that may be seen in a negative light. The label vulnerable may suggest a degree of weakness with no reason for this: furthermore, referring to a person as vulnerable may also ascribe victim status which could disempower the individual. The terms vulnerable and vulnerability are used in statute and policy guidance. Care must be taken when using the terms not to apportion blame; neither must we imply weakness on behalf of the person being described when using the term.

There is no formal definition of vulnerability in health care, although some people may be considered at greater risk from harm than others. This risk may have arisen as a complication of their presenting condition and their individual circumstances (DH 2010). Case study 2.2 demonstrates how a person who may be considered low risk with regards to vulnerability on admission can, because of their presenting condition and individual circumstances, be deemed high risk and subjected to increased vulnerability. Case study 2.2. provides an idea of how a person's health status can change and their risk status can alter, making them more prone to risk and more vulnerable. Recognition of risk and appropriate responses are key if risk and harm are to be minimised.

CASE STUDY 2.2 SANJAY

Sanjay is a 68-year-old married man with four children. He was admitted to hospital to undergo an emergency appendectomy after complaining of lower-right abdominal pain, a history of constipation for three days and pyrexia of 38.2°C. A diagnosis of appendicitis was made and he was admitted to the surgical ward for surgery. Sanjay had previously enjoyed good health with no relevant past medical history.

A laparoscopic appendectomy was performed under a general anaesthetic. While undergoing surgery Sanjay suffered a cardiac arrest and was resuscitated. He was returned to the intensive care unit for three days, was stabilised, made a successful recovery and was transferred to the general surgical ward area.

Post operatively Sanjay's abdominal keyhole incisions became infected and a methicillin-resistant *Staphylococcus aureus* was the causative organism. It was not until two weeks later that Sanjay was discharged home.

Safeguarding adults means (DH 2018):

- Protecting the rights of adults to live in safety, free from abuse and neglect.
- People and organisations working together to prevent and stop both the risks and experience of abuse or neglect.
- People and organisations making sure that the adult's wellbeing is promoted including, where appropriate, taking fully into account their views, wishes, feelings and beliefs in deciding on any action.
- Recognising that adults sometimes have complex interpersonal relationships and may be ambivalent, unclear or unrealistic about their personal circumstances and therefore potential risks to their safety or wellbeing.

Those who provide care (care organisations) must ensure that safeguarding arrangements will always promote the adult's wellbeing. When arrangements are in place, this will impact positively on person centred care and focused outcomes.

Department of Health in its *No Secrets* document (Department of Health and the Home Office 2000), notes that community care services are broader than those services that would usually be considered community care, they will include all care services provided in any setting or context Any adult receiving any form of health care is recognised as vulnerable and the DH (2011b) emphasises that an individual's age does not of itself make the person vulnerable, something external to the individual, according to Martin (2007) creates vulnerability.

The Disclosure and Barring Service (DBS) (2012) describes a vulnerable adult further. In general terms, a vulnerable adult is a person who is aged 18 years or older and is classed as vulnerable when they are receiving one of the following services:

- health care;
- relevant personal care;
- social care work;
- assistance in relation to general household matters by reason of age, illness or disability;
- relevant assistance in the conduct of their own affairs;
- conveying (due to age, illness or disability in prescribed circumstances).

There are similarities in both definitions, however the DBS have amended the term 'vulnerable adult' as it was felt to be inappropriate to label an adult as vulnerable merely based on their circumstances, age or disability. Both definitions provide meaning to this complex concept and both of them indicate that services provided can expose a person to vulnerability. Vulnerability appears to be related to the provision of services. Whether or not a person is vulnerable in the instances that have been described is dependent upon surrounding circumstances and the environment and each case has to be judged on its own merits. Nurses and other health and social care practitioners must strive to ensure that the service they provide are altered and amended if they are causing or are in danger of causing vulnerability, even if this is unintended, as such practitioners need to be vigilant and aware of the potential harm that may be caused.

Safeguarding is about protecting a person's right to live in safety, free from abuse and neglect. Safeguarding requires people and organisations to work together to prevent and stop the risk and the experience of abuse or neglect, while at the same time ensuring that the adult's wellbeing is promoted including, where appropriate, having regard to their views, wishes, feelings and beliefs in deciding on any action. Safeguarding Adults describes all the work that is done to help adults with care and support needs to stay safe from abuse and neglect. It replaces the term 'adult protection'. The term 'adult at risk of abuse and neglect' has been used to replace 'vulnerable adult' as the term 'vulnerable adult' could wrongly imply that some of the reason for the abuse lies with the adult abused and may also assumes that the simple case of being old or having a disability renders one vulnerable. An adult at risk may therefore be a person who:

- is old and frail due to ill health, physical disability or cognitive impairment;
- has a learning disability;
- has a physical disability and/or a sensory impairment;
- has mental health needs including dementia or a personality disorder;
- has a long-term illness/condition;
- misuses substances or alcohol;
- is a carer such as a family member/friend who provides personal assistance and care to adults and is subject to abuse;
- is unable to demonstrate the capacity to make a decision and is in need of care and support.

What constitutes abuse?

Just as it has proved a challenge to define the terms vulnerability and safeguarding, so it is also difficult to define what is meant by abuse. All adults, irrespective of age or mental capacity, have the right to:

- live in dignity and safety, free from maltreatment of any kind;
- have their physical as well as their emotional needs met;
- make their own decisions;
- maintain autonomy (as much as possible within any health constraints).

Abuse, be it physical mistreatment and assault or an abuse that is unseen, that has emotional and psychological impact is always unacceptable. There are not and should not be any hierarchies of abuse (Royal College of Nursing (RCN) 2018), all forms of abuse are potentially damaging, any unwanted or warranted behavior is unacceptable.

It may prove futile to seek a clear and delineated definition of abuse and what it is. Abuse means different things to different people in different settings; abuse is defined by society and as such this will be different for different societies. As the understanding of this complex term advances the definition will change and reflect learning, so what constitutes abuse now will constantly change and develop: any definition is subject to change in time and place. It is therefore essential that at all times the social elements related to abuse are taken into consideration. Despite this it is important that we have a working definition of abuse in order to guide and support, with the caveat that the term abuse is subject to wide variation. A good starting point is the definition provided by the Department of Health and Home Office (2000): 'Abuse is the violation of an individual's human civil rights by any other person or persons'.

This is a broad definition and as such includes a wide range of actions that could be considered abuse. In order to make sense of the definition in a more practical way it is helpful to think of a range of types of abuse. The next section discusses the different types of abuse that can occur.

Kinds of abuse

Abuse can occur as a single act or repeated acts by a single person or a group of people. To recap, abuse may be physical, verbal or psychological, it can be an act of neglect or a failure to act or it may occur where a vulnerable person is persuaded to enter into something which they have not consented to or cannot consent to. It can range from not treating someone with dignity and respect, to extreme punishment, cruelty or torture. There are a range of types and levels of abuse and they can fall into the following categories:

- physical abuse;
- sexual abuse;
- neglect and poor professional practice;
- institutional abuse;
- financial or material abuse;
- emotional/psychological abuse;
- discrimination.

Any list such as the one provided should be treated with caution: as time passes there may be other categories added. Table 2.1 discusses the various categories of abuse; none of the lists provided is exhaustive.

Table 2.1 Types of abuse

Form of abuse	*Description*
Physical	This list highlights what maybe indicators of several different problems. Indicators of physical abuse could be: • History of falls that are difficult to explain • Bruising and injuries that cannot be explained • Bruising at various stages of healing • Teeth marks • Unexplained burns in unusual locations • Unexplained fractures to any part of the body • Cuts, lacerations or abrasions that cannot be explained • Slapping, kicking, punching or finger marks • Injury that is a similar shape to an object, such as a belt buckle • Untreated medical problems • Weight loss that is due to malnutrition or dehydration • Misuse of medications • Restraint or inappropriate sanctions • Deference, the person becomes passive
Sexual	Sexual abuse happens when adults are involved in sexual activities that they do not fully understand, to which they are unable to give their consent, be this verbally or by their behaviour, to which they object or which can cause them harm. They may have been forced into the activity. Some of the indicators of sexual abuse include:

(*Continued*)

Table 2.1 Continued

Form of abuse	*Description*
	• A sudden change in a person's behaviour • Confusion of sudden onset • Incontinence • Withdrawal • The vulnerable adult engages in overt sexual behaviour and inappropriate use of sexual language • Injury that is self-inflicted • Sleep patterns that have become disturbed and periods of poor concentration • Experiencing difficulty in walking or sitting • Torn, stained underwear • Love bites • In the genitalia or anal regions – pain, discomfort or itching, bruising or bleeding • Sexually transmitted infection • Urinary tract infection • Vaginal infection (there may also be a discharge) • Bruising to upper thighs and arms • Severe upset or agitation when being bed bathed or bathed • Pregnancy in a person who is unable to consent
Neglect and poor professional practice	A person may experience neglect because their physical and/or psychological (emotional) needs have or are being neglected by a carer. Failing to keep someone warm, clean and well-nourished or neglecting to provide prescribed medication may be considered neglect. Neglect might also include a failure to intervene in those situations that are dangerous to the person particularly when the individual lacks the mental capacity to assess risk. The following may be indications of many different problems, they could also indicate neglect: • Poor environmental conditions • Insufficient heating and lighting • Poor physical condition of the individual • Person's clothing may be ill fitting, they may be unclean and in a poor condition • Malnutrition • The carer fails to give prescribed medication correctly • Failure to offer appropriate privacy and dignity • Inconsistent or reluctant contact with health and social care organisations • Isolation - refusing access to callers or visitors • Disregarding nursing care/medical needs • Isolated incidents of poor or uncceptable professional practice • Perverse ill-treatment • Professional misconduct
Institutional	Institutional abuse is concerned with who abuses and how that abuse occurs, as opposed to types of harm. Abuse may occur in a number of relationships, family, service or institution and it can be carried out by a specific person or more collectively, by a regime. Possible indicators of institutional abuse can include:

(*Continued*)

Table 2.1 Continued

Form of abuse	*Description*
	• A rigid bedtime routine and/or deliberate waking • Leaving a person on the commode or toilet for longer periods of time than needed • Inappropriate care of a person's possessions, their clothing and the area where they are living • Lack of personal clothes and belongings • Depressing or stark living environments • Deprived environmental conditions and lack of stimulation • Inappropriate use of medical procedures such as enemata, catheterisation • Failure to provide individual care plans/programmes • Unlawful confinement or restrictions • Inappropriate and unacceptable use of power or control • Speaking to or referring to people with disrespect • Service provision that is inflexible and is based on convenience of the provider rather than the individual receiving services • Physical intervention that is inappropriate • The service user being removed from the home or establishment, without discussion with other appropriate people or agencies, because staff cannot manage their behaviours • Inability to make choices
Financial	Many forms in which financial or material abuse can exist, for example, fraud, theft or using the person's property without seeking their permission. This can involve large sums of money or even small amounts from a person's pension or allowance each week. Jumping to the wrong conclusions too quickly should be avoided. The following may be indicators of financial abuse: • A person's sudden inability to pay their bills, particularly after their benefits have been paid on benefits day • Unexpected and unusual withdrawals of money from an account • The individual lacks belongings that they should be able to afford • Power of attorney obtained when the person cannot understand what they are signing, pressure in connection with wills • Unusual interest by family members in the person's assets • Recent change of deeds for property • Misuse or misappropriation of property, belongings or benefits • Carers main interest is financial with little regard for the health and wellbeing of the vulnerable adult • The person managing finances is uncooperative and elusive • Reluctance to accept care services • Purchase of items that the individual does not need or use • Objects of value and personal items going missing • Unreasonable or inappropriate gifts

(*Continued*)

Table 2.1 Continued

Form of abuse	*Description*
Emotional/ psychological	Emotional/psychological abuse may include intimidation, humiliation, shouting, swearing, emotional blackmail and denial of fundamental human rights. Using language that is racist, preventing a person from enjoying activities or meeting friends are all possible indications of emotional/psychological abuse. Other indicators may include: • Uncertainty about carer • Fearfulness, cowering, avoiding eye contact, flinching on approach • Deference • Unable to sleep or need for excessive sleep • An alteration in appetite • Unusual weight loss/gain • Tearfulness • Paranoia that can not be explained • Low self-esteem • Confusion, agitation • Intimidation • Potential violation of human and civil rights • Isolation - no visitors or phone calls permitted • Inappropriate clothing • Sensory deprivation • Access to hygiene facilities restricted • No personal respect • Lack of recognition of a person's rights • Carer fails to offer personal hygiene, medical care, regular food/drinks • Using furniture to restrict movement • Withdrawal from services or supportive networks • The person's choices, opinions and wishes are neglected • Failure to permit the person to follow their own spiritual and cultural beliefs or sexual orientation
Discrimination	These indicators could include: • Racism • Sexism • Insults • Harassment • Discriminatory abuse that is based on a person's disability or age • Low self-esteem • Withdrawal • Fear/rage • Anger • Depression

CASE STUDY 2.3 MRS RAMNATH

Mrs Ramnath, a 68-year-old widow who is partially sighted, was admitted to hospital with crushing chest pain. Mrs Ramnath presented with a history of severe, crushing chest pain that lasted for approximately one and a half hours. Her electrocardiogram (ECG) showed changes consistent with an acute anterior myocardial infarction. Plans were made to transfer Mrs Ramnath to the cardiac care unit, however no bed was available and she was transferred to a medical ward in the hospital at 02:45h.

Analgesia for pain and other essential medications were given 30 minutes after admission to the ward. She was pain-free but anxious, and it was difficult to contact her only daughter as she was abroad. A full blood count was taken and assessment was made of her urea and electrolytes, blood glucose, renal, hepatic and thyroid function – all were normal.

Mrs Ramnath has a history of asthma; she uses a salbutamol inhaler occasionally and the condition is well controlled. She is deaf in the left ear and has poor hearing in the right ear; she speaks little English. Her father died of a myocardial infarction at 52 years of age, her mother is still alive but frail.

Mrs Ramnath is transferred to the cardiac care unit eight days after her original admission to the hospital as her condition has deteriorated. A full nursing assessment is carried out by the nursing staff admitting her. She has developed a grade 3 pressure sore. An investigation is undertaken as to how she developed the pressure sore.

On assessment upon admission Mrs Ramnath was considered to be high risk for the development of a pressure sore and a request was made for a pressure-relieving mattress. During her stay she was transferred three times from ward to ward within her first week. Initial assessment and her subsequent plan of care identified her need for a pressure-relieving mattress, however this never arrived. During her time on the various wards her skin had started to break down. A request was made again for a pressure-relieving mattress, but again due the numerous moves and poor communication between the teams this never arrived and there was a delay in the patient receiving the equipment.

As a result of the above the hospital has instigated a system whereby transferring of patients between wards and departments (regardless of length of stay) will necessitate a full nursing assessment of needs with detailed and appropriate information being given to the receiving nurse from the transferring ward. The movement of high-risk patients from ward to ward has now been reviewed and revised. There is now provision for ward staff to request and receive emergency equipment outside of normal hours as opposed to having to wait for the equipment to arrive.

Classifying in this way can help generate discussion amongst colleagues when considering acts of abuse. When thinking about abuse it is essential that the upholding of a person's human and civil rights are taken into account – these rights are paramount. Case study 2.3 discusses the case of a patient who develops a pressure sore whilst in hospital.

Many of the types of abuse listed in Table 2.1 may be the result of deliberate intent, negligence or ignorance. There are a number of forms of abuse that could constitute a criminal offence and in this instance this should involve the police: vulnerable people are entitled to the same protection of the law as another person. Age UK (2017) provide examples of abuse that may constitute a criminal offence according to the will include:

- assault (physical or psychological);
- sexual assault or rape;

- theft;
- fraud or other forms of financial exploitation;
- discrimination based on gender, race or age.

It can be seen that there are a wide range of actions that can be considered as abuse. The same is also true of those who may abuse.

Who are the abusers?

Family members, relatives, professional staff, paid care workers, other service users, neighbours, friends, strangers, a teacher, a member of the clergy and those who deliberately exploit vulnerable people may abuse. Abusers can be of any gender. Those in positions of power or authority who use their status to the detriment of the health, safety, welfare and general well-being of people in their care are also in a position to perpetrate abuse (see Case study 2.1).

Abuse can take place anywhere:

- in public places;
- in a prison;
- in the person's own home;
- at work;
- in hospital;
- in places of worship;
- in care homes;
- at day care.

What justifies intervention?

The seriousness or extent of abuse is not always clear; therefore it is essential that consideration be given to the appropriateness of intervention and that a comprehensive assessment is undertaken. The Department of Health and Home Office (2000) assessment of seriousness will take into consideration the following:

- the vulnerability of the individual;
- the nature and extent of the abuse;
- the length of time it has been occurring;
- the impact on the individual;
- the risk of repeated or increasingly serious acts involving this or other vulnerable adults.

Taking action and raising concerns

You must act within legal frameworks and also according to local policies in relation to safeguarding those who may be in vulnerable situations. Situations may arise that will necessitate you working with others to implement and monitor any strategies within your work place to safeguard and protect others. Any information that is gained should be shared appropriately with colleagues and advice (you may receive this from a number of sources) should be sought if you have any concerns. Information sharing can be within your sphere of practice or it can include the sharing of information across agency boundaries with the prime aim of safeguarding and protecting the individual and the public. You might also need to make referrals to others: for example, to social workers or the police.

It is important that you remember that the people you care for have a right to confidentiality and you have a duty to ensure that any information you disclose corresponds to local policy and guidance and that the person you are caring for has given their consent. There may be some exceptional circumstances whereby disclosure of information can be made without consent, but these are usually complex and as such you must seek advice prior to disclosing any information. You must also ensure that you have support systems in place that will help you to manage and deal with any emotions that may arise out of the situation (RCN 2017).

Immediate concerns associated with abuse must be dealt with in the first instance under local safeguarding policies and procedures. NHS Improvement (https://improvement.nhs.uk/resources/learning-from-patient-safety-incidents/) has produced information that can help you if you are concerned about patient safety incidents.

When raising concerns this has to be done in an appropriate manner and this includes using local policies, clinical governance and risk-management procedures. Go back to the first case study presented in this chapter and think about how Javelle may have felt when she had to raise concerns about a senior member of the ward team. It may not always be easy to report concerns: you may not know how to do this, you might be afraid of reprisals, you might even feel you are being disloyal. This can appear even more complex and frightening if you are working alone or if you work in remote, small communities. Always keep in mind that the person you care for is your primary concern. Remember that raising issues early has the potential to prevent their becoming more serious and in effect causing more harm to those you care for.

There are a number of sources of advice that you can access to seek assistance if you are unsure. These include your manager, your lecturer or your mentor/supervisor, your trade union (for example, UNISON, UNITE), your professional body (for example, the Royal College of Nursing) or the charity Public Concern at Work (this is an independent whistleblowing charity). These organisations can raise issues formally and sometimes can act for you or on your behalf; they may also be able to offer you personal support. Examples of concern may include (NMC 2018b):

- issues related to health and safety violations where there may be risk to health and safety; unprofessional staff behaviour or attitudes;
- concerns about the standard of care being delivered;
- reservations about the environment in which care is being delivered;
- the health of a colleague and the impact this is having on their ability to practise safely;
- a shortage or lack of the availability of clinical equipment, this may also include a lack of adequate training;.
- any criminal activity, fraud or financial mismanagement.

You have to report your concerns to the appropriate person or authority immediately if you suspect or know of any risk to the safety of those in your care. If there is immediate risk or harm, you should report this without delay.

Silence is not always golden. An everyday aspect of your work is to speak up for the people you care for: to fail to report concerns is unacceptable. Raising concerns and speaking up demonstrates your commitment to the people you care for.

More often than not you will raise your concern directly with the nurse in charge and in most of these cases a satisfactory conclusion will emerge. However, if this fails there may be a need to take your concerns through a formal route, and at this stage you might wish to seek support and advice from a professional body, trade union, mentor/supervisor or lecturer. Figure 2.2 outlines the stages for raising and escalating concerns.

Myths and Facts

Many individuals have a number of misconceived ideas concerning the facts about the abuse and neglect of adults. Mistaken beliefs that are not checked out may be detrimental to the health and well-being of the vulnerable or abused person. Below are some common myths and facts that are coupled with abuse and vulnerability:

Myth: Abuse and neglect of adults is rare.

Fact: It is difficult to determine an accurate percentage of the occurrences of abuse because many of those people who have been abused hide behind a sense of shame and embarrassment. For a variety of reasons some people can find it difficult to speak out about their abuse, because of this the incidence of adult abuse is biased; this also makes it difficult to measure.

Myth: Most abuse of adults occurs in care or nursing homes.

Fact: Abuse can occur just as easily in a person's own home, a busy hospital ward or in day care.

Myth: Abuse in later life only happens to those people who are very frail.

Fact: Abuse can happen to anyone and comes in many forms including physical abuse, emotional abuse and financial abuse. Emotional abuse is just as harmful as physical abuse.

Myth: Adult abuse only occurs to older people, those who are isolated or those with disabilities.

Fact: Anyone can be abused. Often the abuser is a loved one whom the person trusts. It is this bond of trust that can permit the abuser to destroy the person's self-confidence and also challenge their feeling and sense of self-worth.

Myth: Most abuse of adults concerns physical abuse.

Fact: Physical abuse is often the easiest type of abuse to notice as there is easily recognisable physical evidence that can include bruises, scratches, biting or scarring. When verbal, emotional or psychological abuse is present, external indicators can come in the form of behavioural modifications.

Myth: Paid carers and strangers are the ones preying on older people.

Fact: Most vulnerable adults are abused by a known, trusted person – usually a family member.

Ethical considerations

Ethical issues are apparent in all aspects of care and instinctively concluding that something is fair or unfair requires criteria to be called upon to make that judgement. Having an understanding of ethics will help the nurse when caring for patients in acute care settings and will help them make certain judgements that are based on protecting the public from harm. Whatever element of nursing intervention is being undertaken will have the potential to impact positively and also negatively on the patient's physical and psychological well-being. A continuous awareness of this, no matter how short-lived the interaction is with the patient, is required. Nurses are engaged with the ethical practice of nursing and are confronted with ethical issues, challenges and dilemmas almost every day.

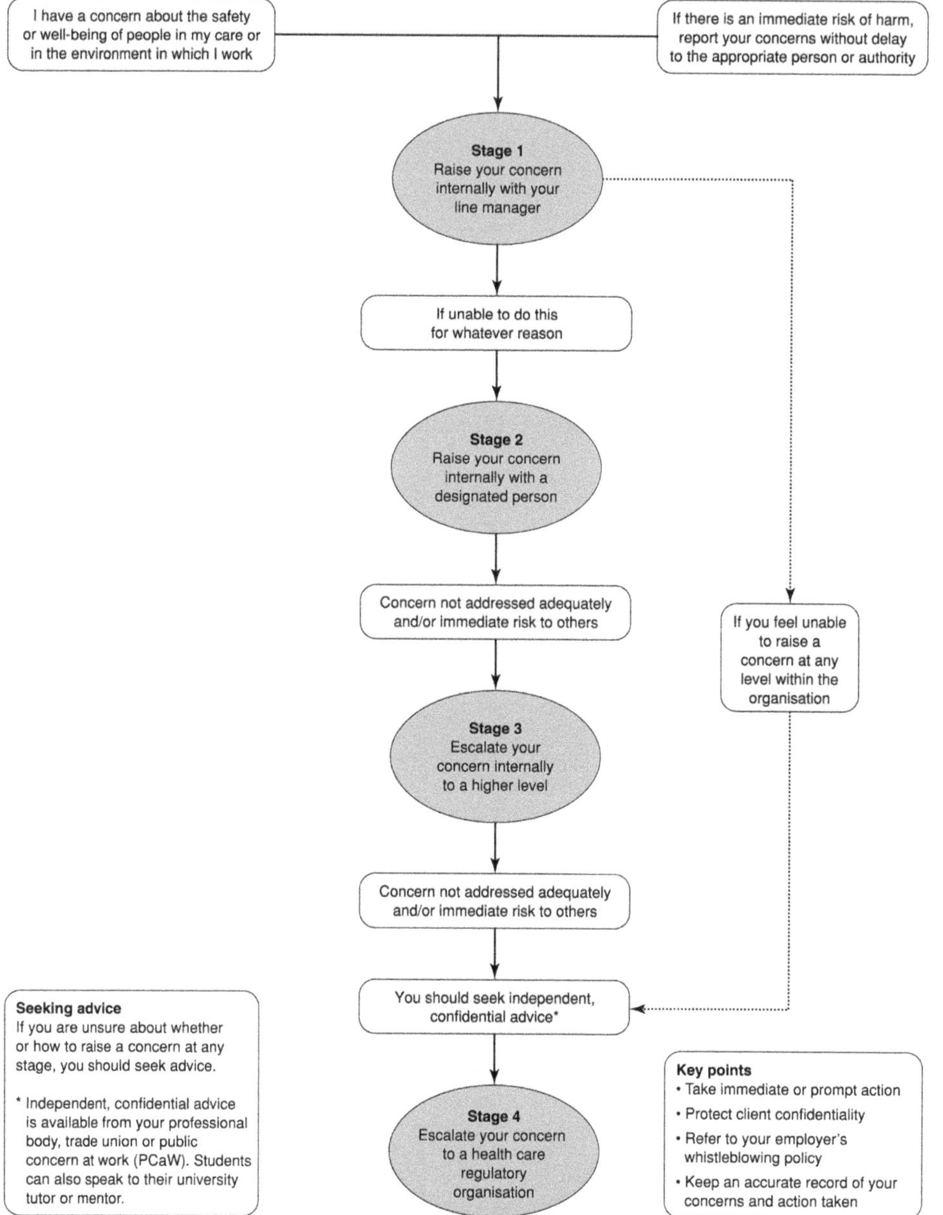

Figure 2.2 Stages in raising concerns. Source: Nursing and Midwifery Council (2018b) Raising Concerns: Guidance for Nurses and Midwives. London: Nursing and Midwifery Council, pp. 12–13. This flowchart should be read in conjunction with the full guidance available at https://www.nmc.org.uk/globalassets/blocks/media-block/raising-concerns-v2.pdf.

Nurses are, at all times, accountable for their own practice (or omissions) regardless of the advice and directions that are given to the nurse by another health or social care professional, for example a doctor (NMC 2018a). If a nurse carries out actions on the directions of another health care professional, this will not relieve the nurse of their personal and professional responsibility if the nurse is acting unethically or unlawfully. It is essential that the nurse is fully aware of the legal and ethical issues that surround patient care. Nurses must have skills in ethical reasoning as well as an understanding of the ethical theories that may inform practice.

The key element of the chapter is associated with ensuring that the patient's best interests and well-being are respected. A number of ethical perspectives have to be considered by the nurse when working with patients in any health and social care setting.

Ethical dilemmas can arise when there is or may be conflict between various interests and interested parties. Decisions need to be taken, care has to be prioritised and resources managed on a daily basis, and undertaking these tasks will unavoidably involve ethical considerations.

Each person is important and is entitled to be treated with respect. The Royal College of Nursing (RCN 2011) suggests that this value, respect, is upheld in law and must underpin all aspects of nursing practice. Ethical theories are complex theories that philosophers use to help consider moral beliefs and practices.

Advocacy

Another ill-defined concept is patient advocacy; it is subject to ambiguity of interpretation. Advocacy has been described in legal and ethical frameworks; nurses often associate this with ethical obligations to act as an advocate for the people they care for and in so doing treat people in a dignified way. Acting as an advocate means that the nurse has to promote the patient's rights to autonomy, free choice and self-determination, Terry (2007) discusses this specifically related to intensive care and cardiac care units. One of the most important roles of the nurse is to act as a patient advocate, to protect the interests of the people they care for when those people cannot because of illness or inadequate health knowledge. There are some patients, however, who may be unable to make independent decisions concerning their health and well-being (LeMone and Burke 2011). People who are, or may be, in vulnerable situations will need an advocate who will be required to help them assert their human rights. You might be this advocate: if this is the case, then you must ensure you are up to date with current legislation and local policy. If you observe any activity that you believe does not safeguard those people in need of support then you have a responsibility to challenge this practice.

According to the Royal College of Nursing (RCN 2014a) advocacy is defined as the act of speaking or acting on behalf of another: an advocate is somebody who expresses and defends the cause of another. Nursing interventions are concerned with helping and empowering people, assisting them to achieve, maintain or recover independence if this is needed. Promotion of a safe environment is also an essential element of advocacy (International Council of Nursing 2002).

The overall role of the advocate is to protect patients' rights (Berman et al. 2016). There are a number of ways in which this role can be accomplished. The role of the nurse is multifaceted, nurses are patient educators and have a responsibility for explaining procedures and treatments to people they care for. Nurses teach patients and their families how to eat more healthily, take medicines, change dressings and use medical equipment.

They also empower patients, directing people toward healthy behaviours and supporting them in times of need. If the patient is able the nurse encourages and teaches them how to be self-caring. Nurses intervene and provide care only when patients cannot do this for themselves.

Nurses provide dignity to individuals near the end of their lives by advocating for sufficient and appropriate pain medication and offering them choice, helping them make decisions concerning the way they wish to die.

Health care systems can be complex and often difficult to navigate; people who are acutely ill may find dealing with this complex system is too much for them, and the nurse is ideally placed to help people here. Berman et al. (2016) suggest that there are three values basic to patient advocacy (see Table 2.2).

There are barriers that can affect or impact on the nurse's ability to act as advocate. These can include:

- apathy;
- disempowerment;
- feelings of inadequacy, preparedness;
- lack of knowledge, education;
- lack of time.

The *Code* (NMC 2018a) states that in order to make people your first concern, treating them as an individual and respecting their dignity may mean that you will have to act as their advocate. This can include helping them to access relevant health and social care, information and support. Rooted in the role of advocate are, according to Maude and Hawley (2007), two moral concepts – fidelity (this is about being honest and truthful) and respect. Respect extends to dignity, privacy, self-determination and choice. When acting as advocate the nurse must be ready to intervene directly on the patient's behalf. This can usually be achieved by influencing others, using interpersonal skills, applying a sound knowledge base and having a desire to ensure that fairness and equity are paramount.

Care with confidence

Providing care has become more complex than ever and this can be in the person's own home or in an acute care setting. Changes in health care have come about for a number of reasons, for example, the increased used of technology, the increased use of a number of specialist practitioners and the provision of more specialist care; this is also coupled with more complex patient needs and the emergence of infectious diseases causing pandemics.

Table 2.2 Values associated with patient advocacy

1	The patient is an holistic being who has the right to make choices and decisions.
2	Each patient has the right to expect a nurse–patient relationship that is based on shared respect, trust, collaboration, solving problems related to health and health care along with consideration of their thoughts and feelings.
3	The nurse has a responsibility to ensure that the patient has access to health care services that meet their health needs.

Source: Adapted from Berman et al. (2016).

Regardless of this the more fundamental aspects of care remain the same; people expect to be safe, to be treated with kindness, courtesy and compassion. Providing these fundamental aspects of care can help the people you care for feel that they are being cared for in a competent way. These issues matter to patients.

Nursing is often described as an art and science. It is essential that nurses 'care for' and 'care about' in equal measures (DH 2008), providing care with kindness takes no more time. The following are cited as confidence creators – patients see these as core to care that is provided:

- a calm, clean, safe environment;
- a positive friendly culture;
- good teamwork and good relationships;
- well-managed care with efficient delivery;
- personalised care for and about every patient.

All of these carry equal importance; there is no one point that matters more than another. Considering them all them will demonstrate that they are all interrelated and require input from the whole health care team. Table 2.3 summarises what patients want from health care providers.

The 6Cs of nursing denote the professional commitment to always deliver excellent care (DH 2012). They are:

1. Care;
2. Compassion;
3. Competence;
4. Communication;
5. Courage;
6. Commitment.

The values associated with the 6Cs are immediately identifiable underpinning all that the nurse does. Nurses assist people in the prevention of illness, in the recovery phase of their illness and when they are ill and this is often when they are at their most vulnerable.

Delirium

Delirium, sometimes also known as acute confusional state, is defined by National Institute for Health and Care Excellence (NICE) (2010) as an acute, fluctuating syndrome

Table 2.3 Summary of what patients want from health care providers

- A healthcare provider who looks and acts professionally; is caring, kind, compassionate and knowledgeable.
- A care provider who offers individualised care that is personalised, holistic, timely, seamless and provides information.
- A champion who puts their interests first and protects them when they are vulnerable.
- A care provider who works with patients and relatives to plan care, offers constant feedback and reports, and assists them to navigate health and social care systems.
- A coordinator who is constant, accessible and accountable for communicating the plan and monitoring the delivery of care. Patients want to know that their care is being actively managed.

Table 2.4 Subtypes of delirium

Subtype	*Description*
Hyperactive delirium	The person may present with behaviour that is inappropriate, they may hallucinate, or be agitated. Impatience, restlessness and wandering can be common.
Hypoactive delirium	May present with tiredness, a reduced ability to concentrate, and appetite. The person may seem quiet or withdrawn.
Mixed delirium	In this subtype signs and symptoms of hyperactive and also hypoactive subtypes are present.

Source: BMJ Best Practice 2015; NICE 2010; Scottish Intercollegiate Guidelines Network (SIGN) 2019

of disturbed consciousness, attention, cognition and perception. The condition generally develops over hours to days, behavioural disturbance, personality changes and psychotic features may occur (Australian and New Zealand Society for Geriatric Medicine 2012).

Usually, delirium occurs in those people with advanced age or multiple comorbidities in critically ill patients, it may develop secondary to multiple precipitating or predisposing causes such as some medications or infection (Kalish et al. 2014). There are three subtypes based on the person's symptoms (see Table 2.4).

Inouye et al. (2014) notes that delirium and its pathophysiology is not fully understood, there are multiple mechanisms that can contribute to its development, for example, cholinergic deficiency, dopaminergic excess and inflammation. Although it can be a transient and reversible syndrome, its occurrence in the acute care setting, for example, in intensive care unit patients, it may be associated with long-term cognitive dysfunction. Delirium is thought to occur in 70–87% of intensive care unit admissions (Raju and Coombe-Jones 2015).

Early identification and risk factor assessment are key if the management of delirium is to be effective. Multidisciplinary collaboration and interdisciplinary team working, together with the use of evidence-based practice guidelines (for example NICE 2010) can minimise the effects of delirium in the acute care setting.

The diagnosis of delirium is mainly clinical, delirium in people with a sudden change in behaviour may be reported by the person, a carer, or relative. Clinical features are summarised in Table 2.5.

NICE (2010) provide evidence-base guidelines regarding the management of delirium. Initial management requires the nurse to identify and manage the underlying causes or combination of causes. Verbal and non-verbal techniques are needed to de-escalate the situation in the person who is distressed or considered a risk to themselves or others.

When de-escalation techniques are ineffective (or inappropriate) consideration should be given to the use of short-term haloperidol (SIGN 2019). Page and Wesley-Ely (2011) suggests that antipsychotic drugs such as haloperidol are used as delirium is associated with an imbalance of neurotransmitters. Haloperidol can be administered orally, subcutaneously, intramuscularly and intravenously, an antiemetic may also be prescribed. At all times the nurse must ensure they are adhering to local policy and procedure and acting in the patient's best interest (NMC 2018a).

Table 2.5 Clinical features – delirium

- Changes in behaviour develop acutely, over hours to days.
- Usually there is clinical evidence of an underlying precipitating factor, such as, infection or an adverse drug reaction.
- Symptoms will often fluctuate. Lucid intervals can occur during the day with the worst disturbance happening at night.
- Behavioural changes may include:
  - Altered cognitive function – the person may be disoriented, experience impairment of memory and language, concentration may worsen, there may be slower responses, and confusion. The person may not be able to recall details of their current illness, instructions or names.
  - Inattention – the person may be easily distracted accompanied with difficulty focusing and shifting attention from one thing to another, they are unable to maintain a conversation or to follow reasonable commands.
  - Disorganised thinking – the person can have disorganised, rambling, or irrelevant conversations, there may be unclear or illogical flow of ideas as well as difficulty expressing needs and concerns.
  - Altered perception – paranoid delusions, misperceptions or visual or auditory hallucinations may be present and these may be distressing.
- Altered physical function (see Table 2.4 subtypes delirium).
- Altered social behaviour – intermittent and labile changes in mood and/or emotions (such as, fear, paranoia, anxiety, depression, irritability, apathy, anger or euphoria). The person's behaviour may be inappropriate, they may not be able to cooperate with reasonable requests, they can become withdrawn.
- Altered level of consciousness – the person may have a clouding of consciousness, a reduced awareness of their surroundings and there may also be sleep-cycle disturbances, for example, daytime drowsiness, night-time insomnia, disturbed sleep or complete sleep cycle reversal.

Falling and a loss of appetite can often be warning signs for delirium.

Source: BMJ 2015; Inouye et al. 2014; NICE 2010; SIGN 2019

Conclusion

There is a growing literature relating to vulnerability and all health and social care providers in all settings should be aware of the developments in this sphere of health and social care. This chapter has defined key terms and has demonstrated that there are challenges present when trying to define terms such as abuse and vulnerability, there are also challenges when attempting to define who is vulnerable or at risk. Vulnerability is a dynamic and ever-changing concept relating to all entities that waxes and wanes.

People being cared for in a variety of care environments are potentially vulnerable. This is applicable to those people you may care for in the acute care setting. There are a number of rights all people have that help to ensure they are safe and free from risk, for example human rights.

Provision exists that provides guidance and support to practitioners to help them identify, protect and monitor those people who are at risk of abuse and who are vulnerable. Professional bodes such as the Nursing and Midwifery Council also provide support, advice and guidance for students, registered nurses, nursing associates and midwives, helping to ensure that the voice of the vulnerable person is heard and acted upon.

Acting as a patient's advocate requires a practitioner who is knowledgeable as well as one who understands ethical theories and how these apply to practice. Understanding ethical behaviour and acting ethically can have an impact on the quality of care.

Glossary

Apathy Lack of interest or concern.

Autonomy The right of patients to make decisions about their health care without the health care provider trying to influence the decision.

Clinical governance A framework through which organisations are accountable for continually improving the quality of services and safeguarding high standards of care.

Coercion Applying either physical or moral force to another.

Cognition Associated with a range of mental processes concerning the acquisition, storage, manipulation and retrieval of information.

Delirium An acute, fluctuating change in mental status comprising inattention, disorganised thinking and altered levels of consciousness.

Dignity Providing dignity in care focuses on three integral aspects: respect, compassion and sensitivity.

Discrimination This can be direct or indirect and is associated with treating a person or a group of people less favourably than others in the same situation.

Disempowerment Processes that lead to a reduction of the power which individuals have to make their own choices and shape their own lives as well making decisions about their own health care and health care needs.

Ethics A system of moral principles, rules of conduct.

Fraud A crime associated with deception deliberately practised in order to secure unfair or unlawful gain.

Harassment Any unwanted or uninvited behaviour which is offensive, embarrassing, intimidating or humiliating.

Health Service Ombudsman Exists to provide a service to the public by undertaking independent investigations into complaints about health services that have not acted properly or fairly or have provided a poor service.

Insomnia Inability to obtain an adequate amount or quality of sleep.

Malnutrition Any condition in which the body does not receive enough nutrients for effective function. Malnutrition may range from mild to severe and life-threatening.

Neglect This is a type of abuse where a person has been remiss in their provision of care or treatment.

Paranoia Unfounded or exaggerated distrust of others.

Physiological needs Physiological needs are those required to sustain life, such as air, water, nourishment and sleep.

Racism Discrimination or prejudice based on race.

Respect To show regard or consideration for another person, respect a person's rights.

Self-esteem Central to a person's survival, the basis of our well-being, the degree of worth and competence one attributes to oneself.

Sensory deprivation Deprivation of adequate and appropriate interpersonal or environmental experience and deprivation of usual external stimuli and the opportunity for development.

Sexism Discrimination or prejudice based on sex.

Statute A law enacted by a legislator.

Wellbeing A broad concept, related to personal dignity, physical and mental health and emotional wellbeing, protection from abuse and neglect.

TEST YOURSELF

1 What is the primary role and function of the Nursing and Midwifery Council?
2 Nurses are accountable first and foremost to the patient. True or false?
3 If you are concerned about the health and well-being of somebody you should:
   a. suspend judgement until you have definitive evidence.
   b. report this immediately.
   c. wait until you get back to university and report it to your lecturer.
   d. say nothing as you are a student.
4 The most vulnerable people in our society are the disabled. True or false?
5 Which of the following may be signs of abuse:
   a. change in a person's behaviour.
   b. unexplained burns in unusual locations.
   c. unexplained fractures to any part of the body.
   d. all of the above.
6 How would you define whistleblowing?
7 An advocate can be defined as:
   a. a person who needs help and assistance.
   b. another name for a midwife.
   c. somebody who acts on behalf of another, somebody who expresses and defends the cause of another.
   d. none of the above.
8 Racism can mean:
   a. abuse of person because of their culture.
   b. belief that one religion is superior to other.
   c. disregarding a person's requests concerning their care.
   d. belief in superiority of a particular race.
9 True or false: Delirium only occurs in those ager 70 years and older?
10 Which of the following might constitute deprivation of liberty:
   a. locking a person in their room as punishment for long periods of time.
   b. excessively restraining a person for long periods of time.
   c. sedating a patient because they are 'causing trouble'.
   d. all of the above.

Answers

1 The primary role and function of the Nursing and Midwifery Council is to protect the public.
2 True
3 b
4 False
5 d

6 Whistleblowing can be defined as enabling staff and employers to identify concerns at work.
7 c
8 d
9 False
10 d

References

Age UK. (2017). *Safeguarding Older People from Abuse and Neglect.* https://www.ageuk.org.uk/globalassets/age-uk/documents/factsheets/fs78_safeguarding_older_people_from_abuse_fcs.pdf. Last accessed September 2019.

Australian and New Zealand Society for Geriatric Medicine. (2012). *Position Statement 13 Delirium in Older People.* Australian and New Zealand Society for Geriatric Medicine. http://www.anzsgm.org/posstate.asp. Last accessed September 2019.

Berman, A., Snyder, S. and Frandsen, G. (2016). *Kozier and Erb's Fundamentals of Nursing. Concepts, Process and Practice*, 10th Edition. Harlow: Pearson.

British Medical Journal. (2015). *Assessment of Delirium.* bestpractice.bmj.com/best-practice/monograph/241.html. Last accessed September 2019.

Care Quality Commission. (2018). *The State of Health Care and Adult Social Care in England 2017/18.* https://www.cqc.org.uk/sites/default/files/20171011_stateofcare1718_report.pdf. Last accessed September 2019.

De Chesnay, M. (2012). Vulnerable populations: Vulnerable people. In De Chesnay, M. and Anderson, B. A. (eds.), *Caring for the Vulnerable: Perspectives in Nursing Theory and Practice and Research*, 3rd Edition. Boston, MA: Jones and Bartlett, pp. 3–14.

Department of Health and Home Office. (2000). *No Secrets: Guidance on Developing and Implementing Multi-Agency Policies and Procedures to Protect Vulnerable Adults from Abuse.* London: Department of Health.

DH (Department of Health). (2008). *Confidence in Caring – A Framework for Best Practice.* London: Department of Health.

DH (Department of Health). (2009). *Safeguarding Adults. Report on the Consultation on the Review of 'No Secrets'.* London: Department of Health.

DH (Department of Health). (2010). *Clinical Governance and Adult Safeguarding: An Integrated Process.* London: Department of Health.

DH (Department of Health). (2011a). *Statement of Government Policy on Adult Safeguarding.* https://assets.publishing.service.gov.uk/government/uploads/system/uploads/attachment_data/file/215591/dh_126770.pdf. Last accessed September 2019.

DH (Department of Health). (2011b). *Safeguarding Adults: The Role of Health Service Practitioners.* London: Department of Health.

DH (Department of Health). (2012). *Compassion in Practice.* London: Department of Health.

DH (Department of Health). (2018). *Care and Support Statutory Guidance Issued under the Care Act 2014.* https://www.gov.uk/government/publications/care-act-statutory-guidance/care-and-support-statutory-guidance. Last accessed September 2019.

Disclosure and Barring Service. (2012). *Referral Guidance and Frequently Asked Questions.* https://assets.publishing.service.gov.uk/government/uploads/system/uploads/attachment_data/file/143692/dbs-referral-faq.pdf. Last assessed September 2019.

Inouye, S. K., Westendorp, R. G. and Saczynski, J. S. (2014). Delirium in elderly people. *Lancet*, 383(9920), 911–922.

International Council of Nursing. (2002). *The ICN Definition of Nursing*. Geneva: ICN.

Kalish, V., Gillham, J. and Unwin, B. (2014). Delirium in older persons: evaluation and management. *American Family Physician*, 90(3), 150–158.

LeMone, P. and Burke, K. (2011). *Medical-Surgical Nursing. Critical Thinking in Clinical Care*, 5th Edition. Old Tappan, NJ: Pearson.

Martin, J. (2007). *Safeguarding Adults*. Lyme Regis: Russell House.

Maslow, A. (1954). *Motivation and Personality*. New York, NY: Harper & Row.

Maude, P. and Hawley, G. (2007). Clients' and patients' rights and protecting the vulnerable. In Hawley, G. (ed.), *Ethics in Clinical Practice: An Interprofessional Approach*. Harlow: Pearson, pp. 54–75.

Mencap. (2007). *Death by Indifference*. London: Mencap.

Michael, J. and The Independent Inquiry into Access to Healthcare for People with Learning Disabilities. (2008). *Healthcare for All: Report of the Independent Inquiry into Access to Healthcare for People with Learning Disabilities*. http://webarchive.nationalarchives.gov.uk/20130105064756/http:/www.dh.gov.uk/prod_consum_dh/groups/dh_digitalassets/@dh/@en/documents/digitalasset/dh_106126.pdf. Accessed September 2019.

Michaels, C. and Moffett, C. (2012). Rethinking vulnerability. In De Chesnay, M. and Anderson, B. A. (eds.), *Caring for the Vulnerable: Perspectives in Nursing Theory and Practice and Research*, 3rd Edition. Boston, MA: Jones and Bartlett, pp. 15–24.

National Assembly for Wales. (2000). *In Safe Hands: Implementing Adult Protection Procedures in Wales*. Guidance Issued by the National Assembly for Wales under s7 of the Local Authority Social Services Act 1970. Cardiff: National Assembly for Wales.

NICE. (2010). *Delirium: Prevention, Diagnosis and Management*. https://www.nice.org.uk/guidance/cg103/resources/delirium-prevention-diagnosis-and-management-pdf-35109327290821. Last accessed September 2019.

NMC (Nursing and Midwifery Council). (2018a). *The Code. Professional Standards of Practice and Behaviour for Nurses, Midwives and Nursing Associates*. https://www.nmc.org.uk/globalassets/sitedocuments/nmc-publications/nmc-code.pdf. Last accessed September 2019.

NMC (Nursing and Midwifery Council). (2018b). *Raising Concerns. Guidance for Nurses and Midwives*. https://www.nmc.org.uk/globalassets/blocks/media-block/raising-concerns-v2.pdf. Last accessed September 2019.

Northway, R. and Jenkins, R. (2018). *Safeguarding Adults in Nursing Practice*, 2nd Edition. London: Sage.

Page, V. and Wesley-Ely, E. (2011). *Delirium in Critical Care*. Cambridge: Cambridge University Press.

Parliamentary and Health Service Ombudsman. (2011). *Care and Compassion? Report of the Health Service Ombudsman on Ten Investigations into the NHS Care of Older People*. London: The Stationery Office.

Peate, I. (2016). Primum non nocere: first do no harm. *Journal of Paramedic Practice*, 8(7), 332–334.

Penhale, B. and Parker, J. (2008). *Working with Vulnerable Adults*. London: Routledge.

Raju, K. and Coombe-Jones, M. (2015). An overview of delirium for the community and hospital clinician. *Progress in Neurology and Psychiatry*, 19(6), 23–27.

RCN (Royal College of Nursing). (2011). *Research Ethics. RCN Guidance for Nurses*. London: RCN.

RCN (Royal College of Nursing). (2014a). *Defining Nursing*. London: RCN.

RCN (Royal College of Nursing). (2014b). *Learning from the Past-Setting Out the Future: Developing Learning Disability Nursing in the United Kingdom. An RCN Policy Statement on the Role of the Learning Disability Nurse*. https://matrix.rcn.org.uk/__data/assets/pdf_file/0007/359359/PosState_Disability_170314b_2.pdf. Last accessed November 2018.

RCN (Royal College of Nursing). (2017). *Raising Concerns*. https://www.rcn.org.uk/professional-development/publications/pub-005841. Last accessed November 2018.

RCN (Royal College of Nursing). (2018). *Zero Tolerance: Where we Stand on Sexual Harassment*. https://www.rcn.org.uk/magazines/activate/2018/may/zero-tolerance. Last accessed September 2019.

Scottish Intercollegiate Guidelines Network. (2019). *Risk Reduction and Management of Delirium. A National Clinical Guideline*. https://www.sign.ac.uk/assets/sign157.pdf. Last accessed October 2019.

Terry, L. M. (2007). Complex care: emergency department, perioperative suite, and ICU and CCU units. In Hawley, G. (ed.), *Ethics in Clinical Practice: An Interprofessional Approach*. Harlow: Pearson, pp. 276–299.

Further reading

Dartington, T. (2011). *Managing Vulnerability: The Underlying Dynamics of Systems of Care*. London: Karnac Books.

Francis, R. (2010). *Independent Inquiry into Care Provided by Mid Staffordshire NHS Foundation Trust January 2005–March 2009*. London: The Stationery Office.

Mandelstam, M. (2017). *Care Act 2014: An A–Z of Law and Practice*. London: Jessica Kingsley.

Care Inspectorate

http://www.gov.scot/Topics/Health/Support-Social-Care/Care-Inspectorate

One of the Care Inspectorate's regulatory and scrutiny functions is to ensure that vulnerable people are safe (Scotland).

Care and Social Services Inspectorate Wales

http://cssiw.org.uk/raiseaconcern/?lang=en

Responsible for inspecting social care and social services to make sure that they are safe for the people who use them (Wales).

Regulation and Quality Improvement Authority

http://www.rqia.org.uk/what_we_do/registration__inspection_and_reviews/safeguarding_vulnerable_groups.cfm

Independent body responsible for monitoring and inspecting the availability and quality of health and social care services (Northern Ireland).

Care Quality Commission

http://www.cqc.org.uk

Monitor, inspect and regulate services ensuring they meet fundamental standards of quality and safety (England).

3 The cell and tissues

John Mears

AIM

The aim of this chapter is to provide an introduction to the structure and function of cells, along with the composition of the main tissue types, their functions, tissue repair and the inflammatory process.

OBJECTIVES

After reading this chapter you will be able to:

- Identify the component parts of a human cell and discuss their function.
- Explain the roles of the plasma membrane and mitotic cell division.
- Explain transmembrane and intracellular transport mechanisms.
- Outline the pathway for the production of adenosine triphosphate (ATP).
- Describe the structure and function of the main types of tissue.
- Describe inflammation and the process of healing and tissue repair.
- Discuss the consequences of the disruption of normal cellular function, particularly the consequences of disrupted ATP production.

Introduction

Understanding how to care for people safely and effectively requires the nurse to appreciate both the microscopic and macroscopic aspects of the human. Studying the human at a cellular level, as described in this chapter, will help you to recognise factors that impact on health and on a person's vulnerability to illness. Observing the person at a cellular level is only one aspect of a wider understanding, as this chapter sets the scene for the following chapters, providing a detailed introduction to the chemical foundations of life and how the body's cells are built and operate. The chapter then explores how the body's tissues function, allowing you to appreciate what occurs when cells, tissues and organ systems fail.

The cell and its environment

Before considering the basic structure of the **cell,** it is important to consider its physiological environment. All human cells contain an **aqueous** fluid (**intracellular** fluid), known as **cytosol**. Apart from the **organelles**, this fluid contains substances such as proteins, other nutrient molecules, metabolic products and also a range of chemicals known as **electrolytes**. Outside the cells, there is the **extracellular** fluid, which is composed of the **interstitial** fluid and the circulating fluid; the latter consists of blood in the vascular system and the lymph in the lymphatic vessels. The extracellular fluid has a similar composition to the intracellular fluid. However, there are important differences in the composition of these fluids, particularly in the type and quantity of electrolytes and in the distribution of protein molecules, as well as the dissolved gases. The intracellular and extracellular environments are separated by the cell membrane, which is **selectively permeable**; it is able to control the movement of electrolytes and other molecules across it. This characteristic will be discussed later in the chapter. The correct balance and movement of these chemicals between the intracellular and extracellular environments is vital to the maintenance of normal function and therefore health (Marieb and Hoehn 2019). A disruption of this balance is one of the factors that can cause homoeostatic imbalance and potentially lead to a medical emergency (Kumar and Clarke 2017).

Electrolytes

Electrolytes are charged atoms or molecules in solution which can conduct electricity. They may be cations, which have lost one electron (or more) and therefore carry a positive charge, or **anions,** which have gained one electron (or more) and therefore have a negative charge. An example of this is common salt, which is composed of sodium (Na) and chlorine (Cl) and is crystalline in structure. When sodium chloride is dissolved in water, the sodium and chlorine dissociate and become sodium cations (Na^+) and chloride anions (note the change of nomenclature) (Cl^-). In so doing, the sodium loses an electron and the chloride gains an electron.

Electrolytes are not evenly distributed through the body. The concentrations of electrolytes (cations and anions) inside and outside the cells are different (see Table 3.1) (McLafferty et al. 2014).

Table 3.1 Common Cations and Anions

	Normal Serum Values and Location
Cations	
Sodium (Na^+)	135–145mmol/L, main extracellular fluid cation
Potassium (K^+)	3.5–5.0mmol/L, main intracellular fluid cation
Calcium (Ca^{2+})	Found in both intracellular and extracellular fluids
Magnesium (Mg^{2+})	Found in both intracellular and extracellular fluids-
Hydrogen (H^+)	Found in both in both intracellular and extracellular fluids
Anions	
Chloride (Cl^-)	95–108mmol/L, main anion in extracellular fluid
Phosphate (PO_4^{3-})	2.5–4.5mmol/L, main anion in intracellular fluid
Bicarbonate (HCO_3^-)	22–28mmol/L, found in both fluid compartments

The key electrolyte differences are that potassium (K^+) is the main **cation** inside the cell and sodium (Na^+) is the main extracellular cation. Phosphate PO_4^{3-} is the main intracellular anion and chloride (Cl^-) is the main extracellular anion. Other electrolytes of significance, such as calcium (Ca^{2+}), magnesium (Mg^{2+}) hydrogen ion (H^+) and bicarbonate (more correctly known as hydrogen carbonate; HCO_3^-), are distributed more evenly but concentrations will vary depending on the actual function of the cell concerned. Changes in the distribution of electrolytes and the ability of the cell to control their concentrations are very significant in disease processes (Kumar and Clark 2017).

Changes in the balance of electrolytes can have a dramatic effect on the functioning of the body. For example, when the myocardial muscle is damaged by **myocardial infarction**, the damaged cells release potassium, which increases the amount of this electrolyte in the interstitial fluid and circulation. This change alters the electrical potential across cells, especially the muscle cells of the heart, and may cause the electrical stimulation to become irregular, leading to **dysrhythmias**. These dysrhythmias may affect the ability of the heart to pump effectively and therefore lead to a decrease in the oxygen supply to the body's cells, which, in turn, will lead to malfunction (Reed et al. 2017).

Acidity, alkalinity and pH balance

All physiological processes in cells are dependent on the correct **pH**. The pH is a measure of the hydrogen ion (H^+) concentration and acidity/alkalinity of the environment, and is represented by a number between 0 and 14 where 0 is the most acidic, 14 is the most alkaline and 7 is neutral. The normal pH of blood, for example, is between 7.35 and 7.45. The pH of the blood, and therefore the pH of the body, is regulated by the lungs and kidneys. This balance is represented by the equation

$$CO_2 + H_2O \rightleftharpoons H_2CO_3 \rightleftharpoons H^+ + HCO_3^-$$

$$(\text{carbon dioxide} + \text{water} \rightleftharpoons \text{carbonic acid} \rightleftharpoons \text{hydrogen ion} + \text{bicarbonate ion})$$

Alteration of this balance can lead to the malfunction of cells. If CO_2 increases because of poor ventilation and gaseous exchange, then the equation will be driven to the left, increasing the amount of H^+ ions and therefore causing an increase in acidity, and *vice versa*. If the kidneys are not able to function properly, then removal of bicarbonate ion will decrease and there will be an increase in alkalinity. The overall process is much more complex than this but these examples are given as indications of the control of the cellular environment (Marieb and Hoehn 2019).

Basic structure of cells

All cells have the same basic structure, with a **plasma membrane**, a nucleus and **cytoplasm**. The cytoplasm consists of an aqueous fluid, the cytosol, which contains a range of organelles (e.g., mitochondria, ribosomes and endoplasmic reticulum), **inclusions** and electrolytes (see Figure 3.1). Exceptions to this general cell structure are erythrocytes (red blood cells) and **corneocytes** (the cells on the surface of the epidermis of the skin), which do not contain nuclei. A third variation is found in cells of skeletal muscle, which are **multinucleate**, i.e., each muscle cell has more than one nucleus. There are significant

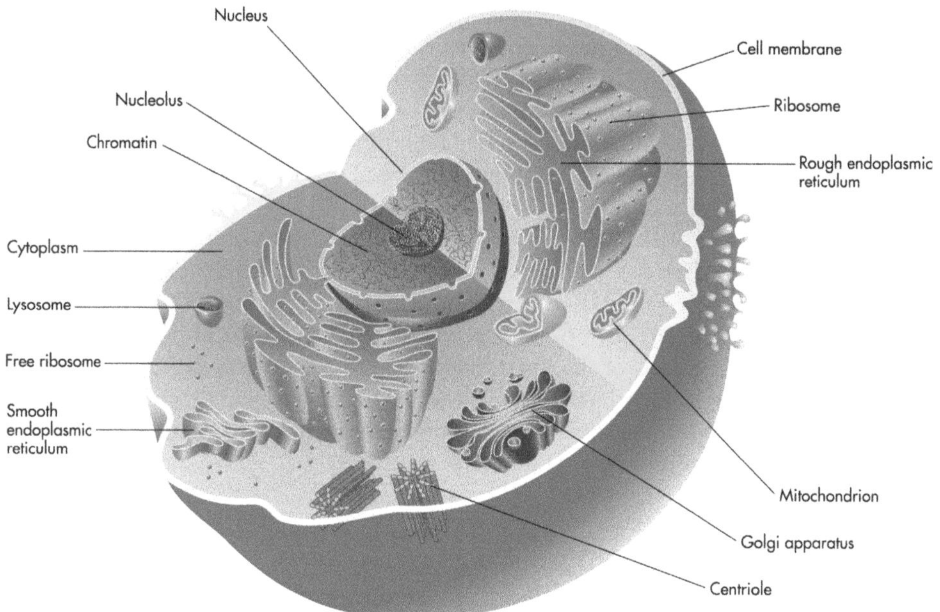

Figure 3.1 Cellular components.

differences in shape and size of cells, depending on the particular **tissue** type and their function. Some neurons (nerve cells) have axons that are over one metre long, whereas red blood cells are only 7μm in diameter and 2μm deep. Some types of cell have more of one type of organelle, e.g., muscle cells have many mitochondria, as they need to produce large quantities of energy.

Plasma membrane

All cells and their organelles are surrounded by plasma membranes (see Figure 3.2). This is a lipid bilayer that also contains a range of proteins and other molecules and is only 5–7nm thick. Some of the proteins in the cell membrane cross the full thickness of the membrane and are integral to it (namely transmembrane or integral proteins), whereas others penetrate only part of the way across the membrane or are on the surface, effectively floating in the lipid layer. There are a range of **glycoproteins** that are attached to the outer surface of the cell membrane, mainly attached to the transmembrane proteins. The phospholipids and proteins of the membranes are not physically connected to each other but are held in place by molecular and atomic attractions. This means that sections of plasma membrane can move into and out of the outer membrane of the cell (see exocytosis and endocytosis in this chapter).

The molecules that make up the lipid bilayer are **phospholipids**. Phospholipids are neutral fats that have had one of the three fatty acids replaced by phosphate (PO_4^{3-}), which is anionic and is therefore compatible with water. The consequence of this is that the molecules have a **hydrophilic** (water-attracting phosphate) end and a **hydrophobic** (water-repelling fatty acid) end. On both layers, the hydrophilic end is on the outer face,

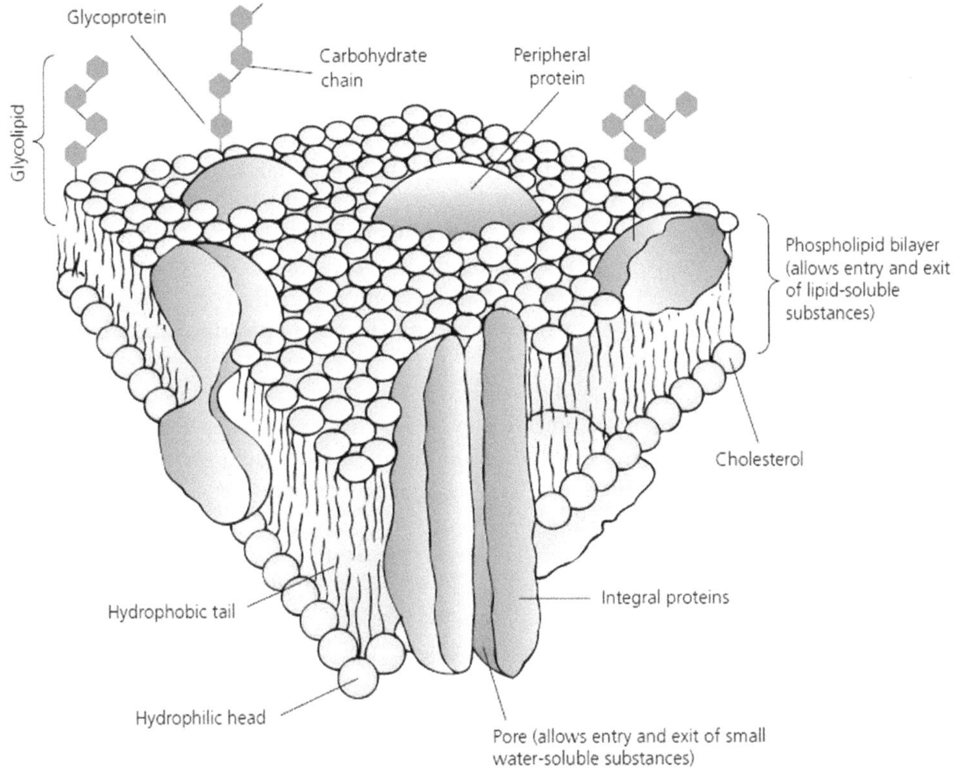

Figure 3.2 The Fluid Mosaic Model of membrane structure. *Source:* Clancy, John and Andrew J. McVicar (2009), Physiology and Anatomy For Nurses and Healthcare Professionals: A Homeostatic Approach Clancy and McVicar, 3rd ed. Taylor Francis. Reproduced by permission of Taylor & Francis.

with the hydrophobic, fatty acid end on the inside of the layer. This means that the outside of the membrane is compatible with the aqueous medium, both inside and outside the cell, but, because of the hydrophobic nature of the interior of the bilayer, water and electrolytes cannot cross the lipid sections of the membrane. The movement of electrolytes through the membrane is facilitated by protein channels.

The structure of the membrane is also the reason why most drugs are fat soluble; this facilitates their transport into the cell in which they will have their action. The hydrophobic barrier is one of the ways in which the differences in concentrations of electrolytes inside and outside the cell are maintained. The membrane also acts as a selectively permeable membrane to help control the movement of both water and electrolytes into and out of the cell.

The cell membrane is stabilised by lipid-soluble molecules, such as cholesterol and vitamin E. Without these stabilising molecules, the cell membrane would not be able to maintain its integrity.

As identified earlier, some of the proteins in the plasma membrane cross the full width of the membrane, whereas others penetrate only part of the way through the membrane.

Some of the membrane proteins form channels through the cell membrane that, under the right conditions, allow the movement or transport of electrolytes and other lipid-insoluble substances into and out of the cell (see Figure 3.3).

Some channels allow passive movement of electrolytes but most of this electrolyte movement is active, dependent on energy supplied by ATP, and also on other transport proteins. In this way, the cell can control the movement of electrolytes and other molecules into and out of the cell. There are exceptions to this mechanism. One is normal and involves the pacemaker cells of the heart, where sodium can passively move into the cells, through gated ion channels, altering the **membrane potential** (Waugh and Grant 2018). The second is an abnormal situation, found in damaged nerves, where the normally stable ion channels are replaced by unstable channels that allow the movement of sodium and therefore set off action potentials that lead to **neuropathic** pain (McCance and Heuther 2018).

Attached to the outside of the plasma membrane, particularly to the protein molecules, there are a number of carbohydrates and glycoproteins that have a wide range of functions. Some are signalling molecules, while others are used for attachment to other cells and for attracting and attaching other cells, such as neutrophils, whereas yet others are part of the immune system, including antibodies.

Each cell in the body, except sperm, has marker molecules on the cell surface that identify them as belonging to that individual. This is part of the **histocompatibility** system of the body and is one of the main reasons why individuals undergoing **organ** transplant need to be immunosuppressed following transplantation. Without the use of

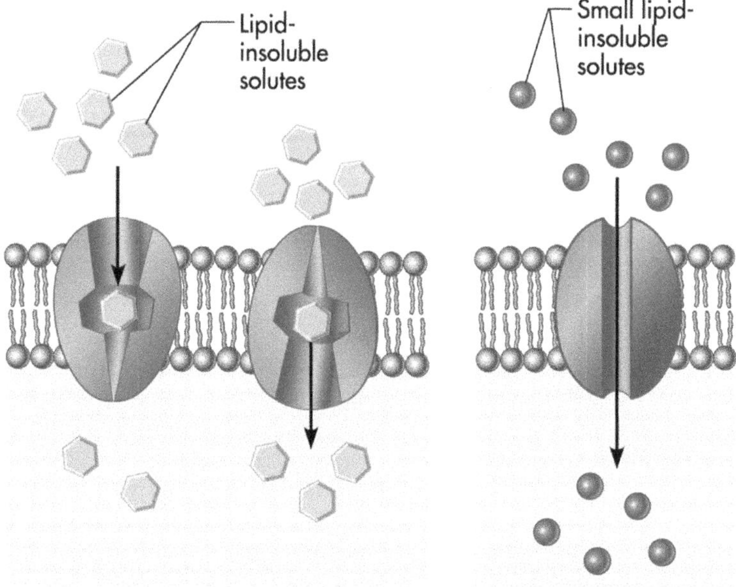

Figure 3.3 Protein channels in the plasma membrane. *Source*: Marieb, E. N. and Hoehn, K. (2010) Human Anatomy and Physiology, 8th edn. Upper Saddle River, NJ: Pearson. Reproduced by permission of Pearson Education, Inc.

immunosuppressive drugs, the donor cells, which do not carry the correct (i.e., the host's) marker molecules, would be attacked by the host's immune system (Norris 2018).

Transmembrane transport

There are two broad types of transport across plasma membranes. The first is passive transport, which, by its very nature, does not require any energy input. Passive transport can be subdivided into four categories; diffusion, facilitated diffusion, **osmosis** and **filtration**.

The second form of transport is **active transport,** and this requires energy input, usually in the form of ATP. This type of transport is energy dependent and requires the continual production of ATP for the mechanisms to work. As the body only has enough ATP available at any time to last a few seconds, if the supply ceases then not only is active transport of electrolytes and other chemicals into and out of the cell compromised, but the normal functioning of the cell is also potentially seriously affected. This is the situation that arises in the decompensating and refractory stages of shock (Norris 2018).

Passive transport

Diffusion is the movement of a substance from an area of higher concentration to an area of lower concentration. Figure 3.4 illustrates this principle. If dye is added to a beaker of liquid, the molecules will gradually spread throughout the liquid (Figure 3.4a). This happens because the molecules of dye move around in the solution and are constantly moving and bumping into each other. The consequence of this is that they gradually spread until they are evenly distributed throughout the solution (Figure 3.4b).

The difference in concentration between areas of high and low concentration is called the concentration gradient. It is this difference in concentration that creates diffusion. The concentration may simply refer to the number of atoms or molecules in a given

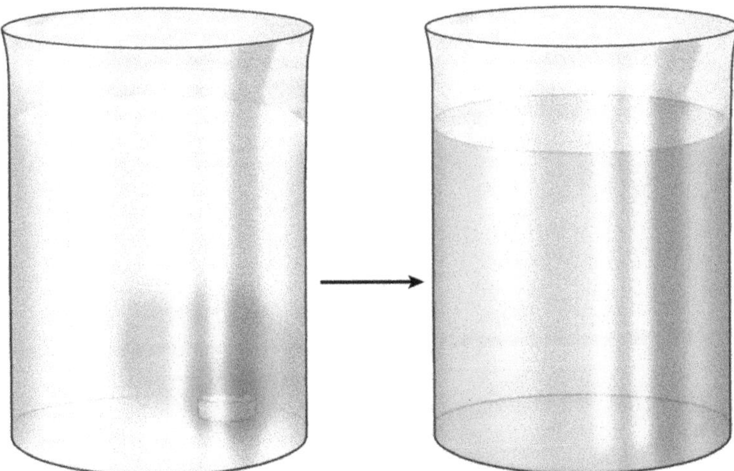

Figure 3.4 Diffusion of a substance from an area of high concentration to an area of lower concentration until the concentration of the substance is uniform throughout the solution.

volume or may refer to the electrical concentration. Examples of diffusion would be the movement of dissolved oxygen from the alveoli of the lungs to the blood in the capillaries surrounding the alveoli. The movement of carbon dioxide in the opposite direction is also achieved by diffusion. The diffusion across the alveoli is dependent on the distance (the diffusion pathway). If this is extended for any reason, e.g., if there is **inflammation** or scarring from previous episodes of injury and healing, then the distance across the diffusion pathway is extended, which can seriously affect the supply of oxygen and the removal of carbon dioxide.

Facilitated diffusion is a process in which molecules are assisted in moving down their concentration gradient across the plasma membrane. A good example of this facilitation is the movement of glucose molecules into the cell. There are receptor molecules on the surface of the cell membrane, which are activated by the attachment of insulin. Once the receptor is activated, it, in turn, activates the carrier molecules in the plasma membrane. The carrier molecules are specifically designed to interact with the glucose molecules. No extra energy is required because the carrier molecules are designed to move into the cell, where they connect with the glucose molecule. There are, in fact, two types of carrier, that operate like taxis. Some are waiting in the cell membrane (taxi rank) and others are cruising waiting to pick up free glucose molecules. If these **transport molecules** are missing or if they malfunction, glucose transport into the cells is reduced. The transport of glucose is also critically dependent on insulin being attached to the cell plasma membrane to enable the glucose transport to take place (see Figure 3.5).

Osmosis is the term used for the movement of water across a selectively permeable membrane (a cell plasma membrane, for example) from an area of lower solute concentration to an area of higher solute concentration, to equalise the concentrations on either side of the membrane (see Figure 3.6). It should be remembered that, in effect, this is water moving along its own concentration gradient.

An example of this in action would be if a person were dehydrated. When we dehydrate, e.g., when we are unwell and sweating or not drinking sufficient fluid, we lose water from the spaces around the cells (interstitial space). This makes the remaining interstitial fluid more concentrated so water moves from inside the cells (intracellular space) into the interstitial space. Unfortunately, this makes the cytosol in the cells more

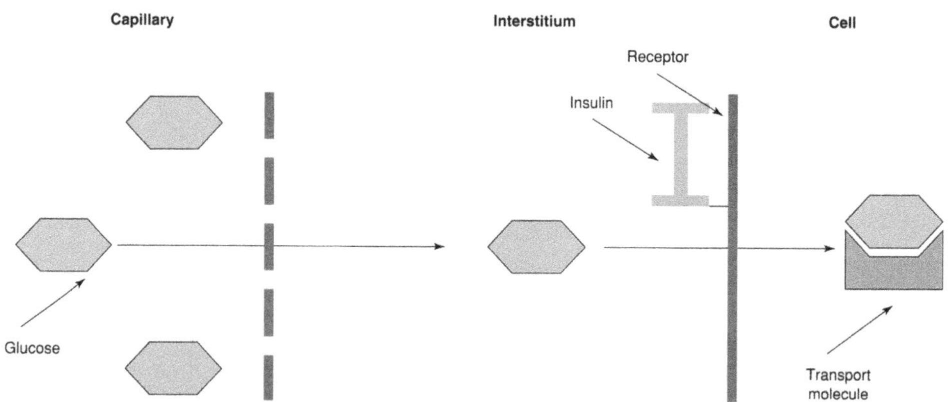

Figure 3.5 The movement of glucose from capillary to cell. *Source*: © Mears Associates 2011.

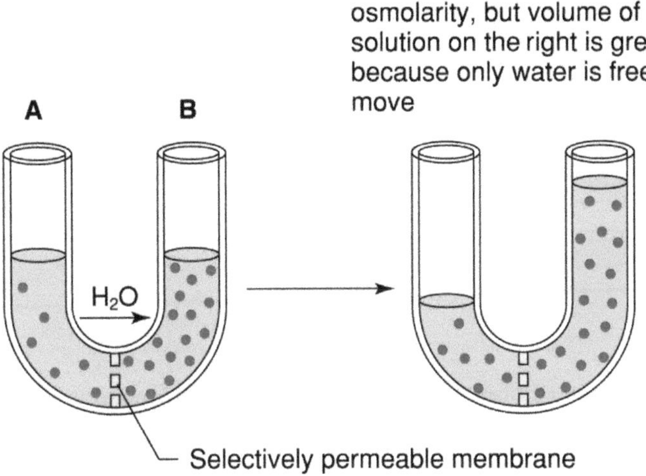

Figure 3.6 Osmosis.

concentrated and affects their ability to function properly. In the central nervous system, this may lead to confusion or loss of consciousness.

Filtration

Filtration is the movement of a fluid under pressure from one space to another through the plasma membrane. An extremely important example of this is the movement of plasma across the arteriolar wall in the systemic circulation, and particularly in the **glomerulus** of the **nephron** in the kidney. Under normal circumstances, approximately 120–125mL of plasma per minute are filtered by the kidney (Marieb and Hoehn 2019). In clinical terms, this is expressed as 120–125mL/minute/1.73m^2 but it does vary with age and sex (Kumar and Clark 2017). If the systemic arterial systolic blood pressure drops below 80mmHg, this filtration ceases and the individual develops acute kidney injury, that may proceed to acute renal failure (Kumar and Clark 2017; Norris 2018).

In the systemic circulation, between three and four litres of fluid are filtered out of the arterioles into the interstitial spaces every day. In healthy individuals, this is returned to the circulation through the **venules** or is cleared by the **lymphatic system**. In some situations, this process is interrupted. For example, if the venous pressure is high, as in cardiac failure, less of the fluid is returned to the circulation. The excess fluid that remains in the interstitial space causes oedema.

This oedema can have a significant effect on the diffusion pathway, creating a problem similar to that in the lungs, identified earlier in this chapter.

Active transport

Active transport pumps require energy input in order to function (see Figure 3.7).

This energy is supplied by ATP, which loses a phosphate group to become adenosine diphosphate (ADP), with the release of energy. This type of transport is involved in moving electrolytes against their concentration gradients, e.g., returning potassium to the cell and removing sodium from the cell to the interstitial fluid. This process is known as primary active transport.

Endocytosis and exocytosis

The two processes involve the formation of a **vesicle,** by pinching off sections of plasma membrane, containing particles or fluid (see Figure 3.7).

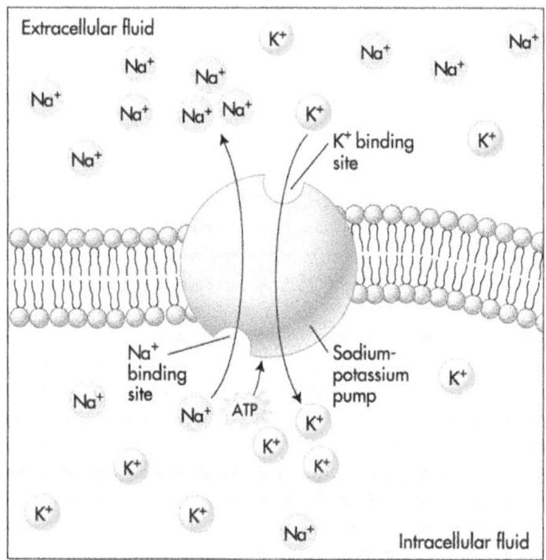

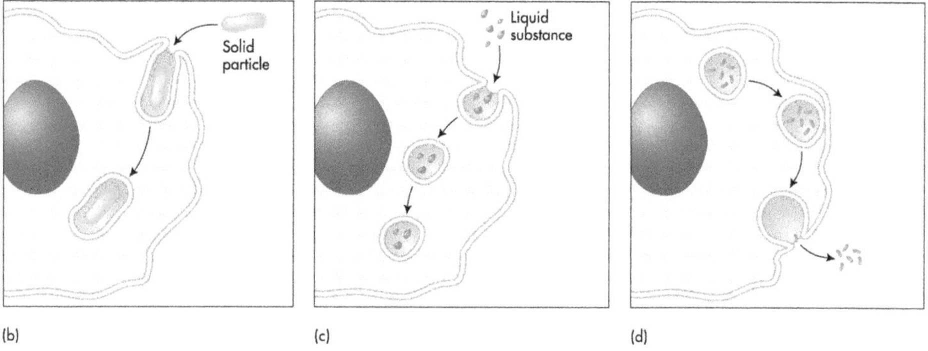

Figure 3.7 Types of active transport in and out of cells: (a) active transport pump; (b) phagocytosis; (c) pinocytosis; (d) exocytosis.

In endocytosis, water, large food particles that are too large to cross the plasma membrane, or microorganisms, such as bacteria, are transported from outside the cell to the inside. If water is being transported, the process is called **pinocytosis**. The same principle is used in **phagocytosis** to engulf bacteria and cell debris (see Figure 3.7).

Exocytosis is the reverse process. Vesicles created by budding from the **endoplasmic reticulum** and **Golgi apparatus** move to the surface of the cell and the vesicle membrane joins the cell membrane and expels its contents into the interstitial space. Always remember that the molecules of the plasma membrane are not physically linked, so this kind of manoeuvre is easily and effectively accomplished.

Cytoplasm

Cytoplasm is the name given to the contents of the cell within the plasma membrane and outside the nucleus. It is composed of an aqueous fluid (cytosol) in which are dissolved or suspended proteins, salts (electrolytes), sugars and other molecules necessary for the function of the cell, as well as metabolic by-products, organelles and inclusions required for the normal function of the cell (see Figure 3.8).

The inclusions will vary from cell to cell but may be glycogen granules in liver and muscle cells, fat globules in fat cells or melanin in epidermal melanocytes.

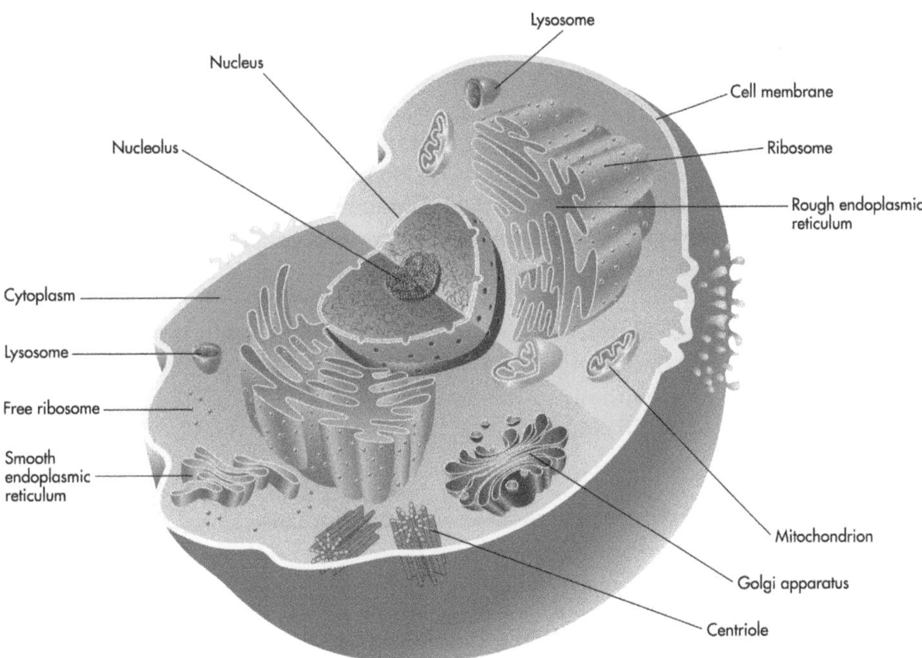

Figure 3.8 The cell membrane, cytoplasm, nucleus, ribosomes, centrosomes, mitochondria, endoplasmic reticulum, Golgi apparatus and lysosomes.

Mitochondria

Mitochondria are small double-walled sausage-shaped structures, in which most of the energy required for **metabolism** and cellular function is produced. It is within these structures that oxygen is utilised to produce **adenosine triphosphate**.

The number of mitochondria within specific types of cells is dependent on the activity of those cells. In liver and muscle cells, there are many mitochondria because these cells are very metabolically active. Bone cells (ostoecytes), on the other hand, have few mitochondria, as they are not very metabolically active.

Mitochondria also contain DNA (mtDNA) which is almost exclusively inherited from the mother. It can be very significant in the development of disease, partly because the quantity of it in the body means that it is subject to significant mutation (McCance and Heuther 2018).

Ribosomes

These small organelles are found attached to the endoplasmic reticulum or floating freely in the cytosol. They are composed of ribosomal ribonucleic acid and proteins and are manufactured in the nucleolus of the nucleus and then transported into the cytosol. Their function is to act as centres for the production of proteins, which include enzymes. The proteins produced are used for metabolism, repair and replication within cells and for transport into the **extracellular matrix**.

Endoplasmic reticulum

The endoplasmic reticulum is a series of tubes and flattened fluid-filled cavities (cisternae) that are continuous with the nuclear membrane. Like all the membranes in the cell, they are lipid bilayers.

There are two distinct types of endoplasmic reticulum. Some of it has **ribosomes** attached and is known as rough endoplasmic reticulum; this is found in all cells. The other is known as smooth endoplasmic reticulum, as it has no ribosomes attached. It is found in a limited number of cells. The two types of endoplasmic reticulum have different roles.

The ribosomes on the rough endoplasmic reticulum produce all the proteins that are secreted from the cells. The various molecules necessary for the production and maintenance of the cell are also produced by this type of endoplasmic reticulum.

Smooth endoplasmic reticulum is composed mainly of loops and is not involved in protein synthesis. Rather, the integral proteins of the membrane have specialist catalytic roles, e.g., cholesterol synthesis in the liver, steroid-based hormone production in the cells of the testes, detoxification of some drugs and of pesticides in the liver and kidney.

Golgi apparatus

The Golgi apparatus is an assemblage of flattened, stacked plasma membranes. This structure is the 'finishing shop' and 'transport centre' for molecules produced in the cell. The Golgi apparatus receives the molecules produced by the endoplasmic reticulum, makes adjustments to the chemical structure and then transports the finished items in vesicles. Some of the products are for use within the cell and its membranes, whereas others are exported. Most of the chemicals produced are transported in vesicles composed of pinched-off plasma membrane. Export from the cell is achieved by exocytosis.

Lysosomes

Lysosomes are small spherical organelles, surrounded by plasma membrane. They contain enzymes that are capable of degrading and breaking down all sorts of material from bacteria and toxins to worn-out organelles. They are therefore abundant in phagocytic cells (cells that engulf and destroy bacteria and cell debris in the inflammatory process), such as macrophages and neutrophils. These small structures create a safe area for the destruction of unwanted material within cells. The digestive environment is very acidic and requires energy in the form of ATP to pump hydrogen ions into these organelles. If the pump fails because of a lack of ATP, associated with poor oxygen supply, then the lysosomes do not function properly and the degradation process is inhibited, leading to a breakdown in cellular function.

Peroxisomes

Peroxisomes are membranous sacs that are similar to lysosomes but are self-replicating and are not produced by the usual endoplasmic reticulum and Golgi apparatus route. They contain a number of enzymes, including oxidases, that are important in the detoxification of substances, such as alcohol, but, just as importantly, they are involved in the quenching of free radicals. These organelles are found in large numbers in kidney and liver cells, which are metabolically very active and are the primary sites for detoxification.

Cytoskeleton

Each cell has a collection of microtubules and filaments that are associated with the cytoplasmic side of the plasma membrane and also form a network throughout the cell. They are composed of proteins, some of which are similar to those found in muscle cells. They help to give the cell shape, attachment for organelles and also enable cell movement. The movement is particularly important in white cells, such as monocytes, macrophages and neutrophils, that have to change shape to pass through capillaries and to be able to move through the pores in capillary walls to reach areas of inflammation and infection.

The **cytoskeleton** is significant in maintaining cell shape and, as a consequence, ensuring that the cell has sufficient volume to remain adequately hydrated. As humans age, connective tissue protein production decreases, reducing the volume of the cell. This can be extremely significant in situations where patients are sitting or lying in one position for a period of time, as the cell can be more easily damaged, which can lead to the production of pressure ulcers. This is a particular problem in the very ill and malnourished and those with significantly reduced mobility (NPUAP/EPUAP/PPPIA 2014).

Centrosome and centrioles

The **centrosome** is an area near the nucleus that contains a pair of rod-like structures called the **centrioles**. This area and the centrioles are associated with the process of cell division. They produce the mitotic spindle in dividing cells. The centrioles also form the basis of cilia and flagella. Cilia are typically found on the columnar epithelium of the lining of the respiratory tract. They are involved in the movement of dust particles and mucus up the respiratory tract. The only example found in humans of a cell with a flagellum is the sperm.

Nucleus

The nucleus is a structure found in all human cells, except those identified earlier in the chapter. It is protected by a double nuclear envelope, the outer layer of which is continuous with the endoplasmic reticulum. The envelope has gaps in it, called pores, that allow the movement of specified molecules into and out of it. Protein molecules enter, and ribosomes and messenger ribonucleic acid (mRNA) exit. Signalling chemicals that can stimulate DNA transcription can also enter through these pores.

Within the nucleus there is an area called the nucleolus. The nucleolus is primarily responsible for the production of ribosomal RNA (rRNA), which combines with proteins imported from the cytoplasm to make the ribosomes, which then leave the nucleus and enter the cytoplasm to attach to endoplasmic reticulum or to attach to the cytoskeleton as individual units.

The nucleus of the cell is where the DNA is mainly stored. The DNA is normally shared out amongst the 46 chromosomes that are the typical karyotype of humans. This number can vary between 45 and 49 depending on events (non-disjunction of chromosomes leading to extra chromosomes in one gamete and less in another) that take place during the production of ova and sperm. In cells that are not undergoing division, the DNA, combined with special proteins called histones, is unravelled and takes the form of long filaments called chromatin. It is only as the cell begins the process of division that the DNA coils up to produce the familiar shapes that we recognise as chromosomes.

DNA is a double helix that carries our genes which, in turn, determine heritable traits, such as what we look like and how we function. DNA carries the code for nearly all the proteins that are produced in the cell by ribosomes. These proteins can be enzymes, surface markers or antibodies. They can also be structural proteins or command molecules, that regulate the production and refinement of other molecules in the cell.

Cell cycle and cell division

Cells, like the organism they form, are mortal, but they are able to postpone their death by asexual reproduction or, in other words, by simply dividing in two. They can do this only a certain number of times before they lose this ability and die. This process of somatic cell division is called **mitosis**. Mitosis, or the mitotic phase, takes up only a small part of the overall life of a cell. Only a proportion of cells are dividing at any time, so most of the cells are not involved in producing new cells but are involved in the normal day-to-day cellular function. This non-dividing phase is called interphase. During interphase, the cells also grow and replicate (double by making exact copies) their DNA and organelles ready for the next mitotic phase. It is during interphase that the DNA in the nucleus does a self-examination and carries out repairs that help reduce the number of mutations in individual genes. The combination of interphase and the mitotic phase is known as the cell cycle (see Figure 3.9) (Marieb and Hoehn 2019).

Mitosis is asexual reproduction, as there is only one cell involved. The process of mitosis is complex and is divided into four phases with the last phase being combined

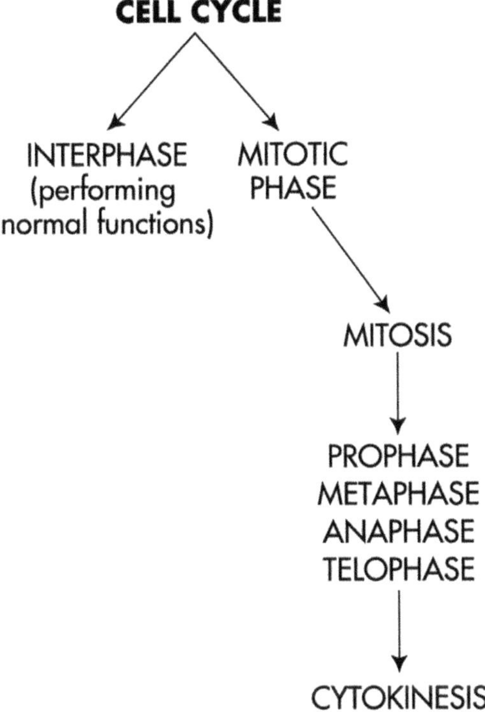

Figure 3.9 Flow chart of the cell cycle.

with cytokinesis, which describes the process of the non-nuclear part of the cell dividing in half. The four phases are prophase, metaphase, anaphase and telophase (see Figure 3.10). These phases are not discrete but are part of a continuous process and indicate the significant stages that can be identified in the overall process.

Prophase

In prophase the nuclear membrane breaks down, the nucleus disappears and the long strands of chromatin condense (become densely coiled) to form the familiar chromosome shapes (remember that the cell has already made duplicate copies of its DNA ready for the two daughter cells). The centrioles, discussed earlier, produce guiding filaments that create a cage-like structure called the spindle. During prophase, the chromosomes begin to migrate towards the middle of the cell.

Metaphase

Metaphase sees the chromosomes, or chromatids as they are more correctly known at this stage, finishing their migration to the middle of the cell and lining up across the middle of the cell. This arrangement is known as the metaphase plate.

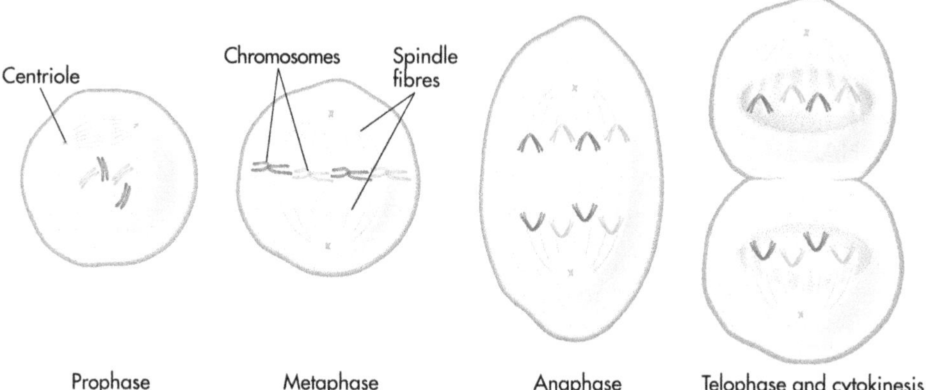

Figure 3.10 Phases of mitosis.

Anaphase

Anaphase is the stage in which the chromatids in each pair become separated and the spindle retracts, pulling and separating the two chromatids in each pair, and moving one towards each end of the cell.

Telophase

In telophase, the chromatids (now known as chromosomes again) complete the journey to each end of the cell, the spindle disappears and the nuclear membranes form around the chromosomes.

Cytokinesis

The division is then completed by the mother cell dividing in two along the midline to create two identical daughter cells, each containing 46 chromosomes.

Energy production in the cell

Normal metabolic function is dependent on the production of energy to drive the reactions and processes of metabolism necessary to maintain homeostasis. The main energy source for cellular activity is ATP. This molecule is key to continued normal function of the cell, and therefore its production needs to be continuous in order to provide the necessary energy.

ATP is required to fuel:

- Energy production itself. It is necessary to initiate glycolysis and fatty acid oxidation.
- Active transport of electrolytes across the plasma membrane, e.g., the Na^+/K^+ pump that restores the resting potential of the heart's pacemaker cells.
- The amplification of the second messenger systems in cells. This process involves small amounts of signalling molecules (for example, water soluble hormones and neurotransmitters) attaching to the surface of the cell and initiating a process involving a

number of membrane and intracellular proteins, that amplify the message to ensure that there is a sufficient response within the cell. This means that a relatively weak signal can produce a significant cellular action. The amino acid endocrines, such as antidiuretic hormone, function in this way.

- Contraction of skeletal, cardiac and smooth muscle cells.
- Phosphorylation of molecules to enable and enhance reactions in the cell.

Any interruption in the production of ATP will have a devastating effect on cell function. ATP can be produced from a number of nutrients including glucose, glycerol and fatty acids, which are the component parts of **triacylglycerols** (also known as triglycerides or neutral fats) and some amino acids. At rest, many cells use glycerol and fatty acids, but this process is relatively slow and only yields 50% of the ATP yielded by glucose under ideal conditions. Therefore, even moderate activity requires the use of glucose. Glucose is found free in the blood or stored as glycogen in the liver and skeletal muscle. If glucose is in short supply, other molecules, including amino acids, are used for the production of glucose. This is a process known as gluconeogenesis and takes place primarily in the liver.

In order to produce sufficient ATP, it is necessary to have an adequate supply of oxygen through the lungs and an effective delivery of oxygen into the cells. This means that any acute or chronic respiratory problem could affect the availability of oxygen for distribution to the cells. Similarly, many cardiovascular problems, such as myocardial infarction, heart failure, stroke, peripheral vascular disease or a significant reduction in systemic arterial blood pressure, as happens in decompensating shock, could also lead to a situation of insufficient oxygen delivery. Where there has been injury, followed by inflammation and consequent scarring following injury in the lungs or the microvasculature, the diffusion pathway can be compromised, potentially reducing oxygen delivery. All of these situations will also affect the removal and disposal of carbon dioxide and other metabolic products, that could alter the blood pH or prove toxic to the cells, further compromising their ability to function effectively.

As identified earlier in this chapter, ATP can be produced from a variety of substrates. The processes are extremely complex, but the pathway is quite straightforward (see Figure 3.11).

The process can be summarised by the following equation:

$$\underset{\text{glucose}}{C_6H_{12}O_6} + \underset{\text{oxygen}}{6O_2} \rightarrow \underset{\text{water}}{6H_2O} + \underset{\text{carbon dioxide}}{6CO_2} + \text{energy (36 molecules of ATP)}$$

Within the cytosol, each molecule of glucose is converted to two pyruvic acid molecules through a number of stages. The process is termed glycolysis. This yields a total of two ATP molecules. There are actually four molecules produced but two molecules are required to initiate the process. The pyruvic acid, therefore, retains much of the chemical energy of the original glucose. The fate of the pyruvic acid molecules is dependent on the availability of oxygen.

Aerobic pathway (oxygen present)

In the presence of oxygen, the pyruvic acid moves into the mitochondria and is converted into acetyl coenzyme A (acetyl CoA) and enters the Krebs or citric acid cycle. This part of the process produces the hydrogen ions that will combine with oxygen in the next phase. It is the Krebs cycle that produces the carbon dioxide that we exhale. During the

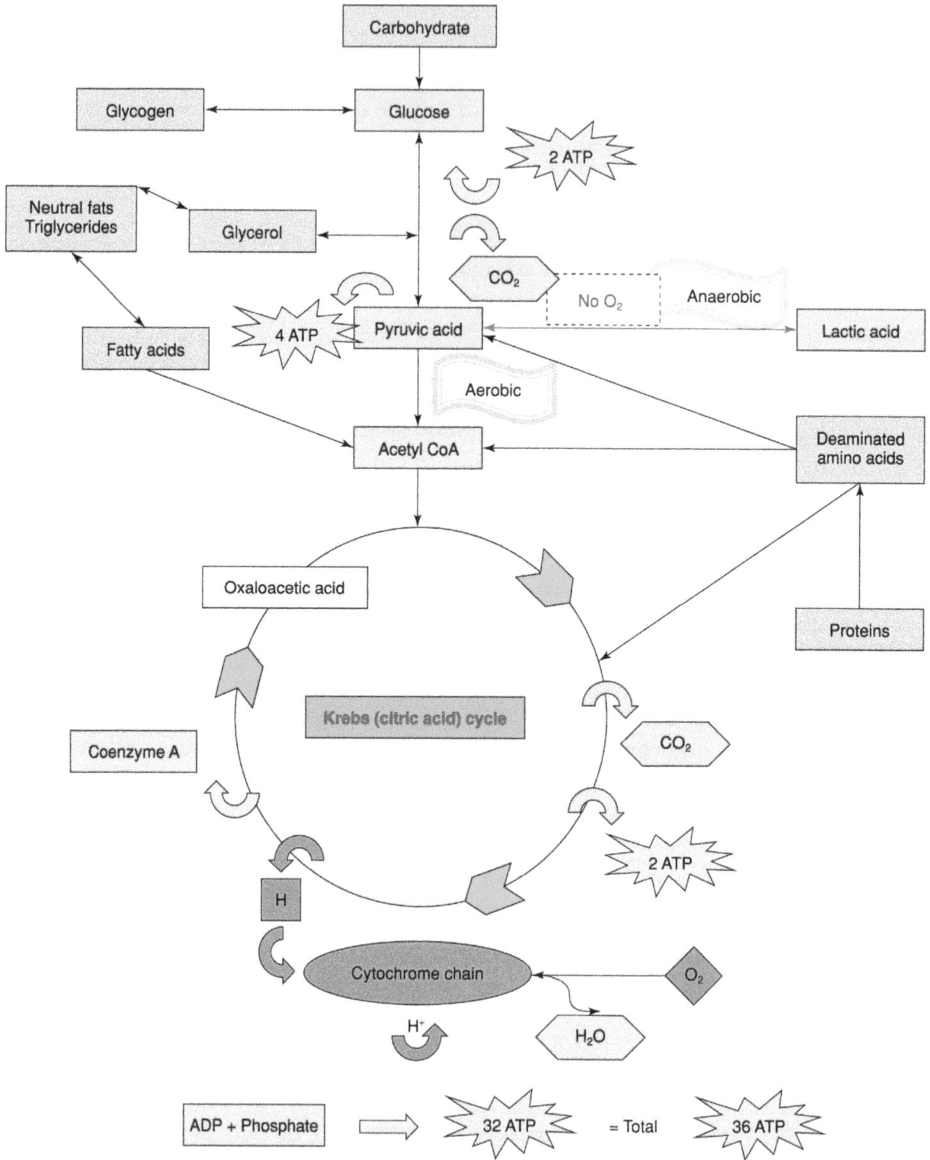

Figure 3.11 Production of ATP through glycolysis and oxidative phosphorylation, showing the aerobic and anaerobic pathways and relation to macronutrients. *Source*: © Mears Associates 2011.

cycle, the coenzyme A is released and the pick-up molecule, oxaloacetic acid, is regenerated, ready for the next cycle. During the cycle, molecules that are the building blocks for non-essential amino acids and fatty acids are produced. It can therefore be seen that this is a very efficient energy production system.

The final phase of ATP production involves a complex system called the cytochrome chain which facilitates the production of water from hydrogen ions and molecular oxygen (see Figure 3.11). It is the energy released from this reaction that is used to produce ATP from ADP and phosphate molecules. The vast majority of the 36 molecules of ATP are produced at this stage. The total output is 38 but we must remember the two molecules needed to initiate the process. The water produced is frequently referred to as the water of metabolism; approximately 250–500mL are produced daily.

To give an illustration of how dependent we are on the process of ATP production, we can turn to the well-known poison, cyanide. Its mode of action is to inhibit the action of one of the proteins (cytochrome A_3) in the cytochrome chain. If given in a large enough dose, death is almost instantaneous, so dependent are we on ATP production.

Anaerobic pathway (oxygen not present)

In the absence of oxygen, the pyruvic acid undergoes a very different fate. It remains in the cytosol and is converted to lactic acid. The total yield is only two molecules of ATP for each molecule of glucose. Initially, the process is faster than the aerobic route but this is only short lived. The cells of the brain, for example, will suffer almost instant failure. A build-up of lactic acid will contribute to acidosis, which will affect the ability of cells to function. This can happen in acute medical emergencies (Kumar and Clarke 2017).

Additional pathways

Both glycerol and fatty acids, the breakdown products of fats, are used as fuel for ATP production under normal circumstances. In fact, the liver and resting skeletal muscle will use them out of preference. The glycerol joins the pathway during glycolysis and contributes to the production of pyruvic acid. Fatty acids undergo a process leading to the production of acetyl coenzyme A.

This process is only effective if there is a sufficient supply of glucose. If there is a deficiency of glucose, cells sequester oxaloacetic acid (the pick-up molecule in the Krebs cycle) for conversion into glucose. This means that acetyl CoA cannot be used. The acetyl CoA is then converted into ketone bodies, which are acidic and contribute to acidosis. This is the situation that arises in uncontrolled diabetes mellitus, with the development of diabetic ketoacidosis (Jerreat 2010).

Amino acids can be converted to a variety of molecules that can be used for energy production. They are essentially converted to pyruvic acid or to other intermediates in the Krebs cycle. Under normal conditions, excess amino acids are converted. Where there is a lack of carbohydrate, there may be breakdown of protein to provide amino acids for ATP production.

Tissues

Cells are the basic building blocks of organisms. At the very simplest level, the cell can actually be an organism, such as a bacterium or an amoeba. Humans are much more complex than this and are composed of many, many cells which have different sizes, shapes and a variety of functions.

Similarly, tissues are very different, and, within each tissue type, there are wide variations in cellular morphology and function. The key is that the tissue types are generally composed of similar cells and carry out related functions, e.g., the epidermis of the face and the lining of the mouth (buccal mucosa) are the same tissue type with related functions, although their appearance is very different to the naked eye. Blood and bone look very different, but both are classified as the same tissue type. At first, it is difficult to reason this out, but, after some consideration, we can see that they both have a support function that involves the whole body.

Four main tissue types are identified:

1. Epithelial;
2. Connective;
3. Nervous;
4. Muscle.

Within these broad classifications, there are many subdivisions.

Epithelial tissue

Epithelial tissue is composed of layers of cells that cover the body surfaces, especially those that are exposed directly to the atmosphere, such as the skin and respiratory tract, or those surfaces that have contact with foreign objects, such as the lining of the gastrointestinal system (the gastrointestinal tract runs from the mouth to the anus). The gastrointestinal tract is effectively a tube that runs *through* the body rather than being *of* the body. Other areas that are protected by epithelial tissue are the vessels of the cardiovascular system, secretory glands and the hollow structures in the liver and genitourinary tract (see Figure 3.12).

All epithelial tissues are composed of cells held tightly together and adhering to a basement membrane, composed mainly of connective tissue. Some form single layers of cells (simple epithelium), whereas others have multiple layers of cells (stratified epithelium). Epithelial tissues are classified as follows.

Simple squamous epithelium

This is a single layer of flattened cells that typically lines the vessels of the cardiovascular system and the alveoli of the lungs. These cells are narrow enough to allow the diffusion of gases and many nutrients. In the small arterioles, capillaries and vennules of the cardiovascular system, they also have adjustable pores between the cells that can be dilated in response to injury, thereby facilitating the inflammatory process.

Stratified squamous epithelium

This is a protective epithelium. Unlike squamous epithelium, it has multiple layers designed to withstand physical trauma. Examples are to be found in the mouth, oesophagus and vagina. The epidermis is a special type of stratified epithelium in that it has a protein called keratin that holds the cells very close to one another, forming a highly effective barrier.

Simple cuboidal epithelium

Cuboidal cells are found in the tubules of the kidney and have an important role in controlling water and electrolyte levels in the body. They are also found in secretory tissues.

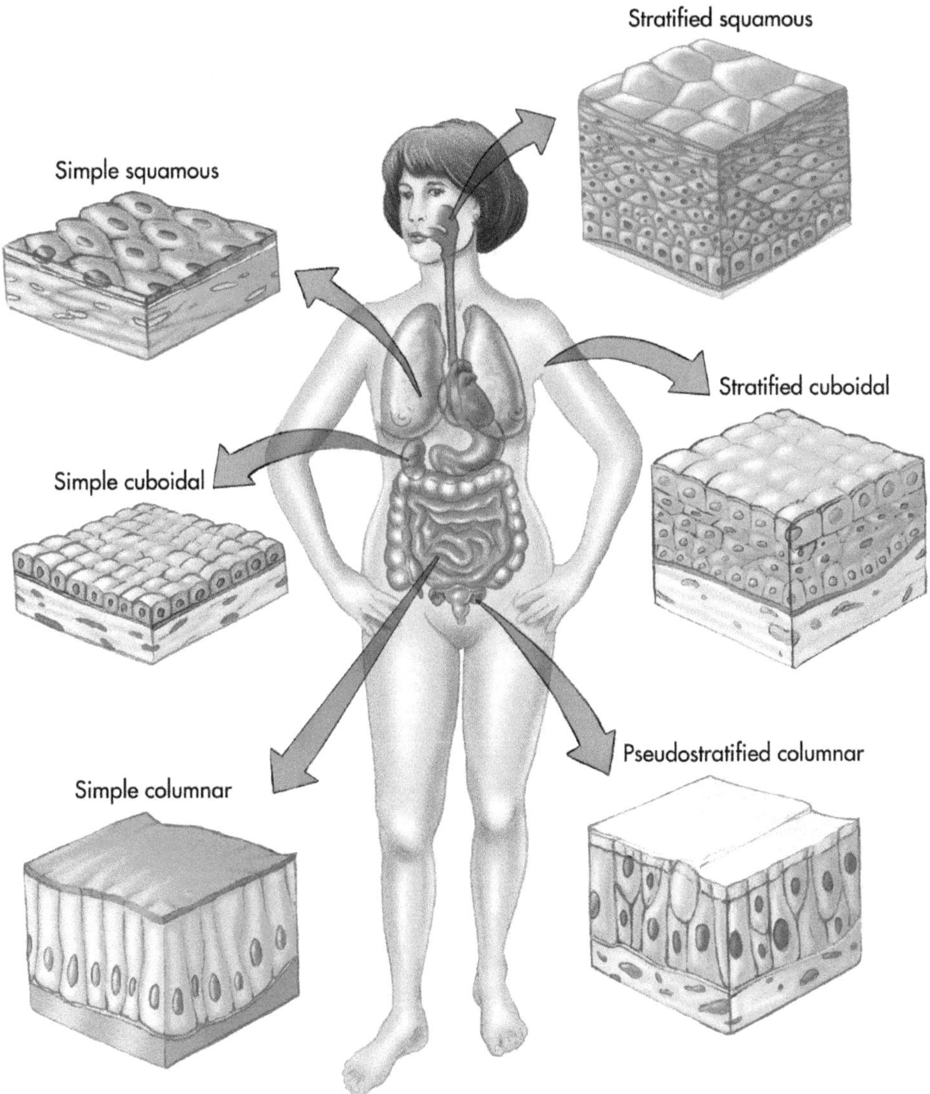

Figure 3.12 Types and location of epithelial tissue.

Because of their shape they are able to control diffusion in and out of each side of the cell more readily than the flat squamous epithelium.

Stratified cuboidal epithelium

The human body contains little of this type of epithelium. It is found in mammary glands and sweat glands.

Simple columnar epithelium

Unciliated versions of this type of epithelium are found in the lining of the gastrointestinal tract. Ciliated versions are found in the small bronchi of the lungs and the reproductive tract. They are frequently secretory. In the bronchi, for example, they secrete the mucus that helps to trap dust particles.

Pseudostratified columnar epithelium

This particular epithelium looks like stratified epithelium but is, in fact, composed of cells of different sizes. These cells are typically found in the respiratory tract and some are known as goblet cells, that produce mucus.

Transitional epithelium

This special epithelium is found in the urinary system. The cells change shape as the bladder fills and empties. In this way, the integrity of the wall is maintained at all times, whether contracted or distended.

Connective tissue

Connective tissue is extremely varied but is all derived from the same embryonic tissue (see Figure 3.13).

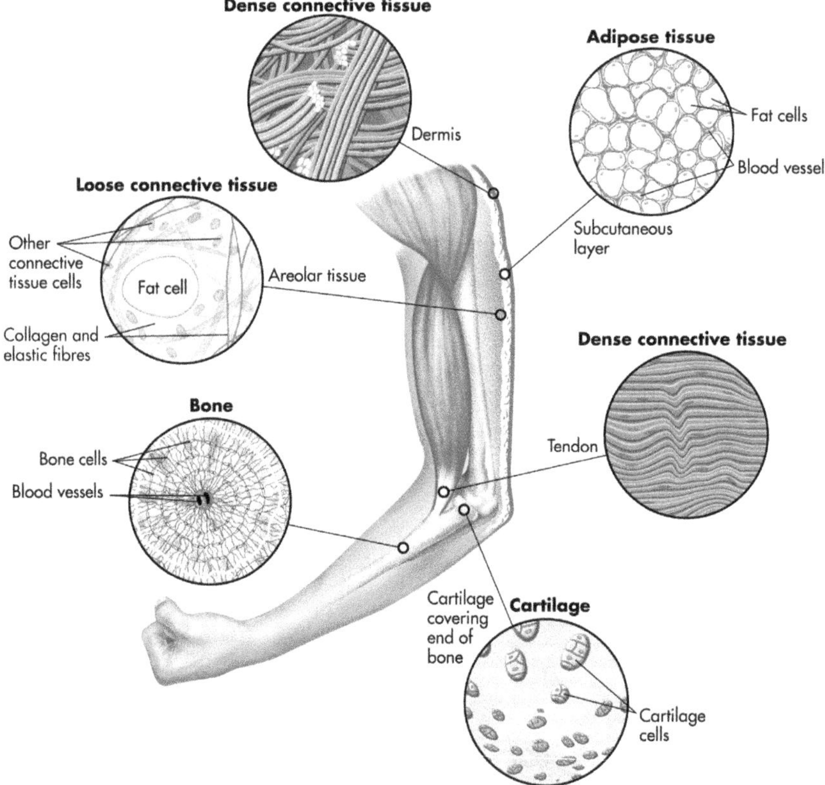

Figure 3.13 Types and location of connective tissue.

This is the commonest type of tissue, found throughout the body, and is intimately connected to the other tissue types. Whereas the other three types of tissue are mainly composed of cells, connective tissue is made up of significant quantities of non-cellular material. It forms the basal membrane that supports epithelial tissue. All blood vessels have an outer support layer of connective tissue that is predominantly made up of filamentous proteins. Ligaments and tendons are structured to provide support for joints and attachment for muscles. Bones provide support for muscles and protection for the more delicate organs.

As with other tissues, connective tissue is constantly being broken down and remade. If there is an imbalance in this process, problems can arise. For example, if there is an imbalance in the production and degradation of the connective tissue proteins that surround and protect blood vessels, so that there is excessive degradation, then there is the possibility of developing aneurysms in arteries and varicosities in veins. The lack of connective tissue can also lead to excessive bruising. This is a particular problem in older people as the production of connective tissue decreases (Waugh and Grant 2018).

Nervous tissue

Nervous tissue is composed of two main types of cell (see Figure 3.14). Neurons are the cells that conduct signals very rapidly to and from the central nervous system. They are primarily composed of a cell body and long extensions called axons. Either at one end of

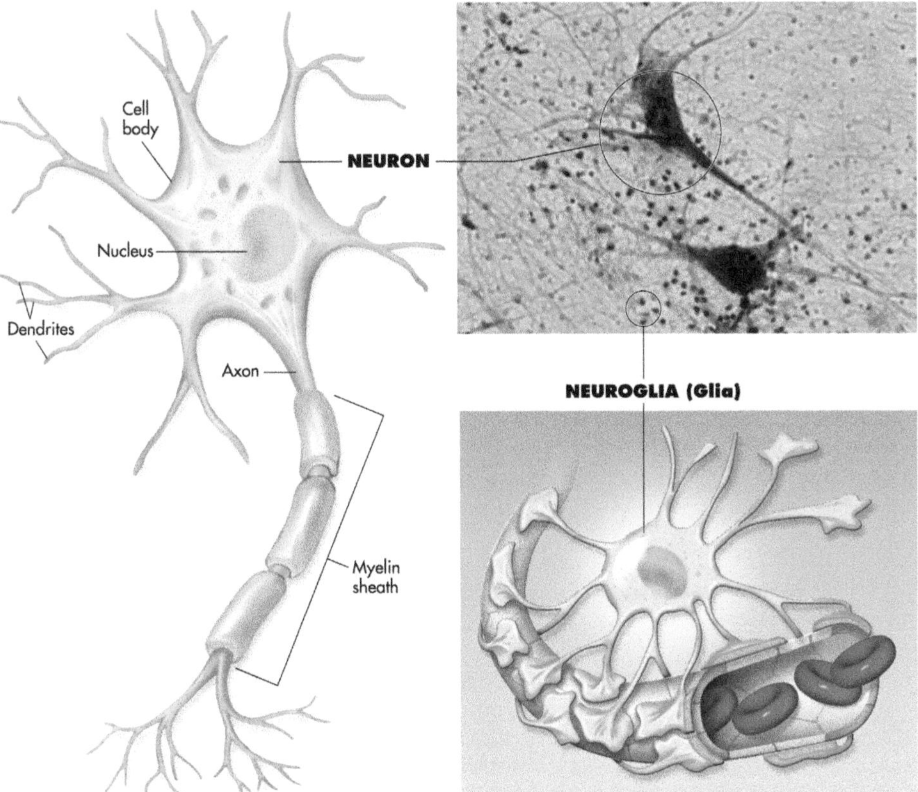

Figure 3.14 The two main types of nerve cell.

the axon or on the cell body are a number of other projections, called dendrites. Neurons conduct impulses in one direction only. The impulses arrive at the dendrites and are then passed along the axon, never the other way round. Unlike many other tissues, the neurons do not touch each other: there is always a small gap known as a synapse between them. The electrical impulse that passes along the axon stimulates the release of chemicals that pass across the synapse to stimulate an electrical impulse in the next neuron. This works as a safety and control mechanism. If the neurons were actually in contact with each other, the whole nervous system could be affected every time one neuron were stimulated.

Neuroglial cells act as the support system, that ensures that the neurons receive nutrients and that they are protected and insulated. The neuroglial cells are non-conducting. The majority of the nervous tissue is found in the central nervous system, namely the brain and the spinal cord. The peripheral part of the nervous system is almost entirely composed of the cranial and spinal nerves, which contain sensory and motor components, both somatic and autonomic. The enteric plexus that innervates the gastrointestinal system is also part of the peripheral nervous system (Marieb and Hoehn 2019).

Muscle tissue

Muscle tissue is the tissue that is involved with movement of and within the body. Every time we move, our heart beats; when we ingest food or pass urine, for example, muscle tissue is involved. Three types of muscle are found in the human body (see Figure 3.15).

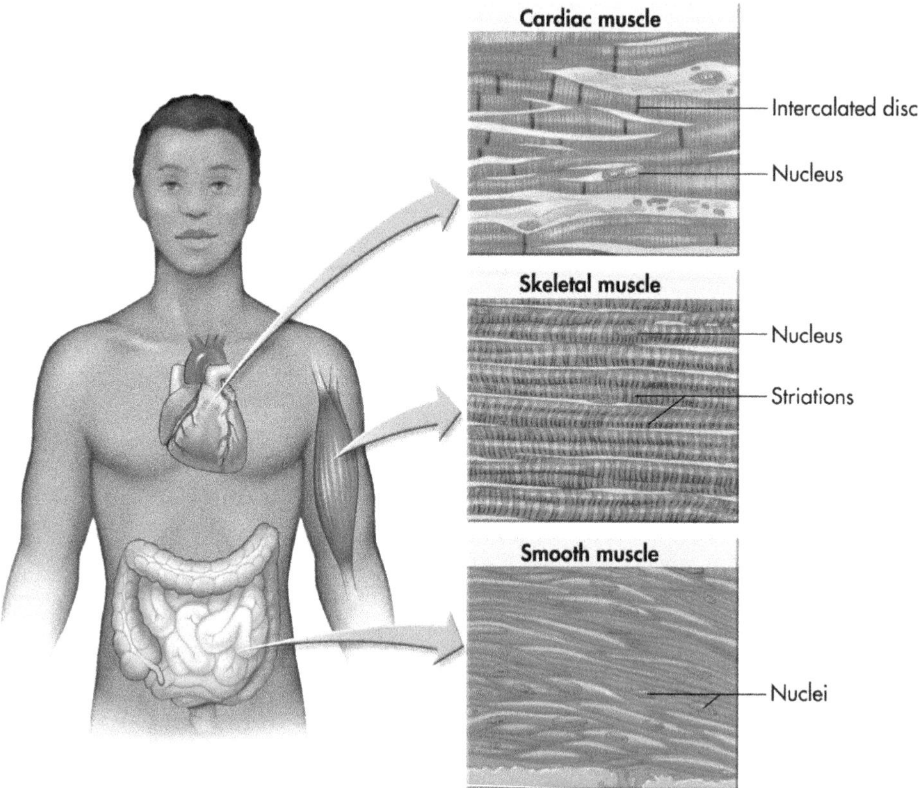

Figure 3.15 The three muscle tissue types.

Skeletal muscle

We are all familiar with skeletal muscle (often referred to as striated muscle because of the patterns that are seen when the muscle is examined under a microscope). This type of muscle is also known as voluntary muscle because we are able to control its activity. The cells of skeletal muscle are long and thin with multiple nuclei. They are gathered into bundles that are then bundled together, similar to multicore electrical cables. The muscle fibres, however, are able to contract and extend. You can easily demonstrate this by looking at the biceps muscle of the upper arm. As you flex your elbow the biceps muscle on the upper arm bulges up and as you straighten your arm the muscle flattens again. This process is complex and involves a number of elastic proteins and a very precise balance and exchange of electrolytes, especially calcium and magnesium.

Cardiac muscle

As its name implies, this is found only in the heart. Indeed, apart from the epithelial lining of the chambers and the outer coat of connective tissue, the heart is made entirely of cardiac muscle. It is similar to skeletal muscle but the muscle fibres interlock with each other. This ensures that, when the muscle is stimulated, all the stimulated fibres contract together and in a programmed, sequential manner. Both atria contract at the same time to force blood through atrioventricular valves into the ventricles. Similarly, the ventricles contract together, starting at the apex, in order to force blood into the aorta and pulmonary artery.

The muscle of the heart is stimulated by impulses from a specialised collection of cells known as the sinoatrial node (pacemaker) and is, therefore, not under voluntary control. The frequency and strength of the contraction of cardiac muscle are controlled by the autonomic nervous system but is also influenced by hormones (endocrines) and a variety of other chemicals, e.g., caffeine.

Smooth muscle

This type of muscle is quite different from the other two types. It is composed of narrow leaf-like mononucleate cells that are held together by connective tissue and have bands of elastic protein wrapped around them. It is the contraction and extension of this protein that lengthens and shortens the muscle.

Smooth muscle is found in the walls of all the hollow structures and vessels of the body, e.g., the blood vessels, bronchioles, ureters, bladder, urethra, uterus and the gastrointestinal tract. It is termed involuntary because we have no conscious control over its function, although we can influence some of its activity by lifestyle changes. Preventing uterine contraction, however, is simply not possible.

Hypertension, which is a permanent upward adjustment of blood pressure and a major factor in the development of atherosclerosis and, consequently, in acute myocardial emergencies, is related to factors that cause continued stimulation and contraction of the smooth muscle of the blood vessels, leading to an increase in total peripheral resistance.

The sudden narrowing of bronchioles in an acute asthma attack is a result of the stimulation of the bronchiolar smooth muscle by the parasympathetic branch of the autonomic nervous system and inflammatory chemicals, causing extreme and prolonged contraction and sensitisation of the muscle (Kaufmann 2011).

Tissue injury

Tissue injury is caused by a range of factors. Some examples are:

- *Mechanical* – blunt force trauma, gunshot and surgery;
- *Chemical* – acids and alkalis, poisons, drugs and alcohol;
- *Heat* – sunburn, sunstroke, flame, hot liquids and gases;
- *Allergens* – pollen, bee sting venom and medications;
- *Pathophysiological* – dehydration, hypoxia and hypercapnia;
- *Microbial* – bacteria and/or their toxins, protozoa and viruses.

When we talk about tissue damage, what we are really talking about is damage to cells. In any tissue injury, it is likely that there will be cells that are damaged beyond repair, others that are injured but are repairable whereas, around the damaged area, there will be cells that are fully functional. Cells and non-cellular material (mainly connective tissue) that are damaged beyond repair and die are termed necrotic.

The process of necrosis is uncontrolled. In extreme conditions, under the influence of bacterial toxins, this situation can progress from the original site of infection at an alarming rate, as in the case of necrotising fasciitis. Necrotic tissue is non-viable, can act as a focus for bacterial growth and inhibits tissue repair. If the necrotic material is not removed, it can spread out from the original site of injury, causing damage elsewhere.

The dead and dying cells, as well as those that are injured but which survive, release and produce a range of chemicals that are designed to try to counteract the insult and to initiate the repair cycle. These will be discussed in more detail in the following section on tissue repair in this chapter.

There is, however, a 'programmed' form of cell death that is called apoptosis. In this process, the cell shrinks and wraps important chemicals and structures in plasma membranes and signals to phagocytic cells to dispose of them. Apoptosis is usually associated with development. The webs between our toes and fingers, found in the embryo, are removed in this way. More significantly, it happens in severely hypoxic cells, particularly in relation to myocardial infarction and stroke (Marieb and Hoehn 2019). This is one of the reasons why patients are very carefully monitored if any hypoxia is suspected.

Tissue repair

There are two possible pathways for healing when tissue is damaged (Dealey 2012).

Regeneration

There are only a limited number of cell types that can regenerate: some liver cells, neurons and epidermal cells (although the range of epidermal cell types which can regenerate is limited, e.g., melanocytes cannot, hence the pale colour of mature scar tissue).

Repair

This includes all other cells and non-cellular material. The damaged area is filled with scar tissue, which is essentially a type of collagen. Collagen is a filamentous protein, which, in scar tissue, is crosslinked with carbohydrate-based molecules to give strength and structure.

The repair process follows a well-identified pathway to healing, provided that there are no obstructing factors, such as necrotic tissue, foreign matter or infection. It is also important that the individual has an acceptable PaO_2 or oxygen saturation within normal limits, an effective circulation and is well nourished. The healing pathway is as follows.

Vasoconstriction

Thromboxane and endothelin are two vasoconstrictor chemicals that are very rapidly released by damaged tissue, particularly the vascular endothelium. They cause vasoconstriction that helps to minimise bleeding at the site of the injury. This response is variable from individual to individual.

Haemostasis

Tissue injury leads to the activation of the intrinsic and extrinsic clotting pathways. These clotting mechanisms reduce blood loss where there is vascular damage. The intrinsic mechanism is activated from within the blood itself. The extrinsic pathway is activated by chemicals released when tissue is damaged.

Inflammation

The inflammatory response is a universal reaction to tissue damage and is characterised by four signs:

1 Rubor – redness;
2 Tumor – swelling;
3 Calor – heat;
4 Dolor – pain.

A fifth sign, loss of function, was later added to the original four. When cells are damaged, there are a number of events that happen almost immediately:

1 Vasodilation;
2 Release of messenger molecules;
3 Activation of complement;
4 Extravasation of vascular components;
5 Phagocytosis;
6 Pain.

Vasodilation

There is a rapid vasodilation of the blood vessels around the site of injury or infection. This causes slowing of blood flow and pooling of the blood in and around the damaged area and is responsible for the redness that is associated with inflammation.

Vasodilation is produced by four main mechanisms:

- First, the kinin system in the cell produces bradykinin, which is a vasodilator. It also stimulates pain receptors that lead to the stimulation of the cerebral cortex and thus the experience of pain.
- Second, the damaged plasma membranes release a fatty acid called arachidonic acid, which is a precursor to prostaglandins. The prostaglandins are vasodilators. They also lower the threshold of the pain receptors, which are then stimulated by bradykinin. The prostaglandins are hyperalgesic (increase pain).
- Third, mast cells (one of the family of white cells) degranulate, releasing histamine. The histamine has the added effect of increasing the pore size between the cells of the capillaries, which allows the movement of macromolecules (mainly proteins) into the interstitial spaces. The abnormal release of histamine in response to allergens and immunoglobulin E causes the massive vasodilation associated with anaphylactic shock.
- Fourth, nitric oxide (NO) is released from vascular epithelial cells. This molecule, which has a lifespan of fractions of a second, is a powerful vasodilator. Macrophages can also release large quantities of NO. However, they generally do not arrive at the site of injury until about 24 hours after injury.

Release of messenger molecules

The key molecule released is interleukin 1, which attracts neutrophils and macrophages to the site of injury. These are the phagocytic cells that will clear the debris from the injured area.

Chemical messengers that attract and activate lymphocytes are also released and thereby initiate the production and release of the antibodies of the immune system.

Activation of complement

Complement is an intriguing group of proteins, that come together to help activate the immune system. It is also responsible for labelling invading microorganisms, to facilitate their destruction by the phagocytic neutrophils and macrophages.

Extravasation of vascular components

Fluid from the vascular system, along with proteins such as thrombin and fibrinogen, move into the interstitial space around the injury. These are rapidly followed by neutrophils. This movement of fluid creates the swelling that we associate with inflammation.

The proteins that are transferred, thrombin and fibrinogen, are involved in the clotting mechanism. When there is a bacterial presence, they are also involved in 'walling-off' the area, classically creating an abscess.

Phagocytosis

The neutrophils arrive at the site of injury quickly and begin the process of removing cell debris and microorganisms, with macrophages arriving later. Macrophages are monocytes that were transformed as they left the vascular system. Phagocytosis is a very metabolically intense activity and accounts for a great deal of the heat produced during inflammation.

Pain

Pain is generated by the action and interaction of bradykinin and prostaglandins. The prostaglandins reduce the threshold of the pain receptors, therefore increasing the sensation of pain at the site of injury. There are a number of other chemicals that can be involved in stimulating pain following injury. Lactic acid, which is produced through anaerobic cellular respiration, is an example, as are hydrogen ions and potassium ions, which are released from damaged cells.

Proliferation

During the process of inflammation, the next stage of healing begins. Fibroblasts are attracted to the site of injury and begin producing the collagen and crosslinking chemicals that make up the bulk of scar tissue. Where there is significant tissue loss, angiogenesis (the production of new blood vessels) also takes place so that the active cells can be supplied with oxygen and nutrients. During this proliferation phase, the swelling decreases as the exuded fluid is reabsorbed.

Maturation

Finally, there is a prolonged period of maturation that may take weeks. During this time the collagen bundles thicken and align, and the new blood vessels, if they were produced, atrophy. Metabolic activity decreases, the damaged area cools and lightens if it is on the surface of the body.

Conclusion

This chapter has introduced the cell and the tissues that are formed from combinations of cells. The structure and function of the cell membrane, the cytosol and the organelles found in the cell have been examined. Transport across the cell membrane has been discussed and the importance of the mechanisms involved has been stressed. The significance of the environment of the cell has been considered, with the introduction of the concept of electrolytes and acidity (pH). Some emphasis has been placed on the production of ATP and the consequences of an interruption of ATP production in the rapid deterioration that can take place in acute illness.

The cell cycle was discussed with an emphasis on mitosis or asexual cell division.

The different types of tissue have been introduced with consideration of the relationship of their structure to their function. There has been a brief examination of the inflammatory process and of tissue regeneration and repair. The significance of inflammation on the ability of cells to continue normal function was identified. There was emphasis on cell function and ATP production by changes in electrolyte balance, pH changes and interruption of oxygen supply.

Finally, the chapter has identified the importance and significance of the cell and its function on the health of tissues, organs and the organism itself. If normal function, particularly ATP production, cannot be maintained, then the cell will malfunction and may even die.

Glossary 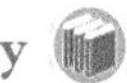

Active transport Any movement of substances across a membrane that requires the input of energy.

Adenosine triphosphate Usually abbreviated to ATP, this is a molecule that stores and provides energy for the metabolic activity of cells.

Anion A negatively charged electrolyte.

Aqueous Pertaining to water or water-based environments.

Cation A positively charged electrolyte.

Cell The basic structural unit of living organisms.

Centriole Rod-like structures in the centrosome that are responsible for the production of the mitotic spindle.

Centrosome An area near the nucleus that contains the centrioles and is involved in mitosis.

Corneocytes The outer cells of the epidermis that are flattened and contain no nucleus. These are the cells that are shed from the surface of the skin.

Cytoplasm The contents of a cell inside the plasma membrane but excluding the nucleus.

Cytoskeleton An array of connective tissue within the cell which helps to give the cell shape and to act as an attachment for organelles and inclusions.

Cytosol The viscous liquid component of the cytoplasm of cells, in which organelles and inclusions are suspended.

Dysrhythmia Any electrical activity in the heart that differs from the normal.

Electrolytes Atoms or molecules in an aqueous solution that have an electrical charge produced by the gain or loss of one (or more) electron(s), and which can therefore conduct electricity.

Endocytosis A process whereby molecules, too large to pass across the cell membrane, can enter the cell. This is achieved by pinching off of a small section of the plasma membrane and forming a vesicle that can then pass into the cell. Water can be transported this way (pinocytosis) as can cell debris and microorganisms (phagocytosis).

Endoplasmic reticulum An array of tubes and discs in the cell that is responsible for production and processing of a variety of molecules in the cell. It has two forms: rough, which has ribosomes attached, and smooth, which does not.

Exocytosis This is the reverse of endocytosis and involves a vesicle formed in the interior of the cell, joining the cell membrane and expelling its contents into the interstitial space.

Extracellular Relating to the internal areas of the body that are not cellular. The extracellular space is usually divided into interstitial and vascular space.

Extracellular matrix The fluid and connective tissue that fills the space between cells in the body.

Filtration The movement of dissolved substances across a membrane. The term implies that some molecules, proteins and other insoluble substances will not be filtered.

Glomerulus The part of the nephron where the blood is filtered as the first step of urine production.

Glycoproteins Molecules that are composed of elements of carbohydrates and proteins.

Golgi apparatus A series of flattened discs that are involved in finishing molecule production in the cell.

Histocompatibility This is the term used to describe the body's identification system and is usually based on molecules attached to the surface of cells, identifying that the cell belongs to that particular person.

Hydrophillic Any substance that interacts with water.

Hydrophobic Any substance that does not interact with water.

Inclusions These are found in cells and are large, unspecified molecules, food particles or cell debris.

Inflammation One of the body's non-specific responses to trauma or infection, involving dilation of blood vessels and the movement of blood components into the interstitial space.

Interstitial This refers to the space around cells that contains fluid (interstitial fluid) or connective tissue.

Intracellular The contents of, or any activity that takes place inside, the cell.

Lymphatic system A collection of capillaries, nodes and duct, that removes excess fluid and cell debris from the interstitial spaces and returns it to the vascular system *via* the subclavian veins.

Lysosome An intracellular organelle that is involved in processing microorganisms and cell debris, entering the cell through phagocytosis.

Membrane potential This is the voltage across the cell membrane, created by the distribution of electrolytes. Changes in voltage across the cell membrane are important for stimulating electrical potential in nerves and muscles, and also for ion pumps.

Metabolism The term that describes all the chemical reactions that take place in the body.

Mitochondrion An intracellular organelle in which oxidative phosphorylation takes place.

Mitosis Asexual cell division involving the production of two daughter cells that are copies of the parent cell. Also known as mitotic cell division.

Mitotic cell division See Mitosis.

Multinucleate Cells that contain more than one nucleus.

Myocardial infarction Death of cardiac muscle usually caused by acute lack of blood supply following blockage of coronary arteries.

Nephron The functional unit of the kidney, where blood is filtered and urine is produced.

Neuropathic pain Pain that is generated by damaged nerves or central nervous system structures, rather than in response to inflammation through pain receptors.

Oedema Excess fluid, above the normal, found in the interstitial spaces that is not rapidly removed.

Organ A combination of two or more tissues adapted to carry out a specific function.

Organelles Structures within the cytosol that are the sites of specific cellular activity.

Osmosis The movement of water from an area of high solute concentration to one of lower concentration.

Peroxisomes Membranous sacs that are involved in intracellular detoxification.

pH A logarithmic scale representing H^+ concentration where '0' is the highest acidity and '14' is the lowest.

Phagocytosis See Endocytosis.

Phospholipid A triacylglycerol (triglyceride) fat that has one of the three fatty acid components replaced by a phosphate molecule.

Pinocytosis See Endocytosis.

Plasma membrane A membrane composed of phospholipids, proteins and cholesterol that surrounds cells and intracellular organelles.

Ribosome An intracellular organelle, composed of protein and ribonucleic acid, which is responsible for protein production in the cell.

Selectively permeable A membrane that is able to control which molecules can cross it. It is usually referred to in connection with the movement of water from an area of high solute concentration to one of lower concentration. This is also known as osmosis.

Tissue Combination of similar cells and extracellular substances that perform a specific function.

Transport molecules These are molecules attached to the surface of the cell or free moving inside the cell, that act as transport or carrier molecules for other molecules, being brought into the cell or transferred from one organelle to another.

Triacylglycerol Known as triglycerides or neutral fats. These molecules are composed of a glycerol molecule joined to three fatty acid molecules.

Vennule Small vessel connecting the capillary bed and vein.

Vesicle A small fluid-filled sac. In cellular terms, it is surrounded by plasma membrane and may also contain particulate matter and a variety of metabolic intermediates and products.

TEST YOURSELF

1 Cells that contain a nucleus are termed:
   a. edentate
   b. prokaryotic
   c. akinetic
   d. eukaryotic

2 Cells join together to form which of the following?
   a. organs
   b. tissues
   c. systems
   d. colonies

3 Which of the following cells is multinucleate?
   a. skeletal muscle
   b. motor neuron
   c. smooth muscle
   d. squamous epithelium

4 Which of the following is involved in protein synthesis in the cell?
   a. peroxisome
   b. centriole
   c. ribosome
   d. lysosome

5 What is the main component of the cell membrane?
   a. protein
   b. phospholipid

   c. cholesterol
   d. vitamin E
6 How many types of muscle tissue are there?
   a. 3
   b. 1
   c. 4
   d. 2
7 Which of the following is the main intracellular cation?
   a. Mg^{2+}
   b. Ca^{2+}
   c. K^{+}
   d. Na^{+}
8 Which of the following are exclusively involved in glycolysis?
   a. fatty acids and glucose
   b. glucose and amino acids
   c. fatty acids and amino acids
   d. glycerol and glucose
9 Which of the following are vasoconstrictors?
   a. endothelin and nitric oxide
   b. nitric oxide and bradykinin
   c. bradykinin and thromboxane A_2
   d. endothelin and thromboxane A_2
10 Which organic acid is produced in anaerobic cellular respiration?
   a. pyruvic
   b. lactic
   c. acetic
   d. succinic

Answers:

1 d
2 b
3 a
4 c
5 b
6 a
7 c
8 d
9 d
10 b

References

Dealey C. (2012). *The Care of Wounds: A Guide for Nurses*, 4th Edition. Chichester: Wiley-Blackwell.
Jerreat L. (2010). Managing diabetic ketoacidosis. *Nursing Standard*, 24(34), 49–56.

Kaufman G. (2011). Asthma: pathophysiology, diagnosis and management. *Nursing Standard*, 26(5), 48–56.

Kumar P and Clark M. (2017). *Kumar and Clark's Clinical Medicine*, 9th Edition. Edinburgh: Elsevier.

Marieb E and Hoehn K. (2019). *Human Anatomy and Physiology*. San Francisco, CA: Benjamin Cummings.

McCance K and Huether S. (2018). *Pathophysiology: The Biologic Basis for Disease in Adults and Children*, 8th Edition. Edinburgh: Elsevier.

McLafferty E, Johnstone C, Hendry C and Farley A. (2014). Fluid and electrolyte balance. *Nursing Standard*, 28(29), 42–49.

National Pressure Ulcer Advisory Panel, European Pressure Ulcer Advisory Panel, Pan Pacific Pressure Injury Alliance and Haesler E. (Ed.). (2014). *Prevention and Treatment of Pressure Ulcers*. Osborne Park, Australia: Cambridge Media.

Norris T. (2018). *Porth's Pathophysiology: Concepts of Altered Health States*, 10th Edition. Philadelphia, PA: Wolters Kluwer.

Reed G, Rossi J and Cannon CF. (2017). Acute myocardial infarction. *Lancet*, 389(10065), 197–210.

Waugh A and Grant A. (2018). *Ross and Wilson Anatomy and Physiology in Health and Illness*, 13th Edition. Edinburgh: Elsevier.

Further reading

Alberts B, Hopkins K, Johnson A, Raff M and Morgan D. (2019). *Essential Cell Biology*, 5th Edition. New York, NY: Garland.

4 Body fluids and electrolytes

John Mears and Michelle Treacy

AIM

The aim of this chapter is to improve your understanding of the factors compromising fluid and electrolyte balance and of the underlying pathophysiology, as well as the essential nursing assessment and management required to prevent further deterioration and a medical emergency.

OBJECTIVES

After reading this chapter, you will be able to:

- Explain the fluid compartments of the body.
- Outline the transport mechanisms of water and solutes which allow them to move between compartments.
- Discuss the mechanisms which help to regulate body fluid balance.
- Describe the nursing assessment of the patient with an acute fluid and/or electrolyte imbalance using an ABCDE approach.
- Critically discuss the nursing management and treatment of a patient with a fluid and/or electrolyte imbalance.
- Understand the reasons for choice of intravenous fluid therapy, based on individual fluid and electrolyte requirements.

Introduction

Blood is a life-maintaining fluid and is the only liquid connective tissue. It comprises approximately 8% of total body weight (5 litres in a normal adult) and consists of red blood cells (erythrocytes), plasma, white cells (leukocytes) and platelets (thrombocytes). Blood helps to transport gases, nutrients and waste products, defends against infections and injury, aids in the immune process and helps regulate temperature, acid-base balance and fluid exchange (Marieb and Hoehn 2019).

Cell function depends on both a stable supply of nutrients and effective removal of waste products, as well as on homoeostasis of the surrounding fluids. Fluctuations in intracellular and interstitial fluids affect blood volume and cellular function, as do changes in nutrients, proteins and electrolytes. Any disturbance of cellular function can be life-threatening. Loss, retention or redistribution of fluid or electrolytes are common clinical problems in many areas of clinical practice (Norris 2018).

Physiology of fluid and electrolyte balance

Distribution of body fluids and electrolytes

Water

Water is the universal **solvent** and is essential for life; body fluids are dilute solutions of water and **electrolytes**. Water accounts for approximately 50% of the body mass, and the total body water mass depends on several factors, including sex, weight, age and relative amount of body fat. Total water content declines throughout life and accounts for only about 45% of body weight in older people, so the risk of suffering from a fluid imbalance increases with age. Whereas a healthy young man is around 60% water, a healthy young woman is about 50% water. This male/female difference is because women have a larger amount of body fat and a smaller amount of skeletal muscle. Skeletal muscle is around 65% water, whereas adipose tissue is only around 20% water (Marieb and Hoehn 2019). People with greater muscle mass have proportionately more body water, whereas an obese person may have a relative water content level as low as 45%.

Body fluids are distributed within two major biochemically distinct fluid compartments, namely inside the cells (**intracellular**) and outside the cells (**extracellular**). In adults, approximately two-thirds of the body's fluid is intracellular fluid (ICF) and is contained within the body's more than 100 trillion cells, amounting to approximately 28 litres in the average 70kg male. As this large number of cells is not a cohesive physical entity, the intracellular fluid compartment is a virtual compartment. However, these discontinuous small collections of fluid have similar behaviours, composition and location so it is physiologically appropriate to discuss intracellular fluid as if it were one single compartment.

The extracellular fluid (ECF) consists of fluid outside the cells, which decreases with advancing age and is more readily lost from the body than intracellular fluid. This fluid is commonly subdivided into smaller compartments, the intravascular and the interstitial compartments or spaces. The intravascular compartment consists of fluid within the blood vessels (i.e., the plasma volume). The average adult blood volume is approximately five to six litres, of which about three litres is plasma (Marieb and Hoehn 2019). The interstitial fluid (sometimes called the 'third space') is water in the 'gaps' between the cells and outside the blood vessels, which includes lymph fluid.

Transcellular fluid is contained within specialised cavities of the body, e.g., pleural, synovial, pericardial fluids and digestive secretions, which are separated from the interstitial compartment by cell membranes of specialised tissue. This fluid is similar to **interstitial fluid** and is often considered to be part of the interstitial volume. At any given time, transcellular fluid is approximately one litre in volume. Figure 4.1 shows how fluids are distributed in the body.

The intracellular and extracellular compartments are separated by the cell plasma membranes, whereas the interstitial and transcellular compartments are separated by the cell membranes of the particular tissues involved. The blood vessel wall separates the blood from the interstitial fluid. It is only at the arteriolar and capillary levels that there is interaction between these two parts of the extracellular compartment. The capillary walls have

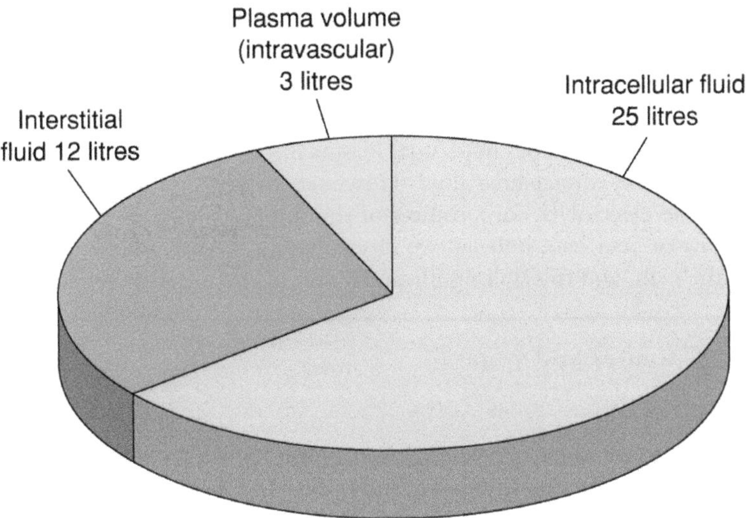

Figure 4.1 Fluid compartments.

a selectively permeable membrane, permeable to most molecules in the plasma except for plasma proteins and red blood cells, which are too large to move through the capillary wall. This selective permeability helps to maintain the unique composition of each compartment, while allowing for movement of nutrients and oxygen from the plasma to the cells, and movement of waste products out of the cells and into the plasma.

Solutes

In addition to water, body fluids contain two types of dissolved substance (solutes): electrolytes and non-electrolytes.

ELECTROLYTES

An electrolyte is a substance which develops an electrical charge when dissolved in water, by gaining or losing one or more electrons. Electrolytes which develop a positive charge in solution, having lost one or more electrons, are called cations. The primary *extracellular cation* is sodium (Na^+) whereas the primary *intracellular cation* is potassium (K^+). Electrolytes which develop a negative charge in solution by gaining one or more electrons are called anions; the primary *extracellular* anions are the chloride (Cl^-) and bicarbonate (HCO_3^-) ions, whereas the primary *intracellular anion* is the phosphate ion (PO_4^{3-}). The number of cations and anions in body fluids, as measured in millimoles per litre (mmol/L), is always equal because positive and negative charges must be equal. All solutions are electrically neutral, and this balance is called electroneutrality. It must be remembered that this is a dynamic homoeostatic state, depending on the acidity of the body; H^+ and HCO_3^- ions will combine and dissociate as needed to maintain a stable pH (Marieb and Hoehn 2019).

NON-ELECTROLYTES

The non-electrolytes have bonds (covalent bonds) which prevent them from dissociating in solution, so that they have no electrical charge. Most non-electrolytes are organic molecules, such as glucose, lipids, creatinine and urea.

The electrolyte content of interstitial fluid is not routinely measured in clinical practice, as it is essentially the same as the values in plasma. Plasma electrolyte values therefore reflect the composition of all the extracellular fluid. However, plasma electrolyte values do not necessarily reflect the electrolyte composition of the intracellular fluid. In situations, such as tissue trauma or acid-base imbalances, electrolytes might be released from or move into or out of the cells, and this will significantly alter plasma electrolyte values.

Transport processes of solutes and water

Fluids

Body fluids, nutrients and waste products are in constant motion within the body's compartments, maintaining healthy living conditions for body cells. The ECF is modified by external factors whereas the ICF remains stable. A change in one compartment can affect all the others, and the continuous shifting of fluid can have important implications for patient care.

Normal movement of fluids through the capillary wall from the vascular system (capillary filtration) into the tissues depends on two forces – like a 'push and pull' mechanism – and it is a delicate balance. Hydrostatic pressure (a pushing force) is created by the pumping action of the heart and the effects of gravity on the blood within the blood vessels. Hydrostatic pressure is the same as capillary blood pressure and it is higher at the arterial end than at the venous end of the capillary bed. When the hydrostatic pressure inside a capillary is greater than the pressure in the surrounding interstitial space, fluids and solutes inside the capillary are forced out into the interstitial space. When the pressure inside the capillary is less than the pressure outside of it, fluids and solutes move back into the capillary. The hydrostatic pressure in the interstitial space ranges from about +2mmHg and −2mmHg. At the arteriolar end of the capillary bed, the pressure is approximately 35 mmHg, whereas, by the time the blood has crossed the capillary bed to reach the venous end, the pressures have fallen to about 15mmHg (Casey 2004). There is therefore a pressure gradient that tends to force plasma water and its solutes from the capillaries to the interstitial space.

Osmotic pressure (the 'pull') is generated by molecules in solution. Osmotic pressure, generated by protein molecules (predominantly albumin), is called colloid oncotic pressure, whereas osmotic pressure, created by electrolytes, is called crystalloid osmotic pressure. Albumin is a large protein molecule, which works like a magnet, attracting water and holding onto it inside the blood vessel. Blood contains more protein than does the interstitial fluid, so that the colloid oncotic pressure of blood is greater than the colloid oncotic pressure of interstitial fluid. The crystalloid osmotic pressure between the two compartments is similar. The 'pull' is about 25mmHg (Marieb and Hoehn 2019), which means that, at the arteriolar end of the capillary, there is a net outward pressure, whereas, at the venular end, there is a net inward pressure. There is, however, an excess of fluid left in the interstitial space, amounting to about three litres per day, which is collected by the lymphatic system and returned to the vasculature at the subclavian veins.

Figure 4.2 demonstrates the direction of push and pull forces, and Table 4.1 summarises the push and pull forces at the capillary bed.

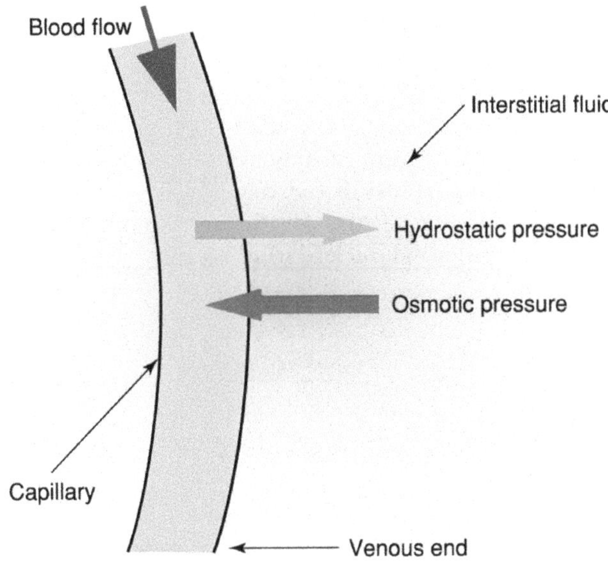

Figure 4.2 Osmotic versus hydrostatic pressure in the capillaries.

Table 4.1 Summary of 'push and pull' forces at the capillary bed

Push	*Pull*
• Hydrostatic pressure, generated by blood pressure.	• Colloidal osmotic pressure, generated by pressure of plasma proteins.
• This pressure forces fluid and solutes through the capillary wall at the arterial end of the capillary bed into the interstitial fluid.	• Osmotic pressure pulls fluid back from the interstitial space into the venous end of the capillary bed.

In health, the overall fluid balance between the intravascular and interstitial fluids is maintained by; blood pressure (approximately 35mmHg at the arterial end of the capillary bed), the osmotic pressure of the plasma (also known as oncotic pressure) of about 25mmHg and the activity of the lymphatic system. If patients are albumin depleted as a result of malnutrition, **sepsis**, **nephrotic syndrome** or injury, such as burns, then generalised oedema can develop. The oncotic pressure reduces with plasma protein loss, reducing the 'pull' at the venous end of the capillary bed. In a healthy person, there are virtually no plasma proteins in the interstitial fluid (Casey 2004).

It is important to note that there is no lymphatic supply to the central nervous system so any situation that leads to increased interstitial fluid in the brain is potentially extremely dangerous, such as the rare but potentially fatal increased intracranial pressure in **diabetic ketoacidosis** (Meaden et al. 2018). Other problem situations include the loss of lymph drainage following radical surgery (e.g., radical mastectomy) and the blockage of lymph ducts in filarial worm infestations, causing **elephantiasis** of the legs, or in **tumour** growth.

Adequate venous return is also aided by the action of the foot and calf muscle pump. This requires the muscles (especially in the legs), to compress the vein and push blood back towards the heart. Good respiratory function is also important; the thoracic cavity generates a relative negative pressure on inspiration, stretching the venae cavae and thereby 'sucking' blood back up to the heart. Valves in the veins help prevent the backflow that would be caused by gravity. Obstructions, such as a tumour, either inside or outside of the veins, can lead to venous **hypertension** and valve failure. This increases hydrostatic pressure in the capillaries and separates the cells in the capillary wall; this causes fluid and proteins to shift into the tissues and can lead to ambulatory venous hypertension and venous leg ulcer formation.

Solutes

There are also several factors which help to maintain the difference in solute composition between the ECF and ICF. Some solutes move freely across the plasma membrane, but most require some form of assistance.

Diffusion is a passive activity, caused by the random movement of particles from an area of high concentration to an area of lower concentration. The movement is dependent on temperature and relative concentrations. It is also constrained by a selectively permeable membrane, such as a cell membrane. In physiology, only small non-polar solutes can diffuse, e.g., oxygen and carbon dioxide.

In health, the overall fluid balance between the intravascular and interstitial fluids is maintained.

Facilitated diffusion is the passive movement of specific molecules, e.g., sodium ions, glucose and **amino acids**, down a concentration gradient (from high to low concentration), passing through the membrane, which requires the assistance of a specific carrier protein. So, rather like **enzymes** and their substrates, each carrier has its own shape and only allows one molecule (or one group of closely related molecules) to pass through, e.g., insulin to facilitate the transport of glucose into a cell (see Figure 3.5 in the previous chapter).

Active transport facilitates particle movement from an area of lower concentration to an area of higher concentration, but this process requires energy to make it happen. The energy required for active transport comes from adenosine triphosphate (ATP), a molecule with high energy bonds that is used by the body to provide physiological energy to facilitate active processes. Many important solutes are transported actively across cell membranes, including sodium and potassium (the sodium–potassium pump). Active transport is vital for maintaining the unique composition of both the ICF and ECF.

Osmosis is the passive movement of water across a selectively permeable membrane, from an area of lower solute concentration to an area of higher solute concentration. The membrane is fully permeable to water but selectively permeable to solutes. Osmosis ceases when there has been enough fluid movement to equalise the solute concentration on either side of the membrane. In clinical practice, you may hear the expression 'water follows salt' (see Figure 4.3). In practice, this means that water can flow easily across cell membranes if the solutions on either side cease to be **isotonic**, as occurs in dehydration.

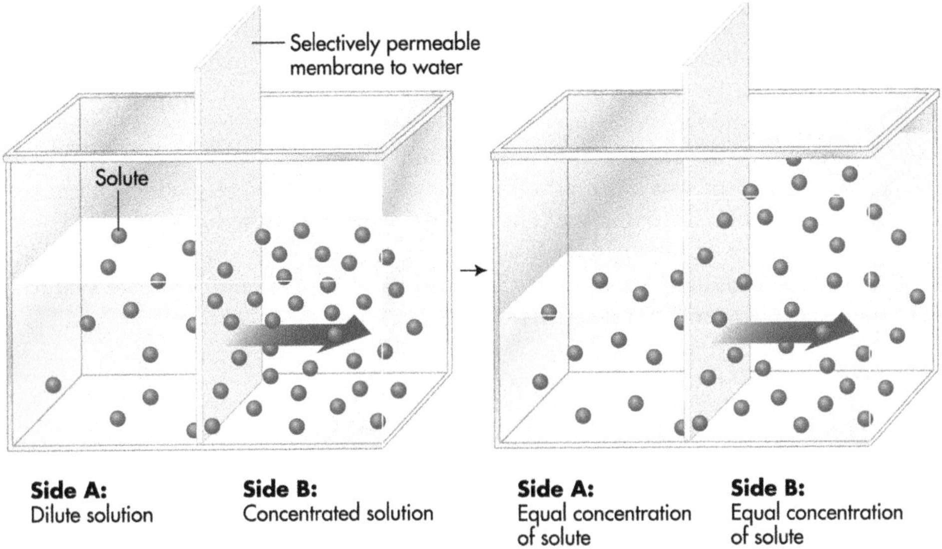

Figure 4.3 Osmosis moves water from an area of low concentration to an area of high concentration.

Table 4.2 Regulation of body fluid and solutes

Osmosis	The passive movement of water through a selectively permeable membrane from an area with a low concentration of solutes to an area with a high concentration of solutes.
Diffusion	Gas or solutes, moving from an area of a high concentration of solute to an area of a low concentration of solute.
Filtration	Movement of a gas or solute through a material that prevents the passage of certain molecules.
Active transport	Movement of gas or solute, particularly into or out of cells and across epithelial layers, resulting directly from expenditure of metabolic energy.

Osmolality: changes in the concentration of body fluids affect the movement of water among fluid compartments by osmosis. The measure of a solution's ability to create osmotic pressure and affect the movement of water is called osmolality. The term 'osmolarity' refers to the concentration of particles in a solution and these terms, 'osmolarity' and 'osmolality' are sometimes used interchangeably. An increase in extracellular osmolality increases movement of fluid from the intracellular space to the extracellular space. Decreased extracellular fluid osmolality moves the water to the cells from the intravascular space.

Filtration is the movement of water and solutes from a region of high hydrostatic pressure to an area of low hydrostatic pressure through a selectively permeable membrane. The pressure is created by the pressure of the fluid. The primary example of this is in the glomerulus of the nephron in the kidney.

A summary of the movement of molecules is given in Table 4.2.

Mechanisms which regulate body fluid balance

Most of the body's major organs work together to maintain body fluid balance. The amount of fluid and electrolytes gained throughout the day must equal the amount lost. Some of the fluid can be seen or measured, such as urine, but fluid loss from the skin through perspiration and from the lungs through water vapour is referred to as 'insensible loss' and is around 800mL per day, although several factors can increase this. When fluid balance is critical, all routes of loss must be taken into consideration, e.g., the loss can be much greater with increased respiratory rate or if the patient is **pyrexial**.

There are a number of organs and physiological systems that regulate body fluid and electrolyte balance, including the kidneys, the **renin–angiotensin–aldosterone system** and hormones such as **antidiuretic hormone.** All of these play a vital role in fluid balance and are discussed in more detail in Chapters 8 and 11.

However, there are also other homoeostatic mechanisms.

Atrial-natriuretic peptide (ANP) and B-type natriuretic peptide (BNP)

Two cardiac hormones, ANP and BNP, also provide short-term assistance to maintain balance.

ANP is stored in the cardiomyocytes in the right atrium and is released when atrial 'stretch' is sensed. It opposes the effect of the renin–angiotensin–aldosterone system, causing vasodilation, increasing glomerular filtration and decreasing antidiuretic hormone (ADH) release from the pituitary gland.

BNP, or brain-type or B-type natriuretic peptide, is secreted by the cardiac ventricles of the heart in response to 'stretch'. Its actions are similar to ANP but with a longer half-life. BNP is an indicator of heart failure because its concentration is raised in the serum of patients who have enlarged hearts (see 'Heart failure' in Chapter 6).

Thirst

The thirst mechanism is the simplest mechanism for maintaining extracellular fluid contents and is experienced when water loss equals 2% of body weight (approximately 700mL) or when there is increased osmolality (Marieb and Hoehn 2019). Volume depletion, increased plasma osmolarity, dry mucous membranes and hypotension stimulate the osmoreceptors (thirst centre) in the **hypothalamus**. All health care workers must be aware that, in older patients, or people unable to ask for water, the thirst mechanism is less effective. This makes these patients more prone to symptomatic hyperosmolarity, i.e., thirst and dehydration. This is a significant problem in those unable to ask for water to drink (McLafferty et al. 2014).

Gastrointestinal (GI) system

The GI system also works to absorb and excrete fluids and electrolytes. Sodium, potassium and chloride are lost from the GI tract and this can increase as a result of vomiting, diarrhoea or **fistulae**. If more water than sodium is lost from the GI tract, hypernatraemia may occur – especially in infants and babies. This may be manifest as increased thirst appetite or nausea but can quickly move to confusion and the consequences of increased intracranial pressure (McCance and Huether 2018).

Fluid and electrolyte balance

In health, there is a dynamic balance between the fluids and electrolytes gained and lost by the body. However, normal fluid and electrolyte balance can be disrupted by illness, and there are situations when the body is unable to cope with fluid deficits or excesses that may be seen in acute care. These common acute problems will now be explored, with a more detailed nursing assessment, and action and management principles described later in this chapter.

Appropriate use of diuretic therapy and intravenous (IV) fluids can help regulate fluid and electrolyte balance, but, if not closely monitored, can produce significant problems. The mechanism of action of commonly used diuretics and a selection of IV fluids is discussed in later sections of this chapter.

Acute fluid balance problems

Dehydration

Loss of body fluids increases the osmolality of the blood. This causes water molecules to shift out of the intracellular space into the more concentrated intravascular compartment. If this is balanced by increasing the water intake and reducing urine output, the body's fluid volume can be restored. However, if there is an inadequate supply of water, or if the kidneys are unable to retain water, the fluid from the cells continues to shift to the intravascular space, causing cell shrinkage and reduced cellular function.

Patients are often unable to drink when they feel thirsty because they have less control over their environment; they rely on health professionals to provide an adequate supply of fluids and food. They may also be confused or unable to express feelings of thirst; they may be tired, frail or unconscious, preventing a normal oral intake, whereas sometimes mental health problems may cause personal neglect. Infants also are unable to drink fluid on their own, and they have immature kidneys, unable to efficiently concentrate urine. Co-existing illnesses may also exacerbate fluid loss, e.g., diarrhoea causing excessive GI loss, pyrexia causing excessive perspiration. Hyper-glycaemia has an osmotic **diuretic** effect, as glucose spills into the urine and takes water and electrolytes with it, leading to **polyuria** and, in turn, dehydration and electrolyte imbalance.

Patient presentation may show changes in mental status as dehydration progresses. The person may complain of weakness, dizziness or excessive thirst. They may be pyrexial, with dry skin or dry mucous membranes. They may be **tachycardic** and **hypotensive**. In severe cases, seizures and coma may result. The patient's urine may be more concentrated, unless they have diabetes mellitus or diabetes insipidus, when large amounts of urine, which is very pale in colour, are passed. Blood results may show an elevated serum sodium level, elevated serum osmolarity and elevated **haematocrit**.

Hypovolaemia

Depletion of extracellular fluid or isotonic fluid loss is termed hypovolaemia. Older people and children are particularly vulnerable to hypovolaemia. It can occur because of

Table 4.3 Common causes of hypovolaemia

• Vomiting and diarrhoea. • Excessive laxative use. • Fistulae. • Abdominal surgery. • Haemorrhage. • Diabetes mellitus with hyperglycaemia (with polyuria). • Pyrexia.	• Excessive sweating. • Renal impairment with excessive urination. • Nasogastric suction. • Excessive diuretic use. • Decreased intake, e.g., anorexia, nausea, inability.

Table 4.4 Common causes of third space fluid shifts

• Acute intestinal obstruction. • Acute **peritonitis**. • Burns (first 24 hours but greatest movement in first 8–12 hours). • Sepsis.	• **Pancreatitis** • Heart failure. • Liver failure. • Hypoalbuminaemia. • Pleural effusion.

abnormal renal, GI or skin losses, bleeding, decreased intake, or fluid movement into the interstitial space, e.g., as a result of pleural effusion, **peritonitis** or burns, as a result of increased permeability of the capillary membrane, or decreased plasma colloid osmotic pressure. Untreated, hypovolaemia (representing less than 40% of intravascular volume loss) can progress to hypovolaemic shock and acute renal failure (Metheny 2012).

Decompensating hypovolaemic shock is a medical emergency, where cardiac output falls and mental status can deteriorate to unconsciousness. The patient will present with supine hypotension, a rapid, thready pulse, flat jugular veins and decreased central venous pressure, with cool and clammy skin (see Chapter 6).

'Third spacing' of body fluids is a unique situation (which may lead to hypovolaemia). This refers to a fluid shift from the intravascular compartment to an interstitial space as a result of an alteration in capillary permeability, secondary to inflammation, injury or **ischaemia**. Whereas this fluid is still technically within the body, it is biologically unavailable for functional use as it is outside of the intravascular compartment. A patient with significant third space loss may appear hypervolaemic (with weight gain and oedema), but they are clinically hypovolaemic (McCance and Huether 2018).

Tables 4.3 and 4.4 outline common causes of hypovolaemia, and of hypovolaemia due to third spacing of fluid.

Hypervolaemia

Excessive isotonic fluid gain in the extracellular compartment is termed hypervolaemia. The volume can increase in either the intravascular or interstitial fluid compartments and can lead to heart failure and pulmonary oedema. Fluid is forced out of the blood vessels and moves into the interstitial spaces, causing tissue oedema. It is caused by excessive sodium or fluid intake, retention of fluid or sodium or a shift from the interstitial space to the intravascular space. It may be a result of renal failure. The body will try to compensate by releasing ANP and decreasing the release of ADH and aldosterone.

Table 4.5 Common causes of hypervolaemia

- Excessive IV administration of normal isotonic 0.9% saline solution, or hypertonic fluids, such as mannitol or hypertonic saline.
- Blood or plasma replacement.
- High intake of dietary sodium.
- Compromised regulatory systems, e.g., heart failure, cirrhosis of the liver, nephrotic syndrome.
- Corticosteroid therapy.
- **Hyperaldosteronism.**

A person with acute hypervolaemia may present with shortness of breath, cough and **orthopnoea**, with an elevated blood pressure, tachycardia and a bounding pulse. Chest auscultation may reveal an expiratory wheeze, and inspiratory crackles may also be audible. The neck veins may be distended. If the patient is being haemodynamically monitored, their central venous pressure (CVP) will be elevated. For causes of hypervolaemia see Table 4.5. If left untreated, hypervolaemia can progress to acute pulmonary oedema, which is a medical emergency (see Chapter 6).

Water intoxication

Water intoxication occurs when excess fluid moves from the extracellular space to the intracellular compartment. The fluid shift happens when there is excess fluid, low in sodium, in the intravascular space, so it becomes **hypotonic** to the cells whilst the cells are **hypertonic** to the fluid. As a result, the fluid moves by osmosis to the cells, which have comparatively more solutes and less water.

Water intoxication can also occur with rapid infusions of hypotonic solutions or if a person continues to drink water or other fluids in large amounts. This can be a result of mental health problems or in situations where the person is perspiring excessively as well as consuming large volumes of fluid, e.g., athletes, or after consumption of amphetamine-type substances such as ecstasy (MDMA). This can be a life-threatening situation.

Water intoxication can be caused by a syndrome of inappropriate antidiuretic hormone secretion (SIADH), which causes the kidneys to retain water, leading to hypervolaemia with a dilutional hyponatraemia (Norris 2018). Signs and symptoms may include headache and confusion, owing to increased intracranial pressure as the cells in the brain expand. Nausea, vomiting, cramps, muscle weakness and thirst may also be experienced. Later signs are those of increased intracranial pressure and may include seizure and coma, bradycardia and widening pulse pressure.

Causes of syndrome of inappropriate antidiuretic hormone secretion

- Neurological injury.
- Central nervous system disorders.
- Malignancy, e.g., small-cell lung cancer, pancreatic cancer.
- Pulmonary disorders, e.g., asthma, chronic obstructive pulmonary disease.
- Certain medications, e.g., some cytotoxic drugs, recreational drugs such as MDMA (methylenedioxymethamphetamine), diuretics, barbiturates, or oral diabetic therapy.

Previously, SIADH has been regarded as the primary mechanism for hyponatraemia, following MDMA ingestion. However, it is now proposed that MDMA has a direct effect on the kidneys *via* the aquaporin-2 channels that carry water molecules across cell membranes, leading to an increase in water reabsorption, regardless of ADH levels (Davies et al. 2018).

In health, the osmolarity of the cerebrospinal fluid (CSF) and extracellular fluid in the brain is slightly lower than that of blood plasma. On ingestion of excessive fluids, dilution of plasma occurs, resulting in hyponatraemia and an increase in ADH stimulation. This disrupts the normal balance as a higher osmolarity (relative to plasma) occurs in the CSF. An abnormal pressure gradient results and movement of water into the brain tissue, resulting in progressive **cerebral oedema,** occurs. Initially, headaches are experienced, then ataxia (affecting co-ordination, balance and speech), seizures and a reduced conscious level. The increase in pressure caused by cerebral oedema may lead to **cerebral herniation**, resulting in death (Davies et al. 2018).

Oedema

Oedema is a result of interstitial compartment expansion, i.e., an excess of fluid in the tissues, and can be caused by an increase in the fluid pushing pressure or by insufficient pulling pressure, causing either excess fluid accumulation or too little removal. Localised oedema can occur where there is obstruction or reduced venous flow in part of the venous system, raising the hydrostatic pressure at the venular end of the capillary. Causes include thrombus, tumour, advanced pregnancy, or reduced activity of the skeletal muscle pump. Generalised oedema is widespread and may be caused by sodium retention or decreased concentration of plasma proteins.

Electrolytes and electrolyte imbalance

A balance of electrolytes is essential for normal cellular function. As previously discussed, a disruption of fluid balance has consequences for serum electrolytes. Electrolyte imbalances can be caused by prolonged vomiting, diarrhoea, sweating or high fever, or hormonal or glucose imbalance, but also by the use of medicines such as diuretics, which influence both fluid and electrolyte balance.

Diuretic therapy

Commonly prescribed medication, such as diuretics, are used to help manage several conditions, including hypertension, heart failure, pulmonary oedema and chronic kidney disease. However, diuretics also have adverse effects, especially on the electrolyte balance as they increase the excretion of sodium, water and other electrolytes. There are four main types of diuretics:

- Loop diuretics.
- Thiazides, including thiazide-like diuretics.
- Osmotic diuretics.
- Potassium-sparing diuretics.

Loop diuretics are one of the most commonly used classes of diuretic, with furosemide being an example of this group. They act on the loop of Henlé in the nephron, where they inhibit the action of the Na-K-2Cl co-transporter in the thick ascending limb. The result is less sodium being extracted from the renal filtrate and less water reabsorbed from the loop of Henlé and the collecting duct. Remember, as water will always follow sodium, if less sodium is reabsorbed, then less water is reabsorbed, with more being lost through the urine. Furosemide has an additional action, blocking the vessel-constricting response to angiotensin and noradrenaline and increasing the secretion of vasodilating **prostaglandins**, resulting in vasodilation. Therefore, a common side effect of furosemide is hypotension (a decrease in BP) as well as an increased urine output (**diuresis**). For this reason, it is used as an anti-hypertensive in those with chronic kidney disease in combination with beta-blockers and angiotensin converting enzyme (ACE) inhibitors (Williams et al. 2018). Unfortunately, the use of loop diuretics results in loss of sodium, chloride and potassium, so serum electrolytes require close monitoring.

Thiazides and *thiazide-like diuretics* have the same pharmacological actions, in that they block the action of the sodium chloride co-transporter in the distal tubules. The distal tubules are located in the last part of the nephron, so most of the sodium has already been reabsorbed. These diuretics are therefore less potent than loop diuretics and the loss of potassium and hydrogen ions is milder. Their action results in a reduction of blood volume due to diuresis, as well as having a mild vasodilator effect. Examples include bendroflumethiazide, hydrochlorothiazide and chlorothiazide.

Potassium-sparing diuretics, as the name suggests, work to preserve potassium. They inhibit sodium reabsorption in the concluding parts of the distal tubule and the early collecting duct. They may be used alongside another type of diuretic to preserve potassium in the body. It is important to note that these diuretics carry a risk of hyperkalaemia, especially for those with chronic kidney disease or individuals taking drugs that also increase potassium concentration, i.e., ACE inhibitors or beta-blockers (Casey 2019).

Osmotic diuretics, such as mannitol, are used primarily for treating cerebral oedema. These are non-absorbable solutes that, after being filtrated in the glomerulus, which acts passively in the nephron. The large molecules create an osmotic gradient along the renal tubule, preventing reabsorption of water. This has a significant effect in increasing diuresis and water loss.

Sodium and sodium imbalance

Sodium is the major extracellular cation, accounting for 90% of extracellular fluid cations, and it exerts significant osmotic pressure. It attracts fluid, and, in turn, plays a vital role in determining the volume and osmolality of the extracellular fluid. It is a key factor in the regulation of body water. It also helps to transmit impulses in nerve and muscle fibres by its reciprocal exchange with potassium across the cell membrane Sodium influences the level of potassium and chloride by exchanging for potassium and attracting chloride. It also combines with bicarbonate (sodium bicarbonate) and chloride (sodium chloride), and assists the acid-base balance (Marieb and Hoehn 2019).

The normal serum range for sodium is 135–145mmol/L. The amount of sodium inside a cell is approximately 10mmol/L. Whereas sodium requirements vary, depending on the size and age of the person, and the average daily intake of sodium far exceeds the body's normal daily requirements, renal and endocrine mechanisms help regulate sodium balance, keeping the levels within normal limits.

Sodium plays a major role in maintaining fluid balance; wherever sodium goes, water will follow. An increase in sodium concentration will increase the osmotic pressure of the fluid and therefore attract more water.

HYPONATRAEMIA

Hyponatraemia is the most common electrolyte imbalance seen in hospitalised patients and refers to a serum sodium below 135mmol/L (Spasovski et al. 2014). It is seen in about 15–20% of emergency hospital admissions. Sodium is lost through the skin, GI tract and genitourinary tract, and, when the concentration of sodium changes, water amount in the extracellular compartment changes accordingly.

Increasingly, patients are on multiple medications and sodium loss can be caused by a number of different drugs. The nurse should be familiar with possible side effects of common medications.

Drugs associated with hyponatraemia

- Diuretics (especially loop and thiazide diuretics).
- Anticoagulants (heparin).
- Anticonvulsants (carbamazepine).
- Desmopressin acetate (DDAVP).
- Recreational drugs (MDMA, ecstasy).
- Antidepressants and antipsychotics (fluoxetine, sertraline, selective serotonin reuptake inhibitors, SSRIs).
- **Antineoplastic drugs** (cyclophosphamide, vincristine).

Clinical indicators and treatment depend on the rapidity of onset of hyponatraemia, its cause and whether it is associated with a normal, decreased or increased ECF volume. Even mild hyponatraemia (126–134mmol/L) can have significant effects on gait stability and in-patient mortality, increasing the risk of falls in the elderly (Dineen et al. 2017).

Hyponatraemia can develop because of a loss of sodium, a net gain in water, or inadequate intake of sodium. Table 4.6 identifies common causes of hyponatraemia. As sodium levels decrease, fluid shifts can occur. The most feared complication of hyponatraemia is cerebral oedema (Narvaez-Rojas et al. 2018), due to the shift of water into the intracellular fluid compartment by osmosis, because the blood vessels contain more water and less sodium than the intracellular compartment.

MDMA (ecstasy) is taken as a recreational drug by some, due its mood-enhancing properties. Unfortunately, whereas many people can take MDMA with few side effects,

Table 4.6 Common causes of hyponatraemia

Causes	*Outcomes*
Hypovolaemic hyponatraemia (both extracellular fluid and sodium are depleted, but the sodium deficit is greater).	• Loss of GI fluids, diuretic abuse, cystic fibrosis, burns, adrenal insufficiency, osmotic diuresis, salt-losing nephritis.
Isovolaemic hyponatraemia (low serum sodium with no evidence of hypovolaemia or oedema).	• SIADH, glucocorticoid therapy, renal impairment.
Hypervolaemic hyponatraemia (both extracellular water and serum sodium levels are increased but water gain is increased to a greater extent).	• Heart failure, liver failure, nephrotic syndrome, hyperaldosteronism, excessive administration of hypotonic IV solutions.

there are potentially life-threatening consequences due to a number of effects, one of those being hyponatraemia. It is thought that the hyperpyrexia, which may occur in response to MDMA, triggers thirst and excessive water intake. The introduction of 'chill out' rooms in clubs, where there are often 'sports' drinks and water readily available, were designed to counteract hyperthermia but may have contributed to an increased fluid intake among drug users. MDMA users may also take other **amphetamine**-type drugs, with a common side effect being a sensation of thirst and dry mouth, exacerbating excessive fluid consumption.

An acute sodium decrease will produce significant neurological changes, whereas chronic hyponatraemia is associated with fewer symptoms, because the brain is able to adapt over time by reducing intracellular solutes, which, in turn, limits the shift of water into the brain cells.

Neurological signs do not usually occur until the serum sodium level falls below 120 –125mmol/L, at which point the patient may complain of nausea and a headache. As the sodium level drops further, irritability, muscle tremors and twitching may develop, or the patient may become disorientated. If the levels fall to 110mmol/L and below, symptoms may progress to **stupor**, **delirium**, psychosis, seizures and possibly coma with permanent neurological damage or even death. Symptomatic hyponatraemia is a medical emergency. The cause needs to be identified, but strategies, such as intravenous hypertonic saline, may be required, with treatment given in a critical care setting to allow for frequent assessment of serum levels, to prevent rapid over-correction (Dineen et al. 2017).

HYPERNATRAEMIA

Hypernatraemia is defined as serum sodium greater than 145mmol/L. In health, the serum sodium rises because of dehydration (i.e., a water deficit) and a rise in serum osmolality, causing the thirst response to be activated and ADH to be released, decreasing renal water excretion. This increases extracellular water to normalise the serum osmolality of sodium. Changes in the serum sodium levels therefore typically reflect changes in the water balance.

Hypernatraemia is much less common than hyponatraemia; it is found in approximately 1–3% of hospitalised patients (Metheny 2012). It is caused by an acute gain in sodium or a loss of water and is always associated with hyperosmolarity. As with hyponatraemia, severe hypernatraemia can lead to seizures, coma and permanent neurological damage or even death. The mortality is around 40–70%, depending on the severity of the underlying diseases (Metheny 2012).

Hypernatraemia usually occurs in people who have lowered osmotic stimulation of thirst and restricted access to water, e.g., confused or elderly people, infants or immobile or unconscious patients. Normally the body protects itself against the development of hypernatraemia by releasing ADH and stimulating the thirst mechanism, but, if there is failure in these responses, hypernatraemia can develop.

As the hypernatraemia develops, the cells shrink as fluid is pulled away from them by osmosis to the hypertonic ECF. As the cells in the brain become dehydrated, the brain tissue can contract on delicate cerebral vessels and lead to vascular trauma and bleeding. As with hyponatraemia, acute, fast-developing hypernatraemia over a period of 24 hours or less is often fatal, whereas slow-developing high serum sodium levels enable the brain to adapt by raising the number of intracellular solutes and, in turn, reducing the water loss.

Hypernatraemia is almost never seen in an alert patient with a normal thirst mechanism and access to water. The signs and symptoms of hypernatraemia include thirst, elevated body temperature, dry mucous membranes, disorientation and confusion, lethargy, muscle irritability and seizures. Someone with severe hypernatraemia may exhibit seizures, coma and permanent neurological damage.

Potassium and potassium imbalance

Potassium is a major intracellular cation (98% of the body's potassium is inside the cells) and plays an important role in many metabolic cell functions. The remaining 2%, which is in the extracellular fluid, is important for nerve impulse transmission. The sodium–potassium pump is critical in maintaining the balance between intracellular and extracellular potassium and even slight changes in potassium concentration can have significant effects on neurons and muscle fibres. Potassium also helps to maintain cells' electrical neutrality and osmolality and assists with skeletal and cardiac muscle contraction and electrical conductivity.

The normal serum potassium level range is 3.5–5mmol/L.

Distribution of potassium between the extracellular and intracellular fluid is affected by extracellular pH and insulin levels. Alterations in the acid-base balance and the shifting of hydrogen ions can have a significant effect on potassium distribution. Potassium ions move into the cells during alkalosis (as hydrogen ions move out) and out of the cells during acidosis (as hydrogen ions move in). Severe cell damage or cell death can also cause potassium to move out of the cells.

Insulin and alkalosis decrease serum K^+ levels, whereas acidosis increases serum K^+.

The kidneys are the primary regulators of potassium balance. About 80% of the potassium excreted daily from the body is *via* the kidneys. The remaining 20% is lost through faeces and sweat (Marieb and Hoehn 2019). As the serum potassium rises after a potassium load, so does the level in the renal tubular cells. This increases the concentration gradient, which promotes the secretion of potassium into the distal renal tubule, to be excreted in the urine. Aldosterone also increases the urinary excretion of potassium because of its reduction of sodium excretion. However, the kidneys are not able to conserve potassium and may continue to excrete it even when the serum potassium level is low. Disturbances in potassium balance are common because they are associated with a number of diseases, injuries and therapies.

HYPOKALAEMIA

Hypokalaemia refers to a below-normal serum potassium concentration. Mild hypokalaemia (between 3.0mmol/L and 3.5mmol/L) is usually asymptomatic in the absence of disease. Moderate hypokalaemia ranges from 2.5mmol/L to 3.0mmol/L, whereas severe hypokalaemia is usually defined as being below 2.5mmol/L.

Hypokalaemia occurs if there is inadequate intake of potassium, a loss of potassium from the body or a movement of potassium into the cells. It is also possible to obtain a false low result owing to a blood sample collection from a vein site or an intravenous infusion where the fluid is low in potassium. However, it is rarely the result of inadequate intake alone, and frequently a combination of factors which leads to hypokalaemia.

The most common causes of hypokalaemia are diuretic treatment and hyperaldosteronism. With hyperaldosteronism, sodium retention is promoted in the distal convoluted tubule, leading to a matched loss of potassium and therefore hypokalemia.

Abnormal GI loss, e.g., vomiting and diarrhoea, laxative abuse, **ileostomies** and nasogastric aspiration, can also cause hypokalaemia. Potassium depletion can also occur when insulin treatment is initiated, because insulin promotes the movement of potassium into the cells. Severe hypokalaemia can lead to death from cardiac or respiratory arrest. Clinical signs are usually not present until the potassium level falls below 3.0mmol/L but patients with liver or cardiac failure are more sensitive to hypokalaemia.

HYPOKALAEMIA DANGER SIGNS:

- Arrhythmias.
- Paralytic ileus.
- Muscle paralysis.
- Respiratory and cardiac arrest.

If your patient is taking **digoxin**, you should check the blood for toxic digoxin levels. Hypokalaemia enhances the efficiency of the drug.

Skeletal muscle weakness and leg cramps are a sign of moderate potassium loss, which can then progress to **paraesthesia**. The patient may also complain of constipation and may present with a paralytic ileus. However, the major cardiac effect of hypokalaemia is atrial and ventricular arrhythmias (see Chapter 6).

HYPERKALAEMIA

How severe is the hyperkalaemia?

Mild: serum K^+ in the range 5.5–5.9mmol/L
Moderate: serum K^+ in the range 6.0–6.5mmol/L
Severe: serum K^+ above 6.5mmol/L, or ECG changes or symptomatic

(GAIN 2014)

Hyperkalaemia can be a serious, life-threatening medical condition. Unfortunately, not all health care professionals appreciate that assessment, treatment and ongoing monitoring of hyperkalaemia is time critical. Cardiac arrest is more frequently associated with hyperkalaemia than with hypokaleamia. Hyperkalamia is present when the serum potassium level rises above 5.5mmol/L. It seldom occurs in patients with a normal renal function,

Table 4.7 Common causes of hyperkalaemia

- Decreased renal excretion; untreated renal failure or renal damage.
- Addison's disease.
- Potassium-sparing diuretics.
- ACE inhibitors.
- Non-steroidal anti-inflammatory drugs.
- Acid-base imbalances.
- Cell injury and cell death, e.g., from infection, crush injury, chemotherapy.
- Donated blood (if close to expiry date).
- High potassium intake, e.g., diet or supplements.

usually being seen in those with acute or chronic renal impairment. An increased intake of potassium, a decreased urinary excretion of potassium or movement of potassium out of the cells may result in hyperkalaemia. Notably, digoxin toxicity can also cause hyperkalaemia. When cells die or are damaged, e.g., after burns, crush injuries, chemotherapy or severe infections, they can release potassium into the extracellular space. Therefore, alterations in serum potassium levels may reflect changes in the ECF potassium, not necessarily changes in the total body levels. See Table 4.7 for common causes of hyperkalaemia.

'Pseudohyperkalaemia' can also occur, and the nurse must always be on guard to be sure that the serum potassium results are accurate. Causes of false readings include haemolysis of blood samples, or an excessively tight tourniquet, or the sample being taken from a site close to an intravenous infusion containing potassium (GAIN 2014). The most common cause of pseudohyperkalaemia is a prolonged transit time to the laboratory or poor storage conditions. False high reading of potassium should be suspected if there is no apparent cause for hyperkalaemia, and there are no changes in the ECG trace, or in muscle strength (UK Renal Association 2014).

Excessive use of salt substitutes may cause hyperkalaemia because most such salt products use potassium as a substitute for sodium.

Most of the signs and symptoms of hyperkalaemia are related to its effect on cellular membrane potential, and, in turn, its neuromuscular and cardiac functions in the body.

By far the most prominent effect of hyperkalaemia is on cardiac conduction (Table 4.7). Whereas the ECG does not always demonstrate changes, the presence of positive ECG findings should trigger urgent action. The earliest changes are a peaked, narrow T wave with a shortened QT interval on the ECG trace. As the serum level rises further, the P wave will flatten, extending the PR interval, and the QRS will widen (see Figure 4.4). Heart block, ventricular arrhythmias and cardiac arrest may occur at any point in this progression. In severe hyperkalaemia, the heart may become dilated and flaccid, with the strength of the myocardial contraction decreasing.

Hyperkalaemia may also cause skeletal muscle weakness and paralysis, related to a depolarisation block of the muscle, although this often does not occur until the serum potassium level is greater than 8mmol/L. The muscle weakness can spread from the large muscles in the lower extremities to the trunk and then to the arms and respiratory muscles. The patient may also complain of abdominal cramps, nausea and diarrhoea. Treatment will be described later in this chapter.

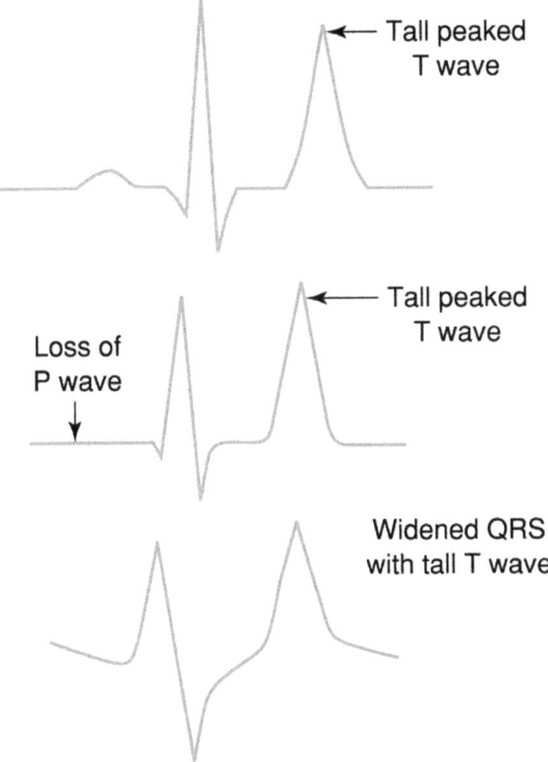

Figure 4.4 ECG trace showing changes with progressive hyperkalaemia.

Magnesium and magnesium imbalance

Magnesium is the body's fourth most abundant cation and, after potassium, the most abundant cation in the intracellular fluid. About 50% of the body's magnesium is in the bone and one-third is in the intracellular fluid. The extracellular fluid only contains about 1% of the body's magnesium (Limaye et al. 2011).

Normal serum level of magnesium is 0.74-1.1 mmol/L.

Magnesium has a role in several important functions in the body and cells. It plays a vital part in helping the body produce and use adenosine triphosphate (ATP) for energy and is implicated in neuromuscular transmission, hormone receptor binding and cardiovascular tone (myocardial contractility). Magnesium also promotes the production of the parathyroid hormone and triggers the sodium–potassium pump, so its effects are closely related to potassium levels inside and outside the cells. Magnesium also influences the body's calcium levels through its effect on the parathyroid hormone, so excretion of magnesium is decreased with increased parathormone (parathyroid hormone, PTH) level or decreased excretion of sodium or calcium.

The body will try to balance the magnesium level. The kidneys are the main route of magnesium excretion, but (unlike potassium) they are also able to conserve magnesium when required. The GI system (mainly the **jejunum** and **ileum**) absorbs dietary magnesium.

Approximately 25–30% of serum magnesium is bound to protein, although a small proportion is combined with other substances and the rest is free (ionised). Whereas it is the free portion which is physiologically important, it cannot be measured alone. Therefore, the serum magnesium level reflects the total amount of circulating magnesium, and the serum albumin levels need to be measured with serum magnesium levels, with a low serum albumin decreasing the total magnesium level, although the amount of free magnesium may be unchanged (Metheny 2012).

HYPOMAGNESAEMIA

Hypomagnesaemia occurs when the serum magnesium falls below 0.75mmol/L. This condition is common among critically ill patients, and, if left untreated, can lead to cardiac arrhythmias, respiratory muscle weakness and seizures. It can occur owing to a shift of magnesium to the intracellular space, decreased GI absorption (e.g., malabsorption syndromes, fistulae, Crohn's disease, bowel resection, cancer) or decreased intake or increased urinary loss (e.g., diabetic ketoacidosis, hyperparathyroidism, loop diuretics). Whereas a healthy balanced diet provides sufficient magnesium, patients who eat a poor diet, e.g., chronic alcoholics and critical care patients, are at risk of hypomagnesaemia.

Hypomagnesaemia is most commonly seen in critically ill patients, even those with normal renal function.

Hypomagnesaemia is often associated with hypercalcaemia and hypokalaemia.

Signs and symptoms of hypomagnesaemia are similar to potassium and calcium imbalance, although some patients may not show any clinical manifestations even if the level is well below 0.75mmol/L. The symptomatic patient may have an altered level of consciousness, exhibit psychosis or vertigo, or develop seizures, they may complain of leg cramps, muscle weakness or tremors. Deep tendon reflexes might be hyperactive, also with a positive Chvostek's and Trousseau's sign (this will be explained in more detail later). Magnesium deficiency is also associated with a high frequency of cardiac arrhythmias (atrial and ventricular) and sudden death. Respiratory muscles may also be affected leading to laryngeal **stridor**. There is also a link between hypomagnesaemia and hypertension.

HYPERMAGNESAEMIA

Hypermagnesaemia is less common than hypomagnesaemia and occurs when the serum magnesium is greater than 1.1mmol/L. It is caused by impaired renal excretion or excessive magnesium intake.

Whereas decreased serum magnesium over-stimulates the neuromuscular system, an increased level diminishes or suppresses it. Therefore, the patient may develop bradycardia, heart block and progression to asystole. Vasodilation may also occur, leading to hypotension, and the patient may appear flushed. Deep tendon reflexes may be hypoactive, and the patient may have generalised weakness. As the serum level increases, the patient's level of consciousness may deteriorate from drowsiness to a coma and finally (with a level at 10mmol/L) cardiorespiratory arrest.

Calcium and calcium imbalance

Calcium is the most abundant mineral in the body and is primarily bound to phosphorus (as phosphate) to form the mineral salts of the bones and teeth. It also has important intracellular functions, such as the development of the cardiac action potential, muscle contraction and relaxation. Less than 1% of the body's calcium is contained within the extracellular fluid and this is regulated carefully by the parathyroid hormone, vitamin D and calcitonin (Beckett et al. 2010).

Calcium is present in three different forms in the plasma: ionised calcium, protein-bound calcium and complex calcium. Almost half of the calcium is free, ionised calcium. Around 40% of calcium is bound to protein, primarily to albumin. The remaining calcium is combined with non-protein anions, such as phosphate, carbonate and citrate. Only the ionised calcium is physiologically important and plasma calcium (Ca^{2+}) refers solely to the concentration of ionised calcium (Metheny 2012).

Serum calcium

- Normal serum levels of total serum calcium in an adult range from 2.1 to 2.6mmol/L.
- Normal serum levels of serum ionised calcium is 1.1–1.3mmol/L.

The percentage of calcium which is ionised is affected by plasma pH, phosphorus and albumin levels, so, if a patient develops alkalosis, causing an increase in arterial blood pH, more calcium becomes bound to protein; as a result, the total serum calcium remains unchanged, but the ionised portion decreases.

Changes in the plasma albumin level affect the total serum calcium level without changing the level of free calcium, so, in cases of hypoalbuminaemia, less protein is available to bind with calcium, and the total calcium level drops but the level of ionised calcium is unchanged. Therefore, when evaluating total calcium levels, these factors, in addition to serum pH, must be taken into consideration.

HYPOCALCAEMIA

Left untreated or poorly managed, hypocalcaemia emergencies can lead to significant morbidity or (more rarely) death.

Hypocalcaemia can be asymptomatic or symptomatic. Asymptomatic hypocalcaemia is often caused by hypoalbuminaemia, and this is sometimes described as 'pseudohypocalcaemia' because there is a reduced total serum calcium concentration but the ionised calcium remains normal.

Symptomatic hypocalcaemia occurs when there is a decrease in the percentage of calcium which is ionised (although the total serum calcium level is normal). Common causes are listed in Table 4.8.

Clinical manifestations of hypocalcaemia include enhanced neuromuscular irritability and tetany (involuntary muscle contractions), tingling of the fingers, muscle cramps, numbness and convulsions. Alterations in mental status might include anxiety or

Table 4.8 Common causes of symptomatic hypocalcaemia (decrease in percentage of ionised calcium)

- Increased calcium loss, e.g., loop diuretics.
- Reduced intake, e.g., inadequate vitamin D consumption or exposure.
- Decreased regulation, e.g., hypoparathyroidism.
- Decreased intestinal absorption.
- Post-partial parathyroidectomy or thyroidectomy.
- Chronic alcoholism.
- Acute pancreatitis.

depression. Sudden drops in plasma calcium levels can lead to decreased myocardial contractility, hypotension and heart failure. Other cardiovascular manifestations may include arrhythmias and bradycardia.

HYPERCALCAEMIA

Hypercalcaemia is a common metabolic emergency which occurs when the serum level of calcium rises above 2.6mmol/L, or when the level of ionised serum calcium rises above 1.3mmol/L, or if more calcium enters extracellular fluid than is removed by the rate of renal excretion of calcium. It has been suggested that the prevalence of hypercalcaemia in the hospital in-patient population ranges from 0.6 to 3.6%.

Any situation which increases the level of total serum or ionised calcium may cause hypercalcaemia. Hyperparathyroidism and malignancy are the two main causes. Cancer (commonly breast and lung cancers and lymphoma), which invades and destroys the bones, may cause more calcium to be released into the bloodstream. Immobility can result in loss of bone mineral leading to an increase in total calcium in the bloodstream.

Hypercalcaemia danger signs:

- Arrhythmias.
- Bradycardia.
- Heart block.
- Cardiac arrest.
- Coma.
- **Stupor**.
- Paralytic ileus.

If the patient develops acute hypercalcaemia, the signs and symptoms are more severe. The patient may complain of fatigue and lethargy or exhibit confusion. Muscle weakness, hyporeflexia and decreased muscle tone may occur. Hypercalcaemia can also alter myocardial muscle function, causing rhythm disturbances, such as bradycardia, heart block and a shortened QT interval. Severe hypercalcaemia can lead to ventricular arrhythmias and cardiac arrest.

Nursing assessment of fluid and electrolyte status in the patient

Nurses are directly responsible for monitoring patients for actual or potential fluid and/or electrolyte disturbances and NMC (2018) requires nurses to be able to carry out accurate assessment of people of all ages, using appropriate diagnostic and decision-making skills. While nurses often keep fluid balance charts and perform vital signs as part of daily practice, it is also important to have a good understanding of normal physiological mechanisms as well as the signs and symptoms of fluid and electrolyte problems. The nurse is responsible for reviewing the patient's history and laboratory data, as well as close clinical observation and assessment, and analysis of the effectiveness of interventions. The nurse should also recognise when specialist knowledge and expertise are required, and to seek advice accordingly.

Airway

The look, listen and feel approach is the best way to assess the airway for obstruction or use of accessory muscles. A patient with fluid volume overload may have wheezing or excessive secretions. (see Chapter 7). If the patent is in shock, the airway must be secured for tissue oxygen delivery, and, in severe situations, endotracheal intubation may be required.

Breathing

Deep, rapid respiration may indicate a change in the acid-base balance, e.g., a compensatory mechanism if the patient is in metabolic acidosis (the lungs attempt to 'blow off' excess carbon dioxide). Slow, shallow breathing may be a compensatory mechanism for metabolic alkalosis (the lungs try to retain carbon dioxide). In situations such as severe hypokalaemia or hyperkalaemia, there may be weakness or paralysis of the respiratory muscles. Crackles or wheezing may be audible or present on auscultation, which may indicate fluid volume overload and pulmonary oedema. The patient might expectorate pink, frothy sputum and they might be using their accessory muscles. Pulse oximetry may also decrease if the patient is developing pulmonary oedema or is hypovolaemic.

Circulation and fluid balance

The look, listen and feel approach is also an important part of assessing your patient's circulatory status. Blood pressure is a sensitive method for assessing fluid depletion. Hypotension may occur as a reduction of stroke volume. Electrolyte disturbances, which can cause arrhythmias, may also then lead to hypotension if heart rate or stroke volume are affected. Lying and standing blood pressures and pulse rate might be recorded to assess for hypovolaemia. Standing from a supine position causes an abrupt drop in venous return, for which the body usually compensates through increasing peripheral resistance and a slight increase in heart rate. However, a fall in systolic pressure of 15mmHg or more and an increase in heart rate greater than 15 beats per minute may suggest fluid volume deficit. Orthostatic changes may also occur with autonomic **neuropathy**, e.g., diabetes mellitus, as well as in response to some antihypertensive medications.

The jugular veins often follow the changes in central venous pressure (CVP), which may help assess fluid status. Normal CVP is in the range 2–8mmHg. Central venous pressure measures the pressure in the right atrium or vena cava and helps to monitor the effectiveness of the heart's pumping mechanism and vascular tone. Flat neck veins when the patient in the supine position may indicate decreased plasma volume and a low CVP, whereas distended neck veins and an elevated CVP may be seen in hypervolaemia.

Elevated blood pressure and a bounding pulse may be present in hypervolaemia as stroke volume increases. The pulse should be palpated manually, and an ECG may show conduction disturbances, e.g., a long or short QT interval, dysarrhythmias or ectopics.

Tachycardia or arrhythmias are usually the earliest sign of hypovolaemia but may also be associated with electrolyte disturbances such as hypokalaemia. Bradyarrhythmias may be present with hypercalcaemia. A bounding pulse may be felt in hypervolaemia, as the strength of the contraction of the left ventricle and the amount of blood it ejects increases, whereas a thready, weak pulse may indicate fluid volume deficit because of a reduced circulating blood volume. At the same time, the patient's skin temperature should be assessed, e.g., is it cold and clammy, or hot and sweaty? The more dehydrated the patient is, the further up the limb the coolness will extend owing to compensatory vasoconstriction.

Palpating the pulse manually can give you vital information about a patient's fluid and/or electrolyte status.

Disability

The ACVPU (RCP 2017) approach should be used to assess for altered mental status, as a change in serum osmolality, acid-base balance or electrolyte balance may affect the patient's level of consciousness, confusion, personality, behaviour or neurological function. The patient may be restless or anxious, or complain of dizziness, if they are dehydrated or water intoxicated. In severe cases, seizures and coma may result. In situations of water intoxication, the patient may develop raised intracranial pressure and may complain of a headache as an early symptom. Later, they may become lethargic and irritable. Late signs of raised intracranial pressure include pupillary changes and a widening pulse pressure.

Patients should also be assessed for neuromuscular irritability if calcium or magnesium imbalances are suspected, by checking for Chvostek's sign (tapping over the facial nerve causes facial muscles to twitch) and Trousseau's sign, a spasm presenting with adduction of the thumb, flexed wrist and extended fingers two and four after inflating a blood pressure cuff on the upper arm (see Figure 4.5); in addition, deep tendon reflexes, which

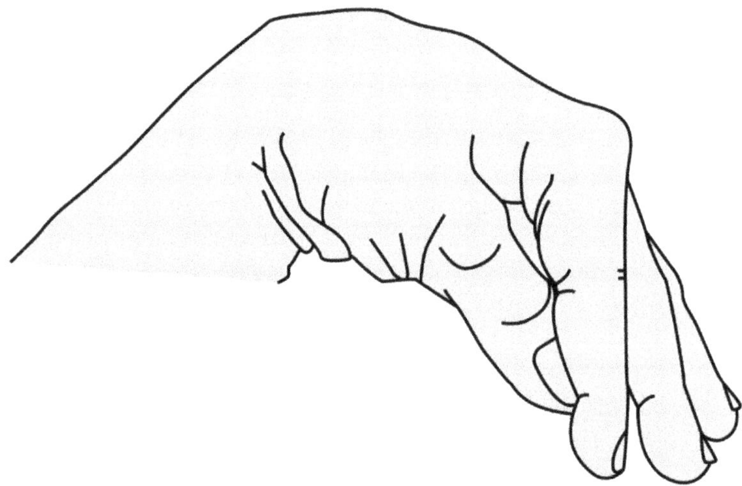

Figure 4.5 Trousseau's sign for hypocalaemic tetany.

may be hypoactive or hyperactive, may be exhibited when imbalances in electrolytes are suspected. Deep tendon reflexes may be altered with some electrolyte disturbances but should be evaluated, considering other clinical signs and laboratory data, such as sensation, neurological status and fatigue level.

The patient may also be complaining of thirst or nausea. They may have absent or reduced bowel sounds as, for example, in hypokalaemia, or may experience diarrhoea. Thirst can be affected by fluid volume and electrolyte changes, such as hypernatraemia, hypercalcaemia and hyperglycaemia. However, patients with altered levels of consciousness, who are debilitated or who have altered mental status, may not be able to respond to thirst.

Exposure and investigations

Oedema formation may be localised, often as a result of inflammation (e.g., thrombophlebitis), or generalised (as a result of water or salt retention), so the nurse may need to examine the whole body. Dependent oedema is when fluid accumulates mostly in the lower extremities (or in the sacral region when the patient is lying down), whereas generalised oedema is spread throughout the body and may accumulate in periorbital and scrotal regions because of the relatively lower tissue hydrostatic pressure in these areas of the body. Pitting oedema can be evaluated by pressing a fingertip into the skin over a bony surface (normally the lower leg or ankle) for a few seconds. Commonly, the amount of pitting oedema is assessed using plus signs although it is a subjective process. A slight imprint can be charted as +1 while a deep, persistent imprint, with the skin slow to return to its original contour, may be documented as +4.

Skin turgor can be assessed by gently pinching the skin over the forearm, sternum or dorsum of the hand (see Figure 4.6). If the patient is adequately hydrated, the skin will return to its original position when released. Skin turgor can also be tested over the clavicle; in patients with hypovolaemia, the pinched skin may remain elevated for several seconds. However, an older patient's skin may have lost elasticity, so this can be an unreliable measure of dehydration.

A dry mouth and flushed dry skin may also signal dehydration. The tongue may have increased **furrowing** if the patient is dehydrated. Hypernatraemia may cause the tongue to become red and swollen. As the tongue turgor is not affected by age, it is considered to be a more reliable physical sign of dehydration than skin turgor.

Acute weight changes may also be indicative of acute fluid imbalances. Each kilogram lost or gained suggests one litre of fluid lost or gained. The weight gain may be as a result of an increase in total body water, which could be in any of the compartments. Ideally, the patient should be weighed daily at the same time in the morning before breakfast using the same scales, wearing similar clothes and after voiding.

Urine is usually straw coloured, but, if the patient is dehydrated, the volume of urine will be reduced, and it will darken in colour. However, there are a number of factors which can alter urinary volume, including fluid intake, blood volume, renal concentrating ability and insensible loss. Some drugs, for example, tuberculosis medication, can alter the colour of urine. In cases of hypervolaemia, the urine will become pale and dilute as the kidneys excrete water to normalise the fluid balance. The patient's urine may be assessed for specific gravity, glucose and protein, and serum blood glucose may also be assessed, if hyperglycaemia is suspected.

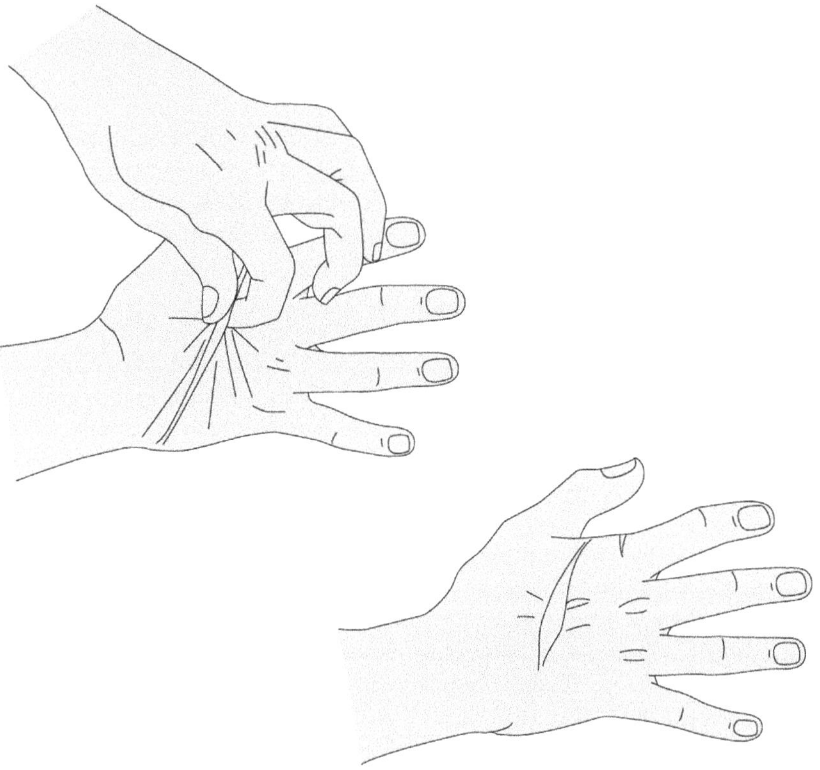

Figure 4.6 Skin with decreased turgor remains elevated after being gently pinched and released.

CASE STUDY 4.1 JYOTI, A PATIENT WITH ELECTROLYTE IMBALANCE: PART 1

SITUATION AND BACKGROUND

Jyoti is an 89-year-old lady admitted onto the acute medical ward yesterday with pneumonia and dehydration; she is being treated with intravenous (IV) antibiotics. Jyoti lives alone, with regular support from her family; she is fully independent. Jyoti admits that she often drinks very little to avoid having to visit the toilet frequently. Jyoti has developed diarrhoea, presumably secondary to her antibiotic treatment, which is a common side effect. Jyoti has been given 3 litres of 5% dextrose in the past 24 hours, to treat dehydration. Since admission, Jyoti has been drinking adequate volumes of oral fluid. Jerome, the health care assistant, alerts the nurse that Jyoti seems confused as he brings her a cup of tea. The nurse goes promptly to assess Jyoti.

Hello, Jyoti, I am the nurse looking after you and I would like to carry out an assessment; is that OK with you? Jyoti consents, therefore, the nurse washes their hands and puts on an apron.

ABCDE ASSESSMENT

Airway: Jyoti is speaking in full sentences, with no additional airway noses. Her lips are pink in colour, with no evidence of cyanosis. The nurse asks if she can cough, and Jyoti demonstrates good airway protection with a strong cough. Therefore, the nurse moves on to assess breathing.

Breathing: On initial observation Jyoti is not using her accessory muscles. Her RR is 21 per minute, and current oxygen saturations are 93%. The nurse checks her drug chart, and oxygen saturations of 94–98% are prescribed. The need for O_2 therapy is explained, and 2L O_2 *via* nasal specs is given as per the BTS guidance (O'Driscoll et al. 2017). Her SpO_2 is now within the target range at 96% and RR reduces to 20. Jyoti reports no secretions on coughing. Bilateral chest rise is identified through palpation, and the trachea is midline.

Breathing NEWS: (2+2+0) = 4
Breathing NEWS: (0+0+2) = 2 (with supplemental oxygen)

Circulation: Jyoti is slightly pale, she feels slightly cool on all limb extremities, and Jyoti reports that she normally has cold hands and feet. Her capillary refill is <3 seconds. There is no evidence of peripheral oedema. Jyoti's pulse on palpitation feels regular, strong and with a rate of 89bpm. Her blood pressure is 138/86mmHg, she has known hypertension, managed with amlodipine 5mg. Her neck veins do not appear distended. Skin turgor is not an accurate assessment measure as Jyoti's skin has decreased elasticity due to her age. Jyoti has had 2 episodes of loose, watery, type 7 stools since this morning as per the bowel chart, but the amount was not recorded. Her mouth appears dry, she reports having passed urine, but unsure as to how much. There is currently no fluid balance chart in place.

Circulation NEWS: (0+0) =0

Disability: Using the ACVPU tool from NEWS, the nurse records Jyoti as being alert. Jyoti, however, is not completely orientated to person, place and time. She keeps forgetting she is in hospital, but recognises the nurse caring for her. She is assessed as having a new confusion; there is no record of previously existing confusion, so this is recorded as C on the ACVPU assessment. Her blood glucose is 6.1mmol/L and she is eating regularly. Her pupils are equal and reactive to light, size 4mm bilaterally. Jyoti is complaining of a mild headache and aching legs.

Disability NEWS: (3+0) =3

Exposure: The nurse assesses her skin for any cuts, wounds, pressure sores, bruises, or rashes. There is no evidence of any abnormalities. Jyoti has a cannula in her left forearm and the VIP score is 0. Her temperature is 36.4°C.

Exposure NEWS: =0

NEWS Score

On the NEWS chart, Jyoti is scoring a 5 with her oxygen therapy, and this warrants review, with the possibility of sepsis being considered. The outreach team is called to escalate care for this patient, using the SBAR format. The outreach nurse reports that they will be there in the next 30 minutes to review the patient. As per NEWS guidance, the medical team providing care for the patient is contacted, and the doctor reports that they will also be on the ward in the next 30 minutes to review the patient. While waiting for the review, blood samples are taken, as per the doctor's recommendation, to assess for electrolyte derangement. This includes a full blood count, urea and electrolytes, liver function tests and a venous blood gas, including lactate.

Maximising fluid and electrolyte balance

The events which lead to fluid volume disturbances often also lead to electrolyte problems. The nurse needs to be alert to the risk of medical care itself precipitating disturbances in fluid or electrolyte balance, particularly in frail elderly or critically ill patents. Therefore, the nurse has an important clinical and professional role to play in the assessment, management and treatment, and for monitoring effectiveness. In most situations, the underlying problems must be resolved, in addition to correcting the fluid or electrolyte imbalance. Fluid, sodium and potassium imbalances are particularly common metabolic abnormalities, caused by a wide variety of conditions, but, if left untreated, they can rapidly become life threatening.

Fluid balance charts are an important part of hydration monitoring. The nurse completing the chart should be aware of the target fluid balance and patient-specific parameters, and report any issues to members of the multi-disciplinary team. However, fluid balance charts are often poorly maintained and inaccurate. This may be due to lack of training or time or poor handover between shifts of staff.

Nurses have a professional responsibility to ensure that their patients have an accurate and adequate fluid balance recorded, when necessary (NMC 2018). The NMC (2018) updated code of conduct emphasises the importance of the personal accountability of the registered nurse in ensuring complete and accurate documentation, and suggests that good record keeping helps to identify risk and to achieve early detection of complications. The RCN (2020) identify key themes related to food, nutrition and hydration care. They identify situations where IV fluids have been prescribed but not given, and where a lack of adequate hydration contributes to formation of deep vein thrombosis. For further information, see https://www.rcn.org.uk/clinical-topics/nutrition-and-hydration/principles-of-nursing-practice/patient-safety. Assessing fluid status, monitoring and keeping accurate records, and implementing strategies to meet fluid requirements are fundamental to safe and effective care.

Maximising fluid status

Hypovolaemia

The type of fluid replacement depends on the type of fluid lost and the severity of the deficit. Acid-base status, serum electrolyte levels and serum osmolality must be taken into consideration.

Table 4.9 Indicators of the need for fluid resuscitation (NICE 2013)

- Systolic BP <100mmHg.
- Heart rate >90 beats per minute.
- Capillary refill >2 seconds or peripheries cold to touch.
- Respiratory rate >20 breaths per minute.
- NEWS ≥ 5.
- 45° passive leg raise suggests fluid responsiveness.

If oral replacement is not enough or if the situation is severe, intravenous therapy solutions are used to replace and restore the circulating blood volume. As the body needs more than water for maintenance, electrolytes are also required. The fluids should be administered at a rate rapid enough and in sufficient quantity to maintain adequate tissue perfusion, taking the patient's cardiac and renal functions into consideration. The patient might require a fluid challenge, when specific volumes are administered at a specific rate and intervals, while monitoring the patient's haemodynamic status and response to ensure that there is an adequate renal result.

NICE (2013, updated 2017) published guidance on intravenous fluid therapy in adults in hospital. Initially, the patient is assessed using the ABCDE approach, considering the patient trends and context. This will enable the nurse to assess if the patient is hypovolaemic and needs fluid resuscitation (see Table 4.9).

Once satisfied that the patient requires fluid resuscitation, treatment must be initiated by identifying the cause of the fluid deficit and responding appropriately.

Once the need for fluid resuscitation has been identified, the following steps should be initiated:

1. Give a fluid bolus of 500mL of crystalloid (containing sodium in the range 130–154mmol/L) over less than 15 minutes.
2. Reassess the patient, using the ABCDE approach.
3. If the patient still requires fluid resuscitation and has currently been given <2000mL of fluid, then another 250–500mL of crystalloid should be given and the patient reassessed. *If 2000mL has already been given*, expert advice needs to be sought.

Intravenous solutions are classified as crystalloids and colloids. Crystalloids are electrolyte solutions and can be described as hypotonic, isotonic or hypertonic, depending on their contents, such as their osmolality. Colloids are colloidal solutions of high molecular weight molecules, such as albumin or dextran, that remain in the circulation as the molecules are too large to cross the plasma membrane. The Surviving Sepsis Campaign (2016) recommends crystalloids as the fluid of choice for initial resuscitation and subsequent intravascular volume replacement in patients with sepsis or septic shock (Rhodes et al. 2017). A recent Cochrane review (Lewis et al. 2018), looking at colloids versus crystalloids for fluid resuscitation in critically ill people, found that using colloids, compared with fluid replacement, probably makes little or no difference to the number of critically ill adults who die. However, evidence is needed from on-going studies to increase confidence in these findings (Lewis et al. 2018).

CRYSTALLOIDS

Water and electrolyte solutions may be given to hydrate, correct electrolyte disturbances, or to expand the intracellular and intravascular volume.

Hypotonic solutions, e.g., 0.45% sodium chloride or 0.18% sodium chloride, provide a basic fluid for maintenance needs, with a small amount of sodium chloride, and are suitable for patients who are hypovolaemic with hypernatraemia. However, care must be taken as excessive use may cause a shift of water into the hypertonic intracellular space, to balance the osmolality of the compartments.

Isotonic fluids, such as 0.9% sodium chloride ('normal saline'), 5% dextrose, Hartmann's, Ringer's lactate or Plamsa-Lyte, remain in the intravascular space and help expand the plasma volume when infused, making the solution suitable for restoring fluid volume. However, owing to the amount of chloride and sodium content, caution should be exercised if the patient has hypernatraemia or renal failure.

Hypertonic solutions, such as 3% sodium chloride or 10% dextrose, are used to treat severe deficits in serum sodium or dextrose. Small volumes must be infused slowly and usually in a clinical area, where the patient is closely monitored, because of the osmotic 'pull' of the solution, which can lead to a shift of fluid into the intravascular space, causing fluid overload.

COLLOIDS

Colloids can be used to increase the osmotic pressure of plasma and increase blood volume. They may be used to help pull fluid from the interstitial to the intravascular space, e.g., in oedematous hypovolaemic patients and/or those with third space fluid shifts.

Colloid solutions, e.g., gelofusine and albumin, contain substances of high molecular weight which do not readily migrate across the capillary walls. They increase the osmotic pressure of the plasma and pull fluid from the other compartments into the intravascular space to increase the volume, and are indicated when there is depletion of circulating plasma proteins or if there has been a movement or loss of fluid into the interstitial space, e.g., in response to septic shock, anaphylaxis or extensive burns.

Hypervolaemia

Reversal of the primary problem is the initial goal of treatment. Administraion of diuretics is typical treatment as well as restiction of sodium and fluids (note, the patient should be monitored for hypokalaemia, if loop diuretics are prescribed). Close monitoring is required as respiratory and circulatory compromise is possible. Renal dialysis may be required if the underlying cause is renal failure.

Maximising sodium balance

Sodium imbalances can cause significant neurological complications. The patient should be nursed in an observable area and a safe environment must be maintained. The person may be confused, agitated, at risk of seizures, or even coma or death.

Hyponatraemia

Treatment depends on fluid volume status and the severity of the condition. In situations of mild hyponatraemia, with hypervolaemia or isovolaemia, water intake is usually restricted to allow the sodium and water to balance naturally. If the patient is hyponatraemic, they may require isotonic IV fluids, e.g., normal saline. Hypertonic saline 1.8% (NICE 2019) or 3% (Spasovski et al. 2014) may be administered but with extreme caution, because this 'pulls' water from the intracellular to the intravascular compartment, owing to the osmotic pull of this highly concentrated solution, and this causes cell shrinkage. In these situations, patients may be moved to high-dependency or intensive care environments. If the shift of water happens too quickly, it can cause the brain cells to contract, with bleeding from damaged blood vessels, and cause the intravascular volume to be overloaded, leading to heart failure. As the patient can develop neurological changes, they must be nursed in an observable position to reduce risk and for any signs of deterioration to be identified and reported immediately.

Hypernatraemia

Sometimes, an inappropriate treatment itself may cause serious consequences – for example, over-rapid rehydration risks cerebral oedema. Therefore, management will depend on the cause and the speed of onset. If it has developed quickly over a few hours, the patient may be given 5% dextrose and this may be given quickly because, in these situations, rapid correction improves prognosis without the risk of cerebral oedema. If it is of longer or unknown duration, the patient may be prescribed hypotonic saline and hypotonic oral fluids. This will need to be administered with caution, as there is a risk of fluid movement to the intracellular space as the body tries to normalise fluid balance. Where there is concurrent renal failure, haemodialysis or filtration may be required.

DIAGNOSIS

The outreach nurse and doctor arrive on the ward to review the patient together; at this stage, the venous blood gas results are available. Jyoti's sodium level has dropped from 135mmol/L yesterday to 125mmol/L today. She is diagnosed with acute-onset moderate hyponatraemia, most likely to have been caused by excessive intravenous administration of 5% dextrose (i.e., water overload), and sodium loss through diarrhoea. She is normovolaemic, as her heart rate and blood pressure are stable, although her confusion is consistent with acute onset of hyponatraemia. Jyoti is in danger of further neurological deterioration and even permanent neurological injury if her sodium levels drop further as cerebral oedema, caused by the shift of water from the extracellular to the intracellular compartment, may occur. The doctor suggests that Jyoti's headache may be due to movement of water into the cerebral cells and her leg pains are being caused by cramps due to the reduced sodium available for conduction of muscle and nerve tissue. All other electrolytes are within normal range, with no other abnormalities in the venous blood gas.

Intervention

Acute hyponatraemia can cause more symptoms than if the level drops slowly, and treatment will usually be based on the presence or absence of symptoms, the rate of onset and the person's volume status. The goal of treatment is to identify the underlying pathology, correct the acute symptoms and gradually return Jyoti's sodium to a normal level. As Jyoti appears to have a normal extracellular fluid volume, but a fluctuation of neurological status, the doctor orders:

- Jyoti's intravenous 5% dextrose to be stopped immediately.
- Fluid intake to be restricted to 500mL for the next 24 hours.
- Consider IV 1.8 % sodium chloride (NICE 2019) if symptoms/serum sodium do not improve.

The doctor considers the treatment option of administration of hypertonic (1.8% or 3%) sodium chloride intravenously, but this must be administered with caution and ideally in a high-dependency or intensive care environment, and is the action to be taken with moderate to severe symptoms. Whereas the fall in sodium has occurred over 24 hours, stopping the 5% dextrose may prevent further hyponatraemia. The doctor decides to review Jyoti's serum sodium in six hours. If the fluid restriction does not increase her serum sodium levels, or if her neurological symptoms have not improved or have deteriorated, hypertonic sodium chloride may be required.

The doctor is aware that the rate of correction of serum sodium concentration in hyponatraemia is still under debate. In Jyoti s case, a target is set of raising the serum sodium by not more than 10mmol/L per 24 hours, but she should be monitored closely. This is because a more rapid correction of serum sodium concentration may cause central pontine myelinolysis (or osmotic demyelination). This is a condition where the brain cells shrink owing to water moving too quickly out of the cerebral cells, causing irreversible brain damage (usually a few days after the serum sodium concentration is corrected).

The outreach nurse asks the nurse to move Jyoti's bed into a position from which she can be closely observed, with suction and artificial airway equipment available. She is at risk of seizures or a coma, if her hyponatraemia worsens. The nurse is asked to record half-hourly neurological observations and to immediately report any worsening in Jyoti's condition. A urinary catheter is inserted by the nurse and a fluid balance chart is begun. Jyoti is allowed sips of water and mouth care to keep her mouth comfortable. The nurse explains in detail why they must restrict her fluid intake. The nurse also communicates to the housekeeping staff and the health care assistant that Jyoti is now on fluid restriction, to ensure that it is maintained.

After the prescribed treatment, Jyoti's urine output has been 200mL over the past two hours and her serum sodium rises to 130mmol/L. Her neurological observations have not deteriorated, she seems more lucid, and her heart rate and blood pressure are within her normal limits. Should Jyoti's diarrhoea continue, isotonic 0.9% sodium chloride intravenously will be prescribed, to avoid intravascular depletion, i.e., dehydration.

The outreach nurse later reassesses Jyoti's serum sodium levels 6 hours after the prescribed therapy and her sodium level continues to rise to 132mmol/L. She is now oriented, bringing her **NEWS** to 2 (due to supplemental oxygen). She is no longer complaining of a headache. She has not had any more episodes of diarrhoea. The outreach nurse communicates this update to the medical team. This is an example of patient deterioration being recognised and treatment escalated appropriately, resulting in prompt and effective management.

Maximising potassium balance

Hypokalaemia

The management of hypokalaemia is usually by potassium replacement, with the urgency of replacement depending on the severity and any underlying problems. The amount of supplementation required depends on the severity of the imbalance. Potassium may be replaced orally or intravenously. Oral replacement is generally preferable to supplementation for mild or low-risk hypokalaemia.

National Patient Safety Agency (NPSA) potassium patient safety alert

Serious adverse effects, due to rapid intravenous potassium chloride (KCl) administered at high concentrations, occur world-wide and may be fatal. In 2002, the first safety alert from the NPSA was released in response to research from the UK and worldwide, which highlighted risks to patients from errors occurring during intravenous administration of potassium solutions (NPSA 2002).

As a result, all NHS trusts and primary care trusts have been required to store, prepare, check and prescribe intravenous potassium in accordance with specific NPSA guidelines to reduce potential harm to patients (NPSA 2002; NHS Improvement 2018).

Patients with severe hypokalaemia will require care in a hospital setting, to establish the cause, and intravenous replacement of potassium *via* an infusion. *Intravenous potassium should never be given as an undiluted solution or as a bolus dose* as a rapid rise in serum potassium causes fatal arrhythmias. Concentrated potassium solution (>20mmol/500mL) can cause extravasation (burning of the vein and surrounding tissues); if higher concentrations are required, it must be administered *via* a central line. Peripheral infusions should be adequately diluted in line with local guidelines (for example, see Table 4.10).

If the patient is taking potassium-non-sparing diuretics, supplements may be prescribed as a preventative measure.

Hyperkalaemia

Treatment will depend on the underlying cause and severity of the situation. Restriction of dietary potassium and/or discontinuation of medications or factors increasing the serum level may resolve the condition. In acute or emergency situations, intravenous administration of agents to antagonise the effects of hyperkalaemia or to shift the potassium into the cells or even dialysis may be required. Steps to be taken in the treatment of hyperkalaemia are shown in Table 4.11.

Table 4.10 Intravenous potassium administration

- Ready-mixed infusion solution should be used, where possible.
- Potassium ampoule containing K+ 20mmol in 10mL can be mixed thoroughly with 500mL sodium chloride 0.9% and given slowly over 2–3 hours, with specialist advice and ECG monitoring as required.
- For peripheral infusion, the concentration of potassium should not usually exceed **40mmol/L.**
- Make sure the peripheral line is patent before administration.
- Higher concentrations of potassium chloride may be given in Intensive Care (Level 2 and Level 3 care, using a central line and continuous cardiac monitoring).
- Monitor IV site closely for signs of local irritation and infiltration.
- Monitor serum potassium every 1–3 hours and monitor for signs of toxic reaction, e.g., paralysis or weakness.
- Monitor urine output and report if less than 0.5mL/kg/hour.
- Potassium can layer in the solution, so it is important that you avoid adding to hanging containers and remember to mix additions thoroughly. Premixed solutions are used where possible; if necessary; to add, invert the container before and after adding the potassium and mix well.

Sources: NPSA (2002); Nakatani et al. (2019); NICE (2019).

Table 4.11 Five key steps in the treatment of hyperkalaemia *(UK Renal Association 2014)*

Step 1: Protect the heart

- Administer IV calcium chloride (10mL10%) or IV calcium gluconate (10mL 10%).

Step 2: Shift K+ into cells

- Administer IV injection of soluble insulin (5–10units) with 50mL glucose 50% given over 5–15minutes; repeat if necessary. An additional option is salbutamol by nebulisation, which may also reduce plasma potassium concentration; caution for patients with cardiovascular disease.

Step 3: Remove K^+ from body

- Although in some clinical scenarios diuretics or intravenous fluids are used in the treatment of hyperkalaemia associated with acute kidney injury, there is no evidence to support this practice.

Step 4: Monitor K^+ and glucose

- Re-check and re-treat if necessary, to ensure blood glucose level >4mmol/L.

Step 5: Prevent recurrence

- Eliminate contributing factors.

The threshold for emergency treatment varies, but most guidelines recommend that emergency treatment should be given if the serum K^+ is $\geq$ 6.5mmol/L, with or without ECG changes. It is also important to note that hyperkalaemia treatment should be initiated if the condition is suspected on the grounds of ECG changes alone (UK Renal Association 2014). Further accumulation should be prevented by immediately stopping treatment with potentially contraindicative medication (e.g., spironolactone, ACE inhibitors).

Calcium imbalances

As with sodium and potassium imbalances, treatment of calcium imbalances depends on the duration, the severity of the imbalance, and the underlying conditions. In acute hypocalcaemia, the symptomatic or high-risk patient should be treated with intravenous calcium gluconate as well as oral calcium preparations. Vitamin D tablets may also be prescribed if the patient is hypovolaemic. If the hypocalcaemia is persistent, the patient may be prescribed oral calcium replacement as well as vitamin D tablets, but, once the serum calcium has stabilised, the calcium supplement may be discontinued.

Hypercalcaemia usually requires the patient to be nursed in hospital under specialist advice. A patient with chronic hypercalcaemia is prone to pathological fractures and may need assistance to reposition, if bedridden. The patient may require intravenous fluids to increase the urinary output of calcium as well as the administration of drugs to inhibit bone reabsorption. Haemodialysis may be required if the condition is secondary to renal failure. Surgery to remove part of the parathyroid gland may also be considered.

Conclusion

Maximising fluid and electrolyte balance is a crucial aspect of nursing knowledge and practice. Nurses should have a thorough understanding of the normal mechanisms which control fluid and electrolyte balance, in order to be able to perform a comprehensive assessment of a patient's fluid and electrolyte status, to identify patients at risk of deterioration and to monitor patients appropriately to prevent further complications. Nurses also have a professional requirement to maintain accurate fluid balance records. Nurses need to be proactive in identifying those at risk, to request/review blood results, containing essential information regarding electrolyte status, and be part of the team that formulate plans to resolve fluid and/or electrolyte imbalances.

Glossary 

Amino acid The building blocks of proteins.
Capillary The smallest of the body's blood vessels.
Delirium Acute brain dysfunction; may present as confusion.
Diuretic A drug that elevates the rate of urine production.
Effusion Excess accumulation of fluid in a space.
Enzyme Proteins causing biochemical reactions.
Fistulae An abnormal connection or passageway between two epithelium-lined organs or vessels that do not usually connect.
Hypertension High blood pressure.
Hypotonic Has a low concentration of electrolytes (a lower osmotic pressure) compared with body cells and can cause cells to swell as a result of osmosis.
Ileostomy A surgical opening in the abdominal wall to allow the end of the ileum through to avoid the remainder of the digestive tract.
Ileum The final section of the small intestine.
Interstitial fluid Consists of interstitial water and its solutes, located outside the blood, lymphatic vessels and parenchymal cells.
Intracellular Inside the cell.
Ischaemia A restriction of blood supply.
Isotonic Solutions that contain the same electrolyte concentration as body cells.
Jejunum The middle aspect of the small intestine.
Neuropathy Damage to nerves.
Node Localised swelling.
Orthopnoea Shortness of breath when lying flat.
Pancreatitis Inflammation of the pancreas.

Paraesthesia An abnormal sensation on the skin i.e. burning, prickling, numbing.
Peritonitis Inflammation of the peritoneum.
Polyuria Condition characterised by the production of large volumes of urine.
Prostaglandins Substances that have hormone-like effects. They affect processes such as inflammation and blood flow by the dilation or constriction of blood vessels
Sepsis A life-threatening illness caused by the dysregulated response infection, resulting in organ dysfunction.
Solvent A liquid that dissolves a solute; an example is water.
Stridor A high-pitched wheezing sound heard on inspiration, caused by collapse/obstruction of the upper airway.
Stupor A reduced level of consciousness.
Tachycardic An elevated heart rate, >100bpm.
Tumour A lump or growth of tissue made up from abnormal cells.
Venule A small blood vessel in the microcirculation.

TEST YOURSELF

1 Which are the correct terms for the fluid compartments of the body?
   a. intracellular, intrastitial, extracellular
   b. intracellular, extracellular, extravascular
   c. intracellular, interstitial, intravascular
   d. intercellular, interstitial, intervascular
2 Hydrostatic pressure
   a. pushes fluid and solutes out of the capillaries
   b. has a pulling power of albumin to reabsorb water
   c. is the pressure generated on the vessel wall by blood flowing through the circulatory system
   d. does not change with blood pressure
3 Osmosis is the passive movement of solutes through a selectively permeable membrane from a region of high osmolality to low osmolality. True or false?
4 Which is not a common cause of hypovolaemia?
   a. haemorrhage
   b. vomiting and diarrhoea
   c. heart failure
   d. excessive diuretic therapy
5 One sign of hypervolaemia is:
   a. acute weight loss
   b. distended neck veins
   c. extreme thirst
   d. weak and thready pulse
6 Signs and symptoms of hyponatraemia include:
   a. flushed skin, thirst, restlessness
   b. abdominal cramping, dysrhythmias, muscle weakness
   c. skeletal muscle weakness, constipation, irregular and weak pulse
   d. changes in level of consciousness, muscle twitching, nausea and vomiting
7 Signs and symptoms of hypokalaemia include:
   a. skeletal muscle weakness, tachycardia, dysrhythmias

b. changes in level of consciousness, muscle twitching, nausea and vomiting
c. chest pain, shortness of breath, cough
d. tetany, anxiety, confusion

8 Blood pressure and pulse are sensitive measures for detecting hypovolaemia. True or false?
9 Intravenous potassium can cause vein irritation and extravasation if it leaks into the tissues. True or false?
10 Colloids are water and electrolyte solutions given to hydrate or correct electrolyte disturbances. True or false?

Answers

1 c
2 a
3 False
4 c
5 b
6 d
7 a
8 True
9 True
10 False

References

Beckett, G., Walker, S. W., Rae, P., Ashby, P. (2010). *Lectures Notes: Clinical Biochemistry*, 8th Edition. Oxford: Wiley-Blackwell.

Casey, G. (2004). Oedema: causes, physiology and nursing management. *Nursing Standard*, 18(51), 45–51.

Casey, G. (2019). 'Understanding diuretics', Kai Tiaki. *Nursing New Zealand*, 25(6), 20.

Crawford, A., Harris, H. (2012). SIADH: fluid out of balance. *Nursing*, 42, 50–58. doi:10.1097/01.NURSE.0000418617.99217.49.

Davies, N., English, W., Grundlingh, J. (2018). MDMA toxicity: management of acute and life-threatening presentations. *British Journal of Nursing*, 27(11), 616–622. doi:10.12968/bjon.2018.27.11.616.

Dineen, R., Thompson, C., Sherlock, M. (2017). Hyponatraemia-presentations and management. *Clinical Medicine*, 17(3), 263–269. Available from http://www.clinmed.rcpjournal.org/content/17/3/263.full.pdf+html.

Guidelines and Audit Implementation Network (GAIN). (2014). *Guidelines for the Treatment of Hyperkalaemia in Adults*. Available from file:///E:/Acute%20NC%202nd%20ed/ACN%202nd%20ed/Chapter%204/reading/Gain%202014%20hyperkalaemia.pdf.

Lewis, S. R., Pritchard, M. W., Evans, D. J. W., Butler, A. R., Alderson, P., Smith, A. F., Roberts, I. (2018). Colloids versus crystalloids for fluid resuscitation in critically ill people. *Cochrane Database of Systematic Reviews*. Edited by Cochrane Injuries Group. doi:10.1002/14651858.CD000567.pub7.

Limaye, C. S., Londhey, V. A., Nadkar, M. Y., Borges, N. E. (2011). Hypomagnesemia in critically ill medical patients. *Journal of the Association of Physicians of India*, 59, 19–22.

Marieb, E., Hoehn, K. (2019). *Human Anatomy and Physiology*. San Francisco, CA: Benjamin Cummings.

McCance, K. L., Huether, S. E. (2018). *Pathophysiology: The Biologic Basis for Disease in Adults and Children*, 8th Edition. Edinburgh: Elsevier.

McLafferty, E., Johnstone, C., Hendry, C., Farley, A. (2014). Fluid and electrolyte balance. *Nursing Standard*, 28(29), 42–49.

Meaden, C., Kushner, B., Barnes, S. (2018). Case report: a rare and lethal complication: cerebral oedema in the adult patient with diabetic ketoacidosis. *Hindawi Case Reports in Emergency Medicine*, 2018, Article ID 504375. doi:10.1155/2018/5043752.

Metheny, N. M. (2012). *Fluid and Electrolyte Balance: Nursing Considerations*, 5th Edition. London: Jones and Bartlett.

Nakatani, K., Nakagami-Yamaguchi, E., Shinoda, Y., Tomita, S., Nakatani, T. (2019). Improving the safety of high-concentration potassium injection. *BMJ Open Quality*. doi:10.1136/bmjoq-2019-000666.

Narvaez-Rojas, A.R., Mo-Carrascal, J., Maraby, J., Satyarthee, G.D., Hoz, S., Joaquim, A.F. Moscote-Salazar, L.R. (2018). Neurocritical care of intracranial brain tumour surgery: An overview. *Journal of Medical Sciences*, 4(1), 4–11.

National Institute for Health and Care Excellence. (2013). *Intravenous Fluid Therapy in Adults in Hospital*, cg 174. Available from https://www.nice.org.uk/guidance/cg174/.

NHS Improvement. (2018). *Recommendations for National Patient Safety Agency Alerts that Remain Relevant to the Never Events List 2018*. Available from https://improvement.nhs.uk/documents/2267/Recommendations_from_NPSA_alerts_that_remain_relevant_to_NEs_FINAL.pdf.

NICE. (2019). *Potassium Chloride*. Available from https://bnf.nice.org.uk/drug/potassium-chloride.html.

NMC (Nursing and Midwifery Council). (2018). *The Code: Professional Standards of Practice and Behaviour for Nurses and Midwives and Nursing Associates*. London: NMC. Available from https://www.nmc.org.uk/globalassets/sitedocuments/nmc-publications/nmc-code.pdf.

Norris, T. (2018). *Porth's Pathophysiology: Concepts of Altered Health States*, 10th Edition. Philadelphia, PA: Wolters Kluwer.

NPSA (National Patient Safety Agency). (2002). *Potassium Chloride Concentrate Solution – Patient Safety Alert 01*. London: National Patient Safety Agency Safety.

NPSA (National Patient Safety Agency). (2007). *Safer Care for the Acutely Ill Patients: Learning from Incidents*. London: NPSA.

O'Driscoll, R., Howard, L., Earis, J., Mak, V., Bajwah, S., Beasley, R., Curtis, K., Davison, A., Dorward, A., Dyer, C., Evans, A., Falconer, L., Fitzpatrick, C., Gibbs, S., Hinshaw, K., Howard, R., Kane, B., Keep, J., Kelly, C., Khachi, H., Asad, M., Khan, I., Kishen, R., Mansfield, L., Martin, B., Moore, F., Powrie, D., Restrick, L., Roffe, C., Singer, M., Soar, J., Small, I., Ward, L., Whitmore, D., Wedzicha, W., Wijesinghe, M., BTS Emergency Oxygen Guideline Development Group On behalf of the British Thoracic Society. (2017). BTS guideline for oxygen use in adults in healthcare an emergency settings. *Thorax*, 72(S1), i1–i20.

Rhodes, A., et al. (2017). Surviving sepsis campaign: international guidelines for management of sepsis and septic shock. *Critical Care Medicine*, 45(3), 486–552. doi:10.1097/CCM.0000000000002255.

Royal College of Nursing (RCN). (2020). *Nutrition and Hydration*. Available at: https://www.rcn.org.uk/clinical-topics/nutrition-and-hydration/principles-of-nursing-practice/patient-safety.

Royal College of Physicians. (2017). *National Early Warning Score (NEWS) 2 Standardising the Assessment of Acute-Illness Severity in the NHS*. Available from http://www.rcplondon.ac.uk/resources/national-early-warning-score-news. Accessed on 14 January 2019.

Spasovski, G., VanHolder, R., Allolio, B., Annane, D., Ball, S., Bichet, D., Decaux, G., Fenske, W., Hoorn, W., Ichai, C., Joannidis, M., Soupsrt, A., Zietse, R., Haller, M., van der Veer, S., Van Bieden, W., Nagler, E., On behalf of the Hyponatraemia Guideline Development Group. (2014). Clinical practice guideline on diagnosis and treatment of hyponatraemia. *European Journal of Endocrinology*, 170(3), G1–G7. Available from https://academic.oup.com/ndt/article/29/suppl_2/i1/1904943.

UK Renal Association. (2014). *Clinical Practice Guidelines. Treatment of Acute Hyperkalaemia in Adults*. Available from https://renal.org/wp-content/uploads/2017/06/hyperkalaemia-guideline-1.pdf.

Williams, B., et al. (2018). 2018 ESC/ESH guidelines for the management of arterial hypertension. *European Heart Journal*, 39(33), 3021–3104. doi:10.1093/eurheartj/ehy339.

5 The patient with acute respiratory problems

Anthony Wheeldon

AIM

The aim of this chapter is to support the reader to respond appropriately where the patient presents with an acute respiratory problem.

OBJECTIVES

- Describe the major structures of the respiratory system.
- Identify the determinants of external and internal respiration.
- Differentiate between oxygen delivery (DO_2) and oxygen consumption (VO_2).
- Describe the functions of the respiratory epithelium including neurohormonal control of the airways.
- Describe how acute respiratory problems may compromise respiratory status.
- Describe the nurse's role in undertaking a respiratory assessment and delivering care to maximise respiratory status.

Introduction

Patients who are acutely ill are in a stressed, hypermetabolic state whereby the body is attempting to cope with crisis and maintain homeostasis. This inevitably results in an increase in the amount of oxygen (O_2) required by the cells for aerobic metabolism. The nurse has a key role in ensuring that oxygenation is maximised, both at pulmonary and cellular level. Where patient assessment is underpinned with a sound knowledge of respiratory and cardiac physiology, then factors possibly compromising O_2 delivery (DO_2) can be detected early and prompt action taken to avoid further deterioration and a medical emergency.

Applied respiratory physiology

Internal respiration

ATP stores energy in the cell, and the aerobic production of ATP is very effective in extracting energy from food sources.

For effective cellar function, an adequate mitochondrial oxygen pressure is important, and **hypoxia** is a cause of cell injury and death. The oxidation of glucose is crucial if energy rich adenosine triphosphate (ATP) is to be released for effective cellular functioning. Although oxidation of glucose can take place in the cytoplasm of the cell (glycolysis), only 2 ATP molecules per glucose molecule are formed. Compare this with inside the mitochondria of the cell where, in the presence of O_2, one glucose molecule can liberate 38 molecules of ATP (a process called oxidative phosphorylation), thus facilitating aerobic metabolism.

The mitochondria can produce ATP without using O_2 (anaerobic metabolism), but this is less efficient, and whilst some cells can function relatively effectively (e.g., skeletal muscle) for short periods, this is not possible in some organs (e.g., brain and heart). Prolonged anaerobic metabolism will result in disruption to cellular function, increased waste products such as lactic acid and possibly irreversible cell damage and death. As a consequence of insufficient oxygen delivery to the cells (possibly due to ischaemia), cellular hypoxia will result in cellular injury, causing destruction of the cell membrane and cell structure.

Factors determining oxygen delivery (DO_2):

- External respiration in lungs (including effective Ventilation/Perfusion).
- Haemoglobin level.
- Cardiac output.
- Micro-circulation.

Oxygen delivery

Oxygen delivery to rapidly metabolising cells must be optimised if cellular demand (VO_2) is to be met. It is useful to think of the steps facilitating O_2 delivery as connecting links in a chain (see Figure 5.1). The first link is at the pulmonary level, where external respiration with gaseous exchange takes place. Additional links include the haemoglobin, which carry O_2 molecules, cardiac function, which must maintain the systemic circulation, and the integrity of the microcirculation, which must facilitate gaseous exchange at cellular level. If any link is weak, then O_2 delivery may well be reduced.

The lungs and chest wall

The lungs are situated in the thoracic cavity, with two lobes on the left and three lobes on the right (see Figure 5.2). The mediastinal cavity is found between the two lungs and accommodates the heart, great vessels, trachea, oesophagus nerves and lymph nodes. The

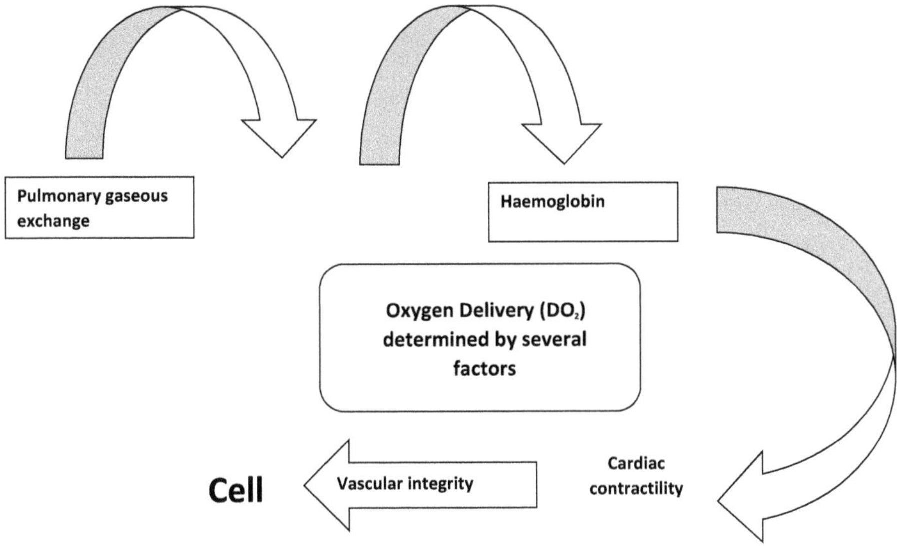

Figure 5.1 Determinants of oxygen delivery.

apices of the lungs extend just above the inner third of the clavicles, a fact that needs to be considered when a central line is being inserted! The bases of the lungs sit on the diaphragm. The anatomical and mechanical relationships of the lungs and chest wall facilitate effective ventilation. Each lung is surrounded by pleural membranes, with the inner membrane (visceral pleura) attached to the lung surface and the outer membrane (parietal pleura) attached to the chest wall (also diaphragm). In the resting state, there is inward recoil of the lungs (also visceral pleura) and outward movement of the chest wall (also parietal pleura). These two opposing forces on either side of the pleural membranes contribute to a negative pressure (less than **atmospheric pressure**) in the pleural cavity, which is important in keeping the lungs inflated. We will return to the significance of this later.

Pressure difference between alveoli and pleural cavity is important in keeping lungs inflated:

Pleural cavity pressure:
Negative (less than atmospheric)

Alveoli:
Positive (atmospheric pressure)

The respiratory tract

The upper respiratory tract (URT) from the nose to the upper trachea has a large surface area and blood supply and for breathing is important in warming, moistening and filtering the air during inspiration. This is by-passed, of course, in patients who have a **tracheostomy** or **endotracheal tube** in place. The lower respiratory tract, from the

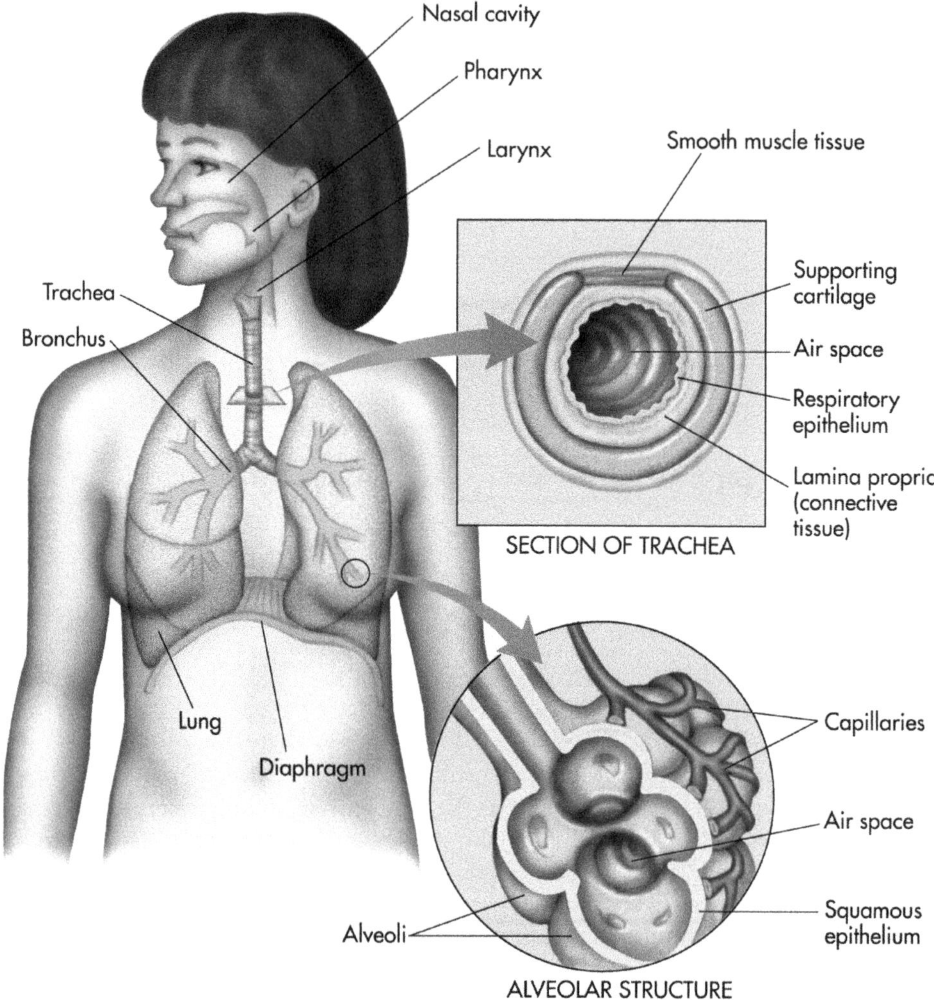

Figure 5.2 The respiratory system.

lower trachea to the respiratory bronchioles, has evolved to conduct air efficiently into the lungs for gaseous exchange during inspiration and to remove air from the lungs during expiration.

Respiratory defence mechanisms:

- Nasal hairs filter air.
- Cough/gag reflex.
- Lymphoid tissue.
- Mucociliary escalator.
- Immunoglobulin A (antibody).
- Alveoli macrophages.

The respiratory tract is described as a tree with different generations of branches (see Figure 5.3). The trachea is the trunk, referred to as generation zero. At the carina, the trachea divides into the right and left major bronchi, referred to as first generation branches. These, in turn, branch again, with each successive branch becoming smaller. The walls of the respiratory tree are made of cartilage to prevent collapse, smooth involuntary muscle and an inner lining of mucous membrane. At generation 16, the bronchi become terminal bronchioles and the cartilage disappears. From generation 16 onwards, the diameter of airways is approximately 1 millimetre. The walls of these bronchioles are made of simple ciliated epithelial cells, secretory Clara cells and smooth muscle. Because there are many of these bronchioles, the total resistance to flow is low, but because they are so small in diameter, the lumen can become further narrowed and obstructed by secretions and inflammation. Generations 20 and onwards of the respiratory tree are the even smaller respiratory bronchioles, which finally merge with the alveolar ducts and alveolar sacs. The respiratory bronchioles, together with the alveolar ducts and sacs, are the site for gaseous exchange.

Clara cells are specialised non epithelial cells in the airways and have both a protective and regenerative role

Functions of the respiratory epithelium

It was once thought that the respiratory epithelial cells simply acted as a barrier to protect the inner layers of the respiratory tree. The respiratory epithelium does indeed have a huge role to play in protection. For most sections of the respiratory tree, each epithelial cell has around 200 tiny hair-like projections called cilia. On top of the cilia sits a blanket of mucus, which is constantly moved upwards by the cilia, all beating in the same direction (1000 beats per minute). Any debris in the air is thus trapped and moved upwards by the muco-ciliary escalator to be expectorated or swallowed. The creation of mucus (up to 100mL each day) is extremely complex, but contributing are goblet cells, which secrete mucus, as well as submucosal glands found throughout the respiratory tract. Pathology, smoking, dehydration and dry gases (including O_2 therapy) can decrease the effectiveness of this protective mechanism. Additional defences include **Immunoglobulin** A (IgA), an antibody produced by B lymphocytes and secreted onto the respiratory surface, irritant receptors and the cough reflex, as well as lymphoid tissue and phagocytic **macrophage** cells in the alveolar wall.

Cytokines are regulatory protein molecules released by a range of cells including lymphocytes.

Examples:

- Interleukins.
- Interferon.
- Tumour necrosis factor.
- Growth factor.

Some cytokines are pro-inflammatory.

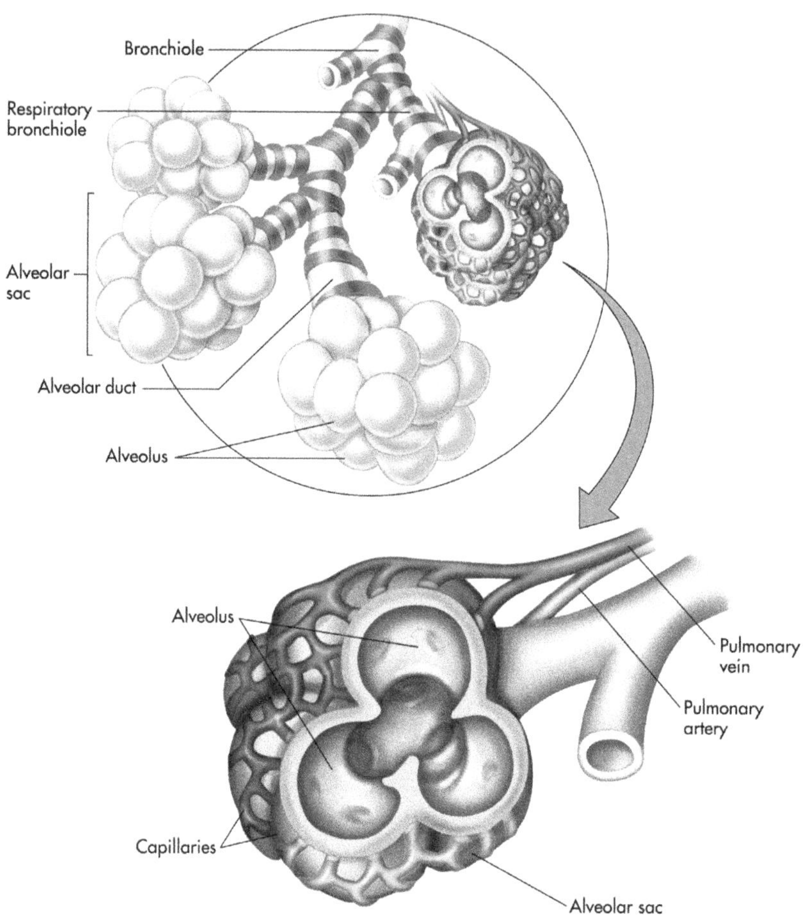

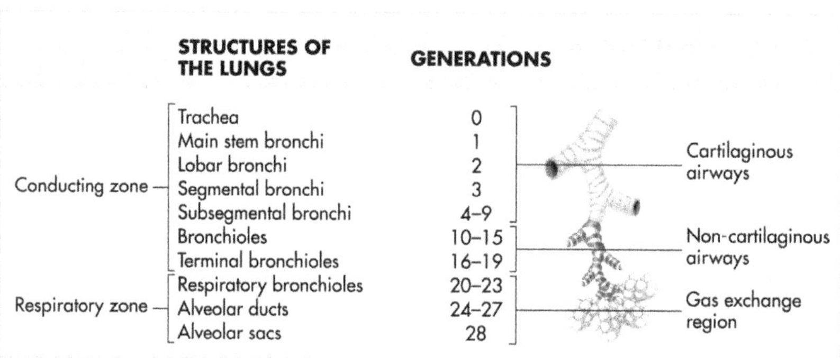

Zone	STRUCTURES OF THE LUNGS	GENERATIONS	
Conducting zone	Trachea	0	Cartilaginous airways
	Main stem bronchi	1	
	Lobar bronchi	2	
	Segmental bronchi	3	
	Subsegmental bronchi	4–9	
	Bronchioles	10–15	Non-cartilaginous airways
	Terminal bronchioles	16–19	
Respiratory zone	Respiratory bronchioles	20–23	Gas exchange region
	Alveolar ducts	24–27	
	Alveolar sacs	28	

Figure 5.3 Conduction and gas exchange structures and functions.

Respiratory epithelial cells are also metabolically active and can produce a range of different substances including nitric oxide and cytokines. Nitric oxide (NO) is a potent bronchodilator, but when produced in excessive amounts, can contribute to inflammation. NO is also released by endothelial cells of blood vessels and is a vasodilator. Cytokines (e.g., interleukins) released by many different cells enable communication between cells, and whilst most are important physiological regulators, some may result in inflammation in a number of respiratory diseases.

Neurohormonal control of the airways

Smooth muscle found in the lining of the respiratory tract enables the airway lumen to dilate and constrict. Each smooth muscle cell is supplied by branches of the **sympathetic** and **parasympathetic** nervous system. Parasympathetic nerves (also called **cholinergic** nerves) from the vagus nerve release acetylcholine and stimulate cholinergic receptors on the cell membrane, resulting in contraction (lumen becomes smaller). These nerves also supply glands and result in increased mucus secretion. Conversely, sympathetic nerves release noradrenaline (a neurotransmitter), which stimulates beta 2 receptors and results in relaxation of the muscle (the lumen dilates). The beta 2 receptors can also be stimulated by adrenaline (hormone) from the adrenal gland. Research has identified additional nerves in the respiratory system which result in bronchodilatation, but the neurotransmitter released is nitric oxide (NO). Although these nerves travel with the autonomic nerves, they are described as non-adrenergic and non-cholinergic (NANC).

Inflammatory cytokines and an increase in parasympathetic (cholinergic) activity narrow the airway lumen, thus increasing airway resistance.

Control of breathing

Fortunately, although breathing can be controlled voluntarily, it becomes automatic, and we do not need to think about it. In a rare congenital disorder (**Ondine's** curse) where autonomic control is lost, breathing then stops during sleep. Air must be replenished in the lungs on a cyclical basis and inspiration and expiration facilitates this. It is carbon dioxide in arterial blood which stimulates the **respiratory centre** in the brain stem, and so powerful is this, that most of us can only hold our breath for a short period of time. As carbon dioxide (CO_2) increases in the blood, it diffuses into the cerebrospinal fluid in the brain and hydrates with water to form weak **carbonic acid**. In turn, this then dissociates into hydrogen and bicarbonate ions, as can be seen in the following chemical equation, which is reversible:

$$\mathbf{CO_2 + H_2O \leftrightarrow H_2CO_3 \leftrightarrow H^+ + HCO_3}$$

$$(\text{carbon dioxide} + \text{water} \leftrightarrow \text{carbonic acid} \leftrightarrow \text{hydrogen} + \text{bicarbonate})$$

In fact, it is the liberated hydrogen (H^+) ions which stimulate special central chemoreceptors in the brain stem as a result of increased CO_2 levels. As a result of being stimulated, nerve impulses in the **medulla oblongata** are generated and pass down the intercostal and phrenic nerves to the respiratory muscles. Peripheral chemoreceptors found in the carotid artery and aortic arch can also stimulate the respiratory centre, but are sensitive to falling O_2 levels (hypoxaemia). As a result of contraction, the external intercostal muscles raise the rib cage upwards and the diaphragm contracts, descending and pushing the abdominal contents out the way. This increases the dimensions of the thoracic cavity, and as gas pressure is inversely proportional to volume, air is drawn into the lungs from the atmosphere.

Muscles used during inspiration in health:

- Diaphragm.
- External intercostals.

Expiration does not require muscle contraction in health.

In quiet inspiration, it is mainly the diaphragm followed by external intercostals which are used. Expiration in healthy individuals is passive and simply involves muscle relaxation and no energy is needed. Energy expenditure for breathing accounts for only 3% of the body's O_2 consumption. This can increase dramatically in breathless patients where the use of accessory muscles for both inspiration and expiration can demand 30% of O_2 consumption.

Lung volumes

Alveolar Ventilation or Volume (AV):

AV = (TV – DS) × RR

At rest:
AV = (500 – 150) × 12 = 4 litres

DS = Anatomical dead space
(Approximately 2mL per kg body weight)

Pulmonary or Minute Volume (MV):

MV = TV × RR

At rest:
MV = 500 × 12 = 6 litres

TV = tidal volume
RR = respiratory rate

At rest, an adult takes in around 500 millilitres of air per breath, and this is called tidal volume. Multiplying the tidal volume with the breathing rate per minute provides the ventilatory volume, referred to as pulmonary or minute volume, and, with a ventilatory rate of 12 breaths per minute, is 6 litres. Increasing tidal volume and rate, as, for example, during exercise, can increase the minute volume to 70 litres per minute. However, of the tidal volume, only 350mL reaches the respiratory bronchioles (generation 17–23) where gaseous exchange takes place. If 350mL is now multiplied by 12 breaths per minute, this is referred to as alveolar volume (ventilation), which in adults is around 4.2 litres. The last portion of the tidal volume (150mL) remains in the larger airways (generations 0–16) and this is called the **anatomical dead space**.

Given that it is alveolar volume that is available for gaseous exchange, this has real significance in clinical practice. There are a number of situations where patients may have reduced tidal volumes, e.g., pain and some respiratory disorders. With anatomical dead space fixed, there is always 150mL of the tidal volume unavailable for gaseous exchange. In this situation, the dead space becomes a larger proportion of the total tidal volume. The body may attempt to maintain effective alveolar volumes by breathing at higher ventilatory rates. However, if this continues for long periods, the patient will utilise a great deal of energy for breathing, and the respiratory muscles may fatigue very quickly.

Types of pneumothorax:

- Primary spontaneous.
- Secondary spontaneous.
- Traumatic.
- Iatrogenic.
- Tension.

Another important lung volume is the **functional residual capacity** (FRC). This is the volume of air in the lungs at the end of expiration and consists of expiratory reserve volume (ERV) and residual volume (RV) (see Figure 5.4). An important aim in clinical practice, particularly where pulmonary status is compromised, is to maintain FRC so that alveolar volume does not fall further. Poor positioning, where patients are nursed flat or not well supported with pillows, can reduce FRC by up to 30% and may precipitate closure of alveoli (**atelectasis**), resulting in reduced oxygenation.

Poor positioning, particularly in older people, will reduce the functional residual capacity and increase the risk of alveoli closure. Where possible position:

- Sitting upright.
- High side lying.
- Sitting in chair.

Fortunately, for most people with good lung function, breathing takes very little effort. Nevertheless, breathing involves work, as muscles must contract to move the lungs and chest wall out (compliance work) as well as move air through the airways (resistance work). Where there are respiratory problems which make the lungs stiffer (e.g., pneumonia/pneumothorax), then compliance is reduced, and the patient becomes conscious of the increased effort needed to move the chest wall and lungs during inspiration. Similarly, where the lumen of the airways is narrowed, then resistance is increased, and once again,

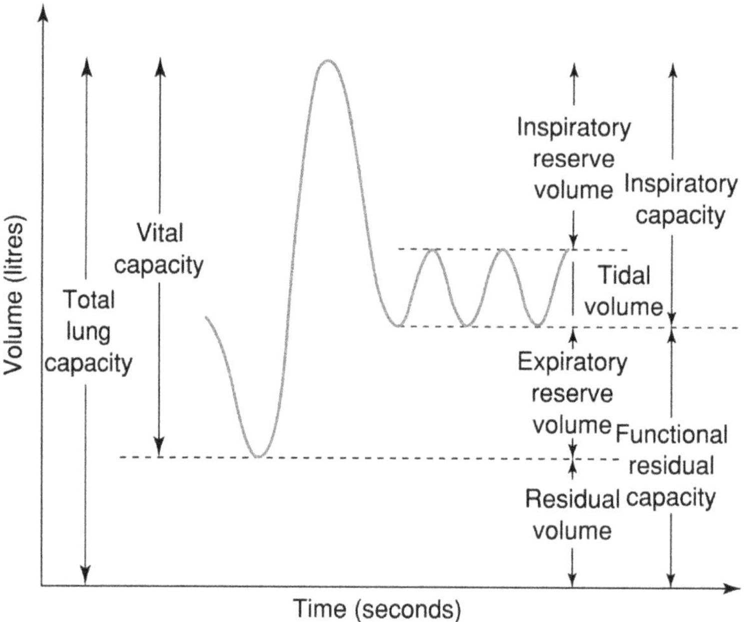

Figure 5.4 Lung volumes.

there is much greater effort required to move air through the airways (e.g., asthma). Try breathing through a drinking straw! Where there is increased work of breathing, then the cause should be established with management aimed at increasing compliance where possible, reducing **airway resistance** – or both.

Lung/chest wall compliance decreased in:

- Pneumonia.
- Atelectasis.
- Pneumothorax.
- Pulmonary fibrosis.
- Pulmonary oedema.
- Chest wall disease.

(Increased, however, in emphysema, where elastic recoil is reduced resulting in air trapping).

Airway resistance increased in:

- Bronchial asthma.
- Chronic obstructive pulmonary disease (COPD).

Gaseous exchange

Composition of atmospheric air:

- Oxygen (20.98%).
- Carbon dioxide (0.04%).
- Nitrogen (76%).
- Other rare gases.

Following inspiration, air is available in the respiratory bronchioles, alveolar ducts and sacs for gaseous exchange (alveolar volume), and there is a huge surface area available for this. Atmospheric air comprises a number of gases, each of which exerts a pressure independent of the others (i.e. each gas has its own partial pressure). Combining the partial pressures of all the gases present gives the atmospheric or barometric pressure, which at sea level is 101kPa (at higher altitudes, pressures decrease). The proportion of O_2 in the air is around 21%, and its partial pressure is approximately 21kPa. However, in alveolar air, the proportion of O_2 is only 14%, and because water vapour also exerts a partial pressure (6kPa), the partial pressure of alveolar O_2 is lower, at 13.5kPa.

Alveolar surfactant:

- Increases compliance.
- Reduces work of breathing.
- Reduces surface tension and prevents alveoli collapse.
- Helps to keep the alveoli 'dry'.

Alveoli are supplied with a vast network of **pulmonary capillaries,** with each alveolus having a single capillary so that alveolar air and pulmonary capillary blood is in close contact. The alveolar wall is extremely thin, and is made up of pneumocyte cells and macrophage cells. Type I pneumocytes are flat squamous cells, whilst type II are larger cells that release **surfactant**. The alveolar lining consists of an interface of water and gas molecules, which increases the surface tension of each alveolus, creating instability and potential alveolar collapse. Surfactant is a detergent-like substance that reduces this surface tension, thereby increasing compliance and reducing the work of breathing.

Pulmonary capillary blood returning from the tissues via the pulmonary arteries is deoxygenated with O_2, exerting a partial pressure of only 5.3kPa. With alveolar O_2 partial pressure at 13.5kPa and pulmonary capillary O_2 partial pressure at 5.3kPa, a pressure gradient exists across the alveolar capillary membrane. O_2 molecules, therefore, diffuse across the membrane into the pulmonary capillary blood until equilibrium is achieved. Similarly, CO_2 moves down a pressure gradient, diffusing from the blood into the alveolar air to be exhaled. Oxygenated blood returns to the left atrium via the pulmonary veins. Diffusion of gases across the alveolar capillary membrane is proportional to pressure gradient, surface area and gas solubility (O_2 is less soluble than CO_2) and is inversely proportional to membrane thickness and molecular weight of the gas (molecular weight of O_2 is less than CO_2).

For effective oxygenation, the relationship between ventilation (V) and perfusion (Q) is crucial. V is the abbreviation for 'volume per unit time' and in this context, refers to alveolar ventilation, the air available for gaseous exchange per minute (4200mL). Q is the abbreviation for 'flow per unit time' and refers to perfusion of blood through the lungs, which is dependent on cardiac output (5L per minute). Overall, perfusion is slightly greater than ventilation, but in health, gravitational forces result in varying V/Q relationships in different areas of the lung. For example, at rest and before inspiration, ventilation is greater than perfusion in the apices of the lung, whereas at the base, perfusion is greater. Pathology can result in abnormal VQ relationships, and this is a common cause of falling oxygen pressures. Where significant numbers of alveoli are not ventilated (low V/Q), as in pneumonia or alveolar collapse, then the blood perfusing these airless units will remain desaturated and result in a right-to-left shunt. It is as if the blood from the right side of the heart has been shunted to the left side of the heart, bypassing the lungs completely. Figure 5.5 shows the different VQ relationships that can exist.

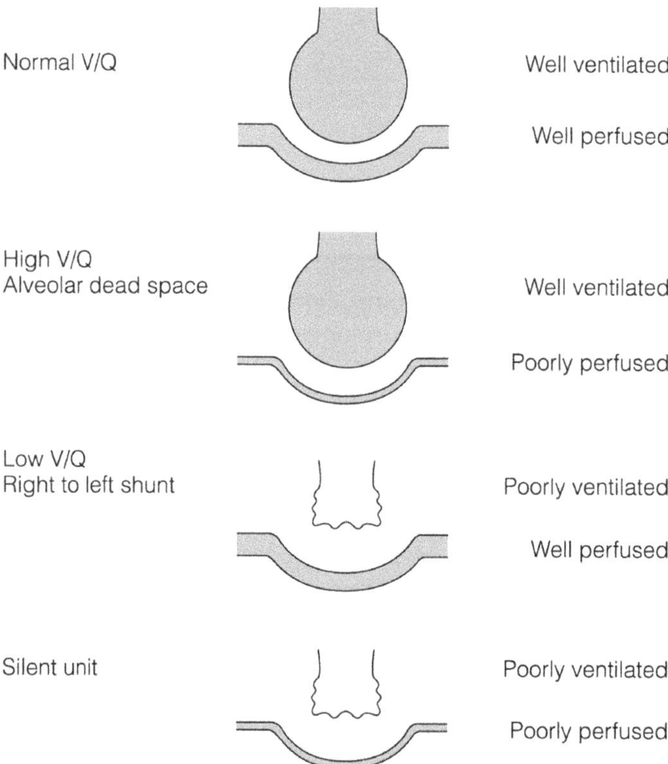

Figure 5.5 Ventilation and perfusion relationships in the lung.

Transport of gases

Normal PaO_2 range:

12–14kPa

Normal $PaCO_2$ range:

4.6–6.0kPa

Once O_2 has diffused across the alveolar capillary membrane into the pulmonary capillary blood, it is transported in two ways. Most (97%) is attached to haemoglobin in the red cells and is transported as oxyhaemoglobin, whilst a small amount of O_2 (3%) is dissolved in plasma. Each molecule of haemoglobin is able to carry four molecules of O_2, and when this is so, the haemoglobin is fully saturated (100%). In clinical practice, this is easily measured by a **pulse oximeter** using a finger probe, with values of 96–100% in health. Where the inspired partial pressure of O_2 is too low, or where there is a problem with gaseous exchange across the alveolar capillary membrane, then the partial pressure of O_2 in arterial blood (PaO_2) will fall (hypoxaemia), and this will be reflected in falling saturations. Where there are increasing levels of reduced haemoglobin (without oxygen), then cyanosis may become evident, where there is bluish discolouration of the skin and mucous membranes.

Each gram of haemoglobin, when fully saturated, is able to carry 1.39mL of O_2, and given a haemoglobin level of 15g/dL, then a little over 20mL of O_2 can be carried in every 100mL of arterial blood, which is called O_2 capacity. Given a cardiac output of 5000mL, then the amount of O_2 carried is approximately 1000mL, and this is referred to as the O_2 delivery or DO_2. From this O_2, which is delivered to the cells each minute at rest, only 250mL is extracted by the cells (for oxidative phosphorylation), and this is called O_2 consumption, or VO_2. This leaves a reserve of O_2 available in arterial blood, which is required when VO_2 needs to increase during exercise or during illness to cope with cellular metabolic demand. The actual O_2 content of arterial blood (CaO_2) for each individual, however, will depend on the saturation, amount of haemoglobin and cardiac output. All these parameters must be considered in ensuring that O_2 delivery (DO_2) is able to keep up with O_2 consumption (VO_2).

Anaemic patients with healthy lungs will have normal saturations, but reduced oxygen content of arterial blood (CaO_2) that may result in hypoxia!

Haemoglobin should be checked.

Just as O_2 moves down a pressure gradient from the lungs to the tissues, carbon dioxide (CO_2) moves down a pressure gradient from tissues to the lungs where it is exhaled (see Figure 5.6). CO_2 is more soluble than O_2 and there is more of it in the body, and, as CO_2 forms carbonic acid (H_2CO_3) in water, then it must be carried in an alternative form. Much of it is carried as bicarbonate (HCO_3^-), and some is carried attached to protein (e.g., haemoglobin) as carbamino compounds. The partial pressure of CO_2 in arterial blood ($PaCO_2$) can be measured through blood gas analysis, which involves obtaining an arterial sample from the radial or femoral artery. Where ventilation is impaired, and the

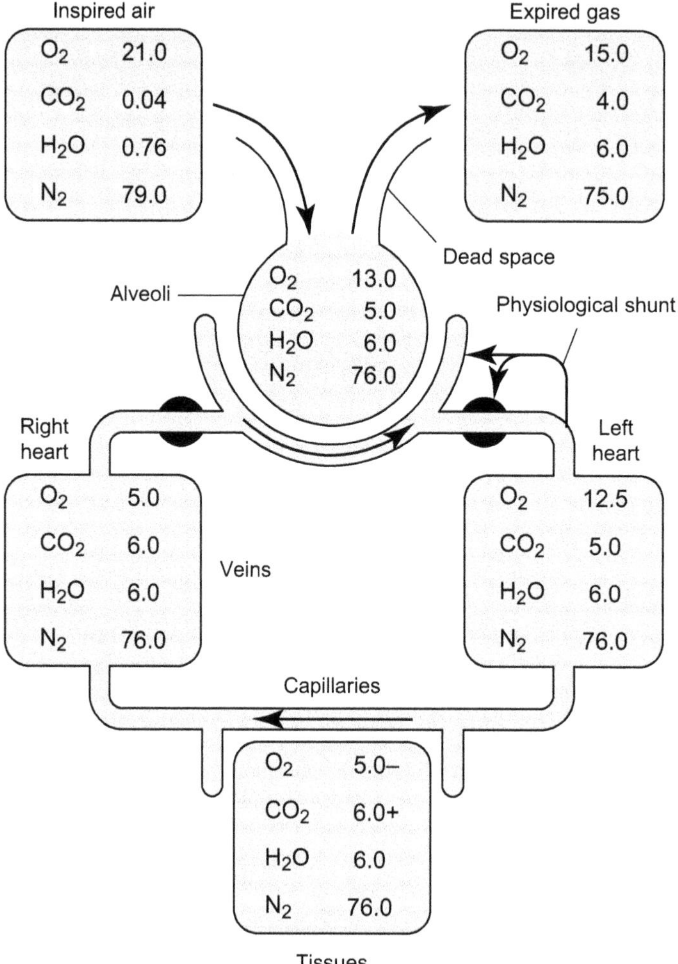

Figure 5.6 Diagram showing movement of gases down a pressure gradient.

lungs cannot remove CO_2 efficiently during expiration, then its partial pressure in arterial blood ($PaCO_2$) will become elevated (hypercapnia), often accompanied by a fall in arterial O_2 (hypoxaemia).

Oxyhaemoglobin dissociation curve

The oxyhaemoglobin dissociation curve is described as S or sigmoid in shape (see Figure 5.7) and illustrates the relationship between PaO_2 (horizontal axis) and haemoglobin saturation (vertical axis). What is evident is that between a PaO_2 of 8–15kPa, the portion of the curve between these two points is relatively flat. That is, despite a fall in PaO_2 from 15kPa, saturations remain high. It is only when the PaO_2 falls to 8kPa (saturation

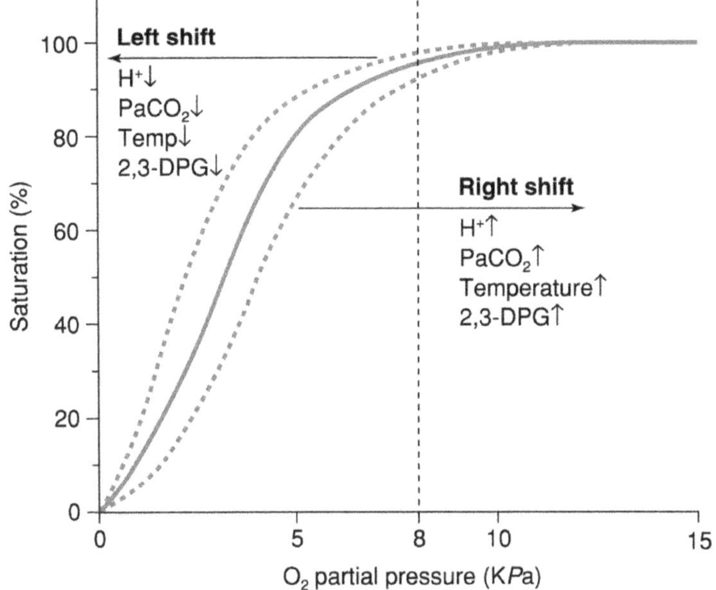

Figure 5.7 Oxyhaemoglobin dissociation curve; the unbroken curve is the normal position.

90%) that the curve then falls steeply, with low saturations. In practice, where PaO_2 falls below 8kPa, then respiratory failure is present, and this has serious consequences for oxygen delivery. The nurse needs to be vigilant so that a trend in falling saturations is detected promptly and appropriate action taken.

The bond between haemoglobin and oxygen can be influenced by a number of factors:

- Temperature.
- 2,3 diphosphoglycerate (2,3-DPG).
- Hydrogen ions or pH status.
- $PaCO_2$.

Where the haemoglobin is affected by an increase in temperature (pyrexia), rising hydrogen ions (acidosis), and/or a rise in CO_2, then the bond is weakened, and oxygen is readily off loaded to the tissues. An increase in 2,3 diphosphoglycerate (2,3-DPG) in the red cells during hypoxia, can also facilitate oxygen release. During these times, the oxyhaemoglobin dissociation curve shifts to the right. Conversely, where the haemoglobin is affected by a fall in temperature, a fall in hydrogen ions (alkalosis) or a fall in CO_2, then the bond is strengthened, and less oxygen is released and the curve shifts to the left. These physiological changes in health ensure that required oxygen is off-loaded easily to metabolising tissues or conserved when metabolism is low (along with oxygen demand). There are clinical situations, however, where abnormalities may shift the position of the curve and compromise the loading and off-loading of oxygen at pulmonary and tissue levels, respectively.

Acute respiratory problems

There are many respiratory disorders, but most fall into one of two groups – obstructive and restrictive disorders, which may increase the work of breathing and result in breathlessness. Restrictive disorders develop when the compliance of the lungs and/or chest wall is reduced and the lungs become 'stiff'. Resistance disorders occur where there is an increase in airway resistance, often due to obstruction. Some people may have mixed pathology, with both restrictive and obstructive features. Breathlessness may be caused by disease affecting the airways, gaseous exchange units, chest wall/pleural membranes or the pulmonary circulation. Breathlessness can also be caused by cardiac problems, as well as anaemia and non-cardiorespiratory causes such as anxiety states. Where there is acidosis, the respiratory system will attempt to restore balance by increasing ventilation, thus removing carbon dioxide (therefore reducing carbonic acid) from the body.

This section will give a brief overview of common respiratory problems which may be seen in an acute care situation. Not only must nurses possess a broad knowledge of the structure and functions of the human body, they must have in-depth knowledge of common physical health problems (Nursing and Midwifery Council 2018a). Later sections will include assessment and general management principles.

Acute airway obstruction

Anaphylaxis is a Type 1 hypersensitivity immune reaction (medical emergency!) where an allergen (e.g., foreign protein), Immunoglobulin E (IgE) and mast cell complex results in a massive release of histamine from the mast cells.

Any part of the upper and lower respiratory tract may become obstructed. Obstruction around the laryngeal and tracheal area will result in high-pitched musical sounds (stridor), particularly on inspiration, and the individual will be acutely distressed. Causes include inhaled foreign bodies, tumour invasion, infection/inflammation and severe allergic reactions such as anaphylaxis. Severe obstruction results in rapid desaturation with respiratory failure and possible cardiopulmonary arrest. Supportive management includes reassurance and positioning the conscious patient upright, well-supporting with pillows, and the administration of high concentration oxygen through a high flow device with a non-re-breathing bag to correct hypoxaemia. It may be necessary for the doctor to perform **tracheal intubation** or tracheostomy with assisted ventilation, and where possible, the cause of the obstruction should be identified and treated, possibly through **fibreoptic bronchoscopy**. Where allergy is the cause, then this will necessitate the administration of drugs such as adrenaline, an anti-histamine and hydrocortisone. If necessary, then cardiopulmonary resuscitation should be performed. Current guidelines, including treatment algorithms for anaphylaxis, have been published by the Resuscitation Council UK (2012).

Pneumothorax

Types of pneumothorax:

- Primary spontaneous.
- Secondary spontaneous.

- Traumatic.
- Iatrogenic.
- Tension.

The difference between sub-atmospheric pressure (negative) in the pleural cavity and atmospheric pressure (positive) in the lungs promotes lung inflation. A pneumothorax occurs when atmospheric air enters the pleural cavity and the pressure becomes positive, resulting in elastic recoil of the lung and either partial or total collapse. It may be spontaneous with no cause, a complication in chronic lung disease, or may follow trauma or occur inadvertently during hospital treatment (e.g., insertion of central line or mechanical ventilation). The visceral pleural membrane in the apices of either lung is usually involved, as a result of gravitational forces and a small tear in the visceral pleura allows air to leak into the pleural space.

Presentation is usually sudden, often with sharp chest pain, but will depend on how large the pneumothorax is, with small volumes of air in the pleural cavity causing relatively few problems. With a larger pneumothorax, perfusion of alveoli that remain non-ventilated may result in significant desaturation, resulting in a greater proportion of the cardiac output leaving the left ventricle without reduced oxygen content. Apart from pain, the individual will be breathless with increasing respiratory rate and tachycardia, and will also be very anxious. There will be reduced chest expansion and breath sounds on the affected side. Cyanosis, a bluish hue on lips and oral mucous membranes denoting significantly reduced oxygenation, may also be present. A pneumothorax may become a tension pneumothorax (a medical emergency) where air that has entered the pleural cavity cannot escape during expiration. The build-up of air will compress the mediastinal space where the heart and great vessels are situated, and this will result in cardiovascular collapse.

In pneumothorax, high concentration oxygen aids reabsorption of air (but not in patients with COPD!).

Depending on the degree of desaturation, a high concentration of oxygen will be prescribed to restore oxygen saturations to within acceptable parameters, although this may be difficult to achieve if the pneumothorax is large. Although small volumes of air will be absorbed, the doctor may decide to withdraw air using a needle and syringe, although, for a large pneumothorax, a chest drain attached to an under-water seal drainage system will be necessary. This facilitates the removal of air during expiration but does not allow air to be drawn in during inspiration, so that eventually all air is removed, with negative pressure restored in the pleural cavity and lung re-expansion.

Guidelines on the management of pleural disease (including pneumothorax) are available from the British Thoracic Society (2010).

Bronchial asthma

Asthma is a chronic inflammatory disorder of the airways, commonly as a result of inhaled allergens leading to hyper-sensitivity. The inflammatory process is extremely complex and involves many different cells in the respiratory epithelium releasing mediators, which are pro-inflammatory. Although there is widespread inflammation throughout the airways, those sections that are particularly vulnerable to this inflammatory process are the terminal and respiratory bronchioles, as there is no cartilage to maintain lumen patency. Swelling as result of inflammation, mucus-plugging and smooth muscle contraction of these airways results in obstruction to airflow and gives rise to wheezing. This airway obstruction in asthma is variable, with symptoms often developing within a very short time frame. Symptom-free periods punctuated with acute episodes may occur in some individuals. Treatment in asthma is very successful, and complete control of symptoms is possible in most cases with appropriate intervention including bronchodilators and steroids as well as health education and the promotion of self-management.

The individual with acute asthma will be distressed and present with chest tightness, increased shortness of breath, wheezing and cough. The work of breathing is increased as a result of increased airway resistance due to narrowing. They must work much harder in order to drive air through these narrowed airways. This is evident by the position adopted to breathe, usually sitting upright and leaning forward, as well as the use of accessory muscles during inspiration and expiration. The positive pressure of expiration can exacerbate/squash the constricted airways, thus making the wheeze during in expiration more prominent. The increased work of the respiratory muscles for breathing will increase their requirements for oxygen at a time when air in the alveoli is reduced. Initially, sufficient reserve may be available for this increased work of breathing, however, this can lead to fatigue and serious compromise of cardiopulmonary status.

Asthma Guidelines are available from the Scottish Intercollegiate Guidelines Network/British Thoracic Society (2019), and these are regularly updated. The severity of asthma attack is characterised by clinical features, and can be classified into moderate asthma, acute severe asthma, life-threatening asthma and near fatal asthma. Features of **acute severe asthma** include the inability to complete sentences in one breath and a **peak expiratory flow rate** (PEFR), which is 33–50% of best or predicted. Known asthmatics will usually know their best PEFR value, which should be recorded, otherwise the nurse will need to refer to a chart with predicted values. The patient with acute severe asthma may not find it easy to measure their peak flow due to breathlessness, but it is useful to assess if possible, to help evaluate effectiveness of treatment given. A respiratory rate greater than 25 breaths per minute (tachypnoea) and a tachycardia of more than 110 per minute are often present. Oxygen therapy should be administered without delay to those who are hypoxaemic, to maintain saturations between 94–98% (as prescribed), and the doctor will usually prescribe nebulised high dose β2 agonist bronchodilators such as salbutamol, with the addition of ipratropium bromide (0.5mg, 4–6 hourly) as required. Bronchodilators are preferably nebulised with oxygen when the target saturations are 94–98%. Steroid medication is important, and oral prednisolone and/or intravenous hydrocortisone should be prescribed for individuals with symptoms of acute asthma to reduce the inflammatory component that contributes to narrowed airways. Where there is no improvement, then the doctor may request additional/continuous doses of β2 agonist bronchodilators (salbutamol). If the desired level of bronchodilation has not been achieved and/or any life-threatening features are present (see below), after consultation with senior medical staff additional, agents such as IV magnesium sulphate (1.2–2g IV infusion over 20 minutes) may be given.

Supplemental oxygen should be used to maintain oxygen saturations between 94% and 98% and titrated to the minimum concentration required in order to maintain SpO_2 above

94%; 15 litres per minute should be given initially if SpO_2 is below 85%. Non-invasive ventilation is **not recommended** for patients with acute asthma (British Thoracic Society/Intensive Care Society Acute Hypercapnic Respiratory Failure Guideline Development Group 2016).

Ongoing monitoring by the nurse is crucial.

Where SpO_2 falls below 92%, then arterial blood gas analysis is required.

Where treatment is unsuccessful, then life-threatening features may be evident, and a discussion with a senior clinician/critical care team is required (BTS 2019). Life-threatening features include oxygen saturation (SpO_2) below 92% and a PaO_2 less than 8kPa, which is often accompanied by central cyanosis. Patients may develop cardiac arrhythmia and hypotension, so nurses should ensure that blood pressure and pulse are carefully monitored. Given the enormous ventilatory effort involved in overcoming airway obstruction, exhaustion eventually ensues, resulting in a poor respiratory effort. Peak expiratory flow rates (PEFR) may drop below 33% of best or predicted, and ventilation may be so weak that breath sounds, including wheeze, may be absent (silent chest). The lack of wheeze may be falsely interpreted as improvement, so vigilance is required with SpO_2 and arterial blood gas monitoring. A significant danger of exhaustion and weak respiratory effort is that the patient will be unable to ventilate sufficiently to remove CO_2. If SpO_2 is below 92%, or the patient appears to be getting tired, arterial blood gas analysis is required to determine whether the $PaCO_2$ is rising (hypercapnia). In acute severe asthma $PaCO_2$ is initially lowered, due to the hyperventilation of any healthy areas of lung and its increased solubility enhancing removal. However, as the patient tires, $PaCO_2$ will normalise. A life-threatening feature of asthma includes $PaCO_2$ levels within the normal safe parameters (4.5–6kPa) as, if the exhaustion and poor respiratory effort continues, CO_2 retention and respiratory arrest may ensue. Raised levels of $PaCO_2$ are a medical emergency(near-fatal asthma), senior clinicians may consider commencing IV β2 agonists (salbutamol), or IV aminophylline. Intensive care admission, possibly with progression to intubation and support with positive pressure ventilation will be required in these circumstances, wth referral to intensive care.

Increasing $PaCO_2$ in acute asthma reflects a near-fatal attack and is a medical emergency.

Exacerbation of chronic obstructive pulmonary disease

Chronic obstructive pulmonary disease (COPD) is also a chronic inflammatory disease of the airways, but the cause and the inflammatory process is different from asthma, with the majority of cases due to the long-term effects of smoking. COPD is an umbrella term for chronic bronchitis and emphysema. In chronic bronchitis, irritation caused by smoking results in inflammation of airways and an increase in mucus-secreting glands as well as an increase in mucus secreting goblet cells. There is increased production of sputum, and the structural changes in the airways as a result of the inflammatory response leads to their narrowing. Emphysema, which often co-exists, affects the respiratory bronchioles, alveolar ducts and sacs where gaseous exchange takes place. There is distension and destruction of the tissue, which may eventually affect gaseous exchange. This loss of elastic recoil of the respiratory bronchioles leads to early airway closure during expiration and air trapping.

As the disease progresses, particularly where smoking continues, then the degree of airway obstruction which is irreversible will become worse. Increasing sputum production, breathlessness and disability, all more severe during winter, are usual. Initially, although there may be mild hypoxaemia, ventilatory drive is sufficient to remove CO_2. Indeed, in some individuals living with severe emphysema the breathlessness can be profound, but ventilatory effort keeps the CO_2 low. In time, some individuals may not be able to maintain this ventilatory drive, and CO_2 excretion may be compromised so that chronic hypercapnia develops. Whilst rising levels of CO_2 will initially stimulate breathing as usual, eventually it is hypoxaemia which stimulates peripheral chemoreceptors in the carotid artery and aortic arch. This is referred to as hypoxic drive and is why caution is exercised when administering oxygen to people living with COPD.

> Where a patient known to have, or is at risk of having chronically elevated $PaCO_2$ levels (hypercapnic failure), then oxygen should be given at 24% initially to maintain SpO_2 at 88–92%, pending result of arterial blood gas analysis (BTS 2017).

People living with COPD often experience exacerbations defined as 'rapid and sustained worsening of symptoms beyond their usual day-to-day variations' (National Institute for Health and Care Excellence [NICE] 2016, p. 5). It is during these times that breathlessness and cough become worse, with an increase in sputum, which is purulent and indicative of infection. In addition, there is often increased chest tightness, wheeze and fatigue with worsening hypoxaemia, often resulting in confusion. With long standing COPD, low levels of O_2 in the lungs can result in hypoxic vasoconstriction, a narrowing of the pulmonary blood vessels, which can increase the work of the right ventricle of the heart, ultimately leading to right-sided heart cardiac failure. Cardiac failure, which develops as a result of chronic lung disease is called **cor pulmonale**, and the patient will have additional problems including fluid retention with swollen ankles and possibly ascites (fluid in the peritoneal cavity).

It is often difficult making the decision as to whether or not the individuals experiencing an acute exacerbation of their COPD should be admitted to hospital. This will depend on what services are available locally. Where there is a community rapid response team or an intermediate care facility, then escalation of treatment at home may avoid hospitalisation. Factors such as breathlessness, impaired level of consciousness, cyanosis, worsening peripheral oedema, confusion, rapid onset, oxygen saturations below 90%, with changes in arterial blood gas readings or chest x-ray, would favour treatment in hospital. However, factors such as an inability to cope at home, poor general condition, limited levels of activity, poor social circumstances and home oxygen therapy, should also be taken into consideration. Treatment would necessitate the administration of inhaled bronchodilators (β2 agonists and ipratropium), nebulised with an air compressor, with any supplemental oxygen requirement given via nasal cannulae. Corticosteroids (e.g., prednisolone) and antibiotics (NICE 2018) are recommended. If fluid retention occurs as a result of right-sided cardiac failure, evidenced by swollen ankles/legs and pitting oedema is present, then diuretic therapy will also be necessary.

During acute exacerbations, the increased work of breathing with inevitable fatigue can result in poor ventilatory drive. The consequence of this is a falling PaO_2 and a rising $PaCO_2$. However, it is important to remember that someone living with COPD may have adjusted to living with chronic hypoxaemia and hypercapnia – this individual's 'normal' state. Arterial blood gasses (discussed in more detail later in the chapter), in those who have adjusted to chronic hypoxaemia and hypercapnia, will reveal smaller reductions in pH in relation to raised $PaCO_2$ levels. The metabolic component of the blood gas will reveal an elevation in the levels of the buffer bicarbonate (HCO_3^-), secondary to the renal compensation response of bicarbonate reabsorption. During acute episodes, great skill is needed in reducing $PaCO_2$ levels without over-correction of PaO_2 oxygen levels. Non-invasive ventilatory support, in the form of bilevel positive airway pressure ventilation (BiPAP) and careful oxygen titration aims to achieve this. This is discussed later in this chapter.

Pneumonia

Pneumonia occurs when inflammatory material (exudate) accumulates in the alveoli. Where the inflammation is confined to the whole of one or more lobes, then it is referred to as lobar pneumonia, or bronchopneumonia when spread more widely throughout the lungs. Similarly, pneumonia can be caused by a range of pathogenic organisms including bacteria and viruses, following the aspiration of vomit or mucus and occasionally following treatment such as radiotherapy. Examples of micro-organisms that can cause pneumonia include:

- Streptococcus pneumoniae.
- Mycoplasma pneumoniae.
- Influenza A viruses.
- Haemophilus influenzae.
- Chlamydia pneumoniae.
- Legionella pneumoniae.
- Pneumocystis carinii.

Host factors (e.g., individual resistance) and agent factors (e.g., virulence of organism) should be taken into account when considering individual susceptibility to infection. Although fit, healthy people can develop pneumonia, the following may increase risk:

- Smoking.
- Excessive alcohol intake.
- Presence of other conditions such as COPD, cancer and heart failure.
- Very young and older people.
- Weak immune system.
- Recent respiratory viral infection.
- Malnutrition/poor hydration.
- Treatment in intensive care.
- Increased susceptibility to inhalation – impaired consciousness, swallowing difficulties.

In previously fit, healthy people who develop pneumonia involving a single lobe, then treatment at home may be appropriate.

Patients with pneumonia typically present with a cough (with or without sputum), breathlessness (respiratory rate >30/minute) and chest pain, and in some there is fever, agitation and confusion. Very often a chest x-ray will reveal abnormalities. Pneumonia can result in rapid deterioration within a short time frame, where ventilation perfusion relationship is seriously compromised and where shunting results in profound hypoxaemia and respiratory failure. Indeed, the degree of shunt may be so severe that high concentration oxygen fails to improve saturations and transfer to intensive care for positive pressure ventilation is necessary. The CURB 65 score can help assess the severity of an episode of pneumonia (NICE 2014). This score is derived from a number of measurements: respiratory rate greater than 30 respirations per minute, new confusion, raised blood urea nitrogen, hypotension and age. It is used to determine mortality risk and prognosis, guiding the admitting clinician regarding the need for hospital admission/requirements for higher level care environments.

CURB-65 score is calculated by giving 1 point for each of the following prognostic features:

- Confusion (abbreviated Mental Test score ≤8 or new disorientation in person, place or time).
- Raised blood urea nitrogen (>7mmol/L).
- Raised respiratory rate (≥30 breaths per minute).
- Low blood pressure (diastolic ≤60mmHg, or systolic <less than 90mmHg).
- Age ≥65 years.

Patients are stratified for risk of death as follows:

- 0 or 1: low risk (<3% mortality risk).
- 2: intermediate risk (3–15% mortality risk).
- 3 to 5: high risk (>15% mortality risk).

(Lim et al. 2003)

Respiratory failure

Acute cardiac and respiratory problems can result in a failure to maintain effective gaseous exchange across the alveolar capillary membrane. Actually, acute respiratory failure is the outcome of one of the following:

Lung failure

This is where there is inadequate gaseous exchange across the alveolar capillary membrane, so that arterial oxygenation cannot be maintained. The PaO_2 will fall (reduced saturations), but effective ventilation (inspiration and expiration) will continue to remove carbon dioxide. Indeed, in the early stages of acute respiratory problems (e.g., pneumonia and asthma), hyperventilation may result in low arterial carbon dioxide levels.

Ventilatory failure

The anatomical structure of the thorax is designed so that the lungs can effectively 'pump' air in and out (i.e. ventilate). This requires the chest wall, ribs, nerves and muscles to work together in order that this can be achieved. There are a number of disorders that can affect this mechanism, which will result in the inability of the lungs to function as a ventilatory pump. When this occurs, carbon dioxide cannot be removed from the lungs effectively, and therefore levels become elevated in arterial blood (hypercapnia). As a result, arterial oxygen levels will also start to fall.

Causes of ventilatory failure:

- Fatigue of ventilatory muscles.
- Problems with the chest wall (e.g., chest injury/deformity).
- Neuromuscular problems.
- Central nervous system depression.

When gas exchange is compromised in the lungs, then the body must compensate to maintain homeostasis. The work of breathing will increase as a result of increased airway resistance, reduced compliance or both. As a consequence, the cardiovascular system will also attempt to restore balance by increasing heart rate, blood pressure and cardiac output. This altered physiology will be reflected in the patient's changing vital signs, and ongoing assessment is crucial so that these developments can be detected early and appropriate corrective measures taken (see respiratory assessment section).

Where there is deterioration in respiratory status with a progressive fall in saturations (SpO_2), then arterial blood gas analysis is required to establish whether or not the patient is in respiratory failure. The following values would confirm the diagnosis:

Type 1 respiratory failure (lung failure)

Profound hypoxaemia with a PaO_2 of less than 8kPa (SpO_2 less than 90%) with normal or low $PaCO_2$ (less than 6.1kPa).

Type 2 respiratory failure (pump or ventilatory failure)

Profound hypoxaemia, with a PaO_2 of less than 8kPa (SpO_2 less than 90%) and an elevated $PaCO_2$ above 6.0kPa (hypercapnia).

In respiratory failure, interventions aim to reduce the work of breathing and restoring arterial blood gas values to within appropriate parameters agreed by the health care team. Where this is not achieved by oxygen administration, then further interventions such as nasal high flow oxygen therapy (HFNOT), continuous positive pressure airways pressure (CPAP), bilevel positive airway pressure (BiPAP) or invasive positive pressure ventilation will be required.

Respiratory assessment

In acute care settings, nurses have a crucial role to play in assessment, so that deterioration in respiratory status is detected as early as possible. In an earlier chapter we saw how concerns regarding competence in this area led to the development of physiological 'track and trigger' systems in order to promote patient safety. A systematic approach should be

Table 5.1 History taking

Personal biography.
Patient perception of major problem.
Medical history – illness, surgery/recent trends.
Allergies.
Medication.
Symptom/systems review.
Psychosocial history.
Risk (e.g., smoking, alcohol).
Functional ability – self-care deficits.

adopted to undertake a respiratory assessment, which involves the gathering of subjective and objective data.

Initial assessment will involve using the ABCDE framework and local protocol should be followed regarding the use of early warning scoring systems. The following discussion has focussed on assessment of breathing. Where the patient's condition dictates, it may be necessary to perform cardiopulmonary resuscitation (see Chapter 7).

Subjective data

The individual's perspective is paramount, and they should be asked what they consider the current problem to be. A great deal of information can be obtained contributing to data analysis and identification of likely problems. This is where a patient history can be taken including the exploration of each symptom that the patient may be experiencing (see Table 5.1). Information should be obtained for each symptom (e.g., pain, breathlessness, cough) the patient has, and PQRSTU can assist here:

P – Provocation and palliation
Q – Quality
R – Region/ Radiation
S – Severity
T – Timing
U – Understanding

Time available for history-taking will depend on the condition of the patient; it may be necessary to move swiftly on to obtaining objective data where there is significant respiratory and haemodynamic instability.

Objective data

Signs of respiratory deterioration:

- Increased respiratory rate.
- Decreased SpO_2.
- Increased oxygen needed to keep SpO_2 in target range.
- Increased physiological trigger score.
- CO_2 retention.

- Drowsiness.
- Headache.
- Flushed face.
- Tremor.

(O'Driscoll et al. 2017)

Objective data obtained should be relatively accurate depending of course on the skill of the nurse and any electronic equipment used. Vital signs including pulse, blood pressure and respiratory rate will be recorded, and a physical examination will be performed with additional diagnostic and laboratory data requested as appropriate.

Nurses spend a great deal of time measuring and recording vital signs, and this is often seen as a routine aspect of nursing care. However, observations need to be contextualised and interpreted as part of a more detailed respiratory assessment. The ability of nurses to recognise early signs of illness and start appropriate and timely management of those who are at risk of clinical deterioration or require emergency care is crucial (Nursing and Midwifery Council 2018a). The frequency of monitoring will depend on the stability of the patient's condition as well any perceived risk of complications developing during or following diagnostic/therapeutic interventions. Where values obtained fall outside of the normal range or agreed parameters, then senior staff should be alerted. No matter how often measurements are recorded, ongoing monitoring of the patient's condition is important, as this can change within a very short time frame (i.e. in between recording observations).

Factors affecting pulse oximetry readings:

- Poor peripheral perfusion.
- Carbon monoxide levels (e.g., smokers) – overestimates!
- Probe site (finger/ear lobe most accurate).
- Nail varnish and false nails.

NB saturations are normal in anaemia, so haemoglobin should be checked.

Pulse oximetry is established as soon as possible. Oxygen saturation is considered the 'fifth vital sign', and measurements (SpO_2) are obtained with a probe, usually attached to the finger. Values in health are 94–98%, with downward trends reflecting worsening hypoxaemia. For readings, there must be capillary blood flow, and this may not be the case where there is haemodynamic instability. Oximeter probes are usually attached to the finger, but the ear lobe may be used and can be useful if fingers are cold and the reading is difficult to obtain. It is important, though, to use the correct probe for each site, as the probes are not interchangeable and could lead to inaccurate readings (up to 50% lower or 30% higher) and therefore, inappropriate therapy (NHS Improvement 2018). Recordings should indicate whether measurements were taken on room air or with oxygen. Saturations alone give no information regarding hypercapnia or oxygen delivery. Where there are normal saturations, the patient can still develop hypoxia due to factors such as low cardiac output or reduced Hb. Nevertheless, saturation values assist in diagnosis and monitoring during interventions to treat hypoxaemia.

Although the pulse rate is usually displayed on the oximeter, it is important to palpate the pulse to obtain further information. During breathlessness with increased work of breathing, heart rate can increase significantly with tachycardia, further increasing oxygen demand with compensatory increases in heart rate and cardiac output. Profound hypoxaemia may result in bradycardia and abnormal heart rhythms, which may be reflected by an irregular pulse. Cardiovascular compensatory changes may cause additional problems, where there are cardiac problems resulting in a weak, thready pulse. Having taken the pulse, and with fingers still on the radial pulse, the nurse can then count the respiratory rate over 1 minute, noting the depth of breathing and chest expansion (see section below on 'Inspection' regarding respiratory assessment).

Blood pressure is recorded, and in the early stages, where there is respiratory compromise, there may be a rise in blood pressure due to activation of the sympathetic nervous system. However, where there is deterioration in respiratory status, this can result in haemodynamic instability, with a fall in blood pressure.

Physical examination

Physical examination

involves the following:

- Inspection (LOOK).
- Palpation (FEEL).
- Percussion (FEEL).
- Auscultation (LISTEN).

Skills utilising LOOK, LISTEN and FEEL are important throughout any patient assessment.

Inspection:

During the recording of vital signs, the nurse is observing the patient (also using the sense of hearing), and this can provide a great deal of information about respiratory status. During inspection, the nurse may hear a stridor if there is an upper airway obstruction, a cough, or may hear wheezes. The level of consciousness and degree of orientation is noted along with whether the patient is unable to complete a sentence in one breath. In a well-lit room, there may be bluish discoloration of mucous membranes in the mouth (central cyanosis) and of the fingers, nose and ear lobes (peripheral cyanosis) if there is desaturation (although this alone is an unreliable sign). Where work of breathing is increased, then there may be signs of distress, and the patient will prefer to sit upright leaning forward where possible. If there is any sputum being expectorated, this should be observed. Blood streaked sputum may suggest haemoptysis and green sputum, bacterial infection.

Note should be made of any accessory muscles used, including the neck muscles (sternocleidomastoids) and scalenes for inspiration and abdominal muscles during expiration. As well as counting the respiratory rate, the nurses should observe the depth of breathing. Remember that for adequate gaseous exchange, alveolar volume is important and determined by respiratory rate and tidal volume. Poor chest expansion will result in reduced tidal volumes, therefore alveolar ventilation (hypoventilation) and increased $PaCO_2$.

Symmetry of chest movement is also important, and reduced expansion on one side may indicate pneumothorax or pneumonia for example. An increase in the Anterior-Posterior (A-P) diameter of the chest is usually seen in patients with chronic obstructive pulmonary disease. Nicotine-stained fingers may be seen in heavy smokers, and chronic hypoxaemia may result in clubbing of the fingers. Patients who are taking bronchodilators, such as salbutamol (beta 2 agonists), may have a fine tremor of the hands, and in those with carbon dioxide retention (hypercapnia), a flapping tremor of the outstretched arms is occasionally seen.

Palpation

Using touch will also provide a great deal of information during the physical examination, and the nurse will already have made a few observations whilst palpating the pulse. The skin, including extremities, may feel warm, suggesting good perfusion, whilst cool skin may indicate reduced cardiac output. Gently palpating the anterior and posterior chest may identify swelling and areas of localised pain. Air can sometimes escape from the lungs and accumulate in the superficial skin layers (following puncture wounds or surgery), and this is called subcutaneous or surgical emphysema, giving rise to a crackling sensation during palpation.

Experienced practitioners may also palpate the position of the trachea just above the supra-sternal notch in the neck. The trachea is usually central, but can shift to one side if air accumulates, as in a tension pneumothorax. Finally, palpation can be used to feel for the vibrations caused by transmission of sounds from the voice. By palpating the chest on both sides and asking the patient to say ‘99’, vibrations may be felt on the practitioner’s hands (tactile fremitus). Solid tissue, such as consolidation in pneumonia, can transmit sounds well (increased tactile fremitus), whereas increased air in a pneumothorax cannot (decreased tactile fremitus).

Percussion

This is where the anterior and posterior chest is percussed. The technique involves placing the middle finger firmly over the surface to be percussed (all other fingers should be off the chest) and then striking it with the middle finger of the other hand. This transmits vibrations through to the underlying chest wall and a note is produced. One side of the chest is compared to the other. Characteristics of the percussion note are as follows:

- Resonant: over normal lung.
- Hyper-resonant: over a pneumothorax.
- Tympanic: over a tension pneumothorax.
- Dullness: over liver and in consolidation e.g., pneumonia.

Auscultation

The areas previously percussed are then auscultated, using the diaphragm of the stethoscope to listen for breath sounds. The sounds produced on one side of the chest are compared to the other side. Normal breath sounds over the anterior and posterior chest wall are vesicular, which are soft, low-pitched sounds where the inspiratory phase is shorter than the expiratory phase. If bronchial sounds are heard, this may suggest an area of consolidation. Bronchial breath sounds are loud and high-pitched, with the inspiratory phase shorter than the expiratory phase. As well as breath sounds, there may be additional breath sounds (adventitious sounds), such as crackles and wheezes. Coarse crackles are usually heard on inspiration with problems such as infection, pulmonary oedema (fluid in the alveoli as a result of left ventricular heart failure) and fine inspiratory crackles in pulmonary fibrosis or in the re-expansion of collapsed alveoli. Wheezes are usually expiratory and can be heard in acute asthma and in chronic obstructive pulmonary disease. Differences in the transmission of voice sounds can also be heard during auscultation. Where there is consolidation, the sounds produced by asking the patient to say '99' will be heard more loudly through the stethoscope as compared to the healthy side; this is called bronchophony. Bronchophony is conversely diminished where there is air present and absent over a pleural effusion or significant pneumothorax.

Nurses mostly use the skills of inspection and palpation, although they are increasingly developing clinical skills in percussion and auscultation to enhance their assessment of patients. However, whilst nurses practise independently, they must be able to recognise the limits of their competence and knowledge, seeking advice from or referring to other professionals when necessary (Nursing and Midwifery Council 2018b). See Table 5.2 for key findings during physical examination relating to specific disorders.

Table 5.2 Physical examination; findings in specific disorders

Disorder	*Inspection*	*Palpation*	*Percussion Note*	*Auscultation*
Pneumonia	Flushed Respiratory rate↑	Fremitus↑ Expansion↓ affected side	Dull over consolidation	Bronchial breath sounds over consolidation Crackles Bronchophony ↑
Atelectasis	Respiratory rate↑	Absent fremitus Expansion↓ affected side	Dull over affected area	Absent
Pneumo-thorax	Breathless Respiratory rate↑	Fremitus↓ or absent Trachea may shift towards the opposite side Expansion↓ on affected side	Hyper-resonant or tympanic	Breath sounds decreased or absent over pleural air Bronchophony↓
Asthma	Breathless Respiratory rate↑ Cough/Tenacious sputum	Fremitus↓	Resonant to Hyper-resonant	Breath sounds obscured by wheezes Possibly crackles Bronhcophony
Acute COPD	Cough/purulent sputum Breathless, pursed-lip breathing Respiratory rate↑ Barrel chest	Fremitus↓	Hyper-resonant	Breath sounds Crackles/wheezes Bronchophony

For further information on physical examination review:

Bickley L, S (2016) *Bates' Guide to Physical Examination and History Taking*, 12th Ed. Philadelphia. Wolters Kluwer/Lippincott Williams & Watkins.

CASE STUDY 5.1 MRS PROCTOR WITH COPD: PART 1

Initial assessment

It is 11:00 and Edith Proctor, aged 71 and a life-long smoker with COPD, has been admitted following referral by her GP with a history of breathlessness. Despite three courses of antibiotics and steroids, there has been no improvement, and for the last few days she has been feeling generally unwell with increased breathlessness, initially on exertion but now at rest.

Airway: on arrival in the ward, the nurse notes that although Mrs Proctor is very breathless and distressed, she is fully conscious and has a patent airway with no stridor audible. The nurse offers reassurance and assists the patient in adopting the most comfortable position, which is sitting upright and leaning forward.

Breathing: responding to questions asked during the initial assessment, it is evident that the degree of breathlessness is quite severe, as Mrs Proctor cannot complete sentences without stopping and gasping for air. Coughing is intermittent, with the expectoration of green, tenacious sputum indicating possible dehydration and/or infection. The respiratory rate is 24 breaths per minute, and although breathing is regular and chest movement symmetrical, contraction of the sternocleidomastoids and abdominal muscles along with poor chest expansion and pursed-lip breathing confirms the increased respiratory effort required for breathing.

The nurse decides to limit the number of questions asked, so as not cause further distress at this stage, and explains to Mrs Proctor that she would like to assess her breathing status and perform a chest examination. Before proceeding, the nurse notes that pulse oximetry shows an SpO_2 of 92%, with 2 litres of oxygen delivered by nasal cannulae, although the level has been falling to 87% without oxygen. Her target saturations have been identified as 88–92%, pending arterial blood gas values, as she is considered a high risk for hypercapnic failure. Scale 2 is used to record her SpO_2 and supplemental oxygen therapy on the National Early Warnings Score (NEWS). Scale 1 has been crossed through on the NEWS chart. On further inspection, it is noted that there is pallor, although there are no signs of cyanosis of the extremities (peripheral cyanosis) or of the tongue/buccal cavity (central cyanosis). The absence of central cyanosis is particularly reassuring, as this indicates that arterial saturation is likely to be satisfactory, and the nurse continues with the assessment in a systematic fashion.

On palpation, Mrs Proctor's equal chest expansion and normal tracheal position is noted, and it is therefore unlikely that a tension pneumothorax is contributing to the current pulmonary compromise. Using palpation skills, the nurse asks Mrs Proctor to repeat '99' and notes that tactile fremitus is decreased bilaterally. Given that transmission of sound is poor through air, this conveys to the nurse that reduced vibration on palpation (fremitus) is possibly due to air trapping in the lungs. Percussion elicits hyper-resonance over the anterior chest.

On auscultation, there are reduced vesicular breath sounds over the anterior and posterior lung fields, and there are some early inspiratory crackles which, again, could indicate infection. Expiratory wheeze was also evident through the lung field.

Breathing NEWS (2 + 0 + 2) = 4 (scale 2)

Circulation

Mrs Proctor's heart rate remains at a regular 110 beats per minute, and a bounding quality is noted. The peripheries are warm, and the capillary refill time is 2 seconds. The 12 lead ECG, requested in light of her tachycardia, reveals sinus tachycardia, possibly caused by the sympathetic activation as a result of hypoxaemia, the stress response to critical illness or perhaps elevated carbon dioxide. However, there are no ectopic beats or other arrhythmias. The nurse reflects on these findings and how unpredictable the overall effect of carbon dioxide on the cardiovascular system can be, and that although hypercapnia and acidosis can have a direct cardiovascular depressant effect, this can often be overshadowed by a sympathetic response resulting in tachycardia, as in Mrs Proctor's case. Elevated $PaCO_2$ levels can also result in a systemic vasodilator effect, giving a flushed appearance and bounding pulse.

Mrs Proctor's blood pressure is elevated, at 154/89mmHg with a mean arterial pressure (MAP) of 110mmHg. There is no pedal oedema, skin is dry with decreased turgor and she has not passed urine since admission. She is also complaining of feeling thirsty. Although renal blood flow and Glomerular Filtration Rate (GFR) are likely to be reduced as a result of hypercapnia, dehydration is also likely to be a contributing factor.

Circulation NEWS (0 + 1) = 1

Disability

Whilst Mrs Proctor is finding it difficult to talk much, you are able to establish that she knows where she is and what time of day it is. You conclude that she is alert (using ACVPU). Neurological status is important as this can be affected by hypoxaemia, hypercapnia and sepsis, leading to drowsiness, confusion and coma. The blood glucose level is checked, as the nurse is aware that this can rise as a result of sympathetic activation, but it is within normal limits, at 5mmols/L.

Disability NEWS = 0

Exposure

The nurse observes that Mrs Proctor is apyrexial, at 37.5°C. She looks underweight, and the nurse calculates her BMI to be 16, which is below normal. She is aware that respiratory status can be affected by poor nutrition and dehydration, and that although breathlessness may have prevented dietary intake, improved nutrition and fluid replacement would be important goals. Weight loss further increases risk and can be a poor prognostic sign. A referral to the dietician will be needed later to optimise nutritional status. Skin, however, is intact, and there are no other abnormalities noted.

Exposure NEWS = 0

Total NEWS = 5, requiring urgent response

The medical team responsible for the patient are on the ward, so they are called to review Mrs Proctor.

Action: given Mrs Proctor's history and presentation, a provisional diagnosis of acute exacerbation Chronic Obstructive Pulmonary Disease (COPD) is made. Given the possible hypercapnia risk, a low oxygen concentration of 24% continues, at 2 litres per minute via nasal cannula to achieve saturations between 88–92%, with a view to promptly assess ABG's. The doctor also prescribes the following drugs:

Nebulised salbutamol: 5mg, 4 hrly prn, driving gas air.
Nebulised ipratropium bromide: 500mcg, 4–6 hrly, driving gas air.
Hydrocortisone: 200mg IV.

Hourly monitoring will be necessary, as she is at risk of deterioration (NEWS 5) and may require a higher level of care if non-responsive to initial therapy. It is also important to consider risk of sepsis as NEWS is 5. It is not unusual for older patients to have an infection without an increase in temperature, but a sputum sample is sent for culture and sensitivity, and a broad-spectrum antibiotic is commenced intravenously.

The nurse documents her findings carefully and is aware that although an initial assessment has been completed, ongoing monitoring of Mrs Proctor is necessary. Once the patient is stabilised and less distressed, the nurse will be able to complete a more comprehensive assessment.

Arterial blood gases

Where there is trend of worsening respiratory status with falling oxygen saturations, the doctor will usually request arterial blood gas analysis. A specimen of arterial blood is obtained usually from the radial artery using a needle and heparinised syringe. An arterialised blood sample may also be obtained from the ear lobe and is useful for measuring pH and $PaCO_2$ (underestimates PaO_2 by 0.5–1kPa). In critical care settings, the patient may have an arterial line temporarily inserted in the radial artery, and this avoids repeated arterial stabs which are somewhat painful (see Table 5.3 for normal values).

If the values obtained from the gas analyser are abnormal, then the problem must be identified (see Table 5.4). In respiratory problems, abnormal blood gas values often reflect a respiratory acidosis, where the $PaCO_2$ is elevated above 6.0kPa (type 2 respiratory failure). The hydration of excess CO_2 in the body results in carbonic acid, which liberates hydrogen ions and increases acidity in the blood. If the patient has ventilatory difficulty, they will not be able excrete sufficient CO_2 during expiration. In acidosis, the pH will be less than the mean of 7.4, and there will be an increase in hydrogen ion concentration

Table 5.3 Normal blood gas values

Normal values	*Arterial blood*	*Venous blood*
pH	7.35–7.45	7.31–7.41
Hydrogen ions	35–45nmol/L	
PO_2	12–14kPa	4.6–5.8kPa
PCO_2	4.6–6.0kPa	5.5–6.8kPa
HCO_3^-	22–26mmol/L	22–26mmol/L
O_2 saturation	95%+	70–75%
Base excess/deficit	-2 to +2	

Table 5.4 Acid-base imbalance

Respiratory acid-base imbalance	*Causes*
↑ $PaCO_2$ = acidosis ↑ hydrogen ions	• Chronic obstructive pulmonary disease (COPD). • Depressed respiratory centre e.g., sedation/head injury. • Neuromuscular disorders. • Acute respiratory infection.
↓ $PaCO_2$ = alkalosis ↓ hydrogen ions	• Hyperventilation e.g., psychogenic.
Metabolic acid-base imbalance	**Causes**
↓ HCO_3^- = acidosis ↑ metabolic acids Loss of HCO_3^- from the body	• Ketoacidosis. • Shock. • Diarrhoea. • Renal disease.
↑ HCO_3^- = alkalosis Loss of H^+ ions (acid) from the body	• Vomiting. • Gastric aspiration. • Excessive bicarbonate intake.

(normal range 35–45nmol/L). If the pH or hydrogen concentration is within normal limits, despite an elevated $PaCO_2$, then compensation is partial or complete, and the bicarbonate level (HCO_3) is likely to be elevated (>26mmol/L). Accompanying the elevated $PaCO_2$ is often hypoxaemia (PaO_2 <8kPa). If the PaO_2 is <8kPa, but the $PaCO_2$ is normal (or low), then this is respiratory failure type 1.

If the abnormal blood gas values reveals a low pH, a $PaCO_2$ within the normal range (or low) with a decreased HCO_3^- (<24mmol/L), then this is likely to be a metabolic acidosis. The pH or hydrogen ion concentration may reflect this acidotic state, but if within the normal range, then once again, the body is compensating. The body will remove some of the hydrogen ions by increasing the ventilatory drive, so that more CO_2 excreted as minute ventilation is increased. In a metabolic acidosis, it is other acids (not carbonic acid) that cannot be removed by the lungs which accumulate, such as lactic acid (cellular hypoxia), or hydroxybutyric acid (ketoacidosis in diabetes). Another cause of metabolic acidosis is a loss of bicarbonate from the body, as in severe diarrhoea where alkaline intestinal fluid is lost.

An alkalosis occurs where either too much CO_2 is expired (e.g., hyperventilation) resulting in a respiratory alkalosis, or where either acids are being lost from the body (e.g., hydrochloric acid through vomiting) or there is a net gain in bicarbonate (intravenous sodium bicarbonate or oral bicarbonate of soda taken as an antacid), resulting in a metabolic alkalosis.

As outlined earlier, acidosis and alkalosis can affect the release of oxygen from the haemoglobin, thus affecting oxygen delivery to the cells. It is important therefore that these acid base disorders are corrected.

Maximising respiratory status

In the acutely ill patient, care is aimed at correcting hypoxaemia by optimising gaseous exchange in the lungs and achieving normal or near normal oxygen saturations, other than in those at risk of hypercapnic failure. Attempts should also be made, where possible, to reduce the work of breathing by increasing compliance or reducing airway resistance.

Position

Ideally, the patient in acute respiratory distress is nursed in an upright position, well-supported with pillows where the condition allows this (in skeletal or spinal trauma this may not be possible). This facilitates effective chest expansion and improves lung volumes. It is important to remember that ventilation and perfusion is affected not only by disease processes, but also by gravitational forces. Moving the patient, where possible, to a high side lying position on alternate sides may improve saturations by encouraging perfusion in healthy lung regions. Where there is disease on one side of the chest, then positioning with the affected side uppermost may improve perfusion through the dependent (healthy) lung.

Frequent re-positioning by the nurse is essential, as the patient may slip down the bed, and this will compromise pulmonary status further by reducing functional residual capacity (FRC) and PaO_2. FRC reduces significantly in patients who are supine and can lead to collapse of small airways with loss of surface area for gaseous exchange.

Oxygen therapy

Oxygen should be prescribed, and saturation target identified by medical staff, but administered immediately in emergencies.

A prescription should show:

- Target saturation.
- Delivery device.
- Flow rate.

Oxygen is administered to correct hypoxaemia, not breathlessness. It is important that nurses recognise that oxygen therapy can increase oxygenation, but does not correct the underlying cause of the individual's hypoxaemia. The aim of oxygen therapy, therefore, is to titrate inspired oxygen concentration to achieve a near-normal oxygen saturation. However, caution is required for patients who are hypercapnic or have had a previous episode of hypercapnia, where excess inspired oxygen can exacerbate respiratory failure. When administering oxygen, nurses must place close attention to the patient's position. Patients receiving oxygen therapy are nursed in an upright position to facilitate ventilation, and the supine position should be avoided unless specifically required, i.e. spinal trauma.

Oxygen therapy

If saturation <85%, then:

- Non-rebreather reservoir mask at 10–15l/min.

Otherwise, meet indicated target saturations with:

- Nasal cannulae 2–6L/min.
- Simple face mask.
- 5–10L/min.

If risk of hypercapnic failure (target stats 88–92%):

- Venturi mask 24% (if history of respiratory acidosis).
- Venturi mask 28%.
- Nasal cannulae at 1–2L/min.

All patients receiving oxygen therapy must have their oxygen saturation levels measured regularly and the concentrations of inspired oxygen titrated accordingly, with extra caution taken with individuals at risk of hypercapnia. While oxygen therapy is not beneficial to non-hypoxaemic individuals, a sudden drop in oxygen saturation of 3% or more is an early sign of acute deterioration, which should prompt further assessment. The target oxygen saturation rate is 94–98% unless the individual is at risk of hypercapnia, in which case the target is 88–92%. In serious illness with milder degrees of hypoxaemia, oxygen can be administered through nasal cannulae at 1–6L/min or by a simple face mask at 5–10L/min (a simple face mask must not be used at flow rates less than 5L/min, as this may result in carbon dioxide rebreathing). The medical team may also prescribe 24%, 28%, 35%, 40% or 60% oxygen via a venturi mask. When administrating oxygen via a venturi mask, it is important that the nurse sets the correct flow rate to ensure the correct percentage. The correct flow rates are indicated on the mask (2L/min for 24%, 4L/min for 28%, 8L/min for 35%, 10L/min for 40% and 15L/min for 60%). For individuals in respiratory distress with RR greater than 30/min, the flow of gas needs to be increased to meet the raised demand for flow. When using the **venturi mask,** this can be achieved by doubling oxygen flow rate; the design of the air entrainment port in the mask means that the percentage of oxygen delivered will remain the same.

Humidification not necessary for:

- Low flow oxygen.
- High flow oxygen for short term use (<24h).

In situations where hypoxaemia remains unresolved and hypercapnic failure is not present, high flow nasal cannula (HFNC) should be considered as an alternative to oxygen delivery via reservoir mask (Roca et al. 2016). This is an innovative treatment for adults with hypoxaemia not comfortable with or not responding well to standard therapy. Heated, humidified gas (an oxygen air mixture) can be delivered at up to 60L/minute via nasal prongs that fit snugly into the nares to prevent entrainment of room air. It is well-tolerated by many patients, as they are able to eat, drink and talk, and the heated humidification prevents oral and nasal dryness. It is suggested that dead space ventilation is reduced with nasal cannula, and that functional residual capacity is increased with a low level of positive end expiratory pressure. HFNC is recommended for moderate, but not severe respiratory failure. Close monitoring of respiratory status is necessary, as escalation to CPAP/intubation and ventilation may be required. CPAP is discussed later in this chapter.

Fixed performance masks, like Venturi masks, provide accurate concentrations of oxygen in situations where a low dose is important, people living with COPD at risk of carbon dioxide retention, for example: where the individual has a history of hypercapnic failure (requiring ventilation) 24% oxygen via a Venturi mask should be initiated, with a target saturation of 88–92%. Where the diagnosis is not known for someone over 50 years of age but who is a long-term smoker and has a complaint of chronic breathlessness then a diagnosis of COPD should be considered. Target saturations of 88–92% may be appropriate pending arterial blood gas analysis (British Thoracic Society Emergency Oxygen Clinical Development Group 2017).

The use of the most appropriate oxygen delivery system is essential if the patient is to receive the correct dosage of oxygen. It is for this reason that prescriptions for oxygen may stipulate a delivery system and the latest National Early Warning Score charts require nurses to document the oxygen delivery system, using the British Thoracic Society device codes (see Table 5.5) (British Thoracic Society Emergency Oxygen Guideline Development Group 2017). This is an essential part of patient monitoring and recording, particularly when increasing oxygen requirements are present clearly.

Where hypoxaemia is not corrected, or where there is hypercapnia, it may be necessary to establish ventilatory support. Nurses need to always practise safely by being aware of the correct use, limitations and hazards of common interventions including the use of medical devices and equipment (Nursing and Midwifery Council 2018b). Oxygen saturation can be a key indicator of acute illness and deterioration. Using the National Early Warning Score (NEWS) enables nurses to use oxygen saturation readings, alongside other vital signs, to establish the severity of deterioration. A competent decision-maker

Table 5.5 Abbreviations for oxygen-delivery systems for bedside charts and NEWS

Codes for recording supplemental oxygen (RCP, 2017)			
Code	*device*	*Code*	*device*
A	air	H28	humidified O_2 28%
N	nasal cannulae	H40	humidified O_2 40%
HFN	high-flow humidified oxygen via nasal	H60	humidified O_2 60%
V24	cannulae	RM	reservoir mask
V28	Venturi mask 24%	SM	simple face mask
V35	Venturi mask 28%	TM	tracheostomy mask
V40	Venturi mask 35%	CPAP	continuous positive airway pressure
V60	Venturi mask 40%	NIV	non-invasive ventilation

(British Thoracic Society Emergency Oxygen Clinical Development Group 2017)

Table 5.6 NEWS scoring system, SpO_2

Physiological Parameter	Score						
	3	2	1	0	1	2	3
SpO_2 (%) Scale 1	≤91	92–93	94–95	≥96			
SpO_2 (%) Scale 2	≤83	84–85	86–87	88–92 ≥93 on air	93–94 on oxygen	95–96 on oxygen	≥97 on oxygen
Air or oxygen		oxygen		air			

- For patients confirmed to have hypercapnic respiratory failure on blood gas analysis, either prior or on their current hospital admission, oxygen scale 2 on the NEWS chart should be used to record and score the oxygen saturation.
- The decision to use SpO_2 scale 2 should be made by a competent clinical decision-maker and should be recorded in the patient's clinical notes.
- In all other circumstances, the regular NEWS SpO_2 scale 1 should be used.
- For the avoidance of doubt, the SpO_2 scoring scale that is not being used should be clearly crossed out across the chart (Royal College of Physicians 2017).

will record the target saturations on the drug chart. However, as the nurse must establish the presence/increased risk of hypercapnic respiratory failure in order to use the NEWS 2 scale correctly, the importance of recording target saturations must not be underestimated. The NEWS 2 assessment tool uses two scales to assess the risk severity of low oxygen saturations, which reflect the different target oxygen saturation levels for patients in respiratory failure type 1 and respiratory failure type 2 (Royal College of Physicians 2017). Table 5.6 shows the two scales currently used on the latest National Early Warning Score (RCP 2017).

For further information on the nursing care of patients receiving oxygen therapy, review Dougherty, L. and Lister, S. (2015). *The Royal Marsden Hospital Manual of Clinical Nursing Procedures*. Student Edition. 9th Ed. Oxford. Wiley-Blackwell.

CASE STUDY 5.2 MRS PROCTOR WITH COPD: PART 2

Recognising deterioration

Following assessment, initial treatment included oxygen administration, IV hydrocortisone and nebulised bronchodilators. However, Mrs Proctor's increased respiratory rate, heart rate, and breathlessness with accessory muscle use reflected the increased work of breathing. The nurse is concerned that there is ongoing respiratory compromise. An arterial blood gas (ABG) analysis is performed at 12:00 and repeated at 12:30.

Observations at 12:00 reveal:

Breathing: RR 30, SpO_2 of 94% with 2 litres oxygen (NEWS 3 + 1 + 2) (note: in scale 2 SpO_2, 94% on oxygen scores 1).

Circulation: BP remains stable. HR: 118 (NEWS 0 + 2).

Disability: alert (NEWS 0).

Exposure: temp: 37.5 (NEWS 0).

NEWS = 8, emergency response:

> **Care escalation; attendance of team at SpR level with critical care competencies. Observations recorded every 15 minutes.**

SBAR is used to clearly communicate urgency of referral. SpR plans to attend immediately and asks the F2 to take an arterial blood gas sample to aid decision-making.

ABG results

Time	*12:00*	*12:30*
Normal Values		
pH (7.35–7.45)	7.31	7.29
PaO_2 (11–13.5kPa)	8.6kPa	8.4kPa
$PaCO_2$ (4.5–6.1kPa)	8.0kPa	8.7kPa
$HCO3^-$ (24–26mmol/L)	32mmol/L	33mmol/L
BE (-2 to +2)	+5	+6
SaO_2 (96–100%)	**94%**	91%
Oxygen	2 litres NS	1 litre NS
Mode	SV	SV

The above ABG analysis reveals a worsening trend. Initially, there is a partially compensated respiratory acidosis (pH 7.31/$PaCO_2$ 8.0kPa). There is an elevation in $PaCO_2$, with more carbonic acid generated (more hydrogen ions). Hypercapnia has resulted in renal compensation, and bicarbonate is reabsorbed (note raised [HCO_3^-] in an attempt to reduce hydrogen ions and acidosis. This renal compensation over time is typical in patients with COPD, who often have an increased bicarbonate (HCO_3^-) and a base excess (greater than +2).

With an acute rise in $PaCO_2$ levels, incomplete renal compensation probably accounts for the ongoing acidosis and symptoms of hypercapnia. An elevated $PaCO_2$ with increased levels in alveolar air can result in falling PaO_2 levels. Given that Mrs Proctor's PaO_2 and SaO_2 are higher than her target saturation, the oxygen is titrated down to 1 litre per minute.

The current National Early Warning Score of 8 requires that the medical SpR and Critical Care Outreach Team are alerted regarding the necessity for urgent review. The team notes the increasing respiratory rate and distress, widespread inspiratory wheezes and rising NEWS. The ABG analysis at 12:30 (worsening respiratory acidosis) confirms the deteriorating respiratory status. The team decide to arrange to transfer Mrs Proctor to a level 2 bed (ICS, 2009) for non-invasive ventilation (NIV) in the form of BiPAP and closer observation. This is in keeping with current guidelines urging such a move within the first 60 minutes of hospital arrival for all patients with an acute exacerbation of COPD who remain acidotic despite maximum standard medical treatment.

The outreach team arrive to support the ward with initiation of Bi-Level Positive Airway Pressure (BiPAP) with an IPAP of 14 and EPAP OF 4 (14/4), with 0.5 litres of entrained oxygen, and supervise the transfer to level 2 care

13:30

After an hour of treatment on BiPAP, in conjunction with the medical treatment:

Breathing: RR 22, SpO_2 of 92% with 0.5L oxygen, on BiPAP (NEWS 1 + 0 + 2).
Circulation: BP remains stable. HR: 105 (NEWS 0 + 1).
Disability: alert (NEWS 0).
Exposure: temp: 37.5 (NEWS 0).
NEWS now = 4.

ABG analysis confirms the clinical improvement, showing now a fully compensated respiratory acidosis, with $PaCO_2$ reducing. The nurse continues to record hourly observations, noting a reduction in her respiratory rate, heart rate and NEWS, and is somewhat reassured that Mrs Proctor is less distressed, stating that she feels a little better. Prompt recognition and appropriate intervention has prevented a medical emergency occurring.

Arterial blood gas results

Time	*13:30*
pH	7.39
PaO_2	9.0
$PaCO_2$	6.7
$HCO3$	29.7
BE	+4
SaO_2	93%
Oxygen	0.5 litre
Mode	BiPAP

Additional diagnostic data becomes available and the nurse is able to check this with earlier findings. The chest X-ray reveals hyper-inflated lungs and a flattened diaphragm, both characteristic of COPD. From the FBC and U&Es, she notes a raised WBC (20 $x10^{(9)}$/L) and elevated CRP (14.9mg/l), confirming the likelihood of a chest infection. Although potassium can rise in metabolic acidosis, this is normal at 4.9mmol/L. She notes a compensatory rise in haemoglobin of 17g/dl as a result of the longer-term hypoxaemia. Blood urea is slightly elevated at 10.6mmol/L and, with a sodium of 146mmol/L, suggests dehydration. Fortunately, creatinine is within normal limits at 84µmol/L, and the nurse is therefore reassured that renal function is most likely to be normal. Magnesium and phosphate are important electrolytes for respiratory muscle function, but these are within the normal range, with magnesium at 0.8mmol/L and phosphate at 1.4mmol/L.

A 12 lead ECG is recorded to rule out possible cardiac involvement; (cor pulmonale) is a concern but the ECG trace is normal.

There is no single diagnostic test for COPD. Therefore, making a diagnosis relies on clinical judgement based on a combination of history, physical examination and confirmation of airway obstruction. Once Mrs Proctor is more stable, she will require further lung function tests, including spirometry. Although the initial focus was on restoring physiological stability, nurses must be able to carry out a comprehensive systematic nursing assessment that takes into account not only physical but social, cultural, psychological, spiritual, and environmental factors in partnership with the patient, relatives and other professionals (Nursing and Midwifery Council 2018a).

Drug therapy

Bronchodilators are often prescribed where there is increased airflow obstruction. Although these are given via a hand-held inhaler, in acute care situations it is often necessary to administer these through a nebuliser.

Drugs such as salbutamol and terbutaline are beta 2 adrenergic agonists, as they stimulate beta 2 receptors on the cell membrane of smooth muscle cells throughout the airways. Activation of these receptors results in relaxation and dilatation of the airway lumen. Additional receptor sites can also be stimulated, however, and this results in a tachycardia with palpitations (beta 1 receptors) and muscle tremors (beta 2 receptors in skeletal muscle) as well as anxiety, headache and nervousness. Another group of bronchodilators is the anticholinergics (ipratropium bromide), which stimulate receptors (cholinergic) on the smooth muscle cell membrane, resulting in relaxation. Both groups are used for their rapid onset.

Bronchodilators will increase lumen size and therefore decrease both airway resistance and the work of breathing. They will also help with airway clearance and facilitate expectoration. By using a nebuliser, drugs can be administered in larger doses by inhalation as an aerosol over a short period of time. Usually a jet-nebulising chamber is used, and the aerosol is generated by using a flow rate of 6–8 litres/minute using piped air or oxygen (in hospital) or an electrical compressor (domiciliary use). Where there is a risk of hypercapnic failure, then nebulisers should be driven with air and, if necessary, low dose oxygen given at the same time through nasal cannulae.

In adults with acute asthma, when high doses of inhaled beta 2 agonists are required, there is no difference in delivery between nebulisers or by using a holding chamber (volume spacer) with a metered dose inhaler.

Magnesium sulphate also acts as a potent bronchodilator, although its precise physiological mechanism is not known. Nevertheless, it is used to reduce airway obstruction in acute cases, where other bronchodilator therapies have not worked, and the patient's life is at risk. It is currently recommended as a front-line treatment in life-threatening asthma when traditional bronchodilators have been ineffective.

Steroids may also be used because of their powerful anti-inflammatory properties. Inhaled steroids are effective in reducing exacerbations in both asthma and COPD. Oral steroids also can reduce airway inflammation and should be prescribed for all patients experiencing an acute asthma attack. Normally, oral doses of prednisolone, 40–50mg daily for up to 5 days, are administered. Intravenous hydrocortisone is a potent anti-inflammatory, but has many common side effects, such as Cushing's syndrome, electrolyte imbalance, fluid retention and cognitive impairment, and therefore is normally reserved for life-threatening respiratory conditions such as airway obstruction secondary to anaphylactic shock or life-threatening asthma (British Thoracic Society Scottish Intercollegiate Guidelines Network 2016).

Ongoing evaluation of prescribed medication is important, and where agreed parameters (including respiratory rate/depth, SpO_2, PaO_2 and $PaCO_2$) are not achieved, the doctor should be informed so that the treatment plan can be reviewed.

Chest drains

A tension pneumothorax is a medical emergency, and once diagnosed, a needle is inserted without delay on the affected side (midclavicular line/second intercostal space) to allow the air to escape (with an audible 'hiss'). Where a chest drain is inserted into the pleural cavity to remove air, pus or blood, it is connected to an underwater seal drainage system. There are a number of devices available, but all provide a one-way valve, allowing the movement of air and fluid in one direction only. Conventionally, a drainage bottle is filled with sterile water and the tube must be below the water level (2cm), otherwise air will enter the pleural cavity during inspiration (see Figure 5.8). In a pneumothorax, air bubbles will be visible, as air is displaced from the pleural cavity during expiration and coughing. The doctor may request low-level suction (e.g., 5kPa) to facilitate removal of air and/or fluid. The drainage bottle must be kept below the level of the chest, and clamping of drains avoided, as this can result in a tension pneumothorax. Clamps should be available, however, in case the system

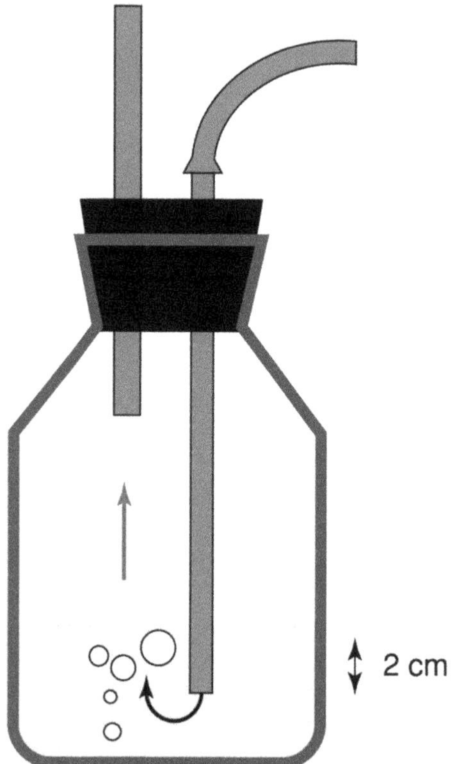

Figure 5.8 Underwater seal drainage.

becomes disconnected. Pain is experienced on insertion, during drainage and on removal of a chest drain, and adequate pain relief must be offered.

Following insertion, it is important to observe the following:

- Respiratory status.
- Fluid level and amount of any drainage.
- Fluid level swing.
- Underwater bubbling (air is removal).
- Dressing and site of insertion.
- Patency of drainage tubing.

For further information on intrapleural drainage see:

Dougherty, L. and Lister, S. (2015). *The Royal Marsden Hospital Manual of Clinical Nursing Procedures*. Student Edition. 9th Ed. Oxford. Wiley Blackwell.

Chest physiotherapy

The nurse and physiotherapist will work collaboratively to reduce breathlessness and the work of breathing, and improve ventilation and the expectoration of secretions. Various techniques may be employed, but the efficacy of physiotherapy may vary depending on the clinical context. Ongoing evaluation is crucial, as some interventions can lead to worsening hypoxaemia. Patients will need encouragement to expectorate and effective pain relief may be necessary before this can be achieved. Active Cycle of Breathing Techniques are often utilised by the physiotherapist, and the nurse should be able to encourage the patients with some of the following exercises:

- Thoracic expansion.
- Breathing control.
- Forced expiratory technique ('huffing').

Where there is difficulty in the expectoration of sputum, then nebulised isotonic saline is often effective.

Non-invasive ventilation

Situations where NIV may be beneficial:

- Pulmonary oedema with hypoxaemia.
- COPD (with respiratory acidosis).
- Hypercapnic failure.
- Obstructive sleep apnoea.
- Pneumonia.
- Post-operative hypoxaemia.

Where hypoxemia and/or hypercapnia are not controlled by other means, then non-invasive ventilation (NIV) may be beneficial. For patients with hypoxaemia in the absence of hypercapnia, continuous positive airway pressure (CPAP) is the treatment of choice, whereas for patients with hypercapnia, where enhanced ventilation is required, bi-level positive airway pressure (BiPAP) is recommended. When referring to NIV, it is important to clarify whether CPAP or BiPAP is being used, as each are used in different clinical circumstances.

Advantages of NIV:

- Increase in tidal volume.
- Recruitment of alveoli.
- Increase in FRC.
- Increased surface area for gaseous exchange.
- Improved oxygenation.
- Increase in lung compliance.
- Reduced work of breathing.
- Reduced risk of infection.
- Sedation avoided.

In health, expiration involves muscle relaxation and elastic recoil with zero airway pressure. By applying positive pressure during expiration (called positive end expiratory pressure, or PEEP), oxygenation can be improved significantly. These techniques utilise a nasal, oral/nasal or full face mask (see Figure 5.9) rather than tracheal tubes and

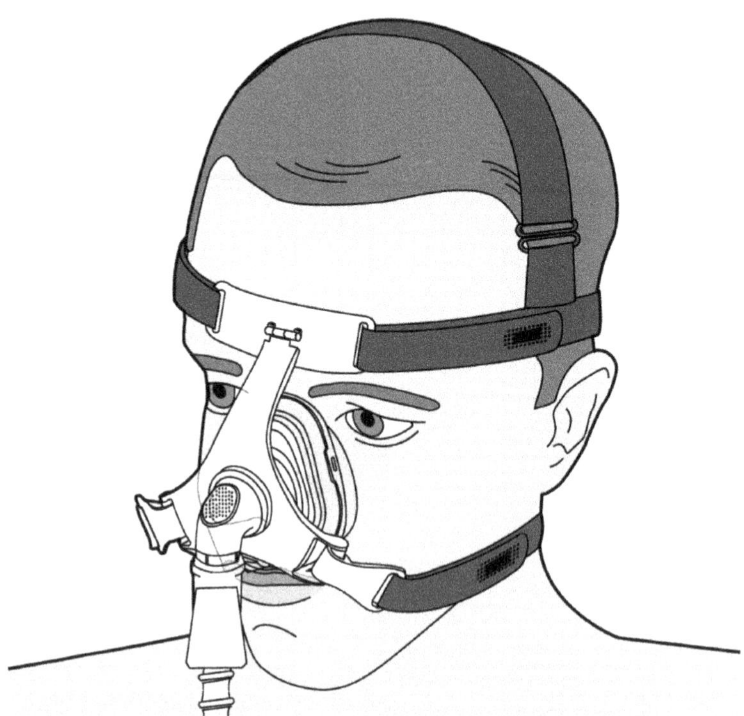

Figure 5.9 Masks for NIV.

tracheostomy, thus minimising the risk of complications. The current BTS guidance recommends that full face masks should be used unless the patient finds them claustrophobic, where nasal masks may be beneficial (British Thoracic Society/Intensive Care Society Acute Hypercapnic Respiratory Failure Guideline Development Group 2016).

Continuous positive airway pressure (CPAP)

CPAP is beneficial for individuals with acute hypoxemic respiratory failure (type 1 failure), post-operative atelectasis, heart failure and pneumonia. Although CPAP does not offer any ventilatory support, it applies a constant positive pressure throughout both inspiration and expiration, with an increase in alveolar recruitment and functional residual capacity. CPAP systems all have a flow generator, which delivers a constant pressure of gas throughout the respiratory cycle. The increased pressure reduces respiratory effort in inspiration and prevents alveolar collapse on expiration by exerting an end expiratory pressure, increasing the surface area for gaseous exchange. An end expiratory pressure of around 10cm H_2O is beneficial, as this facilitates the recruitment of alveoli, improving FRC and oxygenation.

Bi-level positive airway pressure (BiPAP)

BiPAP is beneficial for individuals with acute hypercapnic respiratory failure (type 2 failure). BiPAP enables different pressures to be delivered during inspiration and expiration, therefore providing ventilatory support. A BiPAP machine will not only sense the patient's inspiratory effort and provide an inspiratory volume, but will apply positive pressure during expiration (PEEP). As a result, partial pressures of arterial oxygen and carbon dioxide can be improved, with work of breathing reduced (Shah, 2018).

The main clinical indication for the application of BiPAP is evidence of acute hypercapnic respiratory failure dictated by arterial blood gas analysis. A serum pH of less than 7.35, $PaCO_2$ greater than 6.5kPa and a respiratory rate greater than 23 respirations per minute, all of which persist after bronchodilator therapy and oxygen therapy, indicate that BiPAP is required. Application of positive pressure during breathing can be a little claustrophobic for some, and the patient will need support and encouragement if treatment is to be effective.

Recommended initial pressure settings depend on the underlying cause of the respiratory failure. An EPAP of 3cm of water and an IPAP of 15cm of water is recommended initially, except in cases of respiratory failure secondary to neuromuscular disease, when an IPAP of 10cm of water is more appropriate. Back up rates of 16–20 respirations per minute are recommended, but inspiratory and expiratory (I:E) ratios differ. In most cases, an I:E ratio of 1:1 is recommended, but in respiratory disease I:E ratios of 1:2 or 1:3 may be required.

Contraindications for non-invasive ventilation:

pH less than 7.15 (or less than 7.25 in the presence of one of the following):

- Glasgow coma scale less than 8.
- Confusion/agitation.
- Cognitive impairment that warrants enhanced observation.

(British Thoracic Society/Intensive Care Society Acute Hypercapnic Respiratory Failure Guideline Development Group 2016)

Non-invasive ventilation (NIV) should not be considered in people with severe facial deformity, severe facial burns or a fixed airway obstruction. There are also potential contraindications to NIV, of which nurses must be aware. However, their presence should not automatically lead to a decision to withhold NIV. Rather, the presence of contraindications should lead to a higher level of monitoring/higher level of care. In the main, where nurses are familiar with NIV, trials may be carried out in level 1 areas. In cases where individuals are acutely unwell and where increased monitoring is required, patients trialling NIV should be nursed in level 2 areas. Transfer to a level 3 area must be considered where impending an respiratory arrest is suspected, NIV fails to enhance chest wall expansion, arterial $PaCO_2$ levels remain high with decreasing pH(<7.15) and/or PaO_2 fails to rise above 85% (British Thoracic Society/Intensive Care Society Acute Hypercapnic Respiratory Failure Guideline Development Group 2016).

If nursed in a level 1 area of care, ongoing monitoring of the patient during non-invasive ventilation remains very important, and the following parameters must be monitored:

- Heart rate and respiratory rate.
- Blood pressure.
- Oxygen saturation.
- Cardiac monitoring, where necessary.
- Degree of respiratory distress.
- Accessory muscle use.
- Presence of cyanosis.
- Orientation.
- Risk of aspiration.

If effective, NIV should result in an improvement in oxygenation and a reduction in respiratory acidosis with a decrease in carbon dioxide. In patients with COPD, oxygen saturations of 88–92% will be acceptable.

Nutrition and fluid balance

Insensible water loss will be greater with an increased respiratory rate, pyrexia and an increase in ambient temperature. This can result in decreased mucociliary clearance and secretion retention, which can also be caused by the administration of oxygen. Where low flow oxygen is given, humidification is not required, nor is it necessary for short term use of high flow oxygen (less than 24 hours). However, it is important that fluid intake and hydration status is monitored carefully, including skin turgor, urine output and the condition of oral mucous membranes and tongue. Unless contraindicated, fluid intake should be increased with regular sips encouraged and swallowed during expiration. Poor nutritional status and electrolyte imbalance can also affect respiratory status, and measures should be taken to correct any imbalance.

Psychological care

Breathlessness is extremely frightening and can generate increased anxiety and stress, which in turn will increase the demand for oxygen. Care providers must convey a sense of calmness and efficiency around the bed area, as this will increase patient confidence.

Therapeutic touch as well as procedural touch is important when offering reassurance, and it reduces fear, as does ongoing effective communication and education. Indeed, all nurses must build partnerships and therapeutic relationships through safe, effective and non-discriminatory communication, taking into account individual differences, capabilities and needs (Nursing and Midwifery Council 2018b). Information-giving to patients and, wherever possible, including them in the decision-making process will enable them to remain in control.

Conclusion

The respiratory system is very efficient in ensuring that oxygen delivery is facilitated effectively to meet the demand of the cells. However, in the acutely ill individual, respiratory compromise may occur very quickly, resulting in profound hypoxaemia and possible life-threatening cellular hypoxia. Although primary respiratory disease can be responsible for respiratory compromise, pathology outside the respiratory system can also contribute to problems with oxygen delivery. Physiological responses activated as a result of disease or surgical intervention trigger complex neurohormonal adaptive pathways including the stress response. This will result in increased global oxygen consumption, and the respiratory system may have limited reserves to mobilise an effective response.

The skilled nurse has a sound theoretical knowledge of respiratory physiology and the many factors possibly contributing to respiratory problems. A comprehensive, holistic assessment will facilitate early detection and, through ongoing vigilance in monitoring the patient, potential problems can be anticipated and appropriate measures taken to prevent further deterioration. Before changes are seen in oxygen saturation values, there are often earlier signs of respiratory compromise, and ongoing inspection of the patient and recording of observations is paramount.

Individual risk in relation to the development of respiratory problems can be affected by a host of different factors. Patients admitted into hospital bring with them added risks of deterioration, their general physical health, smoking history, primary diagnosis, age, gender, ethnicity, socioeconomic and mental health status, for example. Following admission, additional contextual and environmental factors can increase risk further. Immobility, poor positioning, suboptimal hydration and nutritional status, increased ambient temperatures, use of sedation, prolonged oxygen administration, invasive procedures, infection control practices and poor communication with increased stress can all increase risk significantly. The nurse has a key role to play in not only assessing individual risk and identifying those who are particularly vulnerable, but also through skilled nursing intervention and management of the care environment in the prevention of respiratory complications.

Glossary 

Acute Severe Asthma A classification of asthma severity. Those with acute severe asthma will have any **one** of a number of symptoms (RR≥25/min, HR ≥110/min, PEF between 35–50 of best or predicted, inability to complete sentence in one breath)Hospital admission may be necessary if they fail to sufficiently respond to treatment given.

Airway resistance Relating to flow of air through the airways where narglossentrying of the lumen increases resistance and therefore the work of breathing.

Atelectasis Collapse of alveoli, which results in loss of surface area for gaseous exchange.

Atmospheric pressure Also called barometric pressure, which is 101kPa at sea level and falls with increasing altitude.

Anatomical dead space The anatomical sections of the respiratory tract, down to and including terminal bronchioles, where air is not available for gaseous exchange (conducting zone).

BiPAPBi-level positive airway pressure ventilation This non-invasive ventilation therapy delivers a pressurised flow of air. BiPAP delivers two different levels, IPAP (inspiratory positive airways pressure) and EPAP (expiratory positive airways pressure), through a face or nasal mask.

Carbonic acid Formed by carbon dioxide in solution and also referred to as a volatile acid which can be removed from the body by increasing ventilation.

Cholinergic Relating to acetylcholine, as in parasympathetic nerves, which release this as a neurotransmitter.

Compliance work Relating to the work involved in distending the lungs and chest wall during inspiration.

CPAP (Continuous positive airways pressure) A form of respiratory support that delivers a constant stream of pressurised air through a fitted face mask, creating a positive pressure to assist inspiration and help keep the alveolar open at the end of expiration though positive end expired pressure (PEEP).

Endotracheal tube A tube which is placed into the trachea to protect the airway. ET tubes are cuffed to prevent inhalation of gastric contents and enable positive pressure ventilation.

Fibre optic bronchoscopy A bronchoscope is passed through the nose or mouth into the air passages. The scope has many small glass fibres that transmit light and enable visual inspection.

Functional residual capacity The amount of air left in the lungs, at the end of quiet expiration, that continues to be involved in gaseous exchange.

Hypercapnia A rise in carbon dioxide in arterial blood as a result of reduced ventilation.

Hypoxia A reduced partial pressure of oxygen in the cells.

Hypoxaemia A reduced oxygen partial pressure in arterial blood.

Immunoglobulin There are 5 sub-classes of immunoglobulins or antibodies – IgA, IgG, IgD, IgM and IgE, which are released by B lymphocytes.

Life-threatening asthma A classification of asthma severity present if any **one** of a number of clinical findings present (PEF<33% predicted, SpO_2<92%, Normal $PaCO_2$, silent chest, poor respiratory effort, arrhythmia. Exhaustion, altered consciousness, hypotension). Admission to critical care is usually indicated.

Macrophages Mature monocytes (type of leucocyte or white blood cell), which mature and leave the circulation.

Medulla oblongata Lower portion of the brain stem which contains the vital centres.

Near fatal asthma A classification of asthma severity present if $PaCO_2$ is raised, or mechanical ventilation is required.

Neurohormonal Relating to nerves and hormones released from endocrine glands. Important communication system in the body.

Ondine A water nymph who, according to German folklore curses her unfaithful husband so that breathing stops if he should ever fall asleep again.

Oxygen delivery (DO_2) The oxygen delivered to the cells which is dependent on oxygen saturation, haemoglobin and cardiac output. This is 1000mL/min at rest.

Oxygen consumption (VO_2) The oxygen utilised by the cells, which will vary according to metabolic demand. This is 250 mL/minute at rest.

Parasympathetic Division of the autonomic nervous system which results, for example, in narglossentrying of bronchioles and slowing of the heart rate.

Pathogenic Resulting in disease (e.g., pathogenic micro-organisms).

Peak expiratory flow The greatest flow rate on forced expiration, starting with a maximum inspiration and measured in litres per minute.

Pulmonary capillaries Tiny blood vessels where the walls are only one cell thick, therefore facilitating gaseous exchange in the lungs.

Pulse oximeter Probe attached to the finger or ear lobe that monitors the percentage of haemoglobin (Hb) saturated with oxygen.

Respiratory Centre Located in the medulla oblongata of the brain stem, close to the fourth ventricle of the brain which contains cerebrospinal fluid.

Surfactant Substance secreted by alveolar cells that helps to stabilise the alveoli, preventing collapse.

Sympathetic Division of the autonomic nervous system which results, for example, in dilatation of bronchioles and an increase in heart rate.

Tracheal intubation Insertion of an endotracheal tube between the vocal cords into the trachea for the administration of oxygen and assisted ventilation.

Tracheostomy An opening made into the front of the trachea so that a tube (temporary or permanent) can be inserted.

TEST YOURSELF 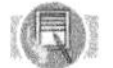

1 Oxygen is required by the cells for which of the following?:
   a. Anaerobic metabolism
   b. Aerobic metabolisms
2 The anatomical relationship between the visceral and parietal pleural membranes creates a pleural pressure that is:
   a. Negative (sub atmospheric)
   b. Positive (atmospheric)
3 The inspiratory muscles include (circle all that apply):
   a. Abdominals
   b. Internal intercostals
   c. Diaphragm
   d. External intercostals
4 The respiratory centre is found in the ________________ of the brain and is stimulated by rising levels of ____________________.
5 Cholinergic nerves in the lungs stimulate cholinergic receptors resulting in:
   a. Reduced airway lumen size
   b. Increased airway lumen size
6 Oxygen delivery to the cells is dependent on (circle all that apply):
   a. Oxygen saturation
   b. Carbon dioxide
   c. Water vapour
   d. Haemoglobin

7 The following respiratory disorders result in increased airway resistance (circle all that apply):
   a. Pneumonia
   b. COPD
   c. Pleurisy
   d. Asthma
8 Atopy results in a hypersensitivity reaction involving which of the following immunoglobulins:
   a. IgD
   b. IgM
   c. IgE
   d. IgA
9 A young patient, aged 30 years, presents acutely ill with an oxygen saturation of 84%. Which one of the following oxygen devices would be appropriate?:
   a. Simple mask at 5L/min
   b. Nasal Cannulae at 6L/min
   c. Non re-breather reservoir mask at 12L/min
   d. Venturi mask at 4L/min
10 Effective positioning of the patient will help to facilitate improved gaseous exchange by increasing the following:
   a. Tidal volume
   b. Inspiratory reserve volume
   c. Functional residual capacity
   d. Residual volume

Answers

1 b
2 a
3 c and d
4 Medulla Oblongata / Carbon Dioxide
5 a
6 a and d
7 b and d
8 c
9 c
10 c

References

British Thoracic Society. (2010). *BTS Pleural Disease Guideline 2010*. Online. Available at: https://www.brit-thoracic.org.uk/document-library/guidelines/pleural-disease/bts-pleural-disease-guideline/ [Accessed 3rd May 2019].

British Thoracic Society/Intensive Care Society Acute Hypercapnic Respiratory Failure Guideline Development Group. (2016). BTS/*ICS Guidelines for the Ventilatory Management of Acute Respiratory*

Failure in Adults. Online. Available at: https://www.brit-thoracic.org.uk/document-library/guidelines/niv/btsics-guideline-for-the-ventilatory-management-of-acute-hypercapnic-respiratory-failure-in-adults/ [Accessed 26th July 2019].

British Thoracic Society Emergency Oxygen Guideline Development Group. (2017). BTS guideline for oxygen use in adults in healthcare and emergency settings. *Thorax*, 72(Supplement 1). Online. Available at: https://www.brit-thoracic.org.uk/quality-improvement/guidelines/emergency-oxygen/ [Accessed 10th June 2019].

British Thoracic Society Scottish Intercollegiate Guidelines Network. (2019). BTS/*SIGN British Guideline on the Management of Asthma*. Available at: https://www.brit-thoracic.org.uk/quality-improvement/guidelines/asthma/ [Accessed August 2019].

Intensive Care Society. (2009). Levels of critical care for adult patients. Available at http://icmwk.com/wp-content/uploads/2014/02/Revised-Levels-of-Care-21-12-09.pdf [Accessed August 2020].

Lim WS, van der Eerden MM, Laing R, et al. (2003). Defining community-acquired pneumonia severity on presentation to hospital: an international derivation and validation study. *Thorax*, 58, 377–382.

National Institute for Health and Care Excellence. (2014). *Pneumonia in Adults: Diagnosis and Management*. Online. Available at: https://www.nice.org.uk/guidance/cg191/resources/pneumonia-in-adults-diagnosis-and-management-pdf-35109868127173 [Accessed 19th July 2019].

National Institute for Health and Care Excellence. (2016). *Chronic Obstructive Pulmonary Disease in Adults*. Online. Available at: https://www.nice.org.uk/guidance/qs10/resources/chronic-obstructive-pulmonary-disease-in-adults-pdf-2098478592709 [Accessed 10th June 2019].

National Institute for Health and Care Excellence. (2018). *Chronic Obstructive Pulmonary Disease in Over 16s: Diagnosis and Management*. Online. Available at: https://www.nice.org.uk/guidance/ng115/resources/chronic-obstructive-pulmonary-disease-in-over-16s-diagnosis-and-management-pdf-66141600098245 [Accessed 10th June 2019].

NHS Improvement. (2018). *Patient Safely Alert: Risk of Harm Form Inappropriate Pulse Oximeter Placements NHS/PSA/W/2018/009*. Available at: https://improvement.nhs.uk/documents/3603/Patient_Safety_Alert_-_Placement_of_oximetry_probes_FINAL.pdf [Accessed August 2019].

Nursing and Midwifery Council. (2018a). *Future Nurse: Standards of Proficiency for Registered Nurses*. Online. Available at: https://www.nmc.org.uk/globalassets/sitedocuments/education-standards/future-nurse-proficiencies.pdf [Accessed 3rd May 2019].

Nursing and Midwifery Council. (2018b). *The Code: Professional Standards of Practice and Behaviour for Nurses, Midwives and Nursing Associates*. Online. Available at: https://www.nmc.org.uk/standards/code/ [Accessed 10th June 2019].

O'Driscoll, BR., Howard, LS., Earis, J., Mak, V. (2017). BTS guideline for oxygen use in adults in healthcare and emergency settings. *Thorax*, 17, i1–i90.

Resuscitation Council UK. (2012). *Emergency Treatment of Anaphylactic Reactions. Guidelines for Healthcare Providers*. Online. Available at: https://www.resus.org.uk/anaphylaxis/emergency-treatment-of-anaphylactic-reactions/ [Accessed 3rd May 2019].

Roca O, Hernandez G, Diaz-Lobato S, Carratala J, Gutierrez R, Masclans J. (2016). Current evidence for the effectiveness of heated humidified high flow nasal cannula supportive therapy in adult patients with respiratory failure. *Critical Care*, 20, 109. Available at: https://link.springer.com/article/10.1186/s13054-016-1263-z.

Royal College Of Physicians. (2017). National Early Warning Score (NEWS) 2. Available at https://www.rcplondon.ac.uk/projects/outputs/national-early-warning-score-news-2 [Accessed August 2020].

Shah NM. (2018). Update: non-invasive ventilation in chronic obstructive pulmonary disease. *Journal of Thoracic Disease*, 10, S71–S79.

6 The patient with acute cardiovascular problems

Helen Dutton and Sharon Elliot

AIM

This chapter aims to give a clear understanding of the normal anatomy and applied physiology of the cardiac and circulatory systems and to explain how altered physiology can lead to acute deterioration. An improved understanding of these principles will enhance nursing assessment and recognition of acute problems, and enable an appropriate response to medical emergencies caused by cardiac and circulatory disorders.

OBJECTIVES

At the end of this chapter you will be able to:

- Describe the major structures and components of the cardiovascular system, the heart, coronary artery circulation and conduction system, and understand the physiological processes that generate and maintain cardiac output.
- Describe the structure and function of blood, mechanisms of clotting and the ABO and rhesus systems.
- Describe the arterial and venous system and the peripheral circulation, and understand common problems of the circulatory system.
- Describe the nurse's role in assessing the cardiovascular system.
- Identify common problems and medical emergencies related to the cardiovascular system, and understand how these are identified and managed.
- Consider the role of haemodynamic monitoring in the assessment and management of therapies that optimise cardiac output and the functioning of the cardiovascular system.

Introduction

The cardiovascular system is responsible for the circulation of blood to and from the organs and tissues of the body. Blood must be transported under a sufficient pressure to facilitate adequate movement of oxygen, nutrients, hormones, electrolytes, water and other blood products to their target locations. In addition to being a transportation system to the tissues of the body, the cardiovascular system facilitates the removal of waste products from cellular activity.

Applied physiology

The cardiovascular system is a continuous circuit that is comprised of three principle components:

- The heart.
- The blood.
- The arterial and venous system.

The heart

The heart is responsible for providing the continuous motion of blood as it travels around the arterial and venous system. The pumping action of the heart is generated by the contraction of the muscle fibres that surround the heart's four chambers. The force of this contraction will remain relatively constant during periods of rest and activity; each time that the heart contracts, a volume of blood (**stroke volume**) will leave the heart and either be distributed around the arterial system or to the lungs for oxygenation, depending on which side of the heart the blood leaves. The heart has a right and a left side. The right side of the heart collects blood that returns from the organs and tissues of the body via the venous system. This blood is deoxygenated and has a relatively high concentration of carbon dioxide. Therefore, the principle function of the right side of the heart is to move this venous blood back to the lungs, where it can remove its carbon dioxide and take on more oxygen from inspired air. After this process, the blood then moves back into the left side of the heart so that it can be distributed around the body via the arterial system. Figure 6.1 provides an overview of the cardiovascular system.

Each side of the heart is comprised of two chambers, an atrium and a ventricle. The atria are the smaller chambers and act as a conduit for blood to be collected and transferred into the ventricles. The ventricles are the larger chambers and move the blood out of the heart. The right ventricular wall has a thinner wall than that of the left ventricle, as it is only required to eject the blood into the pulmonary circulation, whereas the left ventricle is required to send the blood out to the peripheries of the body under sufficient pressure to facilitate the perfusion of the tissues. Hence, the left ventricle has a considerably greater muscle mass in comparison to the right ventricle.

The ventricles are each enclosed by 2 heart valves. These valves are responsible for ensuring that blood is not displaced backwards during ventricular contraction (**systole**) (please see Figure 6.2).

These valves are:

- Tricuspid: separates the right atrium and the right ventricle.
- Mitral: separates the left atrium and the left ventricle.
- Pulmonic: controls outflow of blood from the right ventricle to the Pulmonary artery.
- Aortic: controls the outflow of blood from the left ventricle to the Aorta.

Layers of the heart

The heart is primarily a muscular pump and possesses many muscle fibres. However, there are other structures that allow it to keep its shape and location in the thorax. The heart has 3 primary layers:

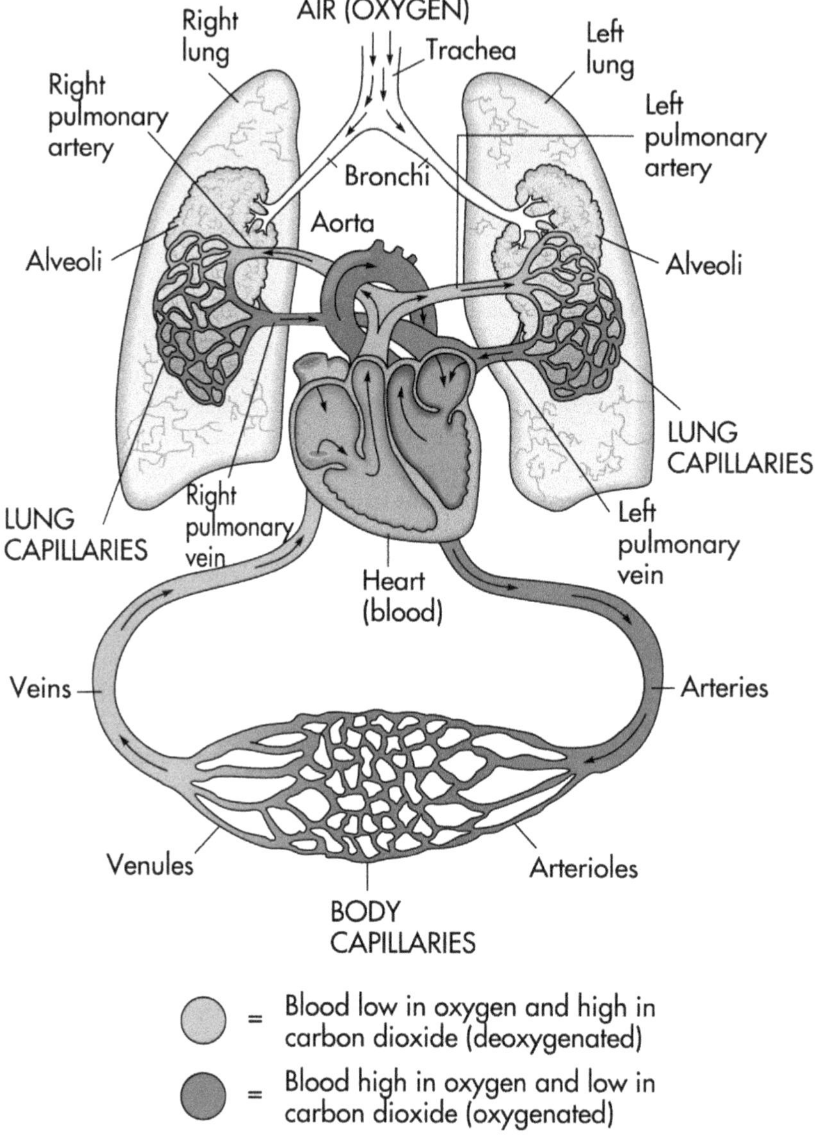

Figure 6.1 Overview of the cardiovascular system.

- The **endocardium**.
- The **myocardium**.
- The **pericardium**.

Endocardium

The innermost layer of the heart is a thin layer of **endothelium** and connective tissue that is continuous with the lining of the blood vessels that supply and are supplied by the

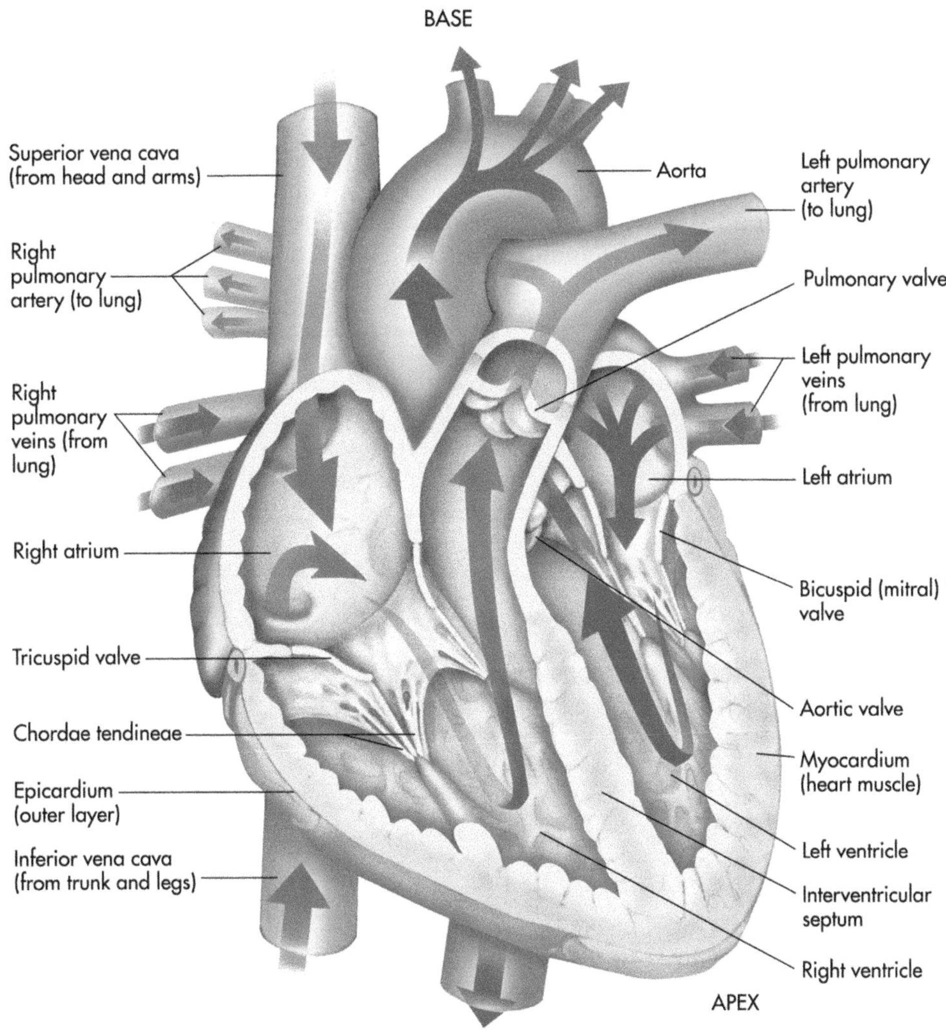

Figure 6.2 The anatomy of the heart, showing direction of blood flow.

heart. The endothelial layer is responsible for expressing anti-thrombotic factors to prevent blood from adhering to the endocardium.

Myocardium

The middle layer of the heart is the myocardium. This is the thickest layer of the heart and is responsible for providing muscular contraction so that blood can be ejected from the chambers that it surrounds. There is a layer of myocardium around the atria and the ventricles. The muscle fibres of the myocardium are laid end-to-end so that they can contract in a wave-like motion when stimulated. The myocardium requires a constant supply of oxygenated blood which is provided by the coronary arteries.

Pericardium

The outermost layer of the heart is the pericardial sack. This is a rigid structure that prevents the heart from over-stretching during systole and helps the heart to maintain its shape. The pericardium is also attached to the chest wall to prevent excessive movement of the heart during activity.

Between the pericardium and the myocardium is the epicardial layer, which covers the surface of the myocardium. These layers are not attached to one another, and there is a small amount of pericardial fluid between them. This fluid prevents friction damage from the rigid pericardium when the myocardium contracts and relaxes.

The coronary circulation

The myocardium and the **conduction system** require a continuous supply of blood for normal function. The heart supplies itself with blood directly from the aorta as it leaves the left ventricle. Two small openings (ostia) are located just above the aortic valve leaflets, and blood flows into the **coronary circulation** during **diastole**, the relaxed phase of the cardiac cycle. The two main coronary arteries are the right coronary artery (RCA) and the left coronary artery (LCA)(please see Figure 6.3).

Individual variance in coronary artery blood supply to the posterior surface of the heart:

- For approximately 70% of the population, this is provided by the RCA.
- For 20% of the population, this is provided by the LCA.
- For the remaining 10%, supply is provided by both.

The right coronary artery tree

The RCA extends round inferiorly and posteriorly across the right ventricle and around to the posterior surface of the heart. Branches called the marginal arteries supply the anterior and lateral surface of the right ventricle. The posterior surface of the heart is supplied by the posterior descending artery (PDA).

Remember

Inferior	underneath
Posterior	back
Anterior	front
Lateral	side

The left coronary artery tree

The LCA divides into two main arteries: the left anterior descending artery (LAD) and the Circumflex (CX). The LAD extends down across the surface of the heart supplying the left ventricle. The LAD has a number of branches that supply the interventricular

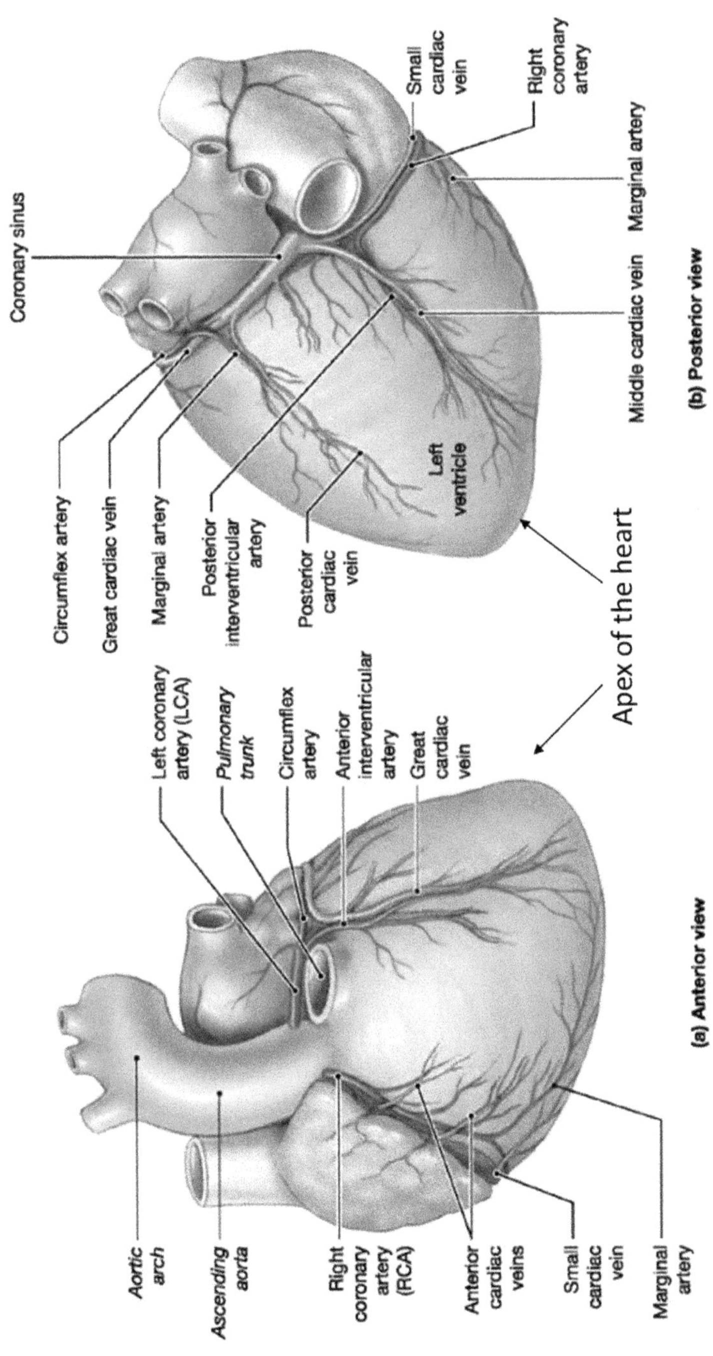

Figure 6.3 Coronary artery circulation.

septum (the septal arteries) and the anterior surface of the left ventricle (the diagonal arteries). The LAD terminates at the apex of the heart.

The circumflex extends around towards the lateral and posterior surfaces of the left ventricle, and in some cases may supply the posterior descending artery.

Cardiac conduction system

The cardiac conduction system is responsible for the maintenance of the correct sequence and timing of events that lead to the movement of blood through the heart. For the cardiac cycle to result in adequate **cardiac output**, the heart's muscular walls need to be activated in the appropriate direction to make sure that the displacement of blood from the atria and ventricles are efficient.

The cardiac conduction system is comprised of conduction cells. These cells are able to generate their own impulse, known as auto-rhythmic cells. They are responsible for the production and transmission of electrical waves that cross the heart and stimulate the myocardium to contract. The conduction cells do not contract themselves but purely provide the stimulus for adjacent myocardial cells to do so. The conduction system is illustrated in Figure 6.4.

Each cell of the conduction system has the ability to spontaneously generate electrical potentials that move in a wave-like motion across the heart. However, the Sinoatrial (SA) node is the primary source of all normal electrical activity in the heart.

Sinoatrial node

The sinoatrial (SA) node is the pacemaker of the heart and can spontaneously become activated (depolarise) at a fixed rate. This inbuilt heartrate is around 100 beats per minute and is referred to as the rate of automaticity. Each cell of the cardiac conduction system has its own rate of **automaticity**, but the further down in the conduction system the cell is, the slower its rate of automaticity. In order for the heart rate to be increased in times of need and for it to slow down at times of rest, the SA node is controlled externally by the sympathetic and para-sympathetic branches of the **autonomic nervous system**. The **sympathetic nervous system** has an excitatory effect on the heart, making it beat faster during exercise, stress, pain or increased metabolic need.

The SA node's rate of automaticity is slightly too fast for normal resting activity or sleeping. Therefore, the SA node is constantly being slowed down, according to the metabolic requirements, via the vagus nerve of the **parasympathetic nervous system**. So, despite the intrinsic rate of automaticity of the SA node being 100 beats per minute, the heart rate that we accept as being normal (60–100) is actually maintained mostly by the autonomic nervous system.

Once the SA node depolarises, the wave of **depolarisation** spreads across the atria via internodal pathways. These ensure that the atria both depolarise at the same time and that the contraction of the atria occurs in a downward motion (allowing the blood to be pushed down into the ventricles).

Atrioventricular node

The **atrioventricular (AV) node** is the only conduit for electrical stimulation to move from the atria through to the ventricles. In this respect, the AV node has an important

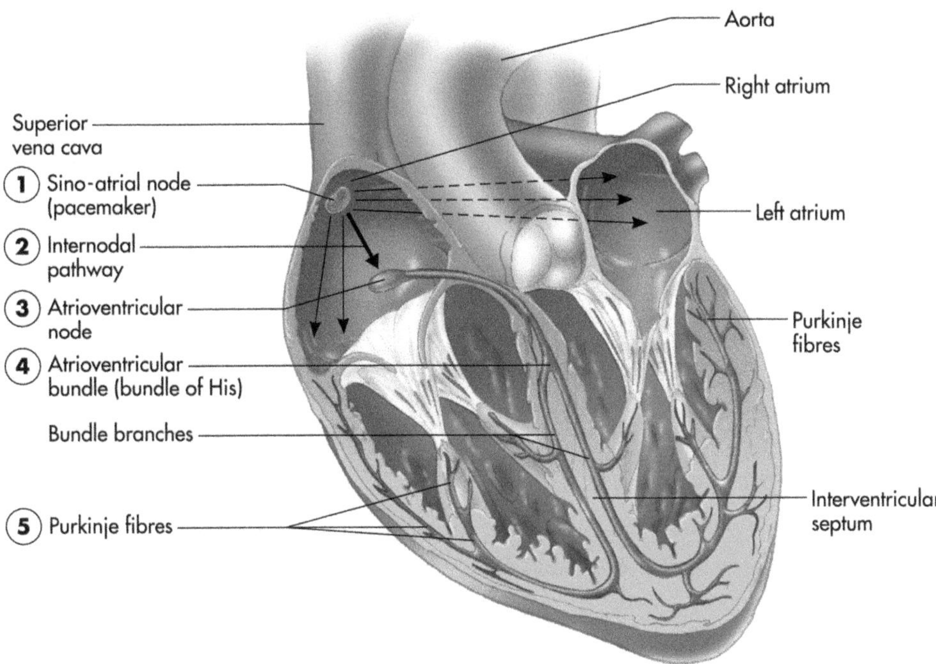

1. The sino-atrial (SA) node fires a stimulus across the walls of both left and right atria, causing them to contract.
2. The stimulus arrives at the atrioventricular (AV) node.
3. The stimulus is directed to follow the AV bundle (bundle of His).
4. The stimulus now travels through the apex of the heart through the bundle branches.
5. The Purkinje fibres distribute the stimulus across both ventricles, causing ventricular contraction.

Figure 6.4 The conduction system of the heart.

regulatory function when the SA node depolarises too quickly or when there is an atrial arrhythmia.

When the wave of depolarisation completes its journey across the atria, it reaches the AV node. Here there is a small delay, before the ventricles become depolarised. This delay lasts only around 0.1 seconds, but is sufficient time for the blood to be ejected from the atria and into the ventricles. The AV node is also under the control of the parasympathetic nervous system, to slow down the heart rate by increasing the period of delay.

Ventricular conduction system

The conduction of the ventricles is co-ordinated by the bundle branches. There are three main conduction fibres that distribute the wave of depolarisation across ventricular myocardium: the right bundle branch, the left anterior fascicle and the left posterior fascicle. When these fibres are depolarised normally, the two ventricular masses contract simultaneously. However, if there is a block or delay in any of these pathways, then there will be a degree of dyssynchrony in the timing between the ventricles, causing an ineffective ejection. The Purkinje fibres are the most distal part of the conduction system. When the wave of depolarisation reaches these fibres, they activate the ventricular myocardial cells to contract.

The ECG complex

Cardiac Monitoring

The cardiac monitor is used for continuous monitoring of heart rate and rhythm of patients that require close observation.

The 12 lead ECG

The 12 lead ECG is performed intermittently and provides a view of the heart from 12 different perspectives (see assessment section).

As the cardiac conduction system becomes activated, the respective parts of the atria and ventricles contract accordingly. As the wave of depolarisation spreads through the muscle fibres of each chamber, an exchange of positively charged ions across the cell membrane of the cardiac myocytes (muscle cells) creates a voltage change that can be recorded on a cardiac monitor as an ECG complex. The process of depolarisation leading to myocardial contraction is known as excitation contraction coupling. The myocardium will only contract in response to depolarisation.

An ECG complex (see Figure 6.5) is comprised of 3 main components:

- P wave.
- QRS complex.
- T wave.

P wave: this is a small rounded wave that is seen on the ECG during atrial depolarisation. P waves should always be present, as this indicates SA nodal depolarisation (sometimes referred to as 'firing') and that the subsequent wave of depolarisation is simultaneously spreading across the atrial myocardium. The PR interval is the time between the beginning of the P wave and the first deflection of the QRS complex. This is 0.2 seconds (or seen as 5 small squares on ECG paper).

QRS complex: the largest part of the ECG complex is the QRS complex. This represents the wave of depolarisation as it spreads across the ventricular myocardium. Providing that the bundle branches are both conducting normally, the QRS should be narrow in configuration, with no visible notches present. The QRS may be upright (positive) or downward (negative), depending on the surface of the heart that is facing the ECG lead. The QRS complex is rapid, at less than 0.12 seconds (seen as 3 small squares on ECG paper).

T wave: once the cells of the ventricular myocardium have been depolarised, they begin the process of returning to their normal resting state. Depolarisation is achieved by

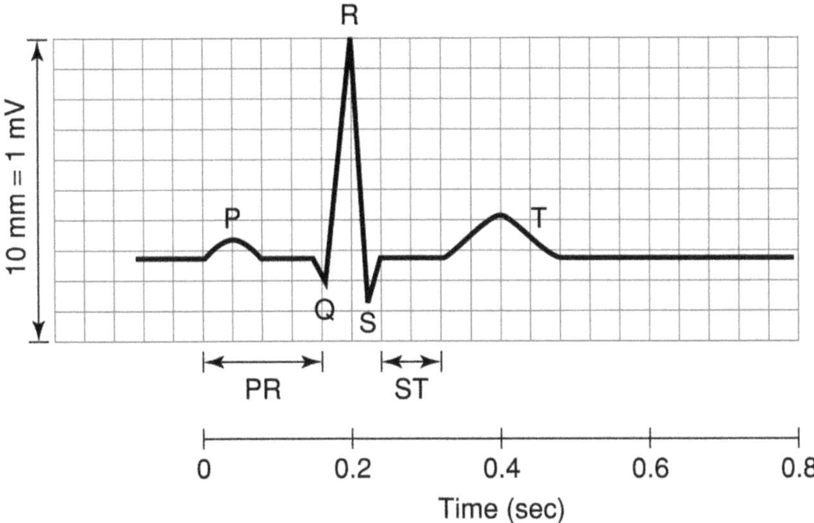

Figure 6.5 The normal PQRST complex.

a rapid influx of positive ions, these need to move back across the cell membrane to reach its resting state in the process of repolarisation. This **repolarisation** phase lasts longer than depolarisation, hence the T wave is wider than the corresponding QRS complex that precedes it. The ST segment sits on the isoelectric line.

The cardiac cycle

The cardiac conduction system is responsible for initiating the chain of events that enables the heart to cycle (see Figure 6.6) between systole and diastole, maintaining a forward flow of blood through the pulmonary and systemic circulations. The ionic changes that occur during depolarisation and repolarisation increase calcium availability in the cardiac myocyte, enabling the **sarcomere** (the basic unit of cardiac muscle) to shorten and contract. Thus, the electrical events are essential for the mechanical events of myocardial contraction to ensue.

The cardiac cycle is the period of time between one contraction and another. The cycle lasts for about 0.8 seconds, with the systolic (contraction phase) being slightly shorter, at 0.3 seconds, than the diastolic (relaxation phase), at 0.5 seconds. This slightly longer diastolic phase enables flow of blood down the coronary arteries to the relaxed myocardium. The following describes stages of the cardiac cycle and is illustrated by Figure 6.6. In *ventricular diastole*, the atria and ventricles are relaxed, the atrioventricular (AV) valves are open and blood is flowing from the atria to the ventricles. Towards the end of ventricular diastole, the SA node and then atria depolarise (viewed as the P wave on the ECG), causing the atria to contract and starting *atrial systole*. The ventricles have received about 80% of their blood already, but the contracting atria push the final 20% through the AV valves; this is sometimes referred to as the 'atrial kick'. The pulmonary and aortic valves remain closed during this phase. The amount of blood in the ventricles at the end of diastole in known as the **end diastolic volume** (EDV).

Rhythm problems where 'atrial kick' is lost include:

- Atrial fibrillation.
- Atrial flutter.
- Third-degree heart block.

This may reduce the cardiac output, with ABCDE assessment revealing breathlessness, hypotension, tachycardia or bradycardia.

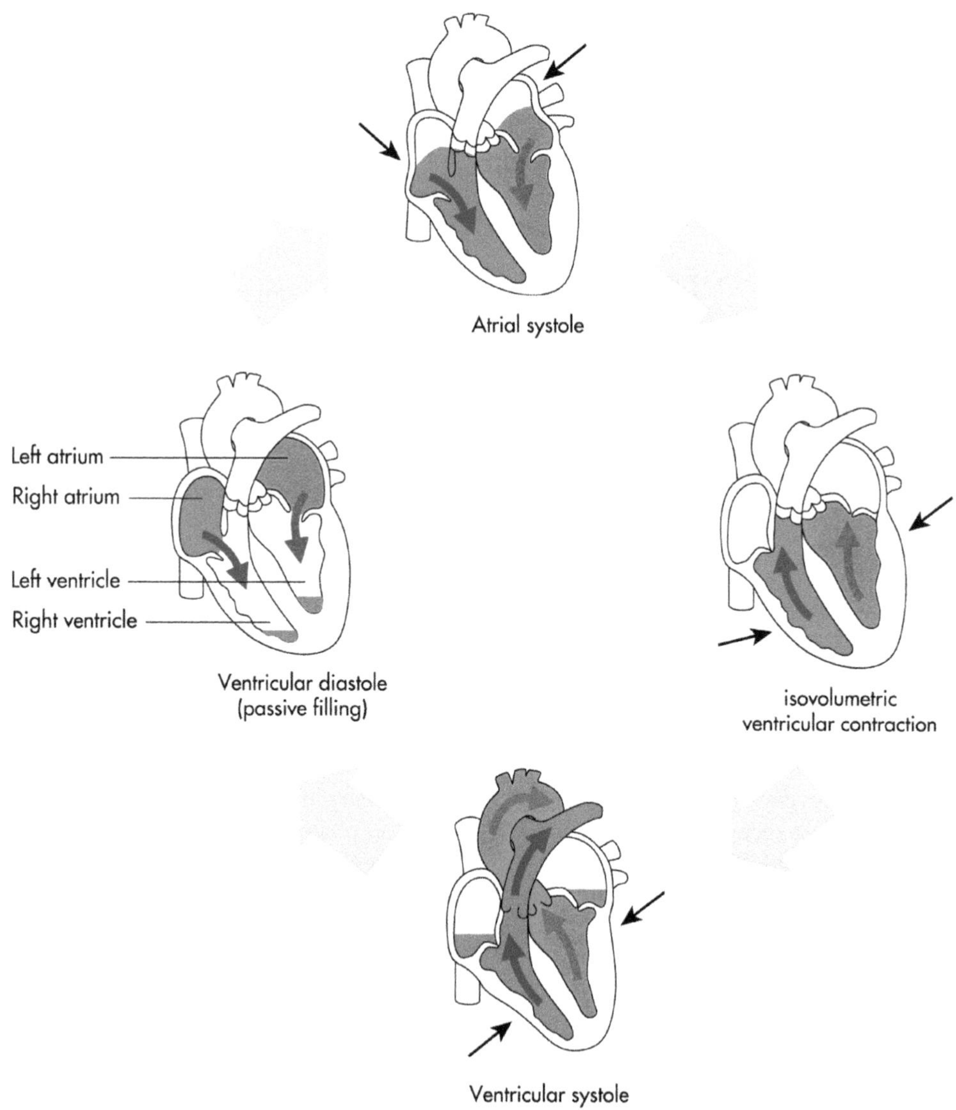

Figure 6.6 Stages of the cardiac cycle.

The electrical impulse passes down the AV node and then through the ventricular conduction system and Purkinje fibres (viewed as the QRS complex on the ECG). This signals the start of *isovolumetric ventricular contraction*, as the ventricles begin to contract. The rising pressure in the ventricles forces the closure of the AV valves generating the **first heart sound**, 'lub'. In the isovolumetric phase, there is a change in ventricular pressure but no change in ventricular volume, because the pressure generated is not yet sufficient to open the pulmonary and aortic valves. At this point, all four valves in the heart remain closed. This phase of the cardiac cycle consumes the most energy, and therefore oxygen, and represents the greatest work of the myocardium. Eventually, the pressure in the ventricles exceeds the pressure in the aorta and pulmonary vessels, the semi-lunar valves are forced open and *ventricular systole* begins.

In ventricular systole, the contents of the ventricle are ejected into the pulmonary and systemic circulations. About 60–70% of the volume of blood in the ventricle at the end of diastole is ejected. End diastolic volume is typically about 120mL, and the amount ejected (stroke volume) is 70mL. This leaves 50mL of blood in the ventricle at the end of systole, which can be ejected if the force of contraction is increased, acting as a cardiac reserve to be used if a greater output is needed. Once the ventricles have finished their contraction, they begin to relax. Pressure in the ventricles fall rapidly, and when it falls below aortic and pulmonary pressure, the aortic and pulmonary valves close. This can be heard as the **second heart sound**, 'dub'. The closure of these valves and then the opening of the AV valves (as the pressure in the atria exceed that of the relaxed ventricles), signals the beginning of ventricular diastole, and the cycle starts once again.

Some useful definitions

Stroke volume: amount ejected in beat (70 mL).
End diastolic volume: the amount in the ventricle at the end of diastole (120mL).
Ejection fraction: the percentage of blood ejected from the left ventricle.

$$(\text{SV/EDV} \times 100)(60-70\%)$$

Cardiac output

An average person has a resting heart rate of 70 beats/minute and a resting stroke volume of 70mL/beat. The cardiac output for this person at rest is:

Cardiac output = 70 (beats/min) × 70 (mL/beat)=4900 mL/minute.

The amount of blood pumped by the ventricles in one minute is the cardiac output.

Cardiac output = heart rate (beats per minute) × stroke volume (mL per beat)

An increase in heart rate will raise cardiac output, but as the rate increases above about 130, there is a reduction in time available for the ventricle to fill (diastole), and cardiac output may fall.

A shortened diastolic time also reduces the time for coronary artery filling, just when the myocardial oxygen demand is increasing.

Cardiac output decreases in sleep and rises during vigorous exercise, increasing in a trained athlete by up to 7 times (up to 35L/minute). In illness, the demand may increase as with sepsis; or the ability to maintain cardiac output may reduce, as with heart failure, and a mismatch of demand and supply may ensue. The cardiac reserve enables the output to increase by increasing the ejection fraction (and therefore stroke volume) and increasing heart rate. Stroke volume depends mainly on three factors:

- **Preload**.
- **Contractility**.
- **Afterload**.

These three factors are crucial for the maintenance of cardiac output and are influenced by the sympathetic nervous system.

Preload

Preload is related to the volume of the blood in the ventricle at the end of diastole, or end diastolic volume. The blood is returned to the heart by the venous circulation and is reduced by problems such as hypovolaemia or vasodilation and increased by hypervolemia and vasoconstriction. This volume exerts a distension pressure on the ventricle at the end of diastole (or preload). **Compliance** refers to the ease at which the muscle can distend or stretch to accommodate the volume returned to the ventricle. A damaged/injured or poorly compliant/stiff ventricle will not stretch easily, and therefore the ventricular end diastolic volume is reduced.

Preload is important, as there is a relationship between the amount of blood in the ventricle at the end of diastole and the amount of blood ejected during systole (stroke volume). This relationship is described by Starling's law of the heart, which states that as the amount of blood returning from the veins to the ventricle at the end of diastole increases, the stretch of the ventricular myocardium increases and therefore the strength of the next contraction is greater. A useful analogy is an elastic band; the further it is stretched, the harder it springs back. This means that the more blood flows into the ventricles, the more blood is pumped out, i.e. as the left ventricular end diastolic volume increases, so does the stroke volume (see Figure 6.7). This relationship is evident in the healthy heart, but for those that have heart failure, the ability to deal with increased preload is reduced. This is discussed later in the chapter.

A non-invasive practical method of clinically assessing ventricular preload is the passive leg raise manoeuvre. This relies on the principle that raising the legs above the level of the heart increases venous return to the heart by about 300–500mL. The increase in ventricular preload will transiently increase the cardiac output in those patients who

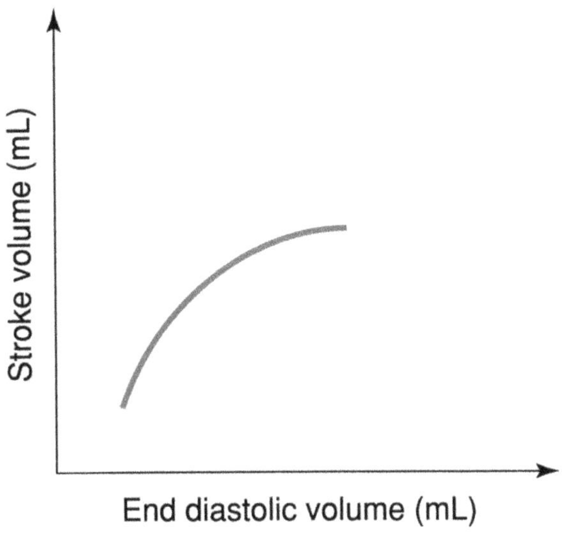

Figure 6.7 A Starling curve showing how the amount of blood ejected from the heart (stroke volume) increases as the amount of blood in the ventricle at the end of diastole (preload) increases.

are fluid-deficient. This approach had the benefits of predicting those patients who will increase their stroke volume when given additional fluid, without the deleterious consequences of fluid overload, as the legs can be returned to the supine position if no improvement is seen. Patients who respond to the passive leg raise manoeuvre can safely be given a fluid bolus/challenge as required (Picket et al. 2017).

For those that are acutely unwell, there is an option to assess ventricular preload by inserting a cannula into the internal jugular or subclavian vein and measuring the central venous pressure (CVP). This is an invasive procedure with associated risks, so it is not appropriate for all situations. Whilst CVP readings are not used in isolation, in general, a lower measurement would be consistent with a lower ventricular preload, with a reduced blood volume returning to the heart. A fluid challenge may be needed to increase ventricular preload. In Figure 6.7, it can be seen that as the ventricular preload (end diastolic volume) increases, so does the stroke volume. If the stroke volume increases, cardiac output and blood pressure will normally increase as well (assuming heart rate remains constant). Invasive haemodynamic monitoring is discussed later in this chapter.

Fluid challenge

This involves giving an intravenous bolus of fluid, usually about 500mL, rapidly, as prescribed.

- Clinical response should be carefully evaluated.
- Increasing ventricular preload (end diastolic volume) should lead to improved stroke volume and cardiac output.
- This should lead to in an improved blood pressure and reduced heart rate.

Table 6.1 Factors that affect myocardial contractility

Increased contractility	Sympathetic stimulation
	Positive **inotropic** drugs
Decreased contractility	Parasympathetic stimulation
	Ischaemia
	Hypoxaemia
	Acidosis
	Electrolyte imbalance

Contractility

Contractility refers to the ability of the myocardium to contract. Healthy myocardium will contract effectively according to how much stretch the volume in the ventricle is exerting on the ventricular myocardium. As with an elastic band, if the myocardium becomes overstretched, it may not spring back so effectively, and so a damaged or failing heart, one with decreased contractility, may not have the capacity to contract so strongly. This is discussed in more detail later when considering heart failure. Factors that affect contractility are summarised in Table 6.1.

Afterload

Afterload is the force opposing ventricular ejection; in the left ventricle, this is the opposition given by the aortic **diastolic pressure**. Changes in **systemic vascular resistance** (SVR) caused by peripheral vasoconstriction or dilation will affect afterload. Systemic vascular resistance will increase with peripheral vasoconstriction, and the patient who feels cool to touch will have an increased left ventricular afterload. The myocardium has to work harder to push the blood out of the ventricle, and will therefore require more oxygen as it uses more energy. In health, this is not a problem, but in the failing heart, pharmacological therapy is aimed at reducing the left ventricular afterload by enabling arteriolar vasodilation in order to reduce the oxygen requirements of the myocardium. Problems with the heart valves, for example, aortic stenosis, increase the work of the left ventricle, as it needs to generate an increased pressure to squeeze blood though the stenotic valve. This, over time, will damage the ventricular myocardium and the damaged heart valves may need to be replaced.

Pharmacology

Drugs used in heart failure to reduce afterload by vasodilation include:

- Angiotensin-converting enzyme inhibitors.
- Angiotensin receptor blockers.
- Calcium channel blockers.

Blood pressure

Blood pressure = cardiac output × systemic vascular resistance

Blood pressure measurement is a familiar activity for the nurse, but it is worth pausing to consider exactly what it is that is being measured. Blood pressure is the pressure the blood exerts on the inner walls of the arteries and is determined by cardiac output (CO) and systemic vascular resistance (SVR). It gives the nurse a good insight into the functioning of the left ventricle's ability to pump blood into the aorta. Blood pressure is a product of cardiac output and systemic vascular resistance. Blood pressure is expressed as a systolic over a diastolic pressure. Normal blood pressure varies but an ideal value is between 120/85mmHg, to a high normal of 140/89 (NICE 2019a). Systolic blood pressure is generated by the strength and the volume of blood pumped by the ventricular contraction. Diastolic blood pressure is related to the tone of the blood vessels. The relationship between the factors that contribute to cardiac output are shown in Figure 6.8. It can be seen that if one of these factors change (for example preload), then stroke volume, cardiac output and blood pressure will all be affected. The sympathetic nervous system can influence each of these factors and contributes to maintaining CO and BP.

Regulation of blood pressure

You may remember that cardiac output varies greatly to meet the physiological demand for oxygen at the cellular level. Despite the wide fluctuation in cardiac output, the blood pressure remains relatively constant to ensure the required perfusion pressure is maintained throughout the system without causing organ damage.

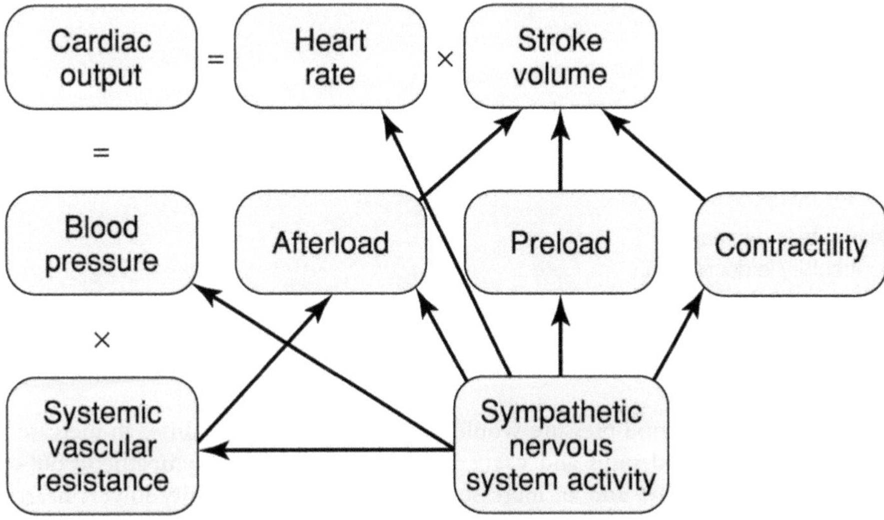

Figure 6.8 Factors contributing to cardiac output.

Adrenergic receptors are:
receptors of the sympathetic nervous system that respond to the neurotransmitter noradrenaline.

- **Beta 1 receptors** are located in the heart and when activated, cause an increase in contractility and heart rate.
- **Beta 2 receptors** are located in bronchial and vascular smooth muscle. SNS activity causes bronchodilation and dilation of vessels supplying skeletal muscles.
- **Alpha receptors** are located in peripheral vasculature and cause vasoconstriction when activated by the SNS.

Neural mechanisms of blood pressure regulation lie predominately within the pons and medulla of the brain. The **cardiovascular centre** (CVC) controls both vessel tone through the vasomotor centre and heart rate through the cardiac centre. Changes in the internal environment are detected by sensors, which communicate with the cardiovascular centre via neural pathways. The cardiovascular centre responds by activation or inhibition of the sympathetic and parasympathetic branches of the autonomic nervous system to maintain homeostasis. The autonomic nervous system is explained in more detail in Chapter 9. Sensor mechanisms include **baroreceptors**, which are sensitive to stretch and are situated in the walls of the aortic arch, and bifurcation of the common carotid arteries, in an ideal position to detect pressure changes. Information from the baroreceptors is transmitted via the carotid sinus and vagus nerves to the CVC, and a falling **mean arterial pressure** will reduce the information flow. A corresponding increase in sympathetic outflow from the CVC causes vasoconstriction via stimulation of alpha-adrenergic receptors in the systemic vasculature and an increase in heart rate and contractility via **beta-adrenergic receptor** stimulation in the heart. These responses will cause an increase in cardiac output and blood pressure (see Figure 6.9).

Pharmacology

Beta-adrenergic receptor blockers (beta blockers) antagonise the receptors and blunt the sympathetic response.

- Heart rate is decreased.
- Contractility is decreased.
- Renin production is decreased.
- Blood pressure will be reduced.

Conversely, an increase in blood pressure would cause the opposite response; an increase in impulses down the carotid sinus and vagus nerves will inhibit the sympathetic outflow, allowing vessels to dilate, and an increase in parasympathetic activity lowers heart rate, thus reducing cardiac output and blood pressure. This regulatory system is rapid and maintains homeostasis during everyday activities, such as moving from a lying to a

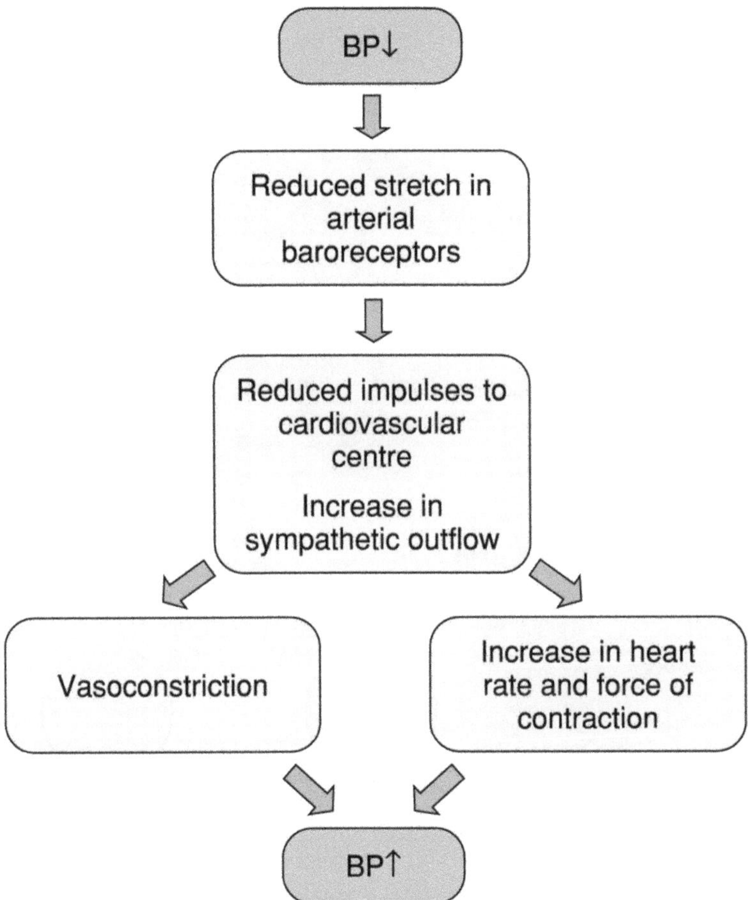

Figure 6.9 Baroreceptor reflex in response to reduced blood pressure.

standing position. Figure 6.10 shows the pathways of transmission to the CVC and the effect of the sympathetic response on the heart (increase in contractility and rate) and blood vessels (vasoconstriction).

Information from chemoreceptors (see also, Chapter 5) also influence the activity of the cardiovascular centre, and the sympathetic response is initiated in response to hypoxaemia. Emotional stress or fear perceived by higher centres in the brain will also be communicated to the CVC, activating the stress response of the SNS and raising heart rate and blood pressure, which are common physical manifestations of stress. When assessing cardiac status, it is important to note clinical signs that indicate SNS activity, as these may be early signs of clinical changes that may lead to acute deterioration.

A number of humoral mechanisms contribute to blood pressure regulation; these are the renin angiotensin aldosterone system (RAAS) **and antidiuretic hormone** (ADH). Other hormones, such as adrenaline, are released from adrenal glands and will have the effect of directly stimulating an increase in heart rate, contractility and vascular tone of

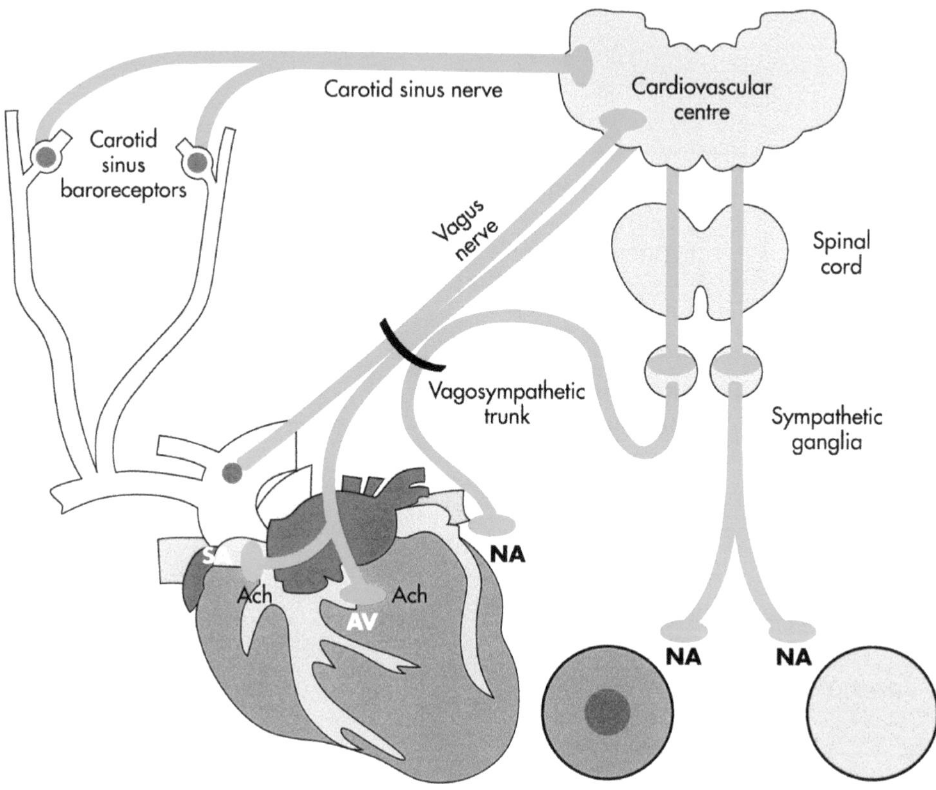

Figure 6.10 Autonomic control of blood pressure NA = noradrenaline; neurotransmitter of the sympathetic nervous system and Ach = Acetylcholine: neurotransmitter of the parasympathetic nervous system.

the gut and skin. However, adrenaline will cause vasodilation of cardiac and skeletal arterioles.

Pharmacology

Angiotensin converting enzyme inhibitors (ACEI) block the conversion of angiotensin 1 to angiotensin 2. This causes:

- Vasodilation, reducing blood pressure.
- A reduction in aldosterone, increasing urine output.

The RAAS is central to blood pressure regulation and involves a chain of events that are activated if mean arterial blood pressure falls. This is discussed in more detail in Chapter 8. The enzyme renin is secreted from the **juxta glomerular cells** in the nephron in response to reduced blood flow. Renin converts angiotensinogen, a naturally occurring **plasma protein**, into angiotensin 1. Angiotensin converting enzyme (ACE), present in the pulmonary endothelium, converts angiotensin 1 to angiotensin 2. Angiotensin 2 is a very powerful vasoconstrictor, which increases systemic perfusion, but also activates **aldosterone** production from the adrenal cortex to reabsorb sodium, and therefore water, in the distal convoluted tubule of the kidney, increasing blood volume.

ADH is released by the posterior pituitary in response to decreased blood pressure and increasing osmolality of the blood. ADH is a vasopressor (increases blood pressure by causing vasoconstriction), but also acts on the collecting ducts in the kidney to increase absorption of water back into the circulation.

Having considered the anatomy and physiology of the heart that provides the pumping force of the circulation, the blood that the heart propels and the vessels through which the blood travels will be discussed.

The blood

The importance of blood in the preservation of life has been a source of interest to scientists, philosophers, writers and artists over many centuries. Due to the relative ease in which blood can be obtained, it has become one of the most studied components of the body (Pallister 1994).

Blood is an organ, and is unique because it comprises the only fluid tissue of the body. It supports the functions of all other body tissues and is, in turn, dependent on other organs, such as the lungs, heart, kidneys and liver. Blood is also one of the body's largest organs: an average 70kg man will have a total blood volume of approximately 5 litres, weighing around 5.5kg.

> Total blood volume is 5–6L, depending on weight. The average adult cardiac output is around 5L; therefore, the severing of a major blood vessel can result in the loss of the entire circulating volume within 1–2 minutes.

Blood is a complex connective tissue and is essentially made up of formed elements (red blood cells, white blood cells and **platelets**) suspended in a liquid called **plasma**. When a sample of blood is placed in a **centrifuge** and spun at high speed, the plasma and formed elements are separated out (see Figure 6.11).

Plasma

Plasma is 90% water and has many elements dissolved within. Approximately 3 litres of the total blood volume is plasma, which is pale yellow in colour, often described as straw-coloured. It contains a small amount of dissolved oxygen and organic compounds such as glucose, electrolytes and proteins. When blood samples are obtained for analysis, the values produced are those of the plasma.

Electrolytes (salts) are substances that, when in solution, conduct an electrical current. This is because when dissolved, they separate into ions. Ions carry an electrical charge that may be either positive (**cations**) or negative (**anions**). Plasma contains extracellular electrolytes, the levels of which are carefully balanced relative to the levels in **intracellular fluids**. If this balance is upset, it causes major disruption to virtually all body functions. The small electrical currents generated by ions are vital for muscle contraction and nerve function. For example, low levels of potassium can result in cardiac arrhythmias

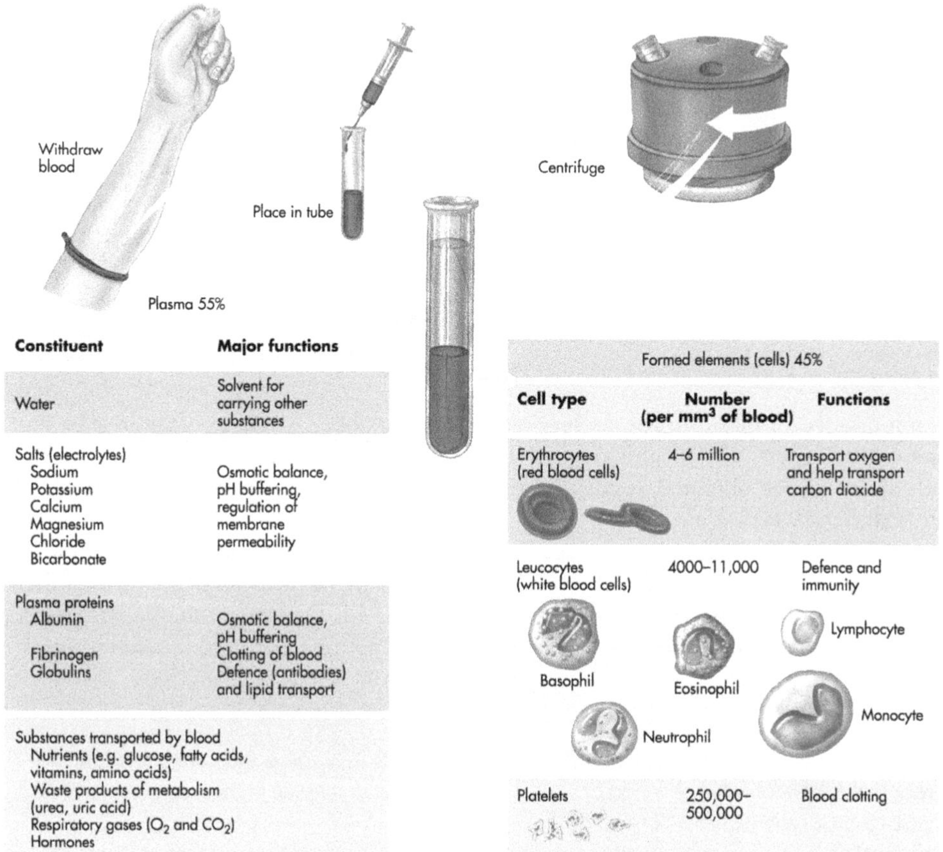

Figure 6.11 Composition of blood.

and ectopic beats as the myocardium becomes more irritable. Plasma is always electrically neutral, in other words, the number of positive charges exactly balances the number of negative ones. Table 6.2 shows the common cations and anions in the body.

Sodium chloride (NaCl) dissolves in water and separates into sodium (Na^+), a cation, and chloride (Cl^-), an anion. A solution containing charged particles is an electrolyte.

Glucose is a non-electrolyte, as the molecules do not dissociate in water. Glucose, therefore, has no effect on the electrical charge of a solution, but provides an energy source.

Water, ions and electrolytes are constantly being exchanged between the plasma and the **interstitial fluid** (the fluid bathing the cells), and therefore the composition of the two is very similar. The main difference is the presence in the plasma of plasma proteins. They do not leave the circulation easily, due to their large size and irregular shapes. Each 100mL of plasma contains 7.6g of protein. Plasma proteins are essential for maintaining **colloid oncotic pressure**, which, in turn, is crucial for ensuring fluid stays within the circulation. Plasma proteins perform additional functions; some act as carrier molecules for drugs and other substances, and some have an important role in blood clotting and the immune response. For a summary of the protein composition of plasma, see Table 6.3.

Table 6.2 Values of common cations and anions

	Chemical symbol	*Normal value in plasma*
Cations		
Sodium	Na^+	135–145mmol/L
Potassium	K^+	3.6–5.1mmol/L
Calcium	Ca^{++}	2.1–2.6mmol/L
Magnesium	Mg^{++}	0.75–1.0mmol/L
Hydrogen	H^+	35–45nanomol/L
Anions		
Chloride	Cl^-	95–107mmol/L
Phosphorous	P^-	2.5–4.5mmol/L
Bicarbonate	HCO_3^-	22–26mmol/L

Table 6.3 Protein composition of plasma

	Functions
Albumin	Colloid oncotic pressure; binds with drugs, hormones.
Globulins	Forms antibodies (immunoglobulins) which attack foreign proteins and pathogens.
Fibrinogen	Essential for the process of blood clotting.

Albumin is the most abundant of the plasma proteins. If albumin levels are low, there is a fall in colloid oncotic pressure, resulting in fluid leaking out of the circulation into the tissues. This is one cause of oedema.

Red blood cells (RBCs) – erythrocytes

These are the most numerous cells in the blood, the principle functions of which are carriage of respiratory gases, as discussed in detail in Chapter 4. Haemoglobin molecules account for more than 95% of the composition of an RBC, and transports oxygen to the tissues and carbon dioxide back to the lungs. **Haemoglobin** is an iron-containing protein. If iron is deficient in the body, then adequate amounts of haemoglobin cannot be made, resulting in **anaemia** and an inability of the blood to carry sufficient oxygen to the tissues (for causes and types of anaemia see Table 6.4). **Erythrocytes** do not have a nucleus, and so are not able to divide to form new cells. They are formed through the process of **haematopoiesis**, principally in the red bone marrow – myeloid tissue. Erythrocytes are among the most abundant cells in the body, accounting for about one-third of all body cells.

Men have 4.5–6.3 million RBCs per mm^3 of whole blood, and women have 4.2–5.5 per mm^3. This is the red cell count reported on a full blood count (FBC) report.

Also reported in the FBC is the haemoglobin (Hb) level.

Whatever the cause of anaemia, there will be a reduced oxygen-carrying ability, and the potential for reduced oxygen delivery to the tissues. For example, sickle-cell disease results from an abnormality in the **haemoglobin**, causing the red blood cell to become fragile, with a tendency to change shape and become crescent- or 'sickle'-shaped. A sickle-cell crisis occurs when large numbers of RBCs assume this sickle shape and is a medical emergency. Sickled cells have a reduced ability to carry oxygen, and due

Table 6.4 Types of anaemia

Direct cause	*As a result of*	*Type*
Decrease in number of RBCs	• Sudden haemorrhage. • Destruction (**lysis**) of RBCs. • Lack of vitamin B[12]. • Bone marrow depression due to cancer, drugs or radiation.	Haemorrhagic **Haemolytic** Pernicious anaemia Aplastic anaemia
Reduced haemoglobin content of RBC	• Lack of iron in the diet necessary for RBC formation. • Slow, prolonged bleeding. .which depletes stores of iron, e.g., heavy menstrual flow	Iron deficiency anaemia
Abnormal haemoglobin present in red cells	• Abnormal haemoglobin in the RBCs becomes sickle-shaped when oxygen use increases. Sickle-cell trait is genetic and mainly occurs in people of African descent. • Large amounts of abnormal haemoglobin present in RBCs due to a genetic abnormality, resulting in a low overall level of Hb.	Sickle-cell anaemia **Thalassaemia**

to their abnormal shape, they obstruct the capillaries, leading to reduced blood flow to organs and therefore ischaemia and organ damage. The most common sites for the action of sickled cells are the lungs, liver, brain, spleen and kidneys, although other parts of the body can be affected. The presenting symptoms are severe pain related to the affected organ(s) and extreme breathlessness. Immediate management includes oxygen and analgesia. A crisis may happen spontaneously with no apparent cause, however, precipitating factors can be hypoxia, hypovolaemia, hypothermia, stress and co-existing illness.

Haemoglobin (Hb) level in the blood is measured in gm per litre (g/L). Normal range is 130–180g/L in men and 115–165g/L in women.

People with chronic anaemia often develop quite a high tolerance for the low Hb levels: however, they have no reserves if they become ill and their oxygen demand increases. In acute situations, a patient with anaemia will commonly display symptoms of breathlessness and pallor. In the immediate term, oxygen saturations should be maximised, while the underlying cause can be found and treated. It is important to remember that an oxygen saturation probe measures the amount of oxygen on the available haemoglobin. Therefore, although the level of haemoglobin may be low, it may be fully saturated with oxygen, so the saturation readings would be within the normal range. However, the overall amount of oxygen transported to the tissues would be significantly compromised. This is a good example of needing a number of parameters when assessing clinical status, rather than just one. Assessment needs to take into account many factors in order to make an accurate interpretation. In contrast to anaemia, some individuals suffer from a condition known as polycythaemia, that causes an abnormally high red cell count resulting in the blood becoming so viscous that it doesn't flow properly. This reduces tissue perfusion and may increase blood pressure and the likelihood of a stroke or myocardial infarction due to **thrombus** formation.

The hormone erythropoietin, which is produced mainly by the kidneys, controls the rate of RBC production. People with renal failure often suffer from anaemia due to the lack of this hormone.

White blood cells (WBCs) – leucocytes

WBCs have an equally vital function to red blood cells in that they defend the body from invading pathogens and are central to the immune response. There are several different types of WBCs which are grouped under two headings: *polymorphonuclear granulocytes* originating from the red bone marrow and *mononuclear granulocytes*, also originating from the red bone marrow but maturing in the lymphoid tissue.

WBCs are like a mobile defence force or army, protecting the body from bacteria, viruses, parasites and tumour cells. Damaged tissues give off certain chemicals that act as 'homing beacons' to the affected area. The ability of WBCs to migrate in response to these chemical signals is known as chemotaxis.

There are three types of polymorphonuclear granulocyte:

- Neutrophils.
- Eosinophils.
- Basophils.

And two types of mononuclear granulocyte:

- Monocytes.
- Lymphocytes.

Neutrophils and monocytes engulf invading organisms and incorporate them into their cell bodies, destroying them by a process called phagocytosis. Neutrophils are the most numerous of the phagocytes and arrive at the site of invasion first. Monocytes arrive later and stay longer, so a raised neutrophil count may indicate a chronic infection. Unlike red blood cells, which carry out their function entirely within the blood, WBCs use blood only as the means of transport to the site where their functions are needed. They are then able to move in and out of the blood vessels.

The normal WBC count in adults is 4–11 $\times 10^9$/L, and when an infection is present, the WBC count may be significantly raised. A white cell count above 11 $\times 10^9$/L is known as leucocytosis. An abnormally low WBC count, below 4 $\times 10^9$/L, is known as leukopenia and can be caused by factors such as corticosteroids and chemotherapy drugs. Leukopenia renders the individual vulnerable to infections of all types. Problems related to infection and sepsis are discussed in Chapter 12.

Leukaemia

Leukaemia is a cancer of the bone marrow that results in huge numbers of immature and ineffective white cells being produced. This makes the patient susceptible to infection and also causes other cells to be 'crowded out', often resulting in severe anaemia and bleeding.

Platelets – thrombocytes

Platelets are responsible for the ability of the blood to clot, and are the smallest of the formed elements of the blood. Platelets also produce a substance called serotonin that causes constriction of the smooth muscle of the blood vessels. This vasoconstriction reduces blood flow and, combined with clotting, helps to minimise bleeding and to achieve **haemostasis**; stopping the bleeding. Platelets, although a vital part of the clotting process, are just one of a number of factors in a complex series of events known as the clotting cascade. The clotting mechanism is initiated by an injury or damage to the blood vessel wall; this roughens the lining of the blood vessel (normally extremely smooth). What follows can be simplified into the following three essential steps.

1 Step 1: platelets become 'sticky' in response to factors released by the injured tissue. The sticky platelets join together or aggregate to form a soft plug at the site of injury. The injured tissue also releases clotting factors that speed up this process.
2 Step 2: a series of chemical reactions occur, culminating in the formation of **thrombin**. Thrombin forms from pro-thrombin, which is produced by the liver and requires vitamin K.
3 Step 3: the final stage in the reaction is between thrombin and fibrinogen (a plasma protein), causing fibrinogen to be converted to fibrin. Fibrin looks like a tangled mass of threads and forms a net in which red blood cells and platelets are trapped: this forms a stable clot.

When we apply pressure with gauze, or similar, to a bleeding wound, the roughened surface of the gauze encourages platelet aggregation and the pressure fractures cells, releasing the tissue factors that further speed the process. If it is possible to raise the site of injury above the level of the heart, this will slow blood flow to the area and reduce bleeding.

Prothrombin time (PT): animal tissue factors are added to the blood sample and the time taken for the sample to clot is the PT. Normal range is 11–16 seconds.
Partial prothrombin time (PTT): activators are added to the sample without tissue factor and the time taken for clotting is measured. Normal range is 25–39 seconds.

As the damaged tissue is repaired, the clot is slowly broken down. This process is called **fibrinolysis** and occurs as a result of an enzyme called plasmin, which causes the fibrin strands to dissolve and the clot to erode. Figure 6.12 summarises the clot formation and dissolution process.

Oral Anticoagulant therapy (NICE 2019)

Aspirin: inhibits the circulating factors which cause platelet aggregation.
Clopidogrel: prevents platelets aggregating and inhibits the ability of fibrin strands to bind the clot together.
Warfarin: inhibits the production of prothrombin. May be used in long term anticoagulation management, such as in the treatment of DVT, and prophylaxis of stroke or embolism in adults with atrial fibrillation.
Apixaban, Edoxaban and Rivaroxaban: may be prescribed instead of warfarin. This group inhibits *activated factor X* (factor Xa, required to covert prothrombin to thrombin).

Parenteral Anticoagulants (BNF 2020)

Heparin: inhibits the conversion of prothrombin to thrombin (inhibits factor Xa). Heparin is a substance which occurs naturally in the body to ensure clots do not form inappropriately.

Low molecular weight heparin – Tinzaparin sodium dalteparin sodium: can be given as a once daily injection.
Fondaparinux sodium: inhibits factor Xa.

Clots can sometimes form inappropriately in blood vessels that are not broken through injury, but are damaged in some way, usually due to the presence of atheroma (discussed in more detail later in this chapter). Clots may form in the coronary arteries (causing a myocardial infarction), the cerebral arteries (causing a stroke) or travel to the pulmonary vasculature (causing a pulmonary embolus), which leads to a potentially catastrophic cessation of blood supply to these organs. A clot that forms and stays in one place is known as a thrombus. A clot that forms and then moves, circulating through the bloodstream either in total or in part, is known as an embolus.

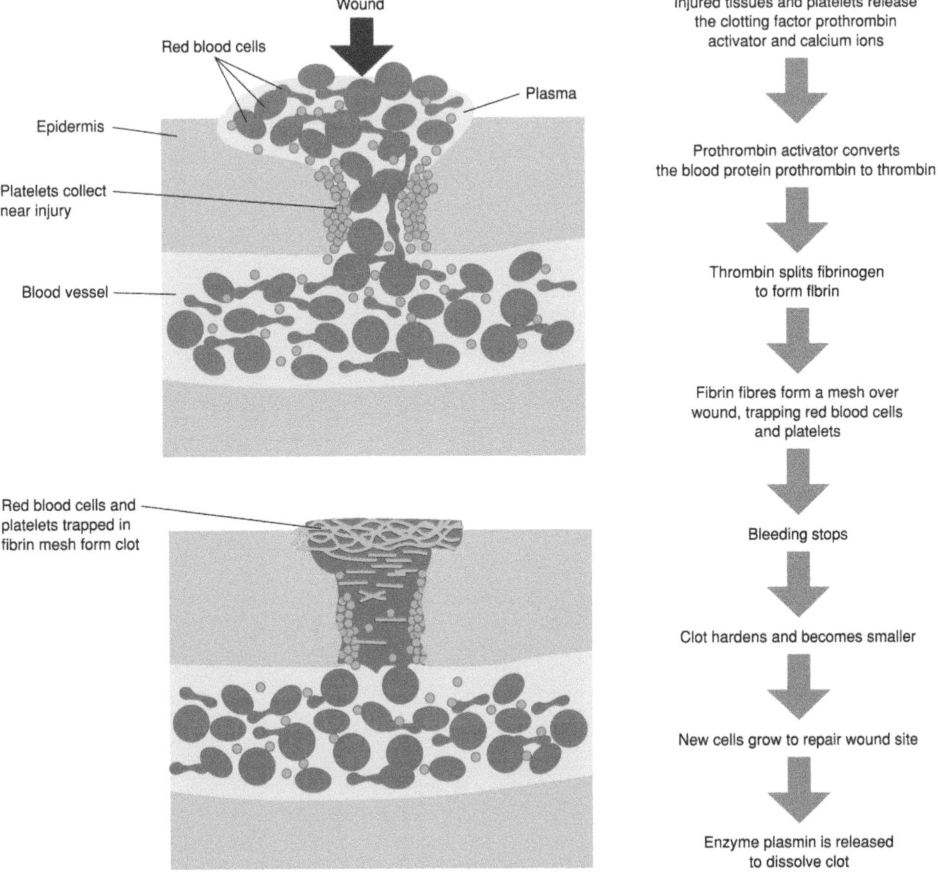

Figure 6.12 Diagram to show clot formation and dissolution.

Disseminated intravascular coagulopathy (DIC)

In DIC, thrombin becomes abnormally active. This may occur due to severe inflammation, infection, or cancer. Small clots form in the blood vessels. Some of these clots impede the blood supply to organs such as the liver, brain, or kidneys. These organs will then be damaged.

Over time, due to the increased activity of the clotting system, the clotting proteins are consumed, or 'used up'. As a result, although the primary problem is abnormal clotting, the most obvious clinical sign is bleeding. The risk, then, is serious bleeding from a minor injury or even without injury.

Blood groups ABO and rhesus factor

There are between 30 and 50 antigens on the plasma membranes of red blood cells, however, the main focus in relation to matching blood for patients who need transfusions is the AB and rhesus antigens. Everyone has only one of the following blood groups:

- Group A (surface antigen A present on plasma membrane).
- Group B (surface antigen B present on plasma membrane).
- Group AB (no surface antigens present on plasma membrane).
- Group O (surface antigens A and B present on plasma membrane).

The majority of the population in the United Kingdom are group O (47%) and group A (40%). Group AB is the least common (3%). There are fluctuations in this among certain ethnic groups, for example, persons of Asian descent are more likely to be group B and in those originating from China and Japan, the incidence of group AB is higher, around 10%.

In early childhood, a person with blood group A will develop antigens to blood group B; conversely, those with blood group B will develop antigens to blood group A. Persons with blood group AB have no antigens, whereas those with blood group O have antigens to both A and B. This is illustrated in Figure 6.13.

Rhesus factor

In addition to the AB antigens, there is one further antigen that is of significance when matching blood for transfusion. This is known as the rhesus factor (Rh): 85% of the population in the UK possess the Rh factor and are therefore termed Rh positive; those in whom the Rh factor is absent are termed Rh negative. In practice, when blood types are talked about, the term rhesus is omitted, and therefore a person's blood group is described, for example, as O positive or negative. Anti-Rh antibodies will not be automatically produced by the body, as is the case for anti-A and anti-B. They are produced in response to a transfusion of Rh positive blood into a Rh negative person. The process of producing antibodies takes time, and therefore the first transfusion is likely to be uneventful, but any subsequent transfusion will result in a typical incompatibility reaction.

Rhesus problems in pregnancy

There can be serious consequences for the foetus if the father is Rh positive and the mother Rh negative.

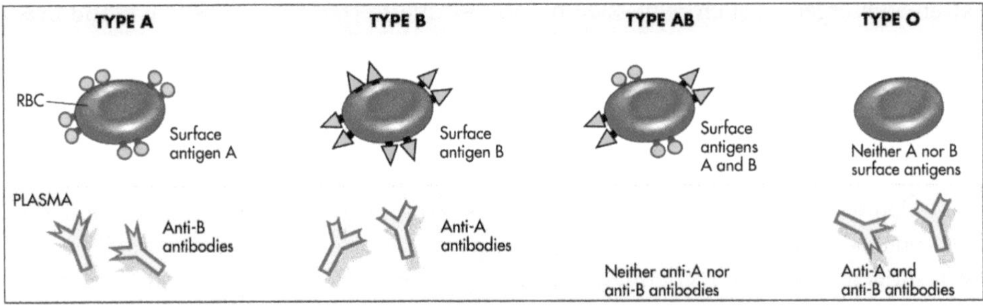

Recipient's blood		Reactions with donor's blood			
RBC antigens	**Plasma antibodies**	**Donor type O**	**Donor type A**	**Donor type B**	**Donor type AB**
None (Type O)	Anti-A Anti-B				
A (Type A)	Anti-B				
B (Type B)	Anti-A				
AB (Type AB)	(None)				

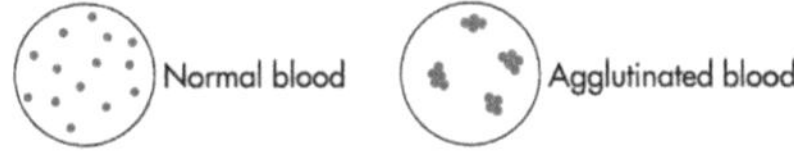

Figure 6.13 Blood groups and results of donor-recipient combinations.

If the first pregnancy produces a child who has developed the father's Rh positive trait, the mother will develop anti-Rh antibodies during her pregnancy.

During the second pregnancy, if that baby is also Rh positive, the mother's antibodies will cause agglutination of the foetal RBCs, resulting in the death of the foetus. This is called erythroblastosis foetalis.

Pregnant women are screened to identify this risk and can then be given medication to prevent the production of antibodies.

If donated blood contains ***no*** A or B antigens, agglutination ***cannot*** occur; therefore blood group O is often referred to as the **universal donor**.

Those with blood group AB do not have antibodies to ***either*** A or B, and therefore agglutination ***cannot occur*** with any donated blood, and group AB is often referred to as the **universal recipient**.

In practice, however, all blood is matched carefully to that of a recipient, although in an extreme emergency, such as massive blood loss due to trauma, O positive blood may be given.

Blood transfusion

The plasma membranes of RBCs carry proteins, as do those of all body cells. These proteins identify us as unique and are known as 'self-antigens'. Antigens that enter the body through wounds, transfusions etc. are 'non-self-antigens'. Because they differ from our self-antigens, they are recognised as foreign by antibodies. Antibodies are produced by the immune system in response to the presence of foreign antigens, or they may be present in the plasma already. The reaction that occurs between the antigen and antibody is the basis of all immune responses. In the case of red blood cells, the antibody antigen reaction that occurs following an incompatible transfusion causes the cells to 'clump' together, or agglutinate. This may result in a blockage of small vessels, causing hypoxia and tissue damage. More devastating is the rupture of red blood cells that also occurs, a process known as lysing. Lysing of red blood cells causes the release of free haemoglobin into the circulation. These freely circulating molecules travel to the kidney and block the glomerulus, resulting in renal failure and possible death.

Transfusion of blood can be a life-saving procedure; however, everyone's blood is different, and transfusing blood that is incompatible with the recipient's blood produces an acute haemolytic transfusion reaction that can be fatal. The hazards of transfusion do not only relate to incompatibility; blood is a complex liquid tissue and transfusion also carries the risk of:

- Febrile non-haemolytic transfusion reactions, which are usually mild.
- Reactions to bacterially contaminated blood, which can range from a mild pyrexia to potentially lethal septic shock.
- Transfusion-related acute lung injury (TRALI).
- Transfusion associated circulatory overload (TACO).
- Acute allergic reaction, ranging from mild urticaria to life threatening angio-oedema anaphylaxis.

Transfusion considerations

Blood transfusion is an essential part of care for many patients in hospital, but transfusions are associated with risk of harm if correct procedures are not followed. Daniels (2013) identified essential considerations before starting a blood transfusion. A transfusion is given after a detailed clinical assessment, along with blood test results, only when the benefits of transfusion outweigh the risks. Reasons for the transfusion are clearly documented and informed patient consent is gained. A timely blood transfusion can improve clinical outcome. The process is enhanced by electronic transfusion monitoring system and bar code technology. The nurse must ensure they are trained and competent and adhere to local guidelines, ensuring:

- Patient identity is checked.
- Wrist identity band, clearly displaying name, date of birth and unique ID number must be present and checked at every stage in the process.

- Patient identifiers on ID band and blood pack must be identical; **if there is any discrepancy, do not transfuse.**
- A safe transfusion involves the right blood being given to the right patient at the right time and in the right place.
- The patient must be monitored during each unit of the blood transfusion. At a minimum, this involves a recording of Respiratory rate, pulse, BP and temperature, initially and after 15 minutes, then regular visual inspections and observation recording as required

Thankfully, serious or life-threatening acute reactions are rare; however, any new symptoms or signs appearing whilst a patient is being transfused must be reported, as they could be the first warnings of a serious reaction. It can be difficult to determine the type of reaction in the early stages, so all those receiving a blood transfusion are monitored carefully, and observations of vital signs are recorded frequently according to local protocols (usually every 30 minutes). Symptoms of transfusion reactions and appropriate actions are detailed in Figure 6.14.

Following a reaction, the unit of blood must be returned to the blood bank and an incident form completed. Severe adverse reactions or events must be reported to SABRE (Serious Adverse Blood Reactions and Events) and SHOT (Serious Hazards of Transfusion), www.shotuk.org. This is done via the blood bank.

The arterial and venous systems

So far we have discussed the heart, cardiac output and the blood. We now move on to how blood is transported around the body, from the heart through the systemic circulation to the tissues and returning back to the heart. This is the circulatory system, a network of blood vessels that can be thought of as having two main components: the systemic circulation and the pulmonary circulation.

Blood is transported away from the heart via arteries, the largest of which is the aorta. Arteries become progressively smaller the further they are from the heart, finally becoming very small vessels known as arterioles. Arterioles feed into capillaries in the capillary bed of all body tissues. Whilst arterioles are very small, capillaries are microscopic, with very thin walls. It is at the capillary bed that the exchange of nutrients and oxygen occurs, from the blood to the tissues, and waste products are exchanged to the blood from the tissues. Blood leaves the capillary bed via small venules that join with others to become veins, the largest of which are the superior vena cava (SVC) and the inferior vena cava (IVC). Veins transport blood to the heart.

The flow of blood down the arterioles can be controlled by regulating the diameter of the vessel. Contraction (vasoconstriction) of the vessels narrows the lumen and reduces blood flow, and relaxation causes dilation of the lumen, increasing the diameter and allowing an increase in blood flow. Control of vascular tone occurs both centrally and peripherally. The autonomic nervous system (ANS) utilises hormones such as adrenaline and nor-adrenaline, which cause vasoconstriction and antidiuretic hormone (ADH) that regulates fluid loss via the kidneys. Vasoconstriction and dilation may occur locally to preserve blood flow to vital organs such as the heart, brain and lungs, but in doing so, divert blood flow from other less essential areas. In addition to collecting blood from the capillary beds and returning it to the heart, veins and venules can expand to act as reservoirs for blood or constrict in order to divert the flow of blood elsewhere.

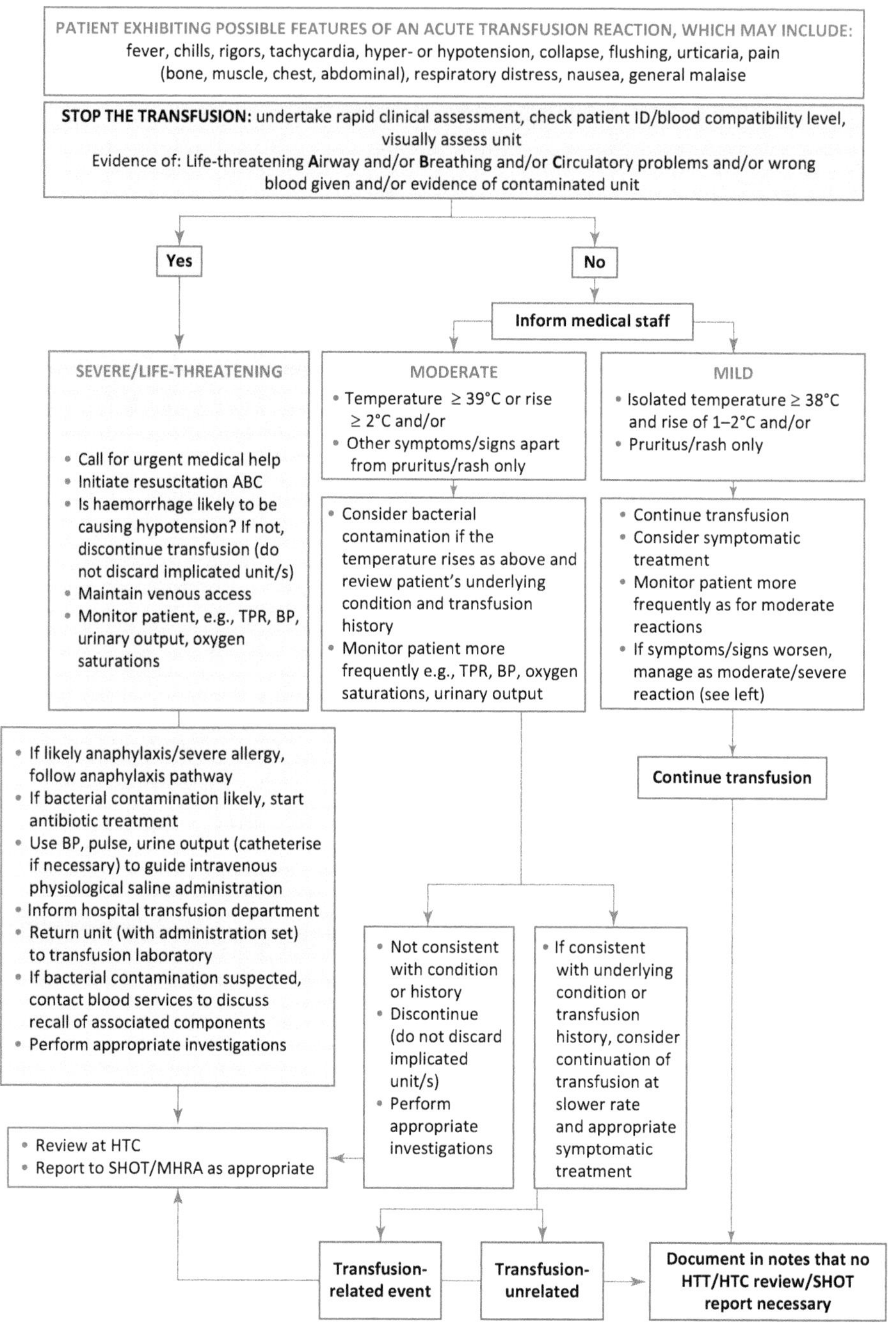

Figure 6.14 Flow chart for the management of transfusion reactions. Norfolk, D. (2013) Handbook of Transfusion Medicine, https://www.transfusionguidelines.org/transfusion-handbook. Produced under the terms of the open Government License.

Structure of blood vessels

The walls of arteries and veins have three layers (see Figure 6.15). The *tunica interna* or *intima* is the innermost layer of the vessels. The surface in contact with the blood is the *vascular endothelium*, and this is present throughout the heart and the vessels of the circulatory system. It is composed of completely flattened cells, providing a very smooth surface to allow uninterrupted blood flow. However, it is not simply an inert lining, but has a number of vital functions, which are controlled by release of vasoactive substances. These functions include regulation of coagulation and platelet adhesion, immune function, fluid distribution through vasoconstriction and dilation and the mediation of the electrolyte content of the intravascular and extra-vascular spaces. Endothelial dysfunction can result from environmental factors, for example smoking, nutritional imbalances and exposure to airborne pollutants, and contribute to several disease processes such as septic shock, hypertension, hypercholesterolaemia and diabetes.

The middle layer, the *tunica media*, is composed of smooth muscle and elastic fibrous tissue that is much thicker in arteries than in veins. This is to enable the arterial wall to expand and contract in response to the pressures generated by the contraction of the left ventricle and plays a crucial role in the control of blood pressure. The venous system is a much lower pressure system, and therefore the elastic muscular middle layer does not need to be as thick.

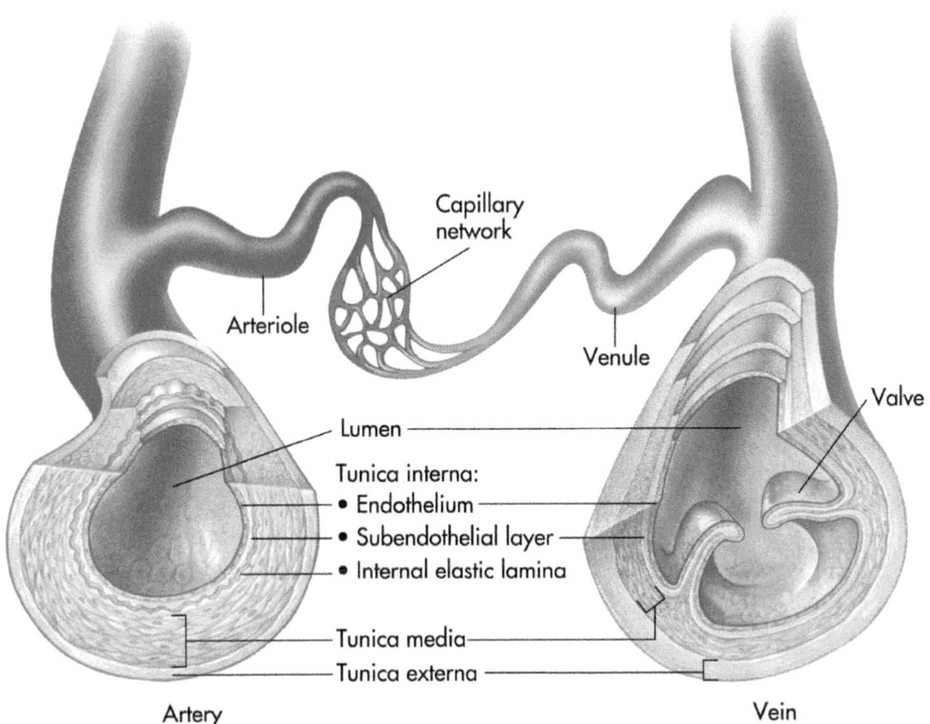

Figure 6.15 Blood vessels and connecting capillaries.

Vascular endothelium

Vascular endothelium actively synthesises and releases vasoactive substances:

- **Angiotensin-converting enzyme**: converts angiotensin 1 to angiotensin 2 in the lungs; **nitric oxide vasodilator** also inhibits platelet activation and clotting.
- **Prostacyclin**: inhibits platelet activation and clotting.
- **Endothelin**: vasoconstrictor.

(Stanfield 2017)

The outermost layer, the *tunica externa* or *adventitia*, is made of connective fibres and provides support and protection to the vessel.

A major difference between arteries and veins in terms of structure is that the larger veins, particularly in the legs, contain valves to prevent blood flowing in the wrong direction. The low pressure in the venous system means that blood needs some assistance on the journey back to the heart. In addition to the valves preventing backflow, the muscles in the legs 'squeeze' the veins and help to push the blood towards the heart. The wall of the capillaries consists solely of the tunica interna and is only one cell thick, to allow exchange of substances between the blood and extracellular fluid.

Venous return to the heart has to defy gravity, so it is aided by:

- The muscular skeletal pump.
- Decreased venous capacitance (vasoconstriction).
- Respiratory pump.

Capillary bed and sphincters – tissue fluid formation and reabsorption

Capillaries, in addition to having very thin walls, have a lumen that is only slightly larger in size than the diameter of a red blood cell. These properties facilitate the efficient movement of substances in and out of the blood at a cellular level. Many capillaries join together to form a web of capillaries, supplying all organs and tissues of the body: this web is known as the capillary bed.

Even at rest, the body requires 250mL oxygen and will produce 200mL carbon dioxide *per minute*, so efficient movement at the capillary level is vital.

The capillary bed is composed of two types of vessel (see Figure 6.16). The vascular shunt is the main route into the network of capillaries and true capillaries where exchange of substances occurs. Within this network are structures known as precapillary sphincters that control the flow of blood from the vascular shunt through into the capillaries. If the blood is stopped at the precapillary sphincters, it continues through the vascular shunt, bypassing the tissues. If the sphincter is open, blood will flow from the vascular shunt into the capillary bed. For example, a muscle at rest may not need blood flowing through the entire capillary network, because its demands for oxygen and nutrients are reduced, as are the production of waste products. If the muscle becomes active due to exercise, the sphincters will open, allowing flow of blood into the capillary networks.

Movement of water, as well as nutrients and oxygen, occurs at the capillary bed to ensure the hydration of cells. This movement is dependent upon two pressures:

SPHINCTERS OPEN

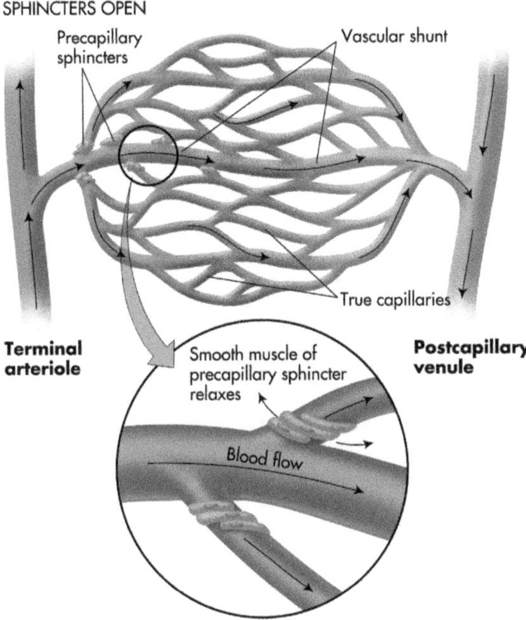

SPHINCTERS CLOSED

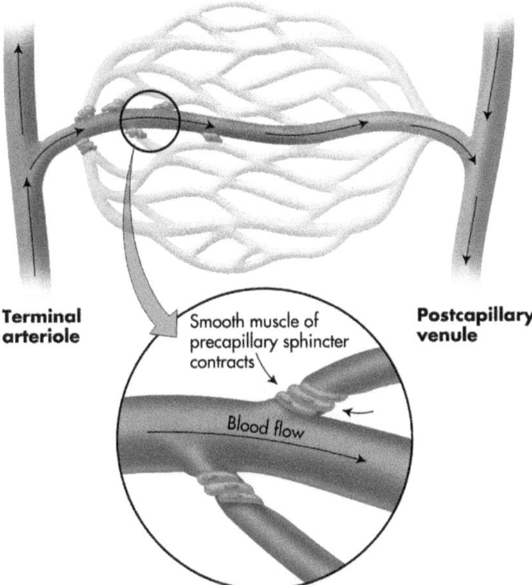

Figure 6.16 Capillary beds and sphincters.

1 *Hydrostatic pressure*: this is best thought of as the 'pushing force' of water and is the pressure generated by the liquid component of the blood against the vessel wall. It therefore tends to force fluid out of the capillary.
2 *Osmotic pressure*: this is generated by the presence of the plasma proteins in the blood and creates a 'pulling' or 'holding' force, which attracts water to and holds it inside the capillary (see, also, Chapter 4).

At the arterial end of the capillary bed, hydrostatic pressure exceeds osmotic, and therefore fluid is forced out of the capillary. At the venous end, osmotic pressure tends to be higher, and fluid from the interstitial spaces is therefore drawn back into the circulation. Changes in either of these pressures can result in oedema, as either too much fluid is forced out or not enough is drawn back in.

Oedema is an abnormally large amount of fluid in the interstitial space and is evidence of fluid imbalance. It may be due to:

- Imbalance of electrolytes, especially sodium (Na^+).
- Increase in capillary blood pressure due to venous congestion, for example, right-sided heart failure.
- Decreased concentration of plasma proteins. This may be due to poor nutrition or 'leakage' into the tissues that can occur in septic shock.

In health, the movement of water solutes and respiratory gases between the intravascular space (blood), the interstitial space (around the cells) and finally, the intracellular space (inside the tissues cells), is controlled by this mechanism.

Fluids that may be given to patients by intravenous (IV) infusion may be:

- Isotonic (having the same concentrations as body cells).
- Hypertonic (having a higher concentration than body cells)
- Hypotonic (having a lower concentration than body cells).

Most fluids given to patients are isotonic, for example, 0.9% saline (normal saline) and 5% dextrose. Hypertonic solutions are sometimes given to patients who have oedema, as due to their high concentration, they will tend to draw fluid out of the tissues and back into the circulation. Hypotonic solutions are rarely given intravenously but may be used in cases of extreme dehydration. Taking these fluids orally is more usual – most rehydrating sports drinks are hypotonic.

IV fluid therapy may be:

- *Crystalloid fluids*: solutions containing molecules that pass freely through the semipermeable membranes of the body fluid compartments, for example, 0.9% saline, 5% dextrose and Hartmann's solution.
- *Colloid fluids*: these contain large protein molecules that tend to remain in the circulation longer. Vascular fluid loss can be replaced with smaller volumes than if crystalloids are used. Colloids tend to be more expensive and do have a higher incidence of adverse effects than crystalloids.

- *Blood and blood products*: these include whole blood, packed red cells, fresh frozen plasma (FFP) and human albumin solution. These should be used to replace the loss of specific fluids, and not for general fluid resuscitation. Caution should be exercised, due to their high potential for causing adverse reactions and their expense.

Having reviewed the components and normal functioning of the cardiovascular system, an overview of some common disorders of this system will be given.

Common disorders of cardiovascular system

Atherosclerosis

Atherosclerosis is a potentially serious condition where there is a progressive build-up of fatty deposits in the subintimal layer of medium and large arteries. It is a chronic inflammatory condition of the arterial wall that can take several decades for the resulting deposits to reach a level where there is significant disruption to the blood flow along the arteries. Atherosclerosis is a major risk factor for many different conditions involving a reduced blood flow. Collectively, these conditions are known as cardiovascular disease (CVD). Examples of CVD include:

- Coronary artery disease and myocardial infarction.
- Peripheral artery disease.
- Stroke.

Risk factors for CHD include:

- Family history.
- Smoking.
- Diet high in saturated fats.
- Lack of exercise.
- Obesity.
- Diabetes.
- Hypertension.

Coronary artery disease

Fatty streaks are non-pathological lesions in the coronary arteries; they are present in most people around the age of 20 and are thought to be the precursors of atheromatous plaques. The progression into pathological lesions is influenced by both genetic and lifestyle factors (Mageed 2018). During the early stages of this disease, lipids are deposited into the sub-intimal space where they combine with monocytes to form large bulky cells called foam cells. As the cells proliferate, the amount of space needed for them is reduced, and they slowly start to force the endothelial layer of the arterial wall out into the lumen of the artery. As a result, the diameter of the lumen becomes slowly more narrow (stenosis) (see Figure 6.17). The patient might be asymptomatic throughout the early phases of atherosclerosis build-up. By the time that symptoms of chest pain (angina) and breathlessness occur during activity, the disease will already be quite advanced in the coronary arteries.

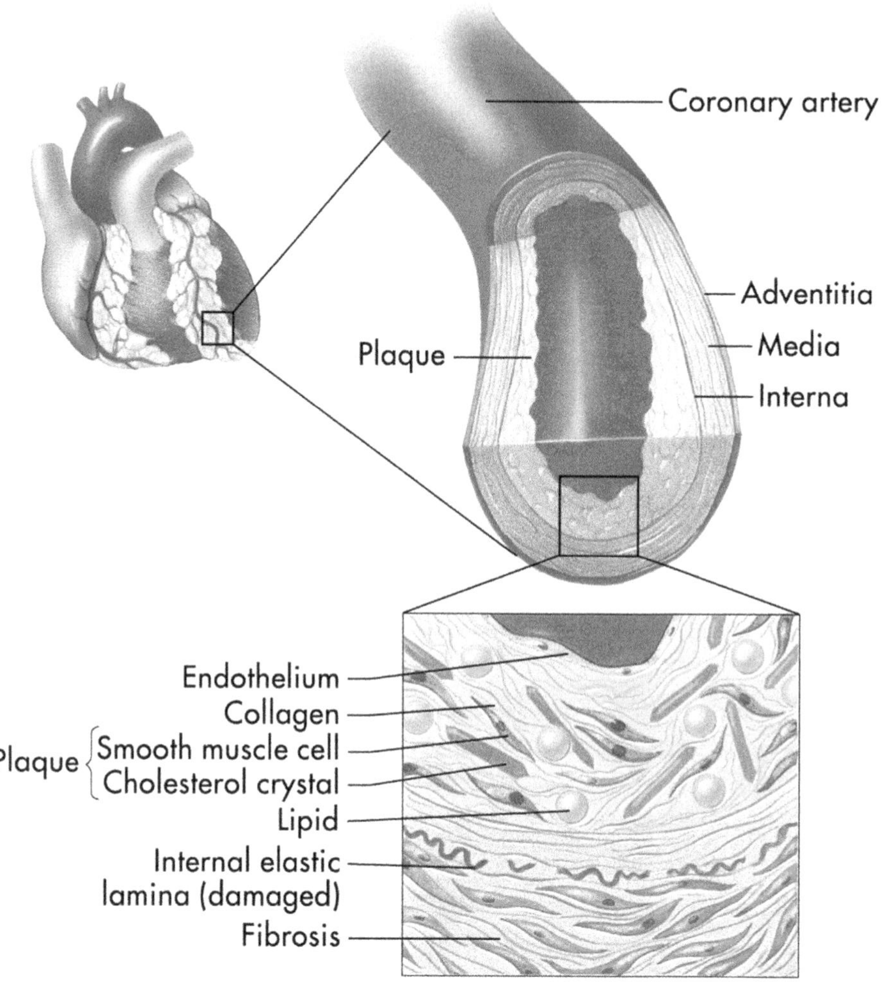

Figure 6.17 Atherosclerosis.

Atherosclerosis alters the efficiency of the endothelium to prevent blood cells and platelets from adhering to the wall of the arterial lumen. In addition to this, the narrowing of the lumen slows down the flow of blood through the artery.

The developing fibrous plaques accumulate large amounts of lipid that disrupt the lining of the coronary vessel (the endothelium). As the lesion progresses, the endothelium is replaced by a fibrous cap, which protrudes in to the artery and may be prone to rupture. Plaque rupture exposes contents that are highly thrombotic, that is, they attract platelets and activate the clotting cascade with thrombus (clot) formation (Badimon et al. 2018). The formation of the thrombus might cause either a partial or complete occlusion, turning coronary heart disease from a chronic disease into an acute coronary event. Where there is a partial occlusion, a small residual blood flow may remain, giving the myocardium a reduced oxygen supply (ischaemia). In this case, the myocardium is not likely to be permanently damaged, but should recover once blood flow is re-established. If the thrombus in the coronary artery causes a complete occlusion, then all of the myocardium that lies beyond the occlusion will firstly become damaged (myocardial injury) and, should the occlusion not be removed quickly, the myocardium will die (causing necrosis), leading to myocardial dysfunction and death. It is this sudden development of a partial or total occlusion by a thrombus that defines **acute coronary syndrome** (ACS), which is discussed in more detail later in this chapter.

Stroke

Embolic strokes typically occur when an occlusive thrombus in a cerebral vessel disrupts blood supply to an area of the brain. Thrombi may occur locally due to atherothrombotic plaques, or may be embolic, travelling through the cardiovascular system to the brain from, for example, a clot from in the atria due to atrial fibrillation (Dutton and Finch 2018). Stroke is considered in more detail in Chapter 9, and atrial fibrillation is discussed later in this chapter

Aneurysm

An aneurysm occurs when an area of the arterial wall has become weakened, possibly by arteriosclerosis or sometimes due to congenital defects. The weakened vessel wall develops into a sac-like protrusion that may predispose to a thrombus formation or may burst. Having an aneurysm increases the risk of damage to the lining of the artery involved; when a small tear occurs, this is called dissection. Damaged vessels are more likely to burst. If an aneurysm bursts, it has potentially catastrophic consequences due to excessive loss of blood. In the case of an abdominal aortic aneurysm, this is a life-threatening emergency. If a vessel in the brain is affected, this is called a haemorrhagic stroke, and a fatal rise in intracranial pressure can occur.

Heart failure

Heart failure is a complex clinical syndrome of symptoms including breathlessness, ankle oedema and fatigue, suggesting there is impairment of the heart working effectively as a pump to support the circulation (ESC 2016a). The heart therefore is unable to adequately perfuse the organs and tissues of the body. The term heart failure should not be confused with cardiac arrest (which is an emergency situation), or 'heart attack' (which normally refers to myocardial infarction). Increases in survival from the chronic diseases that contribute to heart failure has added to the number of people in the UK living with the disease, with a recent increase (2002–2014) of around 23% (Conrad et al. 2017). Common causes of heart failure include ischaemic heart disease, hypertension, heart valve disease and other structural changes to the myocardium (such as cardiomyopathy). Structural changes to the heart occur before symptoms are apparent, so considering risk and treating patients early contributes to a reduced reduce mortality.

There are many reasons why the heart loses the ability to adequately supply oxygenated blood to the target organs, and this is reflected by the type of heart failure that exists and which side of the heart has failed. Acute heart failure occurs when there is a rapid onset of heart failure symptoms that, due to their life-threatening nature, require urgent treatment in hospital, and this is discussed later in this chapter.

There are essentially two types of heart failure (ESC 2016a):

- **Heart failure with reduced ejection fraction** (HFrEF).
- **Heart failure with preserved ejection fraction** (HFpEF).

These were previously known as 'systolic' and 'diastolic' failures, or even the terms 'forward' and 'backward' failures may be used to describe this classification. A good knowledge of the cardiac cycle – concepts such as contractility, the Frank-Starling mechanism, stroke volume, ejection fraction, preload and afterload, discussed earlier in the chapter – will aid understanding of this fairly complex clinical problem!

Heart failure with reduced ejection fraction

Remember

Ejection fraction is the percentage of the blood in the ventricle blood ejected as SV.

In health, this is between 50–70%.

In systolic heart failure (HFrEF), this may fall to:

- 40–49%, 'borderline'
- <40%, low.

Ejection fraction is commonly determined by echocardiography.

HFrEF is rather a mouth full, but describes accurately the nature of the failure, which is essentially a failure of systole. It is characterised by a falling ejection fraction, as the ventricular myocardium is unable to contract effectively during systole. This leads to a reduced stroke volume and cardiac output. This can be due to:

- Reversible causes: including ischaemic heart disease and angina, where blood flow can be restored.
- Irreversible causes: including myocardial infarction, where necrosis of myocardial tissue has occurred, causing a permanent degree of residual heart failure.
- Aortic stenosis and obstructive cardiomyopathy which make it difficult for the blood to be pumped from the ventricle into the aorta.

Heart failure with preserved ejection fraction

Remember

When diastole fails (HFpEF), even though the ventricle can contract effectively, the amount pumped out (SV) is considerably lower. The ventricle has not been able to fill sufficiently in diastole.

HFpEF refers to a failure of diastolic function; the heart is unable to adequately fill with blood during diastole, but is still able to eject a good proportion of this reduced amount as stroke volume. HFpEF can be due to:

- Stenosis of the mitral or tricuspid valve, preventing blood from flowing into the ventricle during diastole.
- Changes in the compliance (or distensibility) of the ventricular myocardium, so that it does not expand as the ventricle fills with blood. A poorly compliant ventricle will have a reduced volume of blood at the end of diastole, and therefore will eject a smaller amount during systole, leading to a reduced cardiac output.
- **Ventricular hypertrophy** may occur in response to some heart problems; the ventricular wall becomes thicker and less compliant. Hypertrophy can occur in patients with a history of hypertension, valve problems and/or renal failure, as the myocardium adapts to increased stress on the ventricular wall.

Left ventricular failure (LVF)

In LVF, the forward flow of blood from the left ventricle into the systemic circulation is reduced. As a result of this impairment, blood pressure and tissue perfusion will decrease. The lowered ejection fraction means that pressure builds up in the ventricle (as more blood is left behind after the ventricular contraction), creating an increase in pressure in the left atrium and pulmonary circulation. This increased pressure in the pulmonary circulation is reflected in the interstitial lung pressures and, if sufficiently raised, may lead to pulmonary oedema, a common sequalae of LVF. Distress and breathlessness are frequently observed; a dry cough may be present (seen with interstitial pulmonary oedema) or, if the pressure is sufficient for fluid to enter the alveoli, pink frothy sputum may be expectorated.

If not resolved, over time the increased pulmonary pressures will extend back to the right ventricle, creating a dysfunction in both sides of the heart. This is commonly referred to as congestive cardiac failure (CCF) or biventricular failure.

Right ventricular failure

Jugular venous pressure

Assessed by measuring the height of the internal jugular vein; observed on the right side of the neck, with the patient at sitting at 30–45°.

Normal range is around 2-4cm from sternal angle, or 9cm above the right atrium (RA) (sternal angle about 5cm above RA).

A raised JVP may be referred to as jugular venous distension (JVD) and can present in heart failure and other cardiac problems

When the right side of the heart fails to provide adequate forward flow through the pulmonary circulation to the left side of the heart, the congestion extends back into the venous circulation. This might be observed as raised **jugular venous pressure** (JVP)

and peripheral oedema. However, because the pulmonary circulation pressure is not increased, there will be an absence of pulmonary oedema, as would be seen in LVF. The reduced flow of blood from the right to the left side of the heart (via the pulmonary circulation) leads to a reduction of preload in the left ventricle. Reduced cardiac output is thus a consequence of RVF and LVF.

Symptoms

We have looked at some of the common conditions of the cardiovascular system that affect the lives of many people. Common symptoms of heart failure are given in Table 6.5. Often, these problems are monitored and managed in primary care, with occasional visits to hospital for additional investigations, or medicine management. The National Institute for Health and Care Excellence have issued guidance on 'Chronic heart failure in adult: diagnosis and management (ng106)', to support the detection and management of heart failure (NICE 2018a). Detailed history-taking, early diagnostic tests with the support of a specialist heart failure, multi-disciplinary team, including a specialist heart failure nurse, are integral to safe and effective care. A plan of care devised for and with the patient should include all aspects of care, aiding communication if referral to specialist heart services is required.

Disordered physiology may give rise to acute clinical deterioration that requires urgent or emergency intervention. The nurse uses assessment skills to evaluate health status and to identify possible problems.

Early diagnostic tests for suspected HF (NICE 2018):

Measure serum NT-ProBNP.

- If NTProBNP>2000ng/L, refer for urgent echocardiography (2 weeks).
- If NTProBNP is between 400ng/l–2000ng/L, refer for echocardiography (within 6 weeks).

Table 6.5 Common symptoms of heart failure

Symptom	*Left ventricular failure*	*Right ventricular failure*	*Biventricular failure*
Dyspnoea	Yes	No	Yes
Reduced cardiac Output	Yes	Yes	Yes
Raised JVP	No	Yes	Yes
Pulmonary Oedema	Yes	No	Yes
Peripheral Oedema	No	Yes	Yes
Pallor	Yes	Yes	Yes
Reduced exercise Tolerance	Yes	Yes	Yes

Pharmacology in heart failure:

ACEI, e.g., Lisinopril
ARB, e.g., Losartan
Beta blockers, e.g., Bisoprolol
Mineralocorticoid receptor antagonists (MRA), e.g., **Spironolactone**

NICE (2018a)

Cardiovascular assessment

In the acute care setting, the nurse has a pivotal role to play in performing a comprehensive assessment of cardiovascular status, so that deterioration can be detected as early possible. Good communication skills are necessary to build a therapeutic relationship with the patient to ensure that care is person-centred and that all nursing activities are understood by the patient (NMC 2018a). These skills are necessary for a sound and comprehensive clinical assessment, and Bickley (2017) advises that all nursing and medical personnel should have skills to perform taking a medical history and performing a physical examination. A medical history involves asking questions ranging from identifying the present complaint through to family and social history. The physical examination involves skills of inspection, palpation and auscultation and will be performed when the patient's clinical condition is sufficiently stable, determined by the ABCDE assessment.

Valuable information can be gained by taking account of both subjective and objective data. The patient's experience and perspective is important and can contribute to the nurse's understanding and identification of likely problems. Taking a brief history can identify relevant past medical history, allergies, risk factors and medication taken. Symptoms should be explored systematically to help identify underlying physiological disturbances.

Objective data includes the vital signs recorded by the nurse as well as information gathered by physical examination and diagnostics test such as Electrocardiograms (ECG), serum electrolyte levels and cardiac biomarkers.

The cardiovascular system is uniquely adapted to maintain homeostasis, ensuring that perfusion of vital organs such as the heart, lungs and brain are maintained for as long as possible. The nurse therefore needs to be aware of subtle changes which indicate that compensation is occurring, in order to maintain oxygen delivery. The development and use of NEWS in response to concerns regarding competence in this area has been discussed at some length in Chapter 1. Whilst NEWS is a useful tool, the nurse also needs to be cognisant of trends over time, to ascertain whether clinical signs of compensation are increasing, signalling deterioration in clinical status that may give rise to a medical emergency.

Assessment utilising the ABCDE framework and incorporating basic physical assessment skills of Look (Inspect), Feel (palpate/percuss) and Listen (Auscultate) identifies the patient at risk. The focus of the following discussion on cardiovascular assessment has integrated aspects of physical assessment (for further information on physical examination, please see Bickley [2017]).

Airway

Any problems identified in the airway assessment should be treated and resolved before moving on to breathing assessment.

Table 6.6 New York Heart Association (NYHA) classification of heart failure

Class I: asymptomatic	No limitations of ordinary physical activity. Ordinary activity will not cause unwarranted fatigue, dyspnoea, palpitation or angina.
Class II: mild	The person is comfortable at rest. There is slight or moderate limitation of physical activity. Ordinary physical activity causes symptoms.
Class III: moderate	Although comfortable at rest, there is marked limitation of physical activity with less than ordinary activity that causes symptoms.
Class IV: severe	Symptoms at present at rest. There is an inability to carry on any physical activity without discomfort, symptoms of cardiac insufficiency evident.

Breathing

Cardiac problems can cause changes in respiratory status, with the sensation of breathlessness or dyspnoea being a key feature of cardiac failure. Looking at the patient can reveal signs of increased work of breathing, such as use of accessory muscles or the inability to complete sentences in one breath. The New York Heart Classification of Heart Failure classifies patients' heart failure according to the severity of their symptoms. Symptoms of dyspnoea should be assessed in relation to level of activity, with dyspnoea at rest being consistent with Class IV failure (see Table 6.6).

Orthopnoea – difficulty in breathing when lying flat – is also often a symptom of heart failure. This may be noticed at night (paroxysmal nocturnal orthopnoea). The patient may complain of being woken at night with extreme breathlessness, which may occur when the patient slips down the bed whilst sleeping. Sitting up or out of bed in a chair may help alleviate the symptoms.

Central cyanosis, a bluish discolouration of the mucous membranes of the mouth, is a late sign of hypoxaemia and is not always reliable, so pulse oximetry should be assessed as soon as possible. Pulse oximetry gives valuable information regarding capillary oxygen saturation levels, which, in health, would be between 94–98%; this is recorded on the NEWS chart in conjunction with the percentage/litres of supplemental oxygen. Peripheral cyanosis, seen as a bluish discoloration of the fingers and toes, indicates vasoconstriction and is related to poor cardiac output, but may also be present in hypoxaemia.

Pulmonary auscultation is a valuable skill in assessing pulmonary status and is now included in the standards of proficiency for registered nurses (NMC 2018a). Pulmonary auscultation of an individual with heart failure may reveal pulmonary crackles. Crackles are non-musical popping sounds heard during inspiration, caused by the re-opening of collapsed alveoli, or by air moving through fluid. Inspiratory crackles will remain even after a cough to clear secretions. Crackles are associated with a number of lung problems (see Chapter 5), including pulmonary oedema secondary to acute left ventricular failure. The expectoration of pink frothy sputum is also a feature of acute pulmonary oedema. This sign of significant deterioration is accompanied by tachypnoea, distress and hypoxaemia, requiring urgent medical review. Respiratory rate is counted over 1 full minute to ensure accuracy, ensuring even small changes, which can be clinically significant, are detected.

Circulation

Skin colour and temperature

Observation of skin for colour and warmth can give a good indication of cardiovascular function. A grey or marble tone to the skin is a late sign of circulatory compromise.

A reduction in cardiac output will activate the SNS, with ensuing vasoconstriction, diverting blood flow from the peripheral circulation and rendering the skin pale and cool to touch. Feeling along a limb, for example, from the toes to foot to calf, detects the degree of vasoconstriction. It may be that just the toes are cool, which would be mild vasoconstriction, but if the leg felt cool up to mid-calf, this would signify more circulatory compromise. In extreme situations, a cold and clammy skim may be felt. This is usually due to the sympathetic nervous system cooling the peripheral skin to the extent that normal sweat evaporation does not occur. This could be due to circulatory collapse, extreme anxiety, pain or low blood glucose and, as such, is a serious concern.

Blood pressure

Blood pressure is kept relatively constant, with homeostatic mechanisms described earlier in this chapter. The nurse needs to be able to interpret blood pressure in the context of a range of parameters, such as heart rate, peripheral warmth and blood flow, level of consciousness and urine output. Changes in all of these parameters may occur prior to significant changes in blood pressure. Normal ranges of blood pressure have been discussed previously; when assessing clinical status, the variation from the patient's normal pressure may be as significant as the actual value. A systolic blood pressure that has fallen suddenly, by more than 20mmHg, or by 30% since the last reading, or that falls below 90mmHg, is indicative of circulatory failure, and tissue oxygen delivery will be impaired. The systolic blood pressure triggers on NEWS at or below 110mmHg. The diastolic pressure is also important, as it determines coronary artery blood flow and needs to be greater than 50mmHg for adequate coronary artery flow and myocardial perfusion. Pulse pressure has been discussed in relation to palpating the pulse, but can be objectively determined by subtracting diastolic pressure from systolic blood pressure, with the normal range between 35–55mmHg. A trend of decreasing pulse pressure signifies worsening cardiac output, and the cause should be ascertained early to maximise appropriate interventions. Acutely, a widening pulse pressure is associated with the vasodilation of sepsis or anaphylaxis. Pulse pressure, though, varies with age, increasing in the over 55's (Gillebert 2018); this value is therefore interpreted in the acute situation in the context of the individual.

Pulse pressure = systolic pressure - diastolic pressure

Examples:
If BP = 120/80, then pulse pressure = 40mmHg.
If BP = 110/90, then pulse pressure = 300mmHg.

This reduction in pulse pressure may indicate hypovolaemia or heart failure.

The majority of people with high blood pressure experience no symptoms, therefore monitoring of blood pressure is vital to detect and treat people early before secondary health problems are experienced.

Mean arterial pressure (MAP) is now commonly recorded in patients who are acutely unwell. Adequate perfusion pressure is essential to enable oxygen delivery at tissue level, and MAP is the best way of determining perfusion pressure throughout the cardiac cycle. You may remember that the time the heart spends in diastole is longer than the time spent in systole, and therefore MAP is skewed towards the diastolic value.

MAP be can be calculated by the following equation:
MAP = 1/3 pulse pressure + diastole
For example:
For a patient with a BP of 100/61

- MAP = (1/3 × 39) + 61
- MAP = 13 + 61

MAP = 74mmHg

A normal MAP is approximately 70–105mmHg. There is some debate as to the lowest acceptable MAP: Woodrow (2019) suggests 70mmHg is necessary for brain, kidney and major organ perfusion, whereas Rhodes et al. (2017) recommends a minimum MAP of 65mmHg is required for management of sepsis/septic shock (discussed further in Chapter 12). A MAP of over 110mmHg signifies hypertension that could have major consequences for the patient and therefore requires close monitoring, with possible pharmacological intervention required. MAP is calculated by both invasive and non-invasive blood pressure measurement devices and, if requested, should be recorded on the chart with the systolic and diastolic pressure. Invasive haemodynamic monitoring is discussed later in this chapter.

Pulse

Palpation of pulses gives valuable information regarding cardiac output. It also involves physical contact, which can be reassuring for the patient, but also aids assessment of peripheral temperature and diaphoresis (sweating). A cold and clammy patient is indicative of sympathetic activation and is a sign of serious circulatory compromise. Help should be sought immediately.

The pulse should be assessed for:

- Rate.
- Volume.
- Rhythm.

A normal heart rate will vary between 60–100 beats per minute, but any changes, even within this normal range, can indicate deteriorating circulatory status. This makes heart/pulse rate an important early warning sign. A steadily rising heart rate is indicative of circulatory problems such as hypovolaemia, cardiogenic shock or sepsis. A rising trend should alert the nurse, even if the trigger threshold for NEWS has not been met. Heart rate will normally be lower than systolic blood pressure, so if it rises beyond this point (or systolic blood pressure falls below heart rate), this is a cause for concern. A falling heart rate is the result of increased **vagal tone**, such as when sleeping, but could be a sign of a conduction problem. Heart rate and rhythm can be continuously assessed with ECG monitoring, so a knowledge of sinus rhythm and the PQRST complex discussed earlier in the chapter is required if abnormalities are to be detected.

Pulses can be palpated at a number of sites:

- Radial.
- Brachial.
- Carotid.
- Femoral.
- Dorsalis pedis.
- Posterior tibialis.
- Popliteal.

When palpating the pulse, the strength of the pulse wave has clinical significance. Pulse pressure is the difference between the pressure in systole (peak pressure) and diastole (lower pressure). A pulse with a large differential will be felt as full, or bounding. Vasodilation increases the pulse pressure and is associated with sepsis and anaphylaxis. A weak and thready pulse has a low pulse volume caused by vasoconstriction and is a sign of poor cardiac output. A pulse pressure which falls significantly during inspiration is called pulsus paradoxus and could be a sign of pericardial effusion or **cardiac tamponade**.

The rhythm of the pulse should be regular, though there may be slight variations within the respiratory cycle. An irregular pulse should always be further assessed with a *12 lead ECG* to ascertain the exact rhythm. People with irregular heart rates may also need to be placed on a cardiac monitor, so the rhythm can be continuously viewed. Problems such as **atrial fibrillation**, ectopic beats and conduction abnormalities will be felt as an irregular pulse, and may need urgent treatment. Although there is no specific place to record an irregular pulse on the NEWS chart, any new irregularity in the pulse is 'a cause for concern' and should be reported and investigated promptly.

The 12 lead ECG

Electrocardiograms (ECG) are used as diagnostic tools for visualising the electrical activity of the heart. The cardiac monitor is commonly used for real-time monitoring of heart rate and rhythm of patients that require close observation for changes in the heart's function. However, the cardiac monitor will usually only show the activity of the heart from one viewpoint at a time. The 12 lead ECG provides 12 different views of the heart, from standardised positions, and would be taken as part of the ABCDE assessment if the patient complains of chest pain or palpations, or an irregular pulse is felt. It is recorded intermittently, as it requires the patient to lie still whilst 10 electrodes are attached to the chest and limbs. Often, a series of 12 lead ECGs are needed to observe for the changes to the conduction pattern that may occur during acute coronary syndromes or following the administration of antiarrhythmic drugs.

Recording a 12 lead ECG

A 12 lead ECG may be taken by a number of different members of the health care team. As with any procedure, the patient needs to be kept at the centre of the process. Informed consent is required, and privacy and dignity must be maintained. Chest hair may need to be removed with a single use razor to ensure good electrode contact. A semi-recumbent position of about 45 degrees is recommended, and the patient should be fully relaxed before the recording is commenced (SCST 2017).

Six electrodes are placed across the front of the chest on the left side; these electrodes give us a series of views of the left ventricle, as observed from the right side of the heart around to the left side (see Figure 6.18). Common errors in lead placement may occur with V1 and V2 frequently being placed too high; they should be each placed over 4th intercostal space, on the right and left sternal border respectively. V4, V5 and V6 are often placed too low; V4 is placed on the 5th intercostal space, with V5 anterior axillary line and V6 mid-axillary line on the same horizontal line as V4 (SCST 2017).

Four electrodes are placed on the limbs. These electrodes may be placed on the extremities (ankles and wrists). Moving the electrodes up the limbs may alter the ECG, so this should only be done as individual circumstances dictate. The important point to note is that these electrodes should be placed symmetrically (see Figure 6.19).

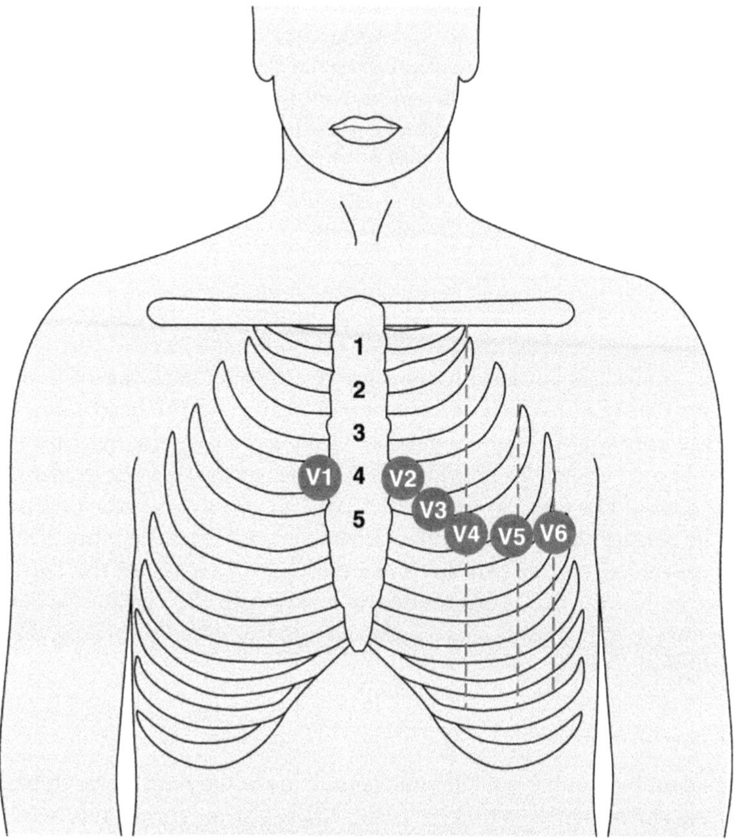

Figure 6.18 Chest lead placement.

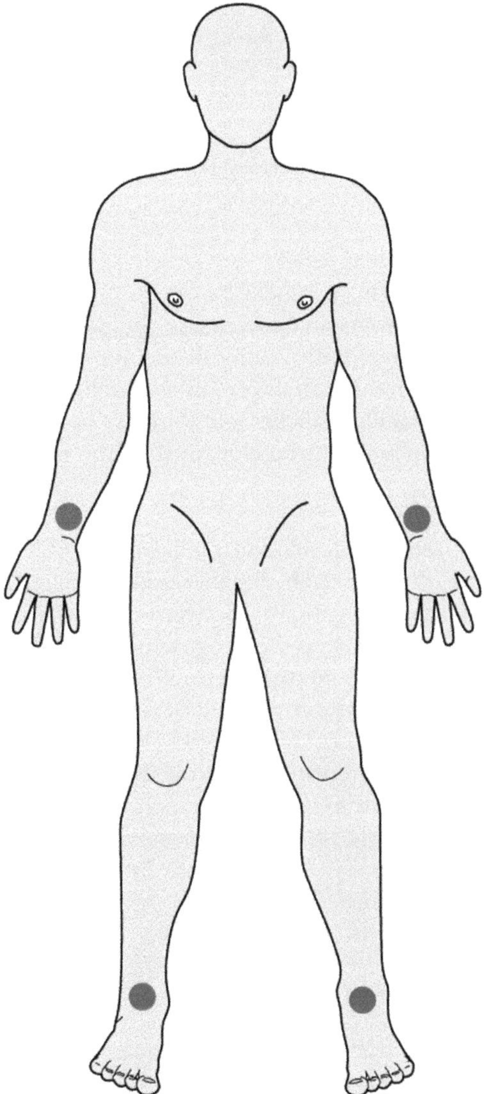

Figure 6.19 Limb lead placement.

Twelve views of the heart are obtained from these ten electrodes: six are views of the heart from the sides, top and bottom (on the vertical plane); six are views of the anterior surface of the left ventricle (on the horizontal plane).

Before recording a 12 lead ECG:

- Explain procedure to patient.
- Ask for consent to proceed (NMC 2018b).

- Check each electrode is attached and correctly placed.
- Ask the patient to lie still and to not speak for a short while, whilst the recording is made.

A normal ECG has been included in Figure 6.20. Recordings should be checked for the following characteristics:

- QRS complexes should be upright in leads I, II, III and aVF.
- QRS complexes should be downwards in leads aVR, V1 and V2.
- In the chest leads (V1 to V6) there should be a progressive increase in the height of the QRS complexes (V1 negative and V6 positive, with a smooth transition from one to the other). This tells us that the conduction through the ventricles is following the normal conduction pathways through the bundle branches and Purkinje fibres.
- The ST segment and the T wave should be level with the baseline in all of the ECG in all leads.

After the ECG has printed, check, before disconnecting the cables, that you have an ECG that is free from artefact (usually appearing as a 'fuzz' through the ECG). Artefact can be caused by any electrical activity, such as shivering, and nearby electrical equipment. If necessary, replace electrodes and repeat the tracing. Check the progression of the R waves in the chest leads. If this is interrupted, recheck the lead placement. Write the date, time and patient identity on the printout (if not automatically completed by the machine) and record any alterations in patient position or lead placement and relevant clinical information, such as recent chest pain, and/or any medications given (Woodrow 2019). Refer to a health care professional who is competent in 12 lead ECG interpretation. For more detailed information on recording the 12 lead ECG, please see guidance from the Society for Cardiological Sciences and Technology (SGOT 2017) (available from http://www.scst.org.uk/resources/SCST_ECG_Recording_Guidelines_2017am.pdf).

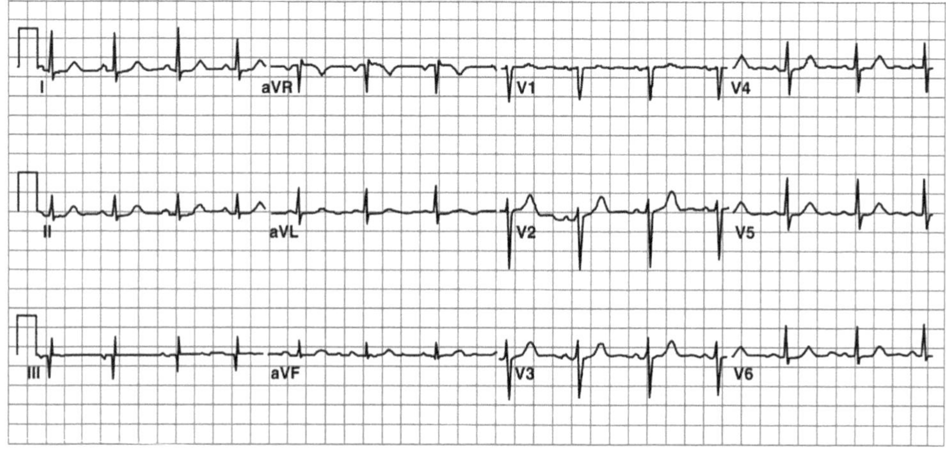

Figure 6.20 A normal 12 lead ECG.

Capillary refill time

Capillary refill time (CRT)

CRT can be used to give an indication of cardiac output.

- Hold hand to level of heart.
- Press the tip of the finger nail for five seconds, and the nail bed will blanch.
- Release the pressure and observe reperfusion (will turn pink).
- Normal refill time will be <2 seconds.

Remember that factors such as temperature will affect capillary refill.

Other clinical signs such as capillary refill time (CRT) are important indicators of cardiac output. A delayed CRT is consistent with a poor cardiac output that has led to reduction in perfusion of the peripheral circulation. It may be associated with hypovolaemia and heart failure. Warm, dilated peripheries with a brisk CRT may be an indication of the increased peripheral flow associated with sepsis.

Urinary output

Urinary output is one of the best indicators of circulatory function, as kidneys receive about 25% of the cardiac output. For accurate hourly measurements, a urinary catheter is required, and as most patients do not have catheters, urine output does not form part of NEWS. Homeostatic mechanisms such as the sympathetic nervous system will reduce blood supply to the kidney in times of low cardiac output, so a reduced urine output is an early sign of cardiovascular compromise. Nurses caring for acutely unwell patients need to closely monitor urine output. Volumes of less than 0.5mL/per Kg, per hour are a cause for concern; renal impairment could ensue. Renal impairment is discussed more fully in Chapter 8.

Skin turgor

Assessing for skin turgor can give information regarding the degree of hydration of the patient. The skin on the back of the hand or forearm is gently pinched, then released. The skin should fall back almost immediately to its previous state. If the fold takes a little time to relax, this could indicate dehydration. Skin elasticity, though, does decrease with age, so this is not always a reliable sign. Other indicators, such as a furrowed tongue, should also be assessed.

Oedema

Oedema is the accumulation of fluid in the interstitial spaces and occurs when interstitial fluid exceeds absorptive capacity. The tissue fluid is mobile and can be moved by finger pressure. Peripheral oedema is assessed for by pressing fingers gently, but firmly for 5 seconds on the lowest part of the body where fluid may accumulate, normally the ankles.

On release of finger pressure, an indentation or pit is left and is evaluated on a scale of +1 (minimal) to +4 (severe). Oedema does not become evident until interstitial volume has increased by 2.5 to 3L (Norris 2019). Right-sided heart failure, fluid/electrolyte imbalance, low albumin levels, venous obstruction, kidney disease and sepsis should be considered if peripheral oedema is present.

If only one leg (often the lower leg) is swollen, is red, warm and painful, this is more likely to be caused by either a deep vein thrombosis (DVT) or cellulitis.

Disability

A poor cardiac output will cause alterations in cerebral perfusion. This may manifest itself as a feeling of discomfort, restlessness, confusion, or even a sense of impending doom, and verbalisation of these feelings should be encouraged by the nurse so that possibly significant changes can be assessed. Anxiety and stress, though, is a normal response when acutely unwell, and questions should be answered honestly and promptly to try and allay fears. Neurological assessment tools such as ACVPU (RCP 2017) detect deterioration in level of consciousness. C is a new addition (RCP 2017) for identifying 'new confusion'. Many acutely unwell patients get a little bewildered with the pace of events, but may not be confused. The nurse should establish orientation to time, place and the level of understanding of recent events, to ascertain whether confusion is present. People with dementia, who have existing levels of disorientation/memory loss, should be assessed for changes and, if necessary, relatives should be used to help the nurse understand what is normal for the individual.

Cardiac pain is intense, and swift nursing intervention is required and is discussed with acute coronary syndromes later in this chapter.

Exposure and physical assessment

Cardiac and circulatory assessment includes an inspection of the patient, looking for signs that indicate cardiovascular problems. Chest wall inspection reveals scars that may indicate previous cardiac surgery or pacemaker implantation. Inspection of the nails may reveal **splinter haemorrhage**, a sign of **endocarditis** or **xanthomata**, which are fatty deposits under the skin associated with raised cholesterol levels. Signs of cardiovascular disease can be observed round the eyes with **Xanthelasma** formation (yellow cholesterol deposits linked to hyperlipidaemia) and a ruddy face flush known as **Malar flush**, suggestive of mitral stenosis. Inspection of the jugular venous pressure (JVP) gives information regarding right-sided heart function, but requires practise to visualise. The patient should be sat at 30–45° for this assessment. The height of the jugular vein can be seen as a double flickering, best visualised on the right side of the neck with the patient looking to the left, but unless raised, may not be visible above the clavicle. A JVP of more than 9cm above the right atrium (5cm above sternal angle) (Bickley 2017) is consistent with right-sided heart failure or fluid overload. An absent or lowered JVP (<4cm at sternal angle) may indicate dehydration. These findings are not interpreted in isolation, but in conjunction with the patient history and a number of clinical variables.

You may see experienced practitioners using skills of cardiac auscultation; this can identify abnormalities of blood flow through the valves in the heart. Closing of the heart valves generates sounds that can be heard when placing a stethoscope in key areas of the chest. The clearest sounds are S1 (1st heart sound), generated by the closure of the mitral and tricuspid valve, signalling the onset of systole, and S2 (2nd heart sound), generated by the closure of the aortic and pulmonary valves, signalling the beginning of diastole. S1 and S2 can be heard in each of the 4 assessment areas (see Figure 6.1). Normal blood flow is not usually heard, but in some instances, for example, with a damaged stenotic and/or leaky valve, the turbulent blood flow through the diseased valve produces murmurs that can be heard in the quiet time between systole and diastole (S1 and S2) (Bickley 2017). Any added sounds (to S1 and S2), systolic or diastolic murmurs should be reported for further evaluation.

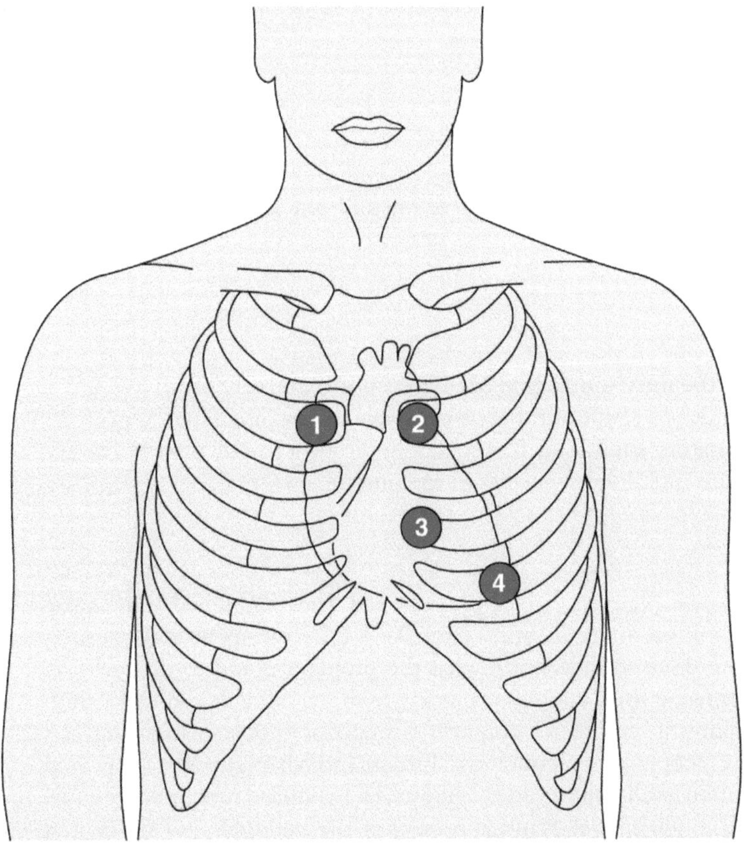

Figure 6.21 Areas for cardiac auscultation.

Nurses mostly utilise skills of observation and measurement, though additional physical assessment skills, such as auscultation and JVP assessment, are increasingly being incorporated into the nurses' skill set. By comprehensively assessing cardiovascular status and identifying problems early, nurses can instigate appropriate interventions and escalate care in a timely manner to prevent further deterioration, or transfer to a higher level of care as necessary.

CASE STUDY 6.1 MR HA NGUYEN

SITUATION

It is 15:00. Mr Nguyen, who is 74 years old, has been admitted to the medical assessment unit (MAU) via the emergency department (ED) with sudden onset of severe shortness of breath and chest pain.

BACKGROUND

Mr Nguyen is a non-smoker who is generally fit and well. He has had extensive orthopaedic surgery in the past, including three hip and one knee replacement.

ASSESSMENT

Airway

On arrival to MAU, the nurse notes that Mr Nguyen is extremely breathless and is finding talking difficult as a result of this, but he is able to vocalise. There is no indication of added inspiratory sounds, such as stridor, indicating partial airway obstruction. No secretions are mobilised when asked to cough.

Breathing

The nurse observes Mr Nguyen is clearly distressed and frightened. The nurse explains what they will be doing in order to make a full assessment and reassures him that this is being done to determine what the problem is and to deal with it. Mr Nguyen is discouraged from talking too much, as this is difficult and makes him more breathless. Talking in complete sentences is impossible due to Mr Nguyen's breathlessness; this is recognised as respiratory distress, and Mr Nguyen is supported into an upright position, well-supported by pillows, to maximise functional residual capacity. There is some peripheral cyanosis present at the nail beds, but no central cyanosis around his lips. Both sides of his chest are moving equally, but there is evidence of activation of the sterno-mastoid and abdominal muscles. His trachea is central.

On auscultation, there are no adventitious sounds, with vesicular sounds through the lung fields. He is currently receiving oxygen via a 60% Venturi mask, with a target oxygen recorded on the NEWS chart of 94–98%, scale 1.

The respiratory rate is 32 breath per minute; breaths are shallow but regular. The nurse attaches a pulse oximeter probe to his finger and reveals an SpO_2 of 94%. This reading is lower than it should be, especially considering the amount of inspired oxygen that Mr Nguyen is receiving.

Breathing NEWS = 3 + 1 + 2 = 6

Circulation

Mr Nguyen looks pale, and his fingers feel cool to touch.

His pulse is regular, but fast, at 108 beats per minute. The blood pressure is 165/90mmHg, with a mean of 112mmHg. His capillary refill time is 3 seconds.

No oedema is noted on Mr. Nguyen's ankles, and his calves do not look swollen. Mr Nguyen passed 450mL of urine in A&E and is complaining of a dry mouth. A mouthwash is offered, but on removal of the mask, the SpO_2 drops to 84% and he becomes very distressed, so it is replaced quickly. The nurse commences recording fluid balance.

Circulation NEWS 1 + 0 = 1

Disability

Although anxious and distressed, Mr Nguyen is fully conscious and oriented to time and place, scoring A on the ACVPU scale. Blood glucose was recorded at 4.7mmol/L. Although there is no known history of diabetes, blood sugars may become elevated due the increased sympathetic activity caused by stress and anxiety.

Disability NEWS 0

Exposure

A low pyrexia of 37.7°C is recorded. The nurse notes that Mr Nguyen appears to be of average weight and build and assesses his skin; she finds this to be intact, with no areas of redness. Immobility and hypoxaemia are factors that increase the risk of skin breakdown. She notes that Mr Nguyen has varicose veins in both legs but no areas of broken skin. She measures his calf circumference in order to fit the correct anti-embolic stockings.

Exposure NEWS 0

Total NEWS 7: Emergency response required: SpR and Outreach are called.

Response: SBAR is used to guide the discussion with the medical SpR, who responded immediately to the call. The relatively low SpO_2 warrants urgent arterial blood gas (ABG) analysis. An IV cannula is inserted in order to be able to administer IV fluids/medication, as Mr Nguyen is unable to drink at present because of his breathlessness and tendency to de-saturate when the mask is removed.

The SpR reviews Mr Nguyen and informs the nurse that the most likely diagnosis is a pulmonary embolism (PE), possibly due to a fragment clot formed in the deep veins of the leg breaking off and circulating to the lungs, where it has become lodged in the pulmonary circulation. This has blocked part of the pulmonary circulation, causing a reduction in gas exchange and hypoxaemia. The lack of clinical evidence of DVT in the calves is not an unusual finding and should not preclude the diagnosis.

Mr Nguyen's heart rate is increased as his sympathetic nervous system is activated due to anxiety, but also as a compensatory response to increase the delivery of oxygen to the tissues. His skin is cool, as blood is being diverted to vital organs to ensure their supply of oxygen. Mr Nguyen's varicose veins and extensive joint replacement surgery have predisposed him to thrombus formation, despite the lack of clinical evidence on assessment. The SpR prescribes a sub-cutaneous dose of Low Molecular Weight Heparin to be given immediately to prevent further clot formation, and Mr Nguyen is prepared for a computerised tomography pulmonary angiogram (CTPA) to provide a definitive diagnosis; the critical care team are informed.

Following the initial assessment, further investigations are ordered, and arterial blood gas is taken. Type 1 respiratory failure is noted. Although the PaO_2 is only just outside normal limits, it must be remembered that the patient is receiving 60% oxygen. A mild compensated metabolic acidosis is present, indicated by the lowered HCO_3^- and BE. His rapid respiratory rate has increased carbon dioxide excretion, thus moving the $PaCO_2$ out of normal range, normalising the pH.

At 15:30, Mr Nguyen seems less responsive and somewhat confused. His respiratory rate has decreased to 16 and his SpO_2 is now 87% on 60% oxygen; she changes Mr Nguyen's Venturi mask for a non-re-breath mask, using a flow rate of 15L/minute and ensuring the reservoir bag is filled before applying the mask. His HR has increases to 122, and his pulse feels thready. **The NEWS is now risen to 9 (B** 0 + 3 + 2, **C** 2 + 0, **D** 3).

Time	*15:00*	*15:30*
Normal Values		
pH (7.35–7.45)	7.39	7.32
PaO_2 (11–13.5kPa)	10.6kPa	8.8kPa
$PaCO_2$ (4.5–6.1kPa)	4.0kPa	6.5kPa
HCO_3^- (24–26mmol/L)	20mmol/L	19mmol/L
BE (-2–+2)	-3	-5
SaO_2 (96–100%)	**93%**	**87%**
Oxygen	60% Venturi mask	60% Venturi mask
Mode	SV	SV

Figure 6.22 Observation 15:00 and 15:30.

The 15:30 ABG analysis indicates further deterioration. The second set of gases is now showing type 2 respiratory failure, as the work of breathing has become overwhelming. Mr Nguyen's respiratory muscles are tiring, it is no longer possible to maintain his PaO_2 and he is too tired to hyperventilate. The $PaCO_2$ is starting to climb as Mr Nguyen's respiratory rate drops and his breathing becomes less effective. The non-re-breathe mask has brought Mr Nguyen's SpO_2 up to 90%. The likely causes of his deterioration are exhaustion leading to type 2 respiratory failure, as the respiratory muscles are unable to maintain the work required and/or a further embolus has occurred. The underlying metabolic acidosis is worsening.

The critical care team are present, and the decision is made to intubate and stabilise Mr Nguyen immediately, then transfer him the Intensive Care Unit for level 3 care and mechanical ventilation. Once intubated, the CTPA is performed and demonstrates several pulmonary emboli. Supportive ventilatory therapy and anticoagulation are required to try and ensure adequate oxygenation and prevent further thrombus formation.

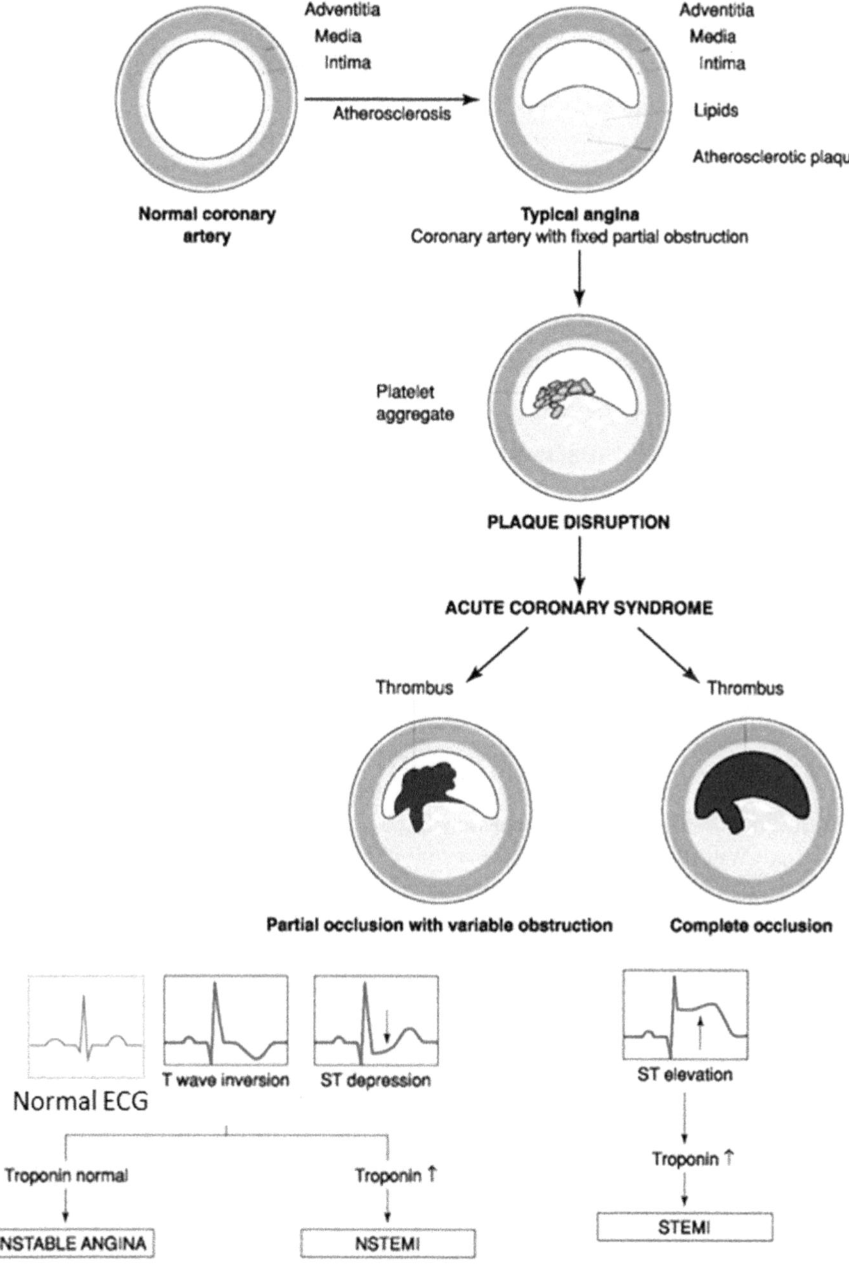

Figure 6.23 Coronary heart disease and acute coronary syndrome.

Acute cardiovascular problems: recognition and treatment

Acute coronary syndromes

Acute coronary syndrome (ACS) (see Figure 6.23) is an umbrella term encompassing a spectrum of clinical presentations all caused by the same disease process, resulting in clot formation in the coronary arterial blood supply. This is triggered by the erosion or rupture of a fibrous plaque, disrupting coronary arterial blood flow to the myocardium. Myocardial injury and/or death is a medical emergency and results from flow disruption. These clinical presentations can be categorised as:

- Unstable angina, ischaemic pain without myocardial death.
- Non-ST segment elevation myocardial infarction (NSTEMI).
- ST segment elevation myocardial infarction (STEMI).

Patient assessment for suspected ACS should include:

- Full clinical history (including age, previous MI and previous medical or surgical intervention for coronary heart disease).
- Physical examination (including heart rate and blood pressure).
- 12 lead ECG.
- Blood tests (such as high-sensitivity cardiac troponin at 1hr and/or 3hrs) glucose, creatinine and Hb.

(ESC 2016c)

The aim of treatment for this group of patients is focused on alleviating symptoms, restoration of blood flow to relieve myocardial ischaemia and the reduction of risk of cardiac arrest. The patient will usually present with severe chest pain, being 'crushing' or 'heavy' in nature, which may cause the patient to experience breathlessness and a drop in blood pressure. When ACS is suspected, immediate actions such as 12 lead ECG, pain relief and oral aspirin 300mg will be commenced prior to (but should not delay) hospital admission (NICE 2019). Oxygen therapy is only recommended if SpO_2 is below target saturations.

Assessing chest pain

Life-threatening problems causing chest pain

- **NTEMI or STEMI.**
- Aortic aneurysm rupture or dissection.
- Tension pneumothorax.
- Pulmonary embolus.
- Pericarditis.

Chest pain is a symptom that is associated with a number of other clinical pathologies; therefore, a detailed patient history, physical examination and clinical assessment of the individual presenting with chest pain is essential to establish the risk of life-threatening problems.

Classically, cardiac chest pain is visceral, which means that it is a deep and diffuse pain rather than a localised and superficial pain. Patient distress is evident, often accompanied by a grey pallor, sweating and nausea. The patient, when asked to locate the pain, will normally indicate a wide area of the chest and will be very unlikely to point to a specific point. Descriptive words such as 'crushing, heaviness/pressure on my chest' are often used by the patient. Cardiac chest pain does vary in location from person to person, but is generally experienced in the centre of the chest (or just to the left of the sternum). It may extend down to the epigastrium or up to the neck and jaw. There is a pattern of referred pain that may extend down the left arm in some cases. It is important to note that women may experience chest pain differently, possibly located in the lower chest/upper abdomen, complaining of fatigue, dizziness and fainting. Not everyone experiences chest pain in ACS. Patients with diabetes mellitus are particularly likely not to complain of chest pain as a result of the neuropathy that accompanies the disease.

NSTEMI and unstable angina

The myocardium cannot survive for long without oxygen and the demand for oxygenated blood is always high in order to maintain the energy required for myocardial contraction. In the presence of even the partial occlusion seen in unstable angina and NSTEMI, the amount of blood and available oxygen diminishes, causing ischaemia. Unstable angina differs from **stable angina** in that the pain is persistent, even at rest. ECG changes associated with ischaemia are variable and include ST depression and/or T wave inversion, though it is possible that no ECG changes are present. In **NSTEMI**, there is an area of infarction within the ventricular wall that does not extend entirely through the full thickness. In this case, there is some tissue surrounding the infarcted area that is ischaemic, and hence, the ECG leads facing this area will show ischaemic changes.

Biomarkers

Biomarkers are used in conjunction with the ECG for diagnosis. The injured myocardium releases troponin, so evidence of heart muscle damage is assessed by measuring cardiac troponin (I or T). Recently, **high-sensitivity cardiac troponin I or T** (hsTnI and hsTnT) assays have been made available, detecting myocardial damage within *1hr of injury*. Troponin is assessed on admission, aiding a speedy provisional diagnosis, with further tests at 3 and 6 hours for confirmation as required.

- If Troponin levels are normal, then there may be a non-cardiac cause of the chest pain, or possibly unstable angina.
- If troponin levels are minimally elevated, this is consistent with unstable angina.
- Mildly or moderately raised troponin is consistent with a non-ST segment elevated MI (NSTEMI). In essence, the higher the level of cardiac troponin, the more likely myocardial infarction has occurred. Some caution is required, though, as troponin can also be raised in pulmonary embolus or aortic dissection.

STEMI

A total occlusion of a coronary artery completely starves the myocardial cells of oxygen, causing myocardial infarction (MI). The extent of the myocardial infarction depends on the location of occlusion; the more proximal the occlusion in the coronary artery, the larger the area of myocardial injury. For example, an occlusion of the left coronary artery at its origin (near the aorta) will affect the entire left ventricle. Whereas an occlusion at the distal end of the coronary artery will affect a small, more localised area. In both cases, the tissue beyond the occlusion will quickly become necrotic if reperfusion is not re-established. In **STEMI**, the full thickness of the ventricle wall is affected and will show up as **ST segment elevation** in the ECG leads facing the infarcted ventricular wall. In STEMI, troponin levels will be significantly raised, as evidence of myocardial infarction, with levels checked on admission and at 3 and 6 hours as required.

Treatments for ACS

HEART score

Risk factors for consideration and scoring include:

- History.
- ECG.
- Age.
- Number of risk factors.
- Troponin.

Risk of Major Adverse Cardiac Event (MACE) (including mortality, AMI or coronary revascularisation)
Low risk: <2%
Medium risk:12 –17%
High risk: 50–65%

(See https://www.mdcalc.com/heart-score-major-cardiac-events)

Treatment for NSTEMI and unstable angina acutely is medication-led, but in some high-risk patients, if adequate blood flow is not re-established, then there is a risk that thrombus will increase in size and progress on to a total occlusion. These high-risk patients need to be identified, so treatment can be escalated. Risk calculators are superior to clinical assessment alone, the Global Registry of Acute Coronary Events (GRACE) score identifies high risk NTEMI patients and is currently recommended by NICE (2014). Guidance is constantly being updated and is available from www.nice.org.uk. Recent studies suggest that the HEART (History-Electrocardiogram-Age-Troponin) score outperforms GRACE (ESC 2016c) in the prediction of adverse cardiac events, and is currently used in many UK trusts.

Priorities of ACS management include:

- Performing a rapid ABCDE assessment and NEWS escalating care appropriately. Chest pain will prompt a cause for concern with urgent clinical review, regardless of NEWS (RCP 2017).
- Sitting the patient upright, assessing SpO_2 and titrating oxygen therapy as prescribed to keep within agreed target saturations. Do not give supplemental oxygen if SpO_2 is within range, as there is no evidence of benefit.

- Obtaining a12 lead ECG and ensuring timely reviews are made.
- Assessing chest pain using an objective scale.
- Establishing IV access and giving morphine, 2.5–5mg IV (the preferred analgesic), with an anti-emetic as required. Intravenous nitrates can be helpful for symptom relief.
- Continuous cardiac monitoring for rhythm changes.

Reducing thrombus size is essential to restoring coronary blood flow. Aspirin limits clot growth through its anti-platelet activity; if given in conjunction with **ticagrelor**, this effect is enhanced. For those with ischaemic ECG changes, additional anticoagulation is required with **fondaparinux**, or **unfractionated heparin** according to bleeding risk and likelihood of angiography. For those with ACS and diabetes mellitus, or with hyperglycaemia >11mmol/L, glucose control is required with a target of between 7–10.9mmol/L.

STEMI

Reperfusion therapy either by:

- Primary percutaneous coronary intervention (PCI).
- Thrombolytic therapy, if PCI contraindicated.

If significant occlusion remains after thrombolysis, angioplasty may be required, after 1–7 days.

High/medium risk NSTEMI

- Coronary angiogram within 72hrs, with possible follow on PCI.

Clinically unstable patients with NSTEMI or unstable angina

- Coronary angiogram within 24hrs, with possible follow on PCI (NICE 2014).

Urgent primary percutaneous coronary intervention (PCI) is the treatment of choice for those with *STEMI.* This involves an invasive procedure and requires further anticoagulation with drugs such as **abciximab** or **tirofiban**. A catheter is inserted through either the radial or femoral artery and advanced into the occluded coronary artery. A balloon is inflated in the artery to compress the clot, often accompanied by the placement of a stent, a metal mesh cylinder that can keep the artery open. NSTEMI patients with high/medium risk also may benefit from this more invasive intervention within 72 hours of admission.

The 12 lead ECG in ACS

A 12 lead ECG should be recorded at the earliest opportunity and will almost immediately show the tell-tale signs of ischaemia and infarction. ECG changes will 'evolve' as the coronary event progresses, so it is important to repeat ECGs as the patient's condition improves or deteriorates. This will give detailed information about the extent, location and evolution of the coronary event.

ST segment elevation occurs when the myocardium is being starved of oxygen and is starting to break down. At this point, the condition is reversible, providing that early intervention to open up the affected artery is established. The location of the myocardial infarction (and hence the artery that is occluded) can be seen by looking at the leads in which the ST elevation occurs.

12 lead ECG features of ***STEMI*** include:

- ST elevation present in at least 2 adjacent leads, depending on the extent of the infarction.
- Q waves greater than 25% of the overall height of the QRS complex. These may be seen simultaneously with the ST segment elevations and indicate that the myocardial injury is progressing on to permanent, irreversible myocardial damage.

12 lead ECG features of ***NSTEMI*** include:

- ST segment depression or T wave inversion located on the leads that are adjacent to the affected area. This shows reduced myocardial perfusion and is reversible; the sooner coronary flow is restored, the less the damage incurred.

Arrhythmias

The electrical conduction system is responsible for initiating and co-ordinating the muscular contraction that pushes the blood through the chambers of the heart, generating the cardiac output. Problems with the conduction system can occur, and these are important because they may directly affect the ability of the heart to maintain adequate blood pressure, cardiac output and organ perfusion. Rhythm problems therefore need to be detected so that action can be taken to treat the arrhythmia or reduce the effects of the arrhythmia on the cardiac output.

Before examining common arrhythmias, it is important that you are confident in recognising sinus rhythm. Whilst the study of arrhythmias can be interesting and challenging, the essential requirement is the ability to recognise deviation from the patient's normal rhythm and evaluate the clinical effect of the arrhythmia (such as changes in blood pressure, breathlessness and/or onset of chest pain), so that early medical review can be requested in the event of rhythm change. For this reason, sinus rhythm and only the most common arrhythmias of sinus tachycardia, sinus bradycardia and atrial fibrillation, will be discussed in this section.

The arrest arrhythmias of ventricular fibrillation, ventricular tachycardia (without a pulse), asystole and pulseless electrical activity have such a devastating effect that the patient becomes unresponsive, with no breathing or pulse (RCUK 2015). These are discussed in Chapter 7.

Sinus rhythm

The PQRST complex has been described earlier in the chapter. Sinus rhythm has the following characteristics (see also Table 6.7):

- Rate of between 60–100 beats per minute.
- Regular.
- P wave is present.

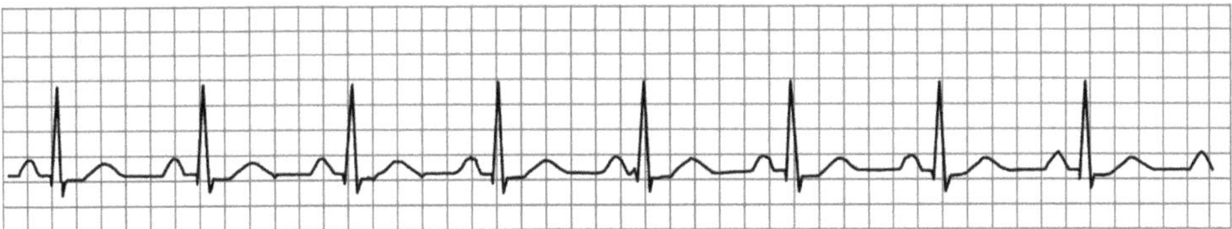

Figure 6.24 Sinus rhythm.

- P-R interval is normal (between 0.12–0.20 seconds or three to five small squares on ECG paper).
- QRS complex follows the P wave (duration less than 0.12 seconds or 3 small squares on ECG paper.
- ST segment on isoelectric line.
- T wave is present.

Sinus arrhythmia refers to the increase in heart rate that occurs during inspiration. This is a normal response, seen more in children than adults, and is not a cause for concern. The rate of sinus rhythm will vary according to parasympathetic and sympathetic activity and will generally change over a period of time, rather then suddenly. You may notice a patient's heart rate rises when talking to relatives or after moving from the bed to the chair, but this should fall back to the resting rate within a few minutes. The complexes look identical and originate from the sinus node. An example of sinus rhythm is given in Figure 6.24.

Sinus bradycardia

Causes of sinus bradycardia:

- Myocardial infarction.
- Hypothyroidism.
- Digoxin, beta blockers.
- Increased intercranial pressure.
- Athletic heart.
- Sleep.
- Hypothermia.

Abnormal parasympathetic stimulation, such as:

- Carotid sinus pressure.
- Tracheal suctioning.
- Valsalva manoeuvre (breath holding and bearing down).
- Reflex actions from the stimulation of PNS terminations in arteries; sometimes seen when arterial cannula sheaths are removed from the femoral artery following cardiac catheterisation.

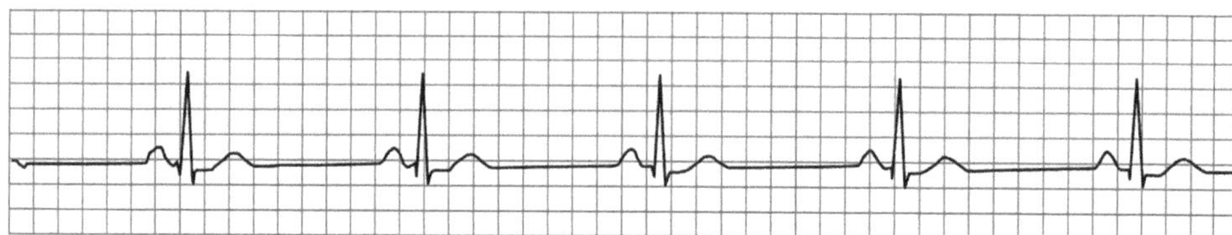

Figure 6.25 Sinus bradycardia.

Sinus bradycardia is a regular heart beat that originates from the sinoatrial node, but at a rate lower than 60 beats per minute (please see Figure 6.24). Whilst in a healthy heart this may not cause problems with cardiac output, as there is a corresponding increase in stroke volume, in the diseased heart, sinus bradycardia may cause circulatory compromise. If the patient becomes symptomatic, feels dizzy, faints, experiences chest pain, has a low blood pressure or becomes breathless, treatment will be required. Supplemental oxygen to maintain saturations between an agreed target range of 94–98% (or 88–92%, if at risk of hypercapnia) should be commenced. IV access will be needed and atropine 500mcg IV may be prescribed, as this inhibits the effect of the parasympathetic vagus nerve and allows the sinus node to increase the heart rate. If the bradycardia is extreme, then a temporary pacemaker may be indicated. It is important that the medications the patient is taking are reviewed, as common cardiac drugs such as beta blockers, digoxin and calcium antagonists such as diltiazem can cause a reduction in heart rate.

Sinus bradycardia will contain the features listed in Table 6.7. It is similar to sinus rhythm in all but rate. If a slow rhythm does not have the features of sinus bradycardia, for example the PR interval is prolonged, or not every P wave is followed by a QRS complex, then the patient has other conduction problems such as heart block, which may require intervention even if the patient in not symptomatic; urgent medical review should be sought. Medical practitioners are guided by the Resuscitation Council (2015) Adult Bradycardia Algorithm (see Figure 6.26) when selecting treatment.

Sinus tachycardia

Causes of sinus tachycardia:

- Fever.
- Stress and anxiety, pain.
- Vagus nerve inhibition.
- Sympathetic stimulation.
- Anaemia.
- Hypovolaemia.
- Sepsis.
- Anaphylaxis.
- Increased thyroxine levels.
- Heart failure.
- Caffeine.
- Salbutamol.

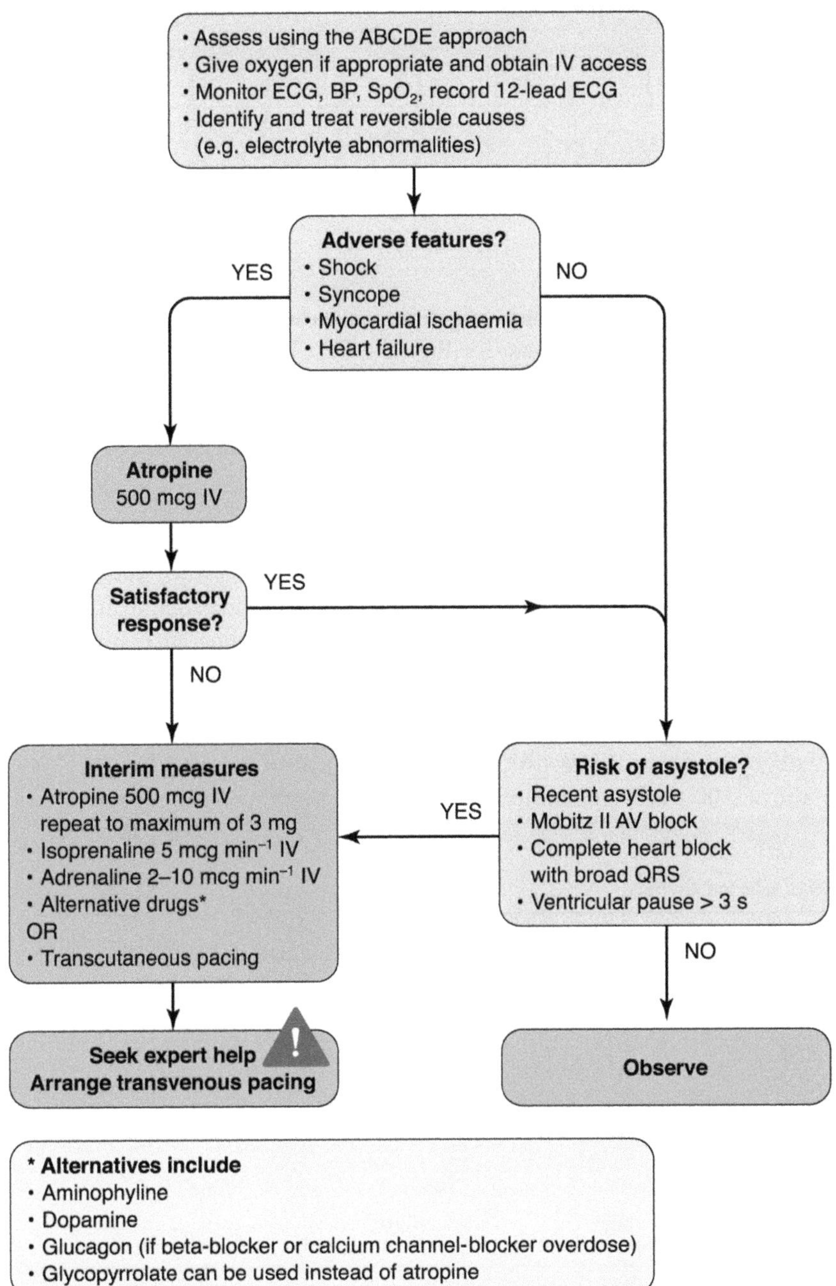

Figure 6.26 Adult bradycardia algorithm (RCUK 2015); reproduced with the kind permission of Resuscitation Council.

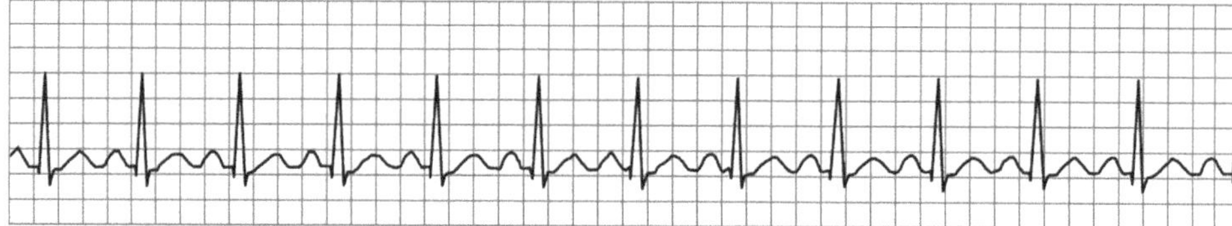

Figure 6.27 Sinus tachycardia.

Sinus tachycardia is a regular heart beat that originates from the sinoatrial node, but at a rate faster than 100 beats per minute (please see Figure 6.27). The resting heart rate will not normally be above 100 beats per minute, so the patient should be carefully assessed to determine the cause of the tachycardia. Sinus tachycardia is non-paroxysmal, that is, it doesn't start or end abruptly, which is a feature of other tachy-arrhythmias. It would seem logical that an increased heart rate would always improve cardiac output and tissue perfusion, but this is not always the case. You may remember that the heart spends a larger proportion of the cardiac cycle in diastole, the filling phase. As the heart rate increases, it is the diastolic phase which shortens, and as the rate moves towards 140, the time for ventricular filling significantly reduces, so cardiac output may fall. Shortened diastole can also lead to a reduction in coronary artery blood flow, resulting in angina, increasing areas of myocardial ischaemia and infarction as the oxygen supply cannot meet the demand of the rapidly contracting myocardium. Ensuring that the patient is not hypoxaemic and is adequately filled, or not dehydrated, is a good starting point.

Sinus tachycardia contains all the features of sinus rhythm, apart from the rate which will be above 100 beats per minute (see Table 6.7). If the patient has a fast

Table 6.7 Features of selected rhythms

	Sinus rhythm	*Sinus bradycardia*	*Sinus tachycardia*	*Atrial fibrillation*
Heart rate	60–100	<60bpm	>100bpm	Any rate, but usually 100180bpm
Heart rhythm	Regular	Regular	Regular	Irregularly irregular
P wave	Present Precedes each QRS complex	Present Precedes each QRS complex	Present Precedes each QRS complex	None Fibrillating wave seen
P–R interval	Normal (3–5 small squares)	Normal (3–5 small squares)	Normal (3–5 small squares)	None
QRS complex	Normal duration (less than 3 small squares) Preceded by P wave	Normal duration (less than 3 small squares) Preceded by P wave	Normal duration (less than 3 small squares) Preceded by P wave	Normal duration (less than 3 small squares)

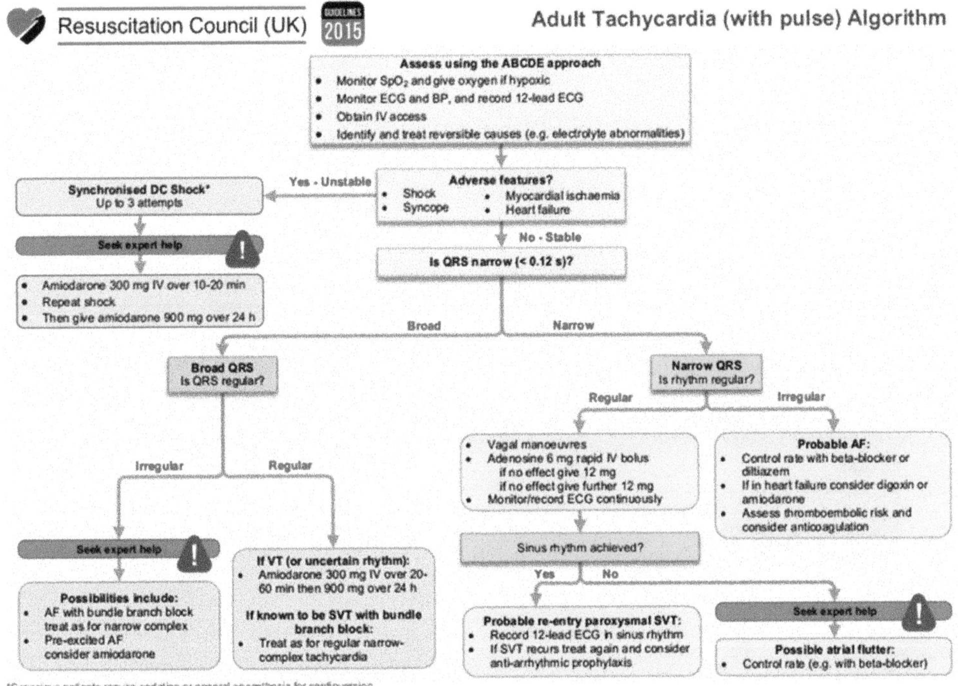

Figure 6.28 Adult tachycardia (with pulse) algorithm (RCUK 2015); reproduced with the kind permission of Resuscitation Council.

heart rate but the features of sinus tachycardia are **not** present, for example, from any of the following: no P waves are visible, PR interval is shorter than 3 small squares, QRS complexes are wider than 3 small squares, the rhythm is irregular or perhaps it has started abruptly, this will not be sinus tachycardia. A rapid assessment should be performed to detect cardiovascular compromise, oxygen therapy should be initiated to maintain saturations between 94–98%, IV access gained as appropriate and urgent medical review is indicated. Treatment for tachycardia (other than sinus tachycardia) will be guided by the RCUK (2015) 'adult tachycardia with a pulse' algorithm (see Figure 6.28).

Atrial fibrillation

Atrial fibrillation (AF) is the most common sustained cardiac arrhythmia (NICE 2014), one most health care professionals will have seen in practice. It is a major cause of stroke, sudden death and cardiovascular morbidity, with AF detected in about a third of all patients with ischaemic stroke. AF will often co-exist, be caused by, cause or exacerbate heart failure. Approximately 30% of patients with AF will have valvular heart disease detected on echocardiogram (ESC 2016b).

Factors contributing to atrial fibrillation:

- Hypoxaemia.
- Hypertension.
- Heart failure.
- Obesity.
- COPD.
- Infection.
- Ischaemic heart disease.
- Age.
- Sympathetic stimulation.
- Drugs.
- Electrolyte disturbance.
- Mitral valve disease.
- Coronary artery disease.
- Diabetes.

AF is an atrial arrhythmia that does not originate from the sinus node. It consists of chaotic atrial impulses, firing at a rate of 400–600 per minute, from different atrial ectopic foci. P waves are absent and fibrillatory waves can be seen, often with a wandering baseline (see Figure 6.29). The AV node receives these impulses, but only allows up to around 180 of these to proceed to the ventricles, to produce the QRS complex and ventricular contraction. The transmission of impulses through to the ventricle, however, is unpredictable, giving rise to a very irregular ventricular response and resulting in an irregularly, irregular pulse being palpated on assessment. Diagnosis will be confirmed by a 12 lead ECG. The atria have no co-ordinated contraction and therefore do not expel their contents into the ventricle in ventricular diastole. This leads to a reduced ventricular preload, especially when the ventricular response rate is high. AF then can give rise to serious haemodynamic problems in the short term, particularly when the ventricular response rate is rapid.

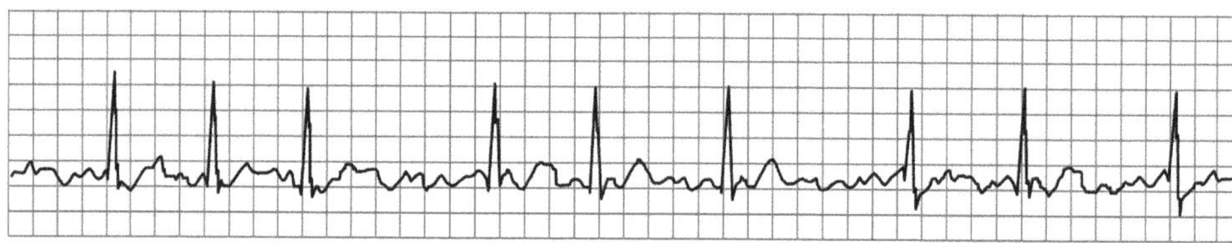

Figure 6.29 Atrial fibrillation.

Atrial fibrillation: serum electrolytes

- Check Serum K^+ (normal range 3.5–5mmol/L) and replace as necessary.
- Check Serum Mg^+ (normal range 0.75–1 mmol/L) and replace as necessary.

Acutely, patients presenting in AF required a detailed assessment to evaluate clinical status and deterioration risk. Triggering factors such as sepsis, anaemia, pulmonary embolism, electrolyte imbalance or hypoxaemia should be considered and addressed. Supplemental oxygenation may be necessary to maintain target oxygen saturation, treating hypoxaemia. Serum electrolytes should be replaced to keep within normal range, as they play a role in cardiac rhythm stability. Many patients present in AF with a tachycardia; NICE (2014) and ESC (2016b) have developed guidance, suggesting two essential treatment approaches:

- Rate control.
- Rhythm control.

Beta blockers or calcium channel blockers may be the agents of choice for rate control, to reduce rate to <110bpm at rest, improving cardiac output. Chemical cardioversion, using medications such as amiodarone or flecainide are aimed at restoring sinus rhythm (rhythm control). Electrical cardioversion by a synchronised electrical shock is the treatment of choice for the acutely unwell, but sedation and monitoring will be required for this procedure. Response to treatment should be evaluated clinically and by 12 lead ECG recordings.

The formation of clots in the atria, due to the stasis of atrial blood in persistent AF (suggested to be longer than 48 hours) can give rise to serious embolic problems. Though embolic episodes can affect many organs, such as the kidney, the gut or even the peripheral circulation, the most serious is a thrombus travelling to the brain and causing a cerebral infarction or stroke. Patients with untreated/undiagnosed AF is a major cause of stroke, raising the question as to whether routine screening for AF would be beneficial (Lown and Moran 2019). Anticoagulation underpins long-term management of AF, guided using risk assessment tools for ischaemic stroke such as $CHADS_2$. Oral anticoagulants such as apixaban and rivaroxaban have largely replaced warfarin. These newer drugs have reduced risks of intracranial bleeding and are often preferred by patients, as there are no requirements for numerous blood tests for coagulation management.

General management of cardiac arrhythmias

If a cardiac arrhythmia is detected, then a full assessment of the patient's condition is required. Table 6.8 outlines the key steps to be taken (RCUK 2015). Often, when the arrhythmia does not affect the patient's cardiovascular status, no immediate treatment is indicated. However, if the arrhythmia results in any change to the patient's cardiac or neurological status, appropriate treatment must be initiated. The action to be taken in the event of a cardiac arrhythmia is detected is given in Table 6.8. Oxygen therapy should be used to maintain SpO_2 between 94–98% (O'Driscoll et al. 2017). A full assessment of the patient is performed immediately, with a focus on circulation to assess compromise. NEWS will help identify the urgency with which to call for medical evaluation and

Table 6.8 Sequence of actions for patients with a suspected arrhythmia

- Assess a patient with a suspected arrhythmia using the ABCDE approach.
- In particular, note the presence or absence of 'adverse features'.
- Give oxygen immediately to hypoxaemic patients and adjust delivery according to observed arterial oxygen saturations.
- Insert an intravenous (IV) cannula.
- Whenever possible, record a 12 lead ECG; this will help identify the precise rhythm, which may guide immediate treatment and/or be crucial to planning later treatment.
- Correct any electrolyte abnormalities (e.g., K^+, Mg^{2+}, Ca^{2+}).

When you assess and treat any arrhythmia, address two factors:

1. *The condition of the patient (stable versus unstable – determined by the absence or presence respectively of adverse features).*
2. *The nature of the arrhythmia.*

(RCUK 2015)

treatment. The extent to which the patient is affected by the arrhythmia will inevitably guide the subsequent management. If the patient becomes unresponsive, then cardiopulmonary resuscitation may be required (see Chapter 7).

Acute heart failure

Factors that may trigger acute heart failure:

- ACS.
- Tachyarrhythmia (AF VT).
- Infection.
- Not taking medication.
- Alcohol, recreational drugs.
- Pulmonary embolus.
- Surgery.

Acute heart failure (AHF) is a rapid onset or worsening of signs and symptoms of heart failure. It can be frightening and distressing for patients and their families and is potentially a life-threatening event. The left ventricle is suddenly overwhelmed with the amount of blood returning to it from the pulmonary circulation, giving rise to increased hydrostatic pressures in the pulmonary vasculature and the rapid formation of pulmonary oedema. Symptoms of breathlessness, tachypnoea, acute anxiety, tachycardia, confusion and the production of frothy sputum are a cause for serious concern. This may be a new event, but often occurs in those with long-term heart failure as an acute exacerbation. AHF may be caused by cardiac a trigger such as ACS or respiratory triggers such as a recent chest infection, but may also be linked to non-compliance with medications. Management of acute heart failure is directed by supporting airway breathing and circulation and includes the following (NICE 2014; ESC 2016a):

- Administer oxygen therapy *if hypoxaemic* to maintain SpO_2 between 94–98% (or as per prescribed target oxygen saturation). Do not give oxygen if not hypoxaemic.

- Position the patient upright to reduce venous return and work of breathing (take care; if the patient is hypotensive, they may need to be in the supine position).
- Administer a diuretic as prescribed (often Furosemide 20–80mg IV) to reduce fluid overload, pulmonary oedema and breathlessness. Monitor response carefully, inserting a urinary catheter if deemed necessary.
- In those whose systolic blood pressure is greater that 90mmHg, vasodilators such as GTN, administered sublingually or as an infusion will be considered. This medication will increase venous capacitance and reduce pulmonary capillary pressure.
- For those with severe dyspnoea and distress, a small dose of IV opiate such as morphine may be considered, but should be used with caution.
- HFNOT can be considered if response to oxygen therapy is poor. CPAP (for type 1 respiratory failure) or BiPAP (for type 2 respiratory failure) further supports breathing by reducing alveolar fluid and respiratory effort and improving oxygenation

Whilst many may respond to initial therapies, those with acute heart failure may need additional circulatory support, requiring transfer to a higher level of care. Where hypotension persists, organ damage can occur. In intensive care, vasoactive medication and or inotropic support can enhance both the circulation and organ perfusion. Intubation ventilation and renal replacement therapy may also be required.

Venous thrombo-embolic (VTE) disorders

Risk factors for VTE:

- Surgery.
- Trauma.
- Critical care admission.
- Immobilisation.
- Oral contraceptives.
- Hormone replacement therapy.
- Lower limb fracture/replacement.
- Spinal injury.
- Cancer.
- Pregnancy.
- Infection.
- Obesity.
- Age.
- Various veins with phlebitis.
- Personal or first degree relative with history of VTE.

A venous thrombo-embolism (VTE) is sometimes referred to as a deep vein thrombosis (DVT) and pulmonary embolism (PE). VTE is a condition in which a blood clot (thrombus) forms in a vein, most commonly in the deep veins of the leg, as a DVT. If the thrombus dislodges from its site of origin to travel in the blood stream, a phenomenon called embolism develops. Thrombi may occur due to damaged blood vessel walls such as with varicose veins, due to stasis of blood in the veins caused by immobility (causing venostasis), abnormalities of the clotting mechanism (hypercoagulability) or vessel wall inflammation.

Part or all of the thrombus in the vein can move through the vena cavae and lodge in the pulmonary vasculature. The likelihood of this occurring has been estimated at around 50%. Pulmonary embolus is a life-threatening medical emergency, therefore prevention and early recognition of DVT is essential. All patients on admission are assessed for their risk of developing a venous thrombo-embolism, balanced against their bleeding risk with anticoagulation therapy. The risk should be assessed on admission, again within 24 hours of admission to hospital and whenever there is a change in clinical condition. Prophylactic therapy is initiated where the risk of harm from DVT is considered greater than the risk of harm from a bleeding event.

Bleeding risk

- Active bleeding.
- Use of anticoagulants.
- Acute stroke.
- Bleeding disorders.
- Expected surgery (within 12 hours) or previous surgery (within 4 hours).

https://www.nice.org.uk/guidance/ng89/resources/department-of-health-vte-risk-assessment-tool-pdf-4787149213

The National Institute for Health and Care Excellence (2018b) have issued guidance for management of specific risk groups that can be found at https://www.nice.org.uk/guidance/ng89. This includes a combination of two approaches to prevention, through the use of mechanical devices and pharmacological intervention. Mechanical devices that have been assessed as appropriate for the individual, include any one of:

- Anti-embolic stockings, thigh- or knee-length.
- Intermittent pneumatic compression devices.
- Foot impulse devices.

The use of anti-embolism stockings requires careful evaluation for the correct size. Staff who have received appropriate training are required to teach patients how to use them. They should be used both day and night until full mobility is restored.

Additionally, one pharmacological agent for prophylaxis is selected, considering the individuals specific circumstances. This should continue until the patient is no longer at risk, examples include:

- Low molecular weight heparin injections or fondaparinux (indicated for acutely ill medical/surgical patients).
- Apixaban, rivaroxaban.

International normalised ratio (INR)

- A measure of coagulation. It is a value derived from the ratio between the patient's actual prothrombin time and the normal value (11–16secs).
- The normal range for INR is 0.8–1.2.

INR monitoring for those on warfarin post DVT

- Target INR is 2.5 (range 2–3). This prolonged clotting time aims to prevent DVT recurrence.

Whilst it should be noted that many people who develop DVT have no symptoms at all, the following signs may indicate its presence:

- A red, swollen calf of affected limb.
- Increase in temperature of affected limb.
- Pain in lower limb on dorsiflexion (moving the ankle joint to bring the toes closer to the leg, pointing upwards).
- Distal venous dilation.
- Pyrexia.

If a DVT is suspected, the use of the two level Wells score is suggested to help assess its probability (available at www.nice.org.uk/guidance/cg144).

Diagnosis is also assisted by ultrasound, contrast venography and D-dimers. D-dimers is a blood test for abnormal levels of clot break down products (fibrinogen degradation products containing D-dimer), indicating, amongst other possibilities, that a clot is present. A negative D-dimer can exclude the presence of a DVT. After acute treatment, longer term anticoagulation with oral drugs such as rivaroxaban or warfarin is required. If warfarin is used, then the INR needs to be frequently monitored and dose adjusted accordingly. The underlying risk factors for those that develop DVT should be assessed carefully, as some hitherto undiagnosed problem may be present (NICE 2018c).

Signs and symptoms of pulmonary embolus

- Breathlessness and tachypnoea.
- Chest pain.
- Haemoptysis.
- Collapse.
- Hypotension.
- Hypoxaemia.

Pulmonary embolism is a major cause of mortality, with about 34% of cases presenting as sudden death (ESC 2014). Fatal pulmonary embolism remains a common cause of in-hospital mortality, with about half of those who develop this doing so whilst an inpatient (NICE 2018b). PE is most commonly associated with VTE, but can also occur as a result of emboli from fat, amniotic fluid, air or sepsis.

PE may be asymptomatic or present with severe symptoms of breathlessness, chest pain and haemoptysis. PE should be suspected in those with sudden otherwise unexplained shortness of breath, particularly in the presence of known risk factors. Risk prediction tools can be used to assist the decision maker. Investigations such as D-dimer are helpful, though D-dimers tend to rise with age >80, so may have less value within this group.

Computerised tomography pulmonary angiogram (CTPA) allows visualisation of the pulmonary vasculature and is now the method of choice for diagnosis. The obstruction of flow out of the right ventricle caused by a large PE can cause right-sided heart failure, detected on echocardiography. Acute right-sided heart failure has a poor prognosis, requiring admission to a higher level of care for complex fluid management, vasoactive medication and inotropes. For the critically unwell/large PE, invasive treatment options such as a surgical removal of the clot or the insertion of a venous filter are available.

The priorities of care are to maximise oxygenation through positioning to facilitate lung expansion, oxygen therapy, comfort to minimise anxiety and to ensure expert help is summoned. Close clinical monitoring is required.

The first line treatment for a non-massive PE is heparin, either IV unfractionated heparin, subcutaneous low-molecular with heparin or subcutaneous fondaparinux. If the suspicion that this is a PE is high, then unfractionated heparin may be given prior to confirmation by CTPA. Otherwise, low molecular weight heparin is preferable, as it is safer and easier to use. The clotting test, activated by partial thromboplastin time (aPPT), is used to adjust unfractionated heparin doses, with a target of 1.5–2 times the control. Once PE is reliably confirmed, oral anti-coagulation (warfarin) can be started with a target international normalised ration (INR) of 2.0–3.0 (ESC 2014). Newer oral anticoagulants (rivaroxaban, dabigatran and apixaban) have also been demonstrated to be safe and effective.

Acute circulatory collapse

The functioning cardiovascular system requires that the heart works as an effective pump, that there is sufficient circulatory volume in the form of blood, a systemic vasculature that enables flow and can constrict/dilate to maintain perfusion pressure. If one of these components fails, then circulation is impaired and acute circulatory collapse will develop. Acute circulatory collapse is a life-threatening medical emergency in which the oxygen supply to the tissues at cellular level is insufficient to meet their demands. The hypoxic tissues metabolise anaerobically, leading to acidosis, organ damage and cellular death (cellular hypoxia is discussed in Chapter 3). The nurse's assessment will help to identify which one of the components of circulation is the likely cause of the circulatory collapse, and this will help guide treatment accordingly.

Classification of shock

Hypovolaemia: loss of blood, plasma or extracellular fluid.
Obstructive: inability of the heart to fill effectively, e.g., tamponade or obstruction to outflow, e.g., PE.
Distributive: lack of sympathetic tone, sepsis, anaphylactic reaction.
Cardiogenic: problem with the pumping ability of the heart.

The problems that can lead to circulatory failure can be categorised according to the aetiology (or mechanism):

- Hypovolaemic.
- Obstructive.
- Distributive.
- Cardiogenic.

Whatever the aetiology of shock, it will normally progress through 3 distinct phases (see Table 6.9) which, unless the causes are identified and successfully treated, will result in an inevitable pathway to death. These stages of shock can be classified into:

- Compensated.
- Progressive.
- Irreversible (refractory).

Hypovolaemic shock

As the name suggests, hypovolaemic shock is a problem with the blood or volume component of the circulation. Hypovolaemia is one of the most common causes of shock and is the most easily reversed. Volume can be lost from the circulation in a number of ways. External blood loss can easily be identified as long as a comprehensive assessment is performed, internal bleeding, though, is not so easily discernible, and information gained from the past medical history and pharmacological therapy contributes to diagnosis. Fluid can also be lost from the circulation into the gut, as with paralytic ileus, or the peritoneal space, as with liver failure (see Chapter 10). Dehydration can occur from excessive vomiting, diarrhoea, sweating, infection, burns and wound exudate/drainage. Hidden losses are not always easy to estimate and may not be obvious, even when accurate fluid balance monitoring is recorded. Insensible losses in health can be 500–900mL per day (Norris

Table 6.9 Summary of physiological and clinical changes in the three stages of shock

Stage of shock	*Response*	*Assessment findings*
Compensated	• Baroreceptor and chemoreceptor activity activates sympathetic nervous system. • RAAS activated. • ADH secreted.	• Blood pressure, heart rate, respiratory rate may have changed, but could still be within normal ranges. • Patient's hands, feet and nose may feel a little cool. • Patient may feel thirsty.
Progressive	• Neurohormonal mechanisms increase their activity. • Non-vital areas may suffer hypoxia. • Impaired flow to vital organs causing organ dysfunction. • Ventilation perfusion mismatch in the lungs, as pulmonary circulation impaired. • Anaerobic metabolism in hypoxic tissues, production of lactic acid. • Cellular function impaired.	• Heart rate and respiratory rate raised, urine output decreasing. • Blood pressure and SaO_2 falling. • Altered level of consciousness. • Further changes in peripheral perfusion (cold in hypovolaemic and cardiogenic, warm in septic, neurogenic and anaphylactic shock). • Metabolic acidosis. • Raised lactate. • Possible pulmonary oedema.
Irreversible	• Severe tissue hypoxia, ischaemia and necrosis • Release of vasoactive mediators and toxic metabolites.	• Severe refractory hypotension, cold clammy skin, tachycardia, respiratory failure, renal failure, alterations in blood clotting. Severe metabolic acidosis.

2019). As they increase with pyrexia, increased respiratory rate and diarrhoea, they need to be taken into account when calculating fluid requirements.

Early signs of hypovolaemic shock

- A trend in rising respiratory rate.
- Changes in peripheral perfusion, hands and nose may feel cool to touch.
- A reduced urine output (if measured hourly).
- A trend in rising heart rate.
- Postural hypotension.
- Patient appears restless and fidgety.

Compensatory mechanisms to regulate blood pressure are effective at preserving pressure in the initial stage of blood/fluid loss. Many people donate about 500mL of blood with few, if any, adverse clinical affects and usually feel fine after a drink and a few minutes rest. However, as the volume loss increases, compensatory mechanisms are not adequate to maintain tissue perfusion. NEWS can be used to alert the nurse to clinical changes, but subtle changes such as trends in HR, RR and increased peripheral cooling may occur prior to key indicators such as the systolic blood pressure starting to fall.

The compensatory response occurs within seconds of volume loss; the sympathetic nervous system-mediated vasoconstriction mobilises blood stored in the venous circulation and spleen to increase blood return (preload) to the heart. Over a little time, fluid from the interstitial spaces moves to the vascular space, enhancing circulating volume. At 10–15% loss (up to 750mL), ADH from the posterior pituitary stimulates the thirst reflex, constricts peripheral arteries and veins, and increases water retention in the kidneys. A decrease in renal blood flow will activate the RAAS, increasing sodium reabsorption and increasing vasomotor tone. Losses of 15–30% cause physiological parameters such as heart rate and respiratory rate to move outside their normal range, pulse pressure may narrow, the skin feels cool and urine output decrease. It is essential that these signs are spotted, as even at this stage the systolic blood pressure may still be within the normal range.

As hypovolaemic shock progresses with a volume loss of greater than 30%, the severity of the vasoconstrictive response reduces blood flow and oxygen delivery, and cells convert to anaerobic metabolism, producing lactic acid (blood lactate may be raised >2mmol/L). As blood pH decreases, the respiratory rate increases, to reduce the acid load by exhaling CO_2. Arterial blood gas analysis at this time will reveal a metabolic acidosis with a lowered pH (<7.35), reduced HCO_3^-, (<22mmol/L) and increased base deficit (more than 2 or BE <-2). Deprived of oxygen, the cell cannot maintain the sodium potassium pump; sodium enters the cell, causing it to swell, and potassium leaves, contributing to a raised serum potassium level. Histamine release increases capillary permeability, causing fluid to leak into interstitial space and further deplete the circulating volume.

The irreversible or refractory stage is reached as cellular breakdown and acidosis rise to critical levels; reperfusion may lead to reperfusion injury, during which oxygen free radicals damage remaining cells and cause microvascular damage. Organ dysfunction and failure will quickly ensue in this refractory stage of shock. The damage sustained by the kidneys, gastrointestinal tract and blood clotting profiles will eventually lead to an irreversible decline and death.

Assessing hypovolaemia

- NEWS≥5.
- RR≥20.
- Systolic BP<100mmHg.
- HR>90b/min.
- Peripherally cool.
- Assess passive leg raise.

Treatment for hypovolaemic shock is centred on oxygenation, fluid resuscitation to re-expand circulating volume and treating the underlying cause (Woodrow 2019). Critically ill hypoxaemic patients should receive oxygen via a non-rebreathe bag at 15L to maximise oxygen delivery (O'Driscoll et al. 2017). If bleeding is overt, then stemming the flow of blood is the immediate priority. This may be achieved by direct pressure or procedures such as embolization or surgical intervention. Insertion of two wide bore cannulae enables rapid fluid administration. Haemorrhagic shock, as seen in trauma or excessive blood loss following emergencies such as a major GI bleed, requires resuscitation with red blood cells, plasma and platelets as soon as possible (Silva, Gonçalves and Sousa 2018).

If volume depletion is suspected, fluid resuscitation is guided by patient assessment and NEWS. NICE (2017) suggest that if NEWS is greater than or equal to 5, with indications of hypovolaemic shock present, then fluid resuscitation is required. The passive leg raise (PLR) manoeuvre is useful to evaluate fluid responsiveness and therefore reduce the risk of excess fluid administration (see Figure 6.30). The purpose of administering a fluid bolus in the hypotensive patient is to increase stroke volume. The PLR recruits the venous

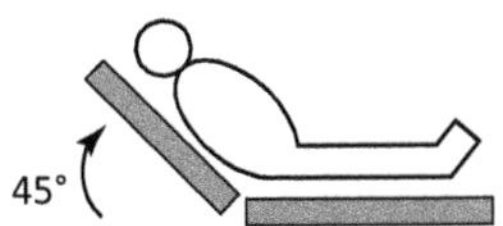

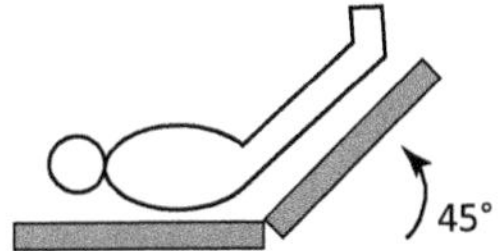

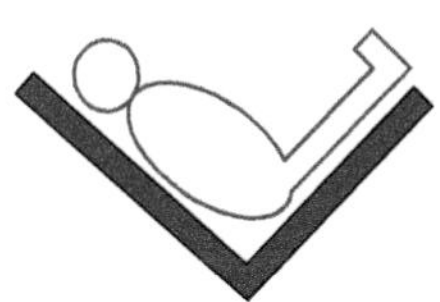

Figure 6.30 Passive leg raise (NICE 2013).

blood in the legs by raising them above the level of the heart, increasing venous return (preload) by about 300–500mL. If the ventricle is operating on the steep rising portion of the Frank-Starling curve, then an increase in SV, cardiac output and BP will be seen (Picket et al. 2017). If, however, the patient is on the flat portion of the curve (e.g., as with heart failure), then there will be no positive response. Any sign of patient deterioration should resolve on moving the legs back to the initial position. This manoeuvre is not appropriate for those with limb surgery or amputations and should be avoided in situations where raised intracranial pressure could cause harm.

Once volume depletion is confirmed, NICE (2013 updated 2017) advocates:

a) A rapid fluid bolus of 500mL of crystalloid (such as 0.9% sodium chloride or Plasma-Lyte) to be given over 15 minutes.
b) Reassessment, using ABCDE approach and NEWS to determine response. If positive, monitor response and continue with maintenance fluid only
c) If no clinical improvement, and signs of shock are present, repeat steps a) and b) up to a volume 2000mL.
d) If no clinical improvement is seen with 2000mL, seek expert advice urgently.

Crystalloids

- Clear solutions containing electrolytes.
- Move freely into interstitial space.
- Only ⅓ to ¼ remain in the vascular space, so large volumes are needed.
- Cheap, easy to store.
- No adverse reactions.
- May increase peripheral oedema.

Whilst crystalloids are often preferred in practice, there currently is no strong evidence to support crystalloids over colloids (Lewis et al. 2018). Colloids can rapidly expand the intravascular space, but are more expensive and carry a low risk of adverse reaction. Crystalloids require larger volumes to be given, as a large proportion moves from the vascular to the interstitial space. Patients with blood loss will need blood replacement; a haemoglobin level of about 8g/dL is generally the threshold for blood transfusion, but this may vary according to age or co-morbidities, such as significant coronary artery disease. Caution should be exercised, though, if there is any history or suspicion of cardiac problems. A reduced fluid challenge of 250mL may be appropriate for this group of patients.

Colloids

- Opaque solutions containing larger molecules, surrounded by water.
- Provide swift volume expansion in intravascular space.
- More expensive.
- May induce clotting disorder, allergic reactions, renal dysfunction.

(Lewis et al. 2018)

In those that are acutely unwell, a central venous catheter is helpful to enable estimation of right atrial filling pressures, and this will be inserted by an experienced medical practitioner in a level 2 environment. Central venous pressure would normally be between 2–8mmHg, but is best interpreted as a series of readings in conjunction with assessment of vascular tone. When hypotension does not respond to fluid alone, it may be necessary to consider vasoactive drugs such as noradrenaline. Haemodynamic monitoring and vasoactive support are discussed later in the chapter.

Obstructive shock

Causes of obstructive shock

- Pneumothorax (large or tension).
- Cardiac Tamponade.
- Pulmonary embolism.

Obstructive shock occurs when there is impedance to the flow of blood through the central circulation. A number of conditions can cause obstructive shock, and treatment is focused on the correction of the disorder causing the obstruction.

A large pneumothorax and, as a medical emergency, a tension pneumothorax, obstructs venous return to the heart by increasing intrathoracic pressure. Treatment is with high concentration oxygen and emergency needle decompression, a cannula usually being introduced in the second anterior intercostal space at the mid-clavicular line (Dutton and Finch 2018), quickly followed by chest drain insertion (see also Chapter 5).

A **tension pneumothorax** results in a large build-up of air in the pleural space, usually due to trauma causing a laceration to the lung or pleura.

On inspiration, air enters the pleural space, but due to a 'one-way valve' effect, cannot leave during expiration.

This is a **medical emergency**, as the raised intrathoracic pressure prevents blood returning to the heart.

Cardiac tamponade (see also Chapter 7) occurs when the normal 30–50mL of fluid between the layers of the pericardium increases to such an extent that diastolic filling is impeded due to the pressure exerted on the heart. A rapid accumulation of as little of 50mL can be sufficient to cause cardiac arrest, though a gradual build-up of a pericardial effusion can accommodate up to 1000mL. Immediate medical intervention of pericardiocentesis is required to relieve the pressure so the ventricle can fill, and cardiac output can be maintained.

Suspect cardiac tamponade with a patient who has:

- Restlessness confusion.
- Decreased stats, raised RR.

- Cool peripheries, tachycardia hypotension, raised CVP or JVP, pulsus paradoxus, low urine output.
- Recent history of cardiac surgery or trauma.
- Recent history of MI.

Distributive shock

Distributive shock is caused by a lack of ability of the vessels to maintain sympathetic tone; thus, systemic vascular resistance falls dramatically, and perfusion pressure is not maintained. Clinically, a patient with distributive shock may feel warm, but the perfusion pressure is not adequate to deliver oxygen to the tissues, so anaerobic metabolism and acidosis swiftly follows. Categories of distributive shock are anaphylactic, septic, (discussed in Chapter 12) and neurogenic (discussed in Chapter 9).

CASE STUDY 6.2 MR PETER FISHER

Situation: Mr Fisher is a 62-year-old patient on the medical ward recovering from an acute myocardial infarction. He has been on the ward for about 12 hours. The nurse notices that since transfer to the ward, he has only asked for the bottle once and passed 100mL of urine. He is complaining of worsening shortness of breath.

Background: Mr Fisher has been transferred from CCU to a general medical ward 48 hours following admission with central chest pain. Mr Fisher had been diagnosed as having an anterior myocardial infarction. At that time, the 12 lead ECG showed ST elevation in leads V1–V4. Following successful reperfusion by stent insertion to his left anterior descending artery, Mr Fisher made an uneventful recovery and was transferred to the ward 12 hours later. He has no past medical history of note. He is normally a fit and active gentleman who plays golf regularly

His medications currently are: simvastatin 40mg daily, ramipril 2.5mg daily, aspirin 75mg daily, clopidogrel 75mg daily and 4L/min oxygen via nasal cannula.

Assessment at 14:45

- Airway: the nurse notes that Mr Fisher has developed a slight cough, which has started only recently; he is not clearing any secretions. His airway is clear; there is no stridor or wheezing. He is complaining of feeling short of breath, but is able to talk in complete sentences.
- Breathing: he is sitting upright, breathing 4L/minute via nasal specs maintaining an SpO_2 of 93%, which is below the target range set by the medical staff of 94–98%. His respiratory rate has increased from 22 to 28 breaths per minute. His breathing is regular, with normal bilateral chest expansion, but with some use of accessory muscles indicating increased work of breathing. The nurse hears basal crackles on chest auscultation and wonders if he may be developing a chest infection. She changes the nasal specs to a venturi mask at 40% and is pleased to see his SpO_2 rise to 95%.

Breathing NEWS 3 + 2 + 2 = ***7****. After increase in oxygen percentage =* ***6****.*

- Circulation: his fingers have a blue tinge, and the nurse notices that they feel cool. The change in peripheral temperature is due to vasoconstriction, and she notes that this could be due to a problem with cardiac output. His heart rate has increased from 90–100 beats per minute and triggers on the early warning score. The cardiac monitor shows a mainly regular rhythm, but with some early broad QRS complexes present, consistent with ventricular ectiopic beats. The nurse makes a note to check his serum potassium levels, as she knows altered levels can contribute to cardiac arrhythmia. He is not complaining of any chest pain. His blood pressure has reduced from 120/70 to 105/65 since his last set of observations. His pulse pressure is calculated to be within the normal range at 40mmHg. His mean arterial pressure is 78mmHg, which is within normal limits. The nurse notes the trends of rising heart rate, falling BP and peripheral cooling and is now a little more concerned. She doubts her first thoughts of a chest infection and starts thinking about his deterioration in cardiovascular status. Capillary refill is sluggish at 3 seconds. A quick check of the fluid balance chart reveals only 100mL of urine has been passed in 12 hours, and a positive balance of 1000mL. She checks his ankles for pitting oedema, and none is present. She completes a 12 lead ECG and is pleased to note there are no new changes, but after labelling it clearly, puts it aside for the doctor to check. The nurse checks the blood results and notes the serum K^+ is 3.4mmols/L.

Circulation NEWS (1 + 1) = ***2***

- Disability: Mr Fisher is restless, but fully conscious and orientated, scoring A on AVPU scale. Blood glucose is assessed and recorded at 5.2mmol/L.
- *Disability NEWS = 0*
- Exposure: his central temperature is recorded at 36.5°C. The nurse notes that Mr Fisher has not been weighed this morning, and reflects that this would have been useful information. As he feels breathless, Mr Fisher does not want to be weighed now, and as his weight would not have been at the same time of day as his previous weight recording, she does not try to persuade him further. She checks his calves for tenderness or pain, and that the antiembolism stockings are correctly fitted. He has a venflon in situ.

Exposure NEWS = 0

Total NEWS = 8 (after increase in supplemental oxygen)

Response: emergency assessment by team with critical care skill (at least SpR level).

Continuous monitoring. Call outreach. Consider transfer to higher level of care.

15:00

The medical team arrive promptly in response to a clear SBAR handover. The nurse is asked to arrange a portable chest X-ray as soon as possible.

- Inspiratory crackles confirmed, chest X-ray reviewed, changes consistent with pulmonary oedema seen.
- 12 lead ECG, no new acute changes.
- 40mg IV furosemide prescribed to increase urine output, reducing the blood volume and therefore ventricular preload. Reducing the volume of blood returning to the failing heart should relieve pulmonary oedema.
- Potassium supplements prescribed.
- ABG's taken:
  pH 7.31
  $PaCO_2$ 4.6kPa
  PaO_2 8.9kPa
  HCO_3^- 19
  BE -5.2
- The reduced pH along with reductions in the metabolic component of the ABG (BE and HCO_3^-) suggest a metabolic acidosis, secondary to reduced tissue oxygenation. This would be consistent with an altered cardiac output, with not all the tissues receiving enough oxygen delivery to ensure aerobic metabolism of glucose. Action needs to be taken to improve cardiac output.

The doctor explains to Mr Fisher that she thinks his heart is not pumping as effectively as it could, probably due to some of the damage that occurred when he had his heart attack.

15:30 assessment reveals

Mr Fischer asks for a bottle and passes 500mL of urine. He says he is feeling better
A: clear.
B: RR reduced to 22, SpO_2 risen to 98% (oxygen 40%) *(2 + 2 + 0)* = *4.*
C BP 110/70, HR 90 *(1 + 0)* = *1.*
D: no change.
E: no change.

NEWS = 5

An echocardiogram is arranged to assess the degree of heart failure. A reduced ejection fraction of 39% with poor left ventricular function is seen, consistent with heart failure with reduced ejection fraction (HFrEF). In light of the satisfactory blood pressure, further actions include:

- Reducing the preload of the heart by starting an infusion of nitrocine (glyceryl trinitrate).
- Measurement of serum NTProBNP and renal function.
- Additional medications to be prescribed when stable, including increasing dose of ACEI, introducing a low dose beta blocker and possibly adding spironolactone to manage his heart failure as per NICE (2018) and ESC (2016a) guidelines.

Mr Fisher responded well to the initial interventions, and as NEWS continued to reduce, it was felt that he could stay in the ward area. After a few days of drug management aiming to decrease extra work on his damaged heart, he was well enough to go home. The heart failure nurse came to see him to discuss the support for him and his family on discharge and advise on medication management.

Cardiogenic shock

Signs and symptoms of cardiogenic shock

- Chest pain.
- Tachycardia.
- Tachypnoea.
- Peripheral shutdown (cold and clammy skin).
- Reduced mental status.
- Reduced or loss of consciousness.
- Hypotension.
- Oliguria or anuria.
- Weak, thready pulse.

Cardiogenic shock occurs when the heart is structurally damaged to the extent that it is no longer able to adequately perfuse the organs of the body. This commonly occurs as a result of major myocardial or valve dysfunction following a myocardial infarction, particularly when a large section of the left ventricle is involved. Cardiogenic shock is a major medical emergency with a poor prognosis. Causes of cardiogenic shock have been summarised in Table 6.10.

Investigations required for the patient with cardiogenic shock are based upon the evaluation of the extent of the damage to the heart and the effect that this has on the major organs of the body and include:

- Echocardiography to reveal the amount of ventricular damage that exists and the functioning of heart valves also affected. The presence of blood in the pericardium can be seen.
- 12 lead ECG to show ST segment elevations in the region of an infarction, which is important for the consideration of the complications that might arise from it. For example, ST segment elevations in the leads V1 to V3 indicate an antero-septal MI, which is implicated in septal wall rupture.
- Cardiac monitoring, used continuously to quickly identify changes to the heart's rhythm. Arrhythmia might occur because of the damage to the ventricular wall, or as a result of changes in blood chemistry caused by renal hypoperfusion.
- Cardiac catheterisation is a commonly used technique for the evaluation of coronary artery blood flow to the affected region of myocardium.

Table 6.10 Common causes of cardiogenic shock

Myocardial infarction	Where a large area of the myocardium has been damaged or has become necrotic. This leads to reduction in ventricular wall movement (hypokinesia) or complete absence of ventricular wall movement (akinesia). Echocardiography reveals the extent of the myocardial dysfunction and the structures involved.
Valvular dysfunction	Where the patency of the heart valves has been severely compromised (allowing blood to be regurgitated during systole), the forward flow of blood from the ventricles is reduced. Mechanisms of valvular dysfunction vary, but sudden acute changes occur as a consequence of damage to the structures that normally prevent the valve leaflets from prolapsing into the atria during systole. These structures are the chordae tendineae that attach the valve leaflets to the endocardium and the papillary muscles that keep the chordae under tension when they are closed.
Rupture of the heart muscle	A complication of myocardial infarction where the ventricular wall becomes so weak that the pressure from within the ventricle during systole forces the wall to disintegrate. Depending on the location, the rupture may lead to cardiac tamponade, whereby the heart becomes constricted by the accumulation of blood in the pericardium. If the rupture occurs in the ventricular septum (between the ventricles) then a shunting of blood from one ventricle to the other will exist, reducing the cardiac output.
Bradyarrhythmias	A slow heart rate reduces the cardiac output if there is no corresponding increase in ventricular contractility. These bradyarrhythmias may be a consequence of AV node block, sinoatrial node disease or overdose of heart-rate-lowering drugs.

Management of cardiogenic shock

The priorities are to restore adequate perfusion to the vital organs and to reduce the workload of the heart. As the primary problem is the inability of the heart to provide sufficient cardiac output to achieve organ perfusion, these priorities are interrelated. By improving cardiac output, there should be a corresponding increase in perfusion pressure. However, the restoration of myocardial function might require a number of supportive therapies that can only be provided in a critical care environment, such as:

- Inotropic drugs.
- Intra-aortic balloon counter pulsation.
- **Ventricular assist device (VAD)**/temporary mechanical circulatory support such as **extra corporeal membrane oxygenation (ECMO)**.

Cardiogenic shock is a complex condition to manage and requires a wide range of monitoring techniques to guide its management. Inotropic drugs to increase ventricular contractility are essential to restore cardiac output in the short-term, but careful titration of these drugs is needed, as they can be harmful. These measurements and treatments require invasive haemodynamic monitoring systems that would normally only be found in an intensive care (level 3) setting for stabilisation, but further assessment may indicate that transfer to a cardiac specialist centre is required.

Interventions to monitor and support cardiovascular status

Haemodynamic monitoring

Assessment of cardiovascular status is looking for clinical indicators of adequate tissue perfusion and can usually be obtained by non-invasive means, such as clinical observations and the measurement of vital signs using equipment such as pulse oximetry sphygmomanometers or automated blood pressure devices. Patients who are acutely ill may benefit from invasive monitoring, giving a continuous 'real time' display of information so that trends can be more easily observed and adverse events can be predicted and averted in a timely manner. This is particularly important for those who require vasoactive/inotropic support for maintenance of perfusion pressure, to enable optimum titration of therapy to meet clinical need. Whilst most patients requiring this level of support will be in intensive care, some will be able to have their needs met in a level 2 area or enhanced care environment such as a post anaesthetic care or higher monitoring area of an acute medical unit.

Invasive pressure monitoring

- Lines must be clearly labelled.
- A continuous pressurised (at 300mmhg) flush system of 0.9% saline maintains cannula patency.
- Transducer to be placed at the level of the right atrium for all measurements.
- Transducer needs to be 'zeroed', i.e. calibrated to atmospheric pressure.
- Dedicated monitoring tubing is used.
- Luer locks for all connections required.
- Alarms should be set appropriately to detect abnormally high and low measurements.
- Insertion sites cleaned and lines changed as per **epic 3** guidance (Loveday et al. 2014).

Invasive haemodynamic monitoring involves the placement of a cannula into an artery (normally the radial) and/or a central vein (often internal jugular). Transducers are small fluid-filled pressure-detecting devices. Pressure changes are conveyed from the cannulated vessel through a fluid-filled line to the transducer, then via an electrical signal to the monitor, which displays the pressure waveform. The advantages of continuous monitoring, though, need to be weighed against the risks. Dislodgement, disconnection, bleeding, inappropriate drug administration, air emboli and sepsis all have the potential to cause severe harm or even death. Catheter-related blood stream infections occur when a systemic infection is identified, and the same organism is cultured from both blood and intravascular catheter cultures (Dutton and Finch 2018).

Nurses are required to be aware of hazards of common treatments, including the use of technology such as invasive monitoring devices (NMC 2018a). Higher staff/patient ratios are required, staff need to be competent at using invasive monitoring systems and in the interpretation of the information gained to ensure safe and effective care.

Hazards of central venous lines

- **Air embolus.**
- Thrombus formation.
- Arrhythmia.
- Pneumothorax.
- Haemothorax.
- Incorrect positioning.
- Infection and sepsis.

Central venous lines are used for continuous medication infusions that cannot be delivered peripherally, parenteral feeding, or for monitoring venous oxygen saturations. They are usually inserted into the right internal jugular vein due to ease of approach, but the subclavian vein may also be used. The lines themselves may be single lumen, but more frequently, multi-lumen catheters are used, facilitating dedicated lumens for each type of infusion. Insertion is a sterile technique using the **Seldinger approach**, with the patient's head placed lower than the heart to prevent air embolus. Placement is confirmed by chest X-ray.

Central venous pressure monitoring (CVP) is helpful for those who have complex fluid management requirements, as they help evaluate fluid status and right ventricular function. The pressure measures right atrial pressure, but also reflects right ventricular end diastolic pressure, as the AV valves open in diastole. Fluid challenges described earlier in this chapter may be repeated if the CVP is low or normal with a reduced BP to ensure circulating volume is adequate. Central venous pressure is normally between 3–8mmHg, but in clinical practice it may be maintained up to 12mmHg to ensure optimum ventricular preload. Those who do not respond to fluid challenge may require inotropic support of the circulation. Factors that may cause a rise in CVP include:

- Heart failure.
- Cardiac tamponade.
- Tension pneumothorax.
- Vasoconstriction (caused by drugs such as adrenaline or as part of the sympathetic response to poor cardiac output).
- COPD.
- Tricuspid valve problems.

Factors that may cause a fall in CVP include:

- Dehydration, bleeding.
- Vasodilation caused by drugs such as nifedipine or by distributive shock.

The CVP waveform varies with the cardiac cycle, and the pressure reading at the end of expiration is recorded (see Figure 6.29 for CVP waveform). It is important to note that 'one off' readings for CVP may not be that useful, as vasoconstriction can raise CVP and mask hypovolaemia. Trends and response to a fluid challenge, evaluating CVP in conjunction with other clinical parameters such as respiratory rate, oxygen saturation, heart rate, blood pressure and urine output is necessary for managing the patient with poor cardiac output.

Central lines may need to be removed once the patient has been stepped down to the ward, so it is important to be aware of the issues around safe removal.

- Patient's bed is tilted so the head is lower than the heart, to prevent air embolus as the catheter is withdrawn.
- Ask the patient to take a deep breath in and hold whilst the catheter is being withdrawn. This maintains positive pressure in the lung and reduces the risk of air being drawn in through the catheter site.
- Apply direct pressure immediately after line removal (the patient may now breath normally), and cover with a transparent occlusive dressing.
- The catheter tip is send for microscopy according to hospital policy.

Arterial monitoring

Hazard of arterial lines

- Bleeding through accidental disconnection. *Luer locks required for each connection.*
- Reduced distal limb perfusion. *Frequent checks for colour and warmth required.*
- Inadvertent administration of drugs. *No drugs should be administered through an arterial line. Labelling arterial lines clearly is essential.*
- Small air bubbles causing tissue damage. *Withdraw small bubbles from circuit with a syringe.*
- Nerve damage.

Intra-arterial cannulation enables real-time monitoring, allowing for rapid evaluation of circulatory compromise that may occur with ectopics and rhythm disturbances. It also enables titrating of vasoactive medication and has the added benefit of giving access for arterial blood gas (ABG) sampling without the need for repeated vessel puncture (arterial stab), which can be distressing for the patient. The radial artery is the preferred site, due to the good collateral supply of the ulnar artery; this can be confirmed by the **Allen test**, or by Doppler ultrasound. ABG analysis is not only useful for assessing oxygenation and ventilatory requirements, but also metabolic problems. An insight into the degree of tissue hypoxia and subsequent anaerobic metabolism can be gained by evaluation of acid base status (pH), metabolic derangement (BE and HCO_3^-) and lactate levels. Trends in acid base status are useful for evaluating response to interventions such as fluid therapy (given for hypovolaemia) or inotropes and vasoactive therapies.

Arterial lines will usually be removed in the critical care area prior to transfer. The higher pressure in the arterial system means that the risk of bleeding is increased. As digital pressure may be required for 5 minutes or more, it may be wise to draw up a chair to sit down comfortably for this procedure! The distal circulation needs to be checked for warmth and sensation after removal, as a clot may form, reducing perfusion. When satisfied that there is no risk of further bleeding, pressure may be removed, and a dressing may be placed.

Pressure waveforms

Figure 6.31 combines the waveforms seen on the ECG, arterial and CV pressure traces. The arterial waveform reflects the change in pressure seen in the arteries through the cardiac cycle. During systole (following the QRS complex on ECG), the pressure rises sharply until the maximum is reached. As the ventricles start to relax (signified by the T wave), pressure starts to fall. The closure of the aortic valve signifies the beginning of diastole and can be seen as the dicrotic notch on the pressure trace. End diastole pressure is reached, prior to the next ventricular contraction. Mean arterial pressure is calculated by the monitor and is often used to guide therapy.

Changes in monitored waveform can be due to patient deterioration or problems with one of the elements of the monitoring system. The monitor alarms will detect changes and alert the nurse. If the loss of waveform is associated with cardiac arrhythmia seen on the ECG trace, this requires urgent escalation. If just one trace has altered or dampened, or blood is tracking up the monitoring line with other clinical parameters remaining stable, it is worth quickly checking:

- Is the flush bag empty?
- Is the flush bag pressure still 300mmHg?
- Are there air bubbles in the line?
- Does an extra flush on the affected line (after removal on bubbles, if present) clear the problem?
- Is the transducer in the correct position?
- Does changing the position of the wrist (arterial) or neck (CVP) fix the problem?
- Are all lines intact and the 3 way taps/connectors all in the correct position?

For further reading on haemodynamic monitoring, please see Adam, Osbourne and Welch (2017). Critical Care Nursing Science and Practice, Oxford: Oxford University Press.

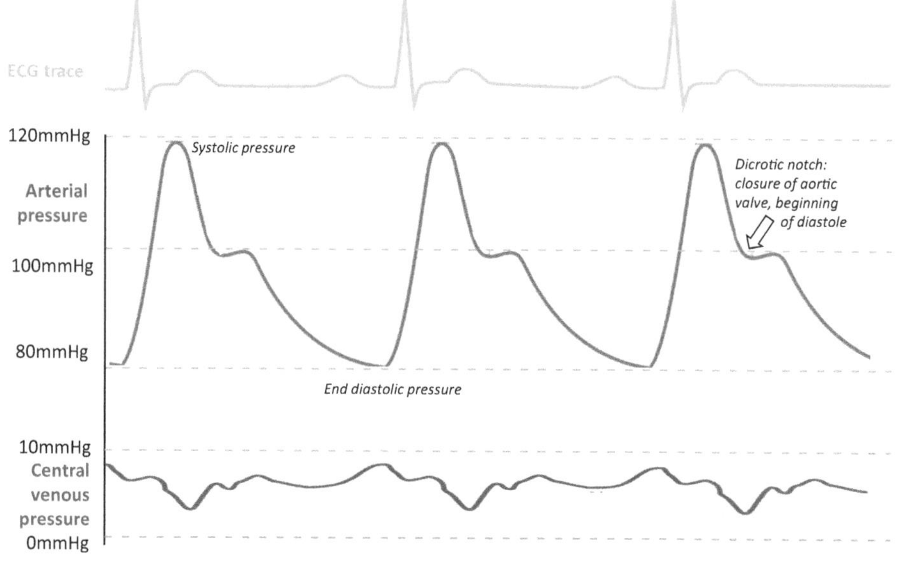

Figure 6.31 Wave forms: ECG, arterial and central venous pressure.

Vasoactive support therapies

Patients with deteriorating cardiac output that do not respond to initial therapy may require the additional support of vasoactive and/or inotropic agents. It is possible that these drugs may need to be commenced in an acute ward area in order to stabilise the patient prior to transfer to a higher level of care. Some acute wards have designated level 2 beds and are able to provide care for patients who require single vasoactive or inotropic support therapy.

Vasoactive: affecting vasodilation or vasoconstriction of blood vessels.
Inotropic: affecting the heart's ability to contract.

Vasoactive dugs affect the degree of constriction (vasoconstrictors) or relaxation (vasodilators) of vessels, thereby eliciting varying effects on vascular resistance. Ventricular preload is increased by constricting agents, thereby increasing stroke volume and cardiac output. Ventricular afterload is also increased, which will raise the MAP. Dilators will reduce preload and afterload, reducing heart work and MAP, but often resulting in an increase in cardiac output as peripheral resistance falls. In practice, the choice of inotropic agent varies between centres and specialities; the following discussion gives an insight only into the mechanisms and use of this complex group of agents.

Inotropic substances are those that alter myocardial contractility. A positive inotrope increases contractility, thereby increasing stroke volume and cardiac output, and a negative inotrope decreases contractility. Many inotropic agents also have chronotropic properties (affecting heart rate) and vasoactive properties and therefore can be somewhat complex to manage. For a summary of inotropic agents and their action, please see Table 6.11.

Specific agent choice is by prescriber preference. Guidelines for choice of agent to support those with septic shock by Rhodes et al. (2017) have been widely adopted (Scheeran et al. 2019), with noradrenaline being the first drug of choice. Noradrenaline may be instituted early in the treatment of sepsis/septic shock if the patient's clinical condition does not improve quickly with fluid resuscitation. This may be initiated in ward areas or the emergency department prior to transfer to a higher level of care. The choice of vasopressor, though, for problems such as low cardiac output states is not a clear one, with a recent Cochrane review unable to demonstrate mortality differences between the various vasopressors (Schumann et al. 2018).

You may find it helpful to refer back to the section on blood pressure control to refresh your memory on beta 1, beta 2 and alpha adrenergic receptors before looking at Table 6.11.

Half-life

The **half-life** of a drug is the time it takes for the plasma concentration to reach half of its original concentration.

Catecholamine (sympathomimetic) inotropic drugs have a short half-life, of 1–2 minutes, and reach maximum plasma concentration in about 10 minutes.

Catecholamine inotropes include:

- Adrenaline.
- Noradrenaline.
- Dobutamine.
- Dopamine.

Intravenous vasoactive and inotropic drugs are normally only administered in areas that are designated for nursing patients of level 2 or 3 dependency (FICM 2019). This is due to several factors, not least of which is that patients who require this type of support are potentially or actually very sick, and require frequent/continuous observations of haemodynamic parameters. Nurses are required by the NMC to act within the limits of their own competence (NMC 2018b). Close supervision and additional preparation may be necessary to equip the nurse with the skills required to safely care for patients requiring vasoactive support and for patients of level 2 and level 3 dependency. These intravenous drugs are very potent and have a very short half-life, so plasma concentrations can fall very rapidly. The short half-life is advantageous in that it allows the experienced clinician to titrate the dose on the basis of required effects (e.g., increase in BP) against the non-required effects (e.g., tachycardia). The nurse needs to understand these physiological effects so that they can be monitored closely in order for the health care team to make appropriate decisions regarding treatment.

Doses are calculated and prescribed in micrograms per kilogram per minute to ensure they are tailored precisely to patient needs. The calculations can be challenging, so even

Table 6.11 Summary of drugs used to support cardiovascular status

Drug	*Action*	*Indication*	*Effect*
Noradrenaline	α agonist	septic shock, given if no early response to fluid resuscitation	vasoconstriction, increase in MAP
Dopamine	β1 agonist, β2 agonist,	Low CO, SBP<90mmHg	increased cardiac contractility, increased CO
Adrenaline	β1 and β2 agonist, high dose:α agonist	cardiac arrest, anaphylactic shock, low CO, post-cardiac surgery	increased CO, vasoconstriction
Dobutamine	β1 agonist, β2 agonist	Low CO, heart failure	increased CO
Levosimendan	increases calcium sensitivity	Low CO state	Increased CO, half-life of 10–20 mins
Milrinone	phosphodiesterase inhibitor, increases calcium availability	Low CO state	Increased CO through a combination of vasodilation and increased inotropy
Metaraminol	α agonist	hypotension *given peripherally* used to stabilise patient for transfer to higher level of care	Half-life of around 20 mins, vasoconstriction, increased BP

experienced nurses may need to update their numeracy skills to ensure that correct doses are given. Standard infusion concentrations are used to reduce risk of harm (FICM 2019) and can be accessed from https://www.ics.ac.uk/ICS/ICS/GuidelinesAndStandards/GPICS_2nd_Edition.aspx. To ensure the delivery of a consistent, even infusion, inotropes will always be administered via a volumetric pump or syringe driver and through a clearly labelled *dedicated* lumen on a central line to prevent accidental bolus doses (RCN 2016). Peripheral lines are not appropriate due to the high risk of necrosis if extravasation occurs. Continuous monitoring of blood pressure via an arterial line will alert the nurse to any changes in flow rate and drug delivery, which may result in significant deterioration. It is important that the patients with hypovolaemic or distributive shock have an adequate circulating volume prior to commencement of inotropic support to ensure organ perfusion is optimised, as many inotropes cause vasoconstriction at higher doses which could actually reduce organ perfusion.

Inotropes and vasopressors can be extremely effective at restoring adequate oxygen to the tissues in the shocked state. There are, though, a number of issues of which the nurse should be aware when caring for a patient receiving such therapy. Vasoconstrictive agents can cause reduced peripheral blood flow, causing ischaemia, a particular problem for patients with existing peripheral vascular disease. Sympathomimetic agents may increase myocardial ischaemia and myocardial irritability, rendering the patient vulnerable to cardiac arrhythmias, so continuous ECG monitoring and maintenance of electrolytes within normal limits is a priority. These agents also decrease serum potassium levels and increase the risk of arrhythmia further. Sympathomimetic agents raise serum glucose levels, so these need to be closely monitored and treated as necessary.

Vasodilators such as glyceryl trinitrate (GTN) reduce preload and afterload and increase myocardial perfusion through dilating coronary arteries and improving collateral flow. GTN is used in decompensated heart failure and ACS.

Inodilators such as milrinone belong to a group of drugs called phosphodiesterase inhibitors (PDI). This group of inotropes have a much longer half-life and also have profound vasodilator properties. PDIs are ideal for management of severe congestive heart failure and are often used in conjunction with other vasoactive/inotropic medication.

Metaraminol is an unusual vasoactive medication in that it can be administered via a peripheral line. It acts as an alpha receptor agonist, causing peripheral vasoconstriction, and is used in the emergency treatment of hypotension. It has a longer half-life than standard medications such as noradrenaline, so small doses can be administered as an IV bolus (NICE 2019). This drug can be useful in situations such as a drop in systemic vascular resistance and BP post-epidural anaesthesia. Cardiovascular monitoring is necessary, but this may be possible with automated non-invasive BP monitoring devices in an enhanced level 1 location if *only short-term* support is required. It is sometimes used as a continuous peripheral infusion, but as yet, there is little evidence to support its longer-term use (Anderson and Chatha 2017). If cardiovascular support requirements continue, it is appropriate to transfer the patient to a higher level of care for the insertion of a central and arterial lines, enabling infusion and close monitoring of drugs such a noradrenaline.

Conclusion

A functioning cardiovascular system is crucial to ensure that oxygen and nutrients are delivered to the body tissues adequately to their needs and to remove potentially harmful waste products. Acute exacerbation of chronic cardiovascular disease and circulatory failure are common and potentially serious problems. This chapter has reviewed physiological concepts of the cardiovascular system and considered some common cardiovascular problems and those that may lead to a medical emergency. The nurses' role in assessment and management has been explored, and concepts relating to the more highly dependent patient with deteriorating cardiovascular function have been introduced. Nurses are required by the Code of Conduct (NMC 2018b) to provide a high standard of care at all times. The code requires nurses to prioritise people, practise effectively, preserve safety and to promote professionalism and trust (NMC 2018b). In order to ensure this, care delivered to patients needs to be underpinned by a sound knowledge base. As can be seen from the case studies presented in this chapter, problems which are primarily of a circulatory nature can have a profound effect on the respiratory system, as the two systems work closely together to ensure adequate oxygen supply to the tissues. Without this understanding, it is not possible to interpret what you observe and therefore to make the full assessment necessary to ensure that the safety and well-being of the patient.

Glossary 

Action potential An event in which the electrical membrane potential of a cell rapidly changes due to ionic movement in and out of the cell. In the cardiac cell this starts the wave of depolarisation, giving rise to the PQRS complex.

Acute coronary syndrome (ACS) An umbrella term encompassing unstable angina, NSTEMI and STEMI.

Adenosine triphosphate (ATP) A high energy molecule that stores the energy created by cellular metabolism; synthesised in the mitochondria.

Adrenergic receptors Receptors of the sympathetic nervous system; subdivided into alpha beta 1 and beta 2

Afterload The load that the (normally left) ventricle has to work against to open the aortic valve and eject its stroke volume. It can also be seen as ventricular wall stress in systole.

Air embolus This occurs when a bubble of air is lodged in the circulatory system. A small arterial air embolus can lead to tissue damage in the limb supplied by the artery. A larger venous air embolus can travel into the pulmonary circulation causing V/Q mismatch, right-sided heart failure and possibly death.

Aldosterone A hormone produced by the adrenal cortex. Aldosterone increases sodium and water reabsorption from the distal convoluted tubule in the kidney and increases potassium excretion.

Allen test A test to evaluate blood flow down both the radial and ulnar arteries. Both radial and ulnar arteries are compressed. The open hand and fingers are observed for pallor, which occurs as the blood flow is interrupted. Release of the ulnar artery only should result in a warm flush and restoration of a healthy pink colour of palms and fingers. This demonstrates that ulnar arterial perfusion of the hand is intact.

Alpha receptor Receptor of the sympathetic nervous system, mainly located in the peripheral vasculature.

Anaemia A lower than normal number of red blood cells, which depletes the ability to transport oxygen.

Angiotensin converting enzyme inhibitors (ACEI) Prevents the production of angiotensin II, a substance that causes vasoconstriction and high blood pressure. By preventing this production, vessels dilate, and blood pressure is reduced.

Anion A negatively charged ion.

Antidiuretic hormone (ADH) Also known as vasopressin, ADH is a hormone secreted from the posterior pituitary which promotes reabsorption of water back into the circulation via the collecting ducts of the kidney. It also causes widespread constriction of arterioles, which leads to increased arterial pressure.

Atherosclerosis Disease of large and medium-sized muscular arteries where the lumen of the vessel is narrowed by build-up of lipid, cholesterol and calcium. This build-up results in plaque formation, abnormalities of blood flow and eventually, diminished oxygen delivery.

Atrial fibrillation Common cardiac arrhythmia in which multiple ectopic foci in the atria cause them to fibrillate, rather than contracting in a co-ordinated manner. AF is characterised by an irregular pulse and lack of p waves on the ECG.

Atrial flutter Cardiac arrhythmia in which a single ectopic focus in the atria fires rapidly, causing abnormal atrial conduction. Atrial flutter is normally regular (or regularly irregular) and is characterised by 'saw tooth' waves replacing the p wave on the ECG.

Atrioventricular block A type of heart **block** in which the conduction between the atria and ventricles of the heart is impaired due to a partial or total lack of transmission of the electrical impulse between the atria and ventricles.

Atrioventricular node The conduit of the electrical impulse from the atria to the ventricles.

Atrioventricular valves The valves between the atria and ventricles (mitral and tricuspid).

Autonomic nervous system The nervous system is divided into the somatic (voluntary) and autonomic (involuntary). The autonomic regulates individual organ function and homeostasis.

Baroreceptors Sensory nerve endings in the carotid bodies and aortic arch that detect stretch and therefore blood pressure changes

Basophil A type of white blood cell that contains histamine and heparin.

Beta receptor A receptor of the sympathetic nervous system subtypes; beta 1 (in myocardium) and beta 2 (in smooth muscle vasculature).

Cardiac output The amount of blood ejected by the ventricle in 1 minute. CO = SV × HR

Cardiovascular centre Part of the brain that regulates heart rate through the nervous and endocrine systems.

Cation A positively charged ion.

Compliance when referring to the heart The ease with which the ventricle expands or stretches to accommodate ventricular filling.

Conduction system Specialised conducting tissue of the heart which transmits an electrical wave across the heart, causing myocardial contraction.

Coronary circulation Arterial supply for the heart, arising from behind the aortic cusps of the aortic valve.

Contractility The ability of the myocardium to contract

Centrifuge A device that separates the components of a liquid by spinning the liquid at a high speed.

Depolarisation A rapid movement of ions across the cell membrane, causing a change in voltage that leads to the action potential. In cardiac muscle, this initiates myocardial contraction.

Diastole The resting phase of the cardiac cycle in which ventricular filling occurs.

Diastolic pressure The pressure exerted (usually in the vessels) during the relaxation phase of the cardiac cycle.

Electrolyte A solution containing solutes that can conduct an electrical charge.

Ejection fraction The amount of blood ejected from the ventricle in systole, divided by the amount of blood that was in the ventricle at the end of diastole.

Embolism Circulating foreign object, such as air, fat or a blood clot, which can lodge in and block a vessel.

End diastolic volume The amount of blood in the ventricle at the end of diastole.

End systolic volume The amount of blood remaining in the ventricle after systolic ejection.

Endocarditis An infection, usually caused by bacteria, of the inner lining of the heart, which can cause damage the cardiac valves.

Endocardium The innermost layer of the heart.

Endothelium A thin layer of cells that lines the blood vessels.

Eosinphils A type of white blood cell so-called because it can be stained with a dye called eosin.

Erythrocyte A red blood cell.

Extra corporeal membrane oxygenation (ECMO) A temporary system where blood is oxygenated as it is pumped round an extracorporeal circuit to provide support for those whose heart and lungs are unable to function sufficiently.

Fibrinogen A substance in the plasma activated by thrombin to produce fibrin necessary for clot formation.

Fibrinolysis The breakdown of a clot also known as thrombolysis.

First heart sound Heard as lub, this is the sound of the atrioventricular valves closing in the onset of systole.

Foam cells Are found in atheromatous plaques and are made up of both macrophages and smooth muscle.

Haemoglobin A red pigment present in red blood cells made of haem, a molecule containing iron, and globin, a protein with oxygen carrying properties

Haemolytic Destruction of red blood cells.

Haemopoiesis Production of red blood cells and platelets from the bone marrow.

Haemostasis The stoppage of bleeding following the formation of a clot.

Hypoxaemia A low level of oxygen in the blood, measured by arterial blood gas analysis or by SpO_2 in pulse oximetry.

Inodilator A drug which has both inotropic and vasodilator properties.

Inotropic (Also inotrope). Has an effect on myocardial contractility. A positive inotrope increases contractility, a negative inotrope decreases contractility.

Interstitial fluid Fluid around and between tissue cells.

Intracellular fluid Fluid inside the cell walls.

Intravascular fluid Fluid within the vascular space.

Isovolumetric contraction Phase of the cardiac cycle after ventricular depolarisation. All 4 valves are closed, as the pressure in the ventricle in increasing, but not yet sufficient to open the aortic and pulmonic valves.

Jugular venous pressure (JVP) The pressure in the jugular veins that can be seen as a pulsating column in the neck. It can be used to estimate whether cardiac filling pressures are high.

Juxta glomerular cells A group of cells situated in the afferent arteries of the nephrons in the kidney that store renin.

Leucocyte A white blood cell containing a nucleus, but no haemoglobin.
Leucopenia A reduced number of white blood cells.
Leukaemia A malignant disease of the blood where large numbers of leucocytes are present.
Lysis Destruction of a cell or the process of breaking up or destruction.
Malar flush A high colour over the cheekbones, often with a bluish tinge; may be indicative of mitral stenosis.
Mean arterial pressure (MAP) The average pressure in the circulation throughout the cardiac cycle.
Mitral valve Valve which separates the left atria from the left ventricle.
Monocyte A white blood cell that can destroy bacteria.
Myocardium The thick muscle layer of the heart that contracts in a wave-like motion.
Neutrophil A type of white blood cell that can attack and destroy bacteria.
Parasympathetic nervous system A branch of the autonomic nervous system.
Pericardium Rigid sack-like structure surrounding and protecting the heart.
Peripheral cyanosis A blue tinge in fingers or extremities due to inadequate circulation.
Plasma Yellow watery liquid that makes up the fluid component of blood.
Plasma protein A protein found in plasma, e.g., albumin, gamma globulin, fibrinogen.
Platelet A small blood cell which multiplies rapidly following injury and encourages clotting of blood.
Pneumothorax A collection of air in the pleural space (between the lung and the chest wall), resulting in collapse of the lung on the affected side.
Preload Left ventricular end diastolic pressure/volume. It can be thought of as the amount of blood returning to the heart from the circulation into the ventricle.
Pulmonic valve Valve which separates the right ventricle from the pulmonary artery.
Pulse pressure The difference in pressure between systole and diastole.
Repolarisation Movement of ions back across the cell membrane, causing the resting potential to be re-established.
Sarcomere The basic functional unit of striated muscle made up of muscle fibres.
Second heart sound Heard as dub, this is the sound of the aortic and pulmonic valves closing at the beginning of diastole.
Seldinger approach Named after Dr Sven Seldinger, this approach to cannulation involves the insertion of a soft, round-tipped guidewire through a hollow needle into the desired vessel. The blunt catheter or sheath can then be placed over the guidewire. Once the catheter is in place, the guidewire is withdrawn.
Sinoatrial node The heart's primary pacemaker, which spontaneously depolarises 100 times per minute.
Splinter haemorrhages Tiny line haemorrhages that can be seen under the nails, indicative of bacterial endocarditis.
Stroke volume The amount of blood ejected by the ventricle during systole, normally about 70mL.
Sympathetic nervous system A branch of the autonomic nervous system.
Sympathomimetic A substance that mimics the sympathetic nervous system (used to categorise inotropic pharmacology).
Systemic vascular resistance The resistance offered to the circulation by the peripheral circulation.
Systole Phase of the cardiac cycle when contraction occurs.

Systolic pressure Pressure, usually systemic, exerted on the walls of the arteries during systole.

Tamponade Compression of the heart by the accumulation of fluid in the pericardial space.

Tension pneumothorax Presence of air in the pleural space that occurs when air escapes into the pleural cavity from a bronchus but cannot regain entry into the bronchus. As a result, continuously increasing air pressure in the pleural cavity causes progressive collapse of the lung tissue.

Thalassaemia A hereditary disorder that causes an abnormality in the protein component of haemoglobin.

Thrombin A substance which converts fibrinogen to fibrin to enable blood clotting.

Thrombocyte Another name for platelet.

Thrombus A blood clot.

Tricuspid valve Valve which separates the right atrium from the left ventricle.

Vagal tone The level of activity in the parasympathetic nervous system, for example, the vagus nerve has an inhibitory effect on the heart rate.

Vasopressor A substance (often a drug) which increases the degree of vasoconstriction of the blood vessels.

Ventricular assist device (VAD) A mechanical device which can be used to assist the pumping action of the heart.

Ventricular hypertrophy A thickening of the muscle layer of the heart, the ventricular myocardium, usually in response to disease, high blood pressure or problems that increase ventricular afterload.

Venturi mask Type of disposable oxygen face mask which delivers a precise, consistent mixture of air and oxygen, regardless of the patient's inspiratory flow rate.

Xanthelasma Yellow/white fatty bumps under the skin around the eye lids, often the upper lid.

Xanthomata A bump in the skin caused by fats building up under the surface. They appear as small white, or larger yellow bumps and may be associated with a high level of lipids in the blood.

TEST YOURSELF

1) Name the two systems that are circulations within the cardiovascular system.
   a) Splenic and hepatic
   b) Pulmonary and mesenteric
   c) Renal and systemic
   d) Systemic and pulmonary
2) Blood flows round heart in the following order:
   a) Right atrium, right ventricle, pulmonary artery, pulmonary vein, left atria, left ventricle, aorta.
   b) Right ventricle, right atrium, pulmonary artery, pulmonary vein, left ventricle, left atria, aorta.
   c) Left atria, left ventricle, pulmonary vein, pulmonary artery, right atria, right ventricle, aorta.
   d) Right atrium, right ventricle, pulmonary vein, pulmonary artery, left atria, left ventricle, aorta.

3) The pressure of 120/80, known as blood pressure, consists of a systolic and diastolic pressure. Which of the following statements is true?
   a) The systolic pressure is generated in the left ventricle as it fills.
   b) The diastolic pressure is the best guide to organ perfusion.
   c) The systolic pressure is pressure generated by the blood on the vessels after ventricular contraction.
   d) The diastolic pressure needs to be below 50mmHg for coronary artery perfusion to occur.
4) There are 3 layers to the heart: endocardium, myocardium and pericardium. Which of the following statements is true?
   a) The pericardial sac is important for the conduction pathway of the heart.
   b) The myocardium is the muscle of the heart and is thickest in the left ventricles.
   c) The endocardium has a rough surface to help the blood to clot if there are any bleeding problems.
   d) The valves of the heart are made out of myocardial tissue.
5) What name is given to acute severe central chest pain due to a decreased blood supply to the heart?
   a) Stroke
   b) Myocarditis
   c) Angina
   d) Hypertension
6) What percentage of your blood volume is plasma?
   a) 1
   b) 55
   c) 70
   d) 90
7) In the ECG, the p wave represents:
   a) Depolarisation of the ventricle
   b) Depolarisation of the atria
   c) Repolarisation of the ventricle
   d) Repolarisation of the atria
8) If a patient's heart rate is 80 and their stroke volume in 60mL, what would their cardiac output be?
   b) 4200mL
   c) 5600mL
   d) 3200mL
   e) 4800mL
9) Increased venous return to the heart causes increases in which of the following:
   b) Preload
   c) Cardiac output
   d) Strength of contraction
   e) All of the above
10) Increased sympathetic stimulation of the heart causes:
    a) Increased force of contraction
    b) Increased heart rate

   c) Increased cardiac output
   d) All of these
11) When arterial blood pressure increases, it is detected by the baroreceptors. These communicate with the cardiovascular centre and the response initiated causes:
   a) Increase in sympathetic outflow to the heart
   b) Increase in parasympathetic outflow to the heart
   c) Increase in sympathetic outflow to the peripheral vasculature
   d) Decrease in sympathetic outflow to the peripheral vasculature
   e) a and c only
   f) b and d only
12) Clinical findings of raised respiratory rate, raised heart rate, cool peripheries and low blood pressure are consistent with:
   a) Hypovolaemic shock and cardiogenic shock
   b) Septic shock
   c) Early neurogenic shock
   d) Late hypovolaemic shock and early anaphylactic shock
13) Which of the following is not a reason for a cardiac arrhythmia to develop?
   a) Hypoxia
   b) Hypokalaemia
   c) Central venous pressure below 5mmHg
   d) Infection
14) On noticing a cardiac arrhythmia, the nurse should:
   a) Put out an arrest call immediately.
   b) Check ABCDE assessment and refer for medical help quickly if the patient is compromised.
   c) Not be overly worried, cardiac arrhythmias are very common.
   d) Give oxygen, do a 12 lead ECG and wait for the doctor to review on the next ward round.
15) Acute coronary syndrome refers to:
   a) A situation where there is disrupted blood flow down the coronary artery due to obstruction of a thrombus.
   b) A situation where there has been death of the heart muscle due to lack of blood flow.
   c) A rapid irregular heartbeat, which requires emergency action.
   d) A situation where the patient has chest pain, but no changes on the 12 lead ECG recording.
16) Identify the functions of 3 plasma proteins below:
   a) Albumin
   b) Globulins
   c) Fibrinogen
17) The following are true about erythrocytes
   a) They contain haemoglobin.
   b) They have a large nucleus and can divide rapidly.

    c) There are only a few cells functional at one time.
    d) They are phagocytes and help engulf pathogens.
18) Which blood group is described as the universal donor and which the universal recipient?
    a) O positive is the universal recipient and B negative is the universal recipient.
    b) O negative is the universal recipient and 0 positive is the universal donor.
    c) O negative is the universal donor and AB positive is the universal recipient.
    d) A positive is the universal recipient and AB negative is the universal recipient.
19) Which type of shock may be characterised by vasoconstriction and tachycardia?
    a) Septic and hypovolaemic
    b) Cardiogenic and anaphylactic
    c) Obstructive and cardiogenic
    d) Neurogenic and hypovolaemic
20) The ABCDE approach to assessment is important because:
    a) It is a recognised pain assessment tool.
    b) It help to identify problems with breathing and circulation.
    c) It provide a systematic approach to assessment.
    d) It provides a systematic approach to assessing neurological status.

Answers

1 d
2 a
3 c
4 b
5 c
6 b
7 b
8 e
9 e
10 d
11 f
12 a
13 c
14 b
15 a
16 Albumin: maintains colloid oncotic pressure, binds with drugs and hormones.
Globulin: forms antibodies.
Fibrinogen: essential for blood clotting.
17 a
18 c
19 c
20 c

References

Anderson K and Chatha H. (2017). Peripheral metaraminol infusion in the emergency department. *Emergency Medical Journal*, 34(3), 190–192. Available from: https://emj.bmj.com/content/emermed/34/3/190.full.pdf#page=1&zoom=auto,-82,800. Accessed August 2019.

Badimon L, Peria E, Arderiu G, Padro T, Slevin M, Vailahur G and Chiva-Blanch G. (2018). C-reactive protein in atherothrombosis and angiogenesis. *Frontiers in Immunology*, 9, 430. doi:10.3389/fimmu.2018.00430.

Bickely S. (2017). *Bates' Guide to Physical Examination and History Taking*, 12th Edition. Philadelphia, PA: Wolters Kluwer.

British National Formulary-NICE. (2020). Available from: https://bnf.nice.org.uk/treatment-summary/parenteral-anticoagulants.html.

Conrad N, Judge A, Tran J, Mohseni H, Hedgecott D, Crespillo A, Allison N, Hemingway H, Cleland J, McMurray J and Rahimi K. (2017). Temporal trends and patterns in heart failure incidence: a population-based study of 4 million individuals. *The Lancet*, 391(10120), 572–580.

Dutton, H and Finch, J. (eds.) (2018). *Acute and Critical Care Nursing at a Glance*. Chichester: Wiley-Blackwell.

European Society of Cardiology (ESC). (2014). 2014 ESC guidelines on the diagnosis and management of acute pulmonary emobolism. *European Heart Journal*, 35, 3033–3080. doi:10.1093/eurheartj/ehu283.

European Society of Cardiology and Ponikowski P, et al. (2016a). 2016 ESC guidelines for the diagnosis and treatment of acute and chronic heart failure. Developed with special contribution of the Heart Failure Associated (HFA) and the ESC. *European Heart Journal*, 37, 2129–2200. doi:10.1093/eurheartj/ehw128.

European Society of Cardiology (ESC). (2016b). 2016 ESC guidelines for the management of atrial fibrillation developed in collaboration with EACTS. *European Heart Journal*, 37(38), 2893–2963. doi:10.1093/eurheartj/ehw210. Available from: https://academic.oup.com/eurheartj/article/37/38/2893/2334964. Accessed August 2019.

European Society of Cardiology (ESC). (2016c). 2015 ESC guidelines for the management of acute coronary syndromes in patients presenting without persistent ST-segment elevation. *European Heart Journal*, 37(3), 267–315. doi:10.1093/eurheartj/ehv320.

European Society of Cardiology (ESC). (2017). 2017 ESC guidelines for the management of acute myocardial infarction in patients presenting with ST-segment elevation: the task force for the management of acute myocardial infarction in patients presenting with ST-segment elevation of the European Society of Cardiology (ESC). *European Heart Journal*, 39(2), 119–177. doi:10.1093/eurheartj/ehx393.

Faculty of Intensive Care Medicine. (2019). *Guidelines for the provision of intensive care services*. Available from: https://www.ics.ac.uk/ICS/ICS/GuidelinesAndStandards/GPICS_2nd_Edition.aspx. Accessed September 2019.

Gillebert T. (2018). Pulse pressure and blood pressure: is the sum more than the parts? *European Journal of Preventions Cardiology*, 25(5), 457–459.

Intensive Care Society. (2016). *Medication Concentration in Critical Care Area*. Available from: ics-standard-medication-concentrations-2016. Accessed August 2019.

Lewis S, Pritchard M, Evans D, Butler A, Alderson P, Smith A and Roberts I. (2018). Colloid versus crystalloids for fluid resuscitation in critically ill people (Review). The *Cochrane Collaboration*: Wiley and Sons. Available from: https://www.cochranelibrary.com/cdsr/doi/10.1002/14651858.CD000567.pub7/epdf/abstract. Accessed August 2019.

Loveday H, Wilson J, Pratt R, et al. (2014). Epic 3: national evidence-based guidelines for preventing healthcare associated infections in NHS hospitals in NHS hospital in England. *Journal of Hospital Infection*, 8651, S1–S70. Available from: https://www.journalofhospitalinfection.com/article/S0195-6701(13)60012-2/pdf. Accessed August 2019.

Lown M and Moran P. (2019). Should we screen for atrial fibrillation? *BMJ*, 364, 143. doi:10.1136/bmj.l43.

Mageed L. (2018). Coronary artery disease: pathogenesis, progression of atherosclerosis and risk factors. *Open Journal of Cardiology & Heart Diseases*, 2(4), 1–7. Available from: https://crimsonpublishers.com/ojchd/pdf/OJCHD.000545.pdf. Accessed August 2019.

National Institute for Health and Care Excellence. (2013 updated 2017). *Intravenous Fluid Therapy in Adults in Hospital*, cg 174. Available from: https://www.nice.org.uk/guidance/cg174/.

National Institute for Health and Care Excellence. (2014a). *Acute Coronary Syndromes in Adults. Quality Standard*. Available from: www.nice.org.uk/guidance/qs68. Accessed August 2019.

National Institute for Health and Care Excellence. (2014b). *Atrial Fibrillation: Management CG180*. Available from: www.nice.org.uk/guidance/cg190. Accessed August 2019.

National Institute for Health and Care Excellence. (2018a). *Chronic Heart Failure in Adult: Diagnosis and Management*, ng 106. Available from: https://www.nice.org.uk/guidance/ng106/resources/chronic-heart-failure-in-adults-diagnosis-and-management-pdf-66141541311685. Accessed August 2019.

National Institute for Health and Care Excellence. (2018b). *Venous Thromboembolism in Over 16s: Reducing the Risk of Hospital-Acquired Deep Vein Thrombosis or Pulmonary Embolism (NG89)*. Available from: https://www.nice.org.uk/guidance/ng89. Accessed August 2019.

National Institute for Health and Care Excellence. (2018c). *Deep Vein Thrombosis Scenario: Management of Deep Vein Thrombosis*. Available from: https://cks.nice.org.uk/deep-vein-thrombosis#!scenario. Accessed August 2018.

National Institute for Health and Care Excellence. (2019a). *Assessment and Immediate Management of Suspected Acute Coronary Syndrome* (NICE Pathway updated June 2019). Available from: http://pathways.nice.org.uk/pathways/chest-pain. Accessed August 2019.

National Institute for Health and Care Excellence. (2019b). *Metaraminol Indication and Use*. Available from: https://bnf.nice.org.uk/drug/metaraminol.html.

National Institute for Health and Care Excellence. (2019c). *Hypertension in adults: diagnosis and management NG10054*. Available from: https://www.nice.org.uk/guidance/indevelopment/gid-ng10054. Accessed August 2019.

Norfolk D. (2013). *Handbook of Transfusion Medicine*. Available from: https://www.transfusionguidelines.org/transfusion-handbook.

Norris T. (2019). *Porth's Pathophysiology, Concepts of Altered Health States*, 10th Edition. London: Wolters Kluwer.

Nursing and Midwifery Council. (2018a). *Future Nurse: Standards of Proficiency for Registered Nurses*. Available from: https://www.nmc.org.uk/globalassets/sitedocuments/education-standards/future-nurse-proficiencies.pdf. Accessed August 2019.

Nursing and Midwifery Council. (2018b). *The Code: Professional Standards Practice and Behavior for Nurses, Midwives and Nursing Associates*. Available from: https://www.nmc.org.uk/globalassets/sitedocuments/nmc-publications/nmc-code.pdf. Accessed August 2019.

O'Driscoll R, Howard L, Earis J, Mak V, Bajwah S, Beasley R, Curtis K, Davison A, Dorward A, Dyer C, Evans A, Falconer L, Fitzpatrick C, Gibbs S, Hinshaw K, Howard R, Kane B, Keep J, Kelly C, Khachi H, Asad M, Khan I, Kishen R, Mansfield L, Martin B, Moore F, Powrie D, Restrick L, Roffe C, Singer M, Soar J, Small I, Ward L, Whitmore D, Wedzicha W, Wijesinghe M and BTS Emergency Oxygen Guideline Development Group On behalf of the British Thoracic Society. (2017). BTS guideline for oxygen use in adults in healthcare an emergency settings. *Thorax*, 72(S1), i1–i20.

Pallister C. (1994). *Blood physiology and pathophysiology*. Oxford: Butterworth-Heinemann.

Picket J, Bridges E, Kritek P and Whitney J. (2017). Passive led-raising and prediction of fluid responsiveness: a systematic review. *Critical Care Nurse*, 37(2), 32–48.

Resuscitation Council UK. (2015). *Advanced Life Support*, 3rd Edition. UK: Resuscitation Council (UK).

Rhodes A, Evans L, Alhazzani W, Levy M, Antonelli M, Ferrer R, Kumar A, Sevransky J, Sprung C, Nunnally M, Rochwerg B, Rubenfeld G, Angus D, Annane D, Beale R, Bellinghan G, Bernard G, Chiche J, Coopersmith C, De Backer D, French C, Fujishima S, Gerlach H, Hidalgo J, Hollenberg S, Jones A, Karnad D, Kleinpell R, Koh Y, Lisboa T, Machado F, Marini J, Marshall J, Mazuski J, McIntyre L, McLean A, Mehta S, Moreno R, Myburgh J, Navalesi P, Nishida O, Osborn T, Perner A, Plunkett C, Ranieri M, Schorr C, Seckel M, Seymour C, Shieh L, Shukri K, Simpson S,

Singer M, Thompson B, Townsend S, Van der Poll T, Vincent J, Wiersinga W, Zimmerman J and Dellinger R. (2017). Surviving sepsis campaign: international guidelines for management of sepsis and septic shock: 2016. *Intensive Care Medicine*, 43(3), 304–377. doi:10.1007/s00134-017-4683-6.

Royal College of Nursing. (2016). *Standards for Infusion Therapy*, 4th Edition. RCN. Available from: https://www.rcn.org.uk/clinical-topics/infection-prevention-and-control/standards-for-infusion-therapy.

Royal College of Physicians. (2017). *National Early Warning Score (NEWS) 2 Standardising the assessment of acute-illness severity in the NHS*. Available from: http://www.rcplondon.ac.uk/resources/national-early-warning-score-news._ Accessed January 2019.

Scheeren T, Bakker J, Backer D, Annane D, Asfar P, Boerma E, Cecconi M, Dubin A, Dünser M, Duranteau J, Gordon A, Hamzaoui O, Hernández G, Leone M, Levy B, Martin C, Mebazaa A, Monnet X, Morelli A, Payen D, Pearse R, Pinsky M, Radermacher P, Reuter D, Saugel B, Sakr Y, Singer M, Squara P, Vieillard-Baron A, Vignon P, Vistisen S, van der Horst I, Vincent J and Teboul J. (2019). Current use of vasopressors in septic shock. *Annals of Intensive Care*, 9(20), 1–12. doi:10.1186/s13613-019-0498-7.

Schumann J, Henrich E, Stobl H, Prondzinsky R, Weiche S, Thiele H, Werddan K, Frantz S and Unverzagt S. (2018). Inotropic agents and vasodilator strategies for the treatment of cardiogenic shock or low cardiac output syndrome (Review). *Cochrane Database of Systematic Reviews*, 2018(1), CD009669.

Silva J, Gonclaves L and Sousa P. (2018). Fluid therapy and shock: an integrative literature review. *British Journal of Nursing*, 27(8), 449–454.

Society for Cardiological Science and Technology. (2017). *Clinical Guidelines by Consensus Recording a Standard 12-Lead Electrocardiogram: An Approved Method by the Society for Cardiological Science & Technology (SCST)*. Available from: http://www.scst.org.uk/resources/SCST_ECG_Recording_Guidelines_2017am.pdf.

Stanfield CL. (2017). *Principles of Human Phsyiology*, 6th Edition. Harlow: Pearson Education.

Woodrow P. (2019). *Intensive Care Nursing: A Framework for Practice*, 4th Edition. Oxon: Routledge.

Further reading

Adam S, Osborne S and Welch J. (2017). *Critical Care Nursing Science and Practice*, 3rd Edition. Oxford: Oxford University Press.

7 Recognition and management of cardiopulmonary arrest

Sharon Elliott

AIM

The aim of this chapter is to improve your recognition and management of the patient who has problems with maintaining airway patency and/or suffers cardiopulmonary arrest, and to explore the issues surrounding the end of life, that accompany many of these emergencies in acute care.

OBJECTIVES

At the end of this chapter you will be able to:

- Recognise partial and complete airway obstruction, and identify appropriate airway support manoeuvres.
- Understand in detail the chain of survival, its application to in-hospital resuscitation and the advanced life support algorithm.
- Differentiate between shockable and non-shockable rhythms and explain the safe use of defibrillation.
- Identify the drugs most commonly used during a cardiac arrest.
- Identify the important aspects of post-resuscitation care and staff debriefing.
- Describe the role of the nurse in caring for the family during and after a resuscitation attempt, and explore and evaluate the ethical issues involved in resuscitation attempts and "Do not attempt resuscitation" (DNAR) orders.

Introduction

The UK National Cardiac Arrest Audit (NCAA) indicates that in-hospital cardiac arrest occurs in 1.6 per 1000 hospital admissions, with a rate of survival to discharge of 18.4 % (Nolan et al. 2014). Whilst this figure might appear relatively low, recent international data suggests that survival rates for cardiac arrests, occurring inside or outside hospital, are improving (Girotra et al. 2012; Wissenberg et al. 2013; Chan et al. 2014).

It is well established that adults who experience cardiac arrest usually display adverse clinical signs, usually related to airway, breathing or circulation (Kause et al. 2004;

NCEPOD 2005; Findlay et al. 2012). This physiological deterioration has been shown, in many cases, to have developed over time, often involving unrecognised or inadequately treated hypoxaemia or hypotension (Kause et al. 2004; Findlay et al. 2012).

There is strong evidence correlating higher ratios of registered nurse staffing with lower rates of pneumonia, shock and cardiac arrest (Needleman et al. 2002; Aiken et al. 2014). The preceding chapters in this book have aimed to equip you with the knowledge needed to recognise and identify changes in a patient's condition that could precede a cardiac arrest. Early recognition and effective management will prevent cardiac arrest from occurring in many instances (Soar et al. 2015), although, even with optimal assessment and monitoring, some patients will suffer cardiopulmonary arrest.

This chapter outlines airway management and the actions required, along with the underpinning rationale in the event of a cardiopulmonary arrest, based on the latest published guidance from the Resuscitation Council (Resuscitation Council UK 2015). These guidelines are updated regularly and can be accessed at https://www.resus.org.uk.

Airway assessment and management

Airway assessment and management requires determining whether the airway is open, closed or at risk, and includes the measures taken to reduce the risk of obstruction or to relieve it.

A partially or completely obstructed airway may be the primary event leading to a **cardiopulmonary arrest**. A reduced level of consciousness is often the cause, but loss of gag reflex and inability to clear secretions are also important factors. In order to ensure the best chance of a successful outcome, prompt assessment, protection of the airway and adequate oxygenation are essential.

Causes of airway obstruction

Obstruction can occur at any level from the nose/mouth to the bronchi. Potential causes are:

- Lack of muscle tone of the epiglottis, soft palate and tongue, which may be the cause in a person with reduced consciousness levels.
- Vomit, blood, foodstuff or other foreign bodies.
- Oedema due to burns, anaphylaxis or inflammation.
- Inhalation of an irritant or stimulation of the upper airway, such as during intubation, which may result in laryngeal spasm.

Recognising airway obstruction

The best approach is to **look**, **listen** and **feel**:

- **Look** for chest and abdominal movement.
- **Listen** for breath sounds.
- **Feel** for air movement at the nose and mouth.

Partial airway obstruction is **noisy** and may be indicated by:

- **Inspiratory stridor** – caused by obstruction at, or above, the larynx.
- **Expiratory wheeze** – suggests constriction or spasm of the lower airways.
- **Gurgling** – suggests liquid in the upper airway.
- **Snoring** – the pharynx is semi-occluded by the tongue.
- **Crowing** or **stridor** – caused by laryngeal spasm or obstruction.
- **Partial airway obstruction** will involve the use of accessory muscles such as those of the neck, shoulders and abdomen, as well as the intercostal and subcostal muscles.

Complete airway obstruction is **silent** and may result in paradoxical or 'see-saw' breathing. As attempts are made to draw in air, the chest is drawn in and the abdomen distends. The opposite occurs on exhalation.

Obstruction of the airway with a foreign body

This can occur due to inhalation of foodstuffs. Sudden airway obstruction results in choking. Foreign body airway obstruction (FBAO) is very frightening and occurs acutely, so the patient is often unable to explain what is happening to them. If the obstruction is severe, it can result in rapid loss of consciousness and death. Therefore, effective life-saving measures are required quickly. Immediate recognition and response are of the utmost importance.

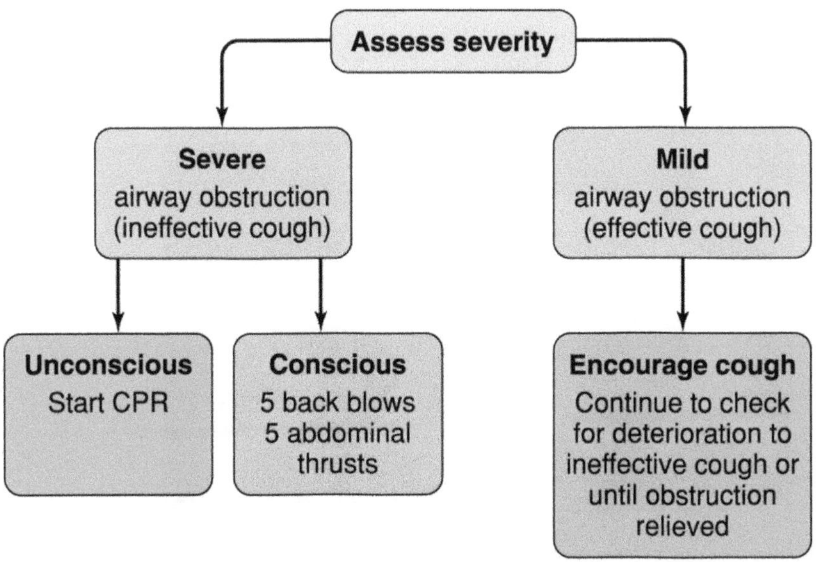

Figure 7.1 Adult choking treatment algorithm. *Source*: Resuscitation Council UK (2015) *2015 Resuscitation Guidelines*. Reproduced with the kind permission of Resuscitation Council (UK).

The Resuscitation Council UK (2015) has compiled the adult choking treatment **algorithm** (see Figure 7.1), which is a helpful guide in the recognition and treatment of airway obstruction.

The key stages are:

- Recognition.
- Assessment of the severity of the obstruction.
- Management.

Opening the airway

Oropharyngeal airway

The basic techniques of head-tilt, chin-lift and jaw-thrust manoeuvres will be discussed later. Simple airway adjuncts, such as the oropharyngeal airway (OPA) and nasopharyngeal airway (NPA), can be helpful in maintaining an open airway, but should only be inserted if you have been trained to do so.

Oropharyngeal airways come in a variety of sizes, from infant to adult, and ensuring the correct size is important. If it is too big it can obstruct the airway or cause trauma. Figure 7.2 shows OPAs which are colour-coded, according to size.

To ensure the correct size, the bite block should be placed at the level of the incisors and should reach to the angle of the jaw (see Figure 7.3).

The airway is inserted upside down and then turned 180° once contact has been made with the back of the throat (see Figure 7.4).

OPAs should only be used on an unconscious casualty. In a conscious person, their insertion can stimulate the gag reflex and induce vomiting.

Figure 7.2 Oropharyngeal colour-coded airways.

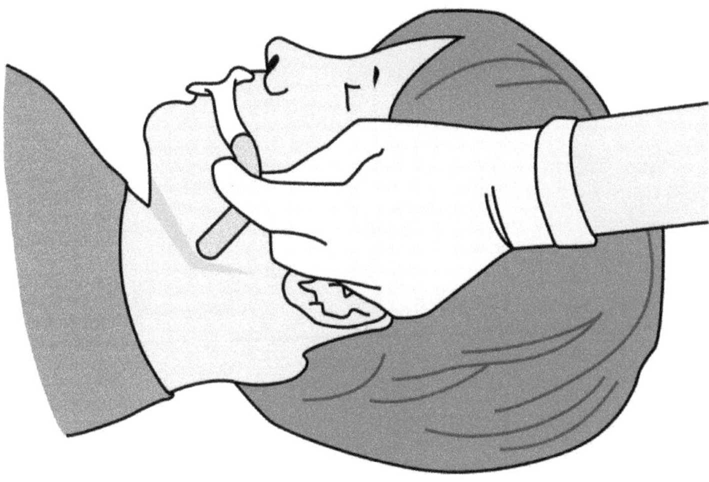

Figure 7.3 The correct sizing of OPAs.

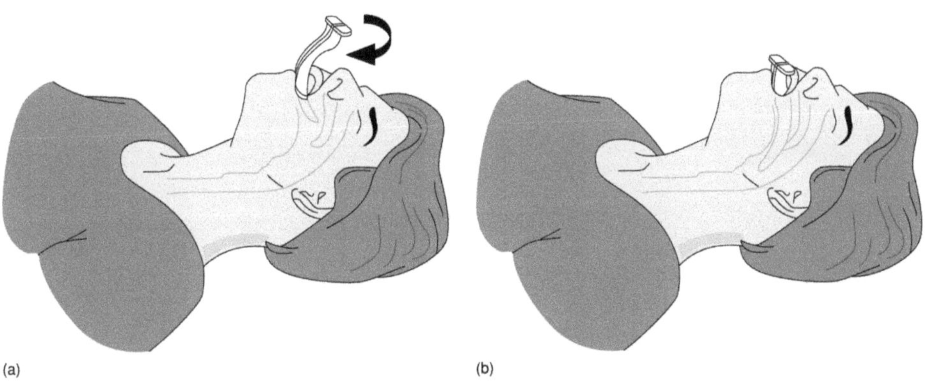

Figure 7.4 (a) Inserting the OPA, (b) the OPA *in situ*.

NASOPHARYNGEAL AIRWAYS

Nasopharyngeal airways are inserted into the nasal passageway to secure an open airway (see Figures 7.5 and 7.6). An NPA can facilitate removal of secretions, as a suction catheter can be passed down it. They can be used in a conscious casualty but should not be used in cases of head trauma until a fractured base of skull has been ruled out.

Remember

Once the airway is open, the priority is to maintain it and ensure adequate ventilation and oxygenation. Obstruction of the airway and/or lack of oxygen for more than a few minutes can cause injury to the brain and other vital organs.

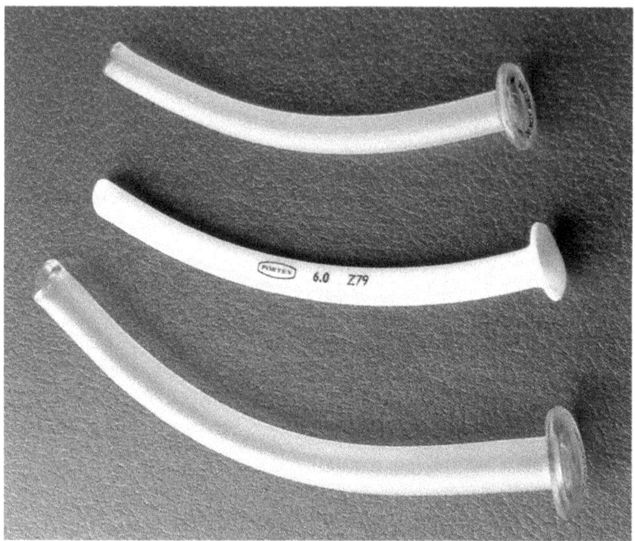

Figure 7.5 Nasopharyngeal airways.

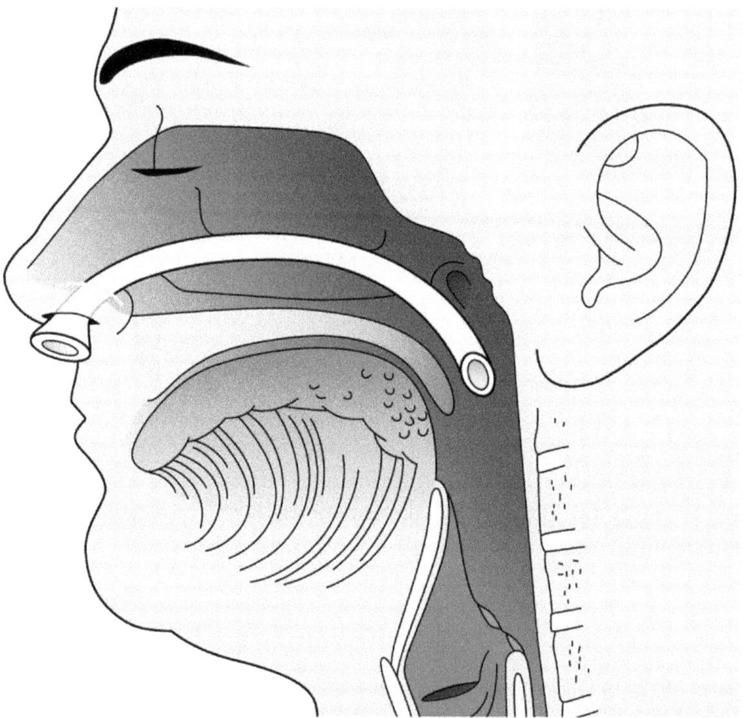

Figure 7.6 NPA *in situ.*

Once inserted, oropharyngeal or nasopharyngeal airways can be used to help maintain the airway and can be used in conjunction with the pocket mask or **bag valve mask** devices as an aid to ventilation. Even with an OPA or NPA *in situ*, the airway can obstruct if the head is not correctly positioned.

ENDOTRACHEAL TUBE AND SUPRAGLOTTIC AIRWAY

The gold standard for securing a safe airway is generally considered to be the endotracheal tube (ETT) (Benoit et al. 2015). However, considerable experience and expertise in the placement of ETTs is required if potentially catastrophic complications are to be avoided, such as unrecognised oesophageal intubation and accidental dislodgement (Nolan and Soar 2008; Lyon et al. 2010). It is necessary to stop chest compressions during attempts to intubate if attempts are prolonged, as this can lead to reduced coronary and cerebral perfusion.

Supraglottic airways (SGAs) are a group of airway adjuncts inserted into the pharynx, to enable ventilation, oxygenation and, if necessary, administration of anaesthetic gases. They consist of a wide-bore tube and an elliptical cuff designed to seal around the laryngeal opening (Resuscitation Council UK 2015). SGAs are easier to insert, usually while chest compressions continue. SGAs result in less gastric distension, when compared with facemask or bag valve mask ventilation, and offer an efficient, alternative way of securing and protecting the airway during a resuscitation attempt.

There are two main types of SGAs:

- Laryngeal Mask Airways (LMAs).
- I-Gel.

The I-Gel is similar in appearance and function to an LMA, but the cuff does not require inflation; in addition, a bite block is integral to the stem and a narrow oesophageal drainage tube is included. It is ideal as an airway device during resuscitation attempts, due to the ease of insertion, again without interruption to chest compressions, but with the added advantage of providing a good cuff seal.

Suction

A wide-bore rigid suction device (Yankauer) can be used to remove blood, vomit and secretions from the mouth. Caution should be used if the patient is semi-conscious as it can stimulate the gag reflex and therefore vomiting. Fine-bore flexible suction catheters can be passed, *via* an oropharyngeal or nasopharyngeal airway, to remove secretions.

Chain of survival

In a hospital setting, it could be patients or relatives who are the victims of a cardiac arrest. Ideally, patients at high risk should be cared for in an area that enables monitoring and facilities for immediate resuscitation, although cardiac arrests may occur in non-clinical areas, such as bathrooms, corridors and car parks. In the event of a cardiac arrest, time is of the essence. If the person who has collapsed is not found quickly and/or cardiac arrest is not recognised, the chances of survival diminish significantly as each minute passes. There will be varying skill levels amongst staff, and you should only attempt what you

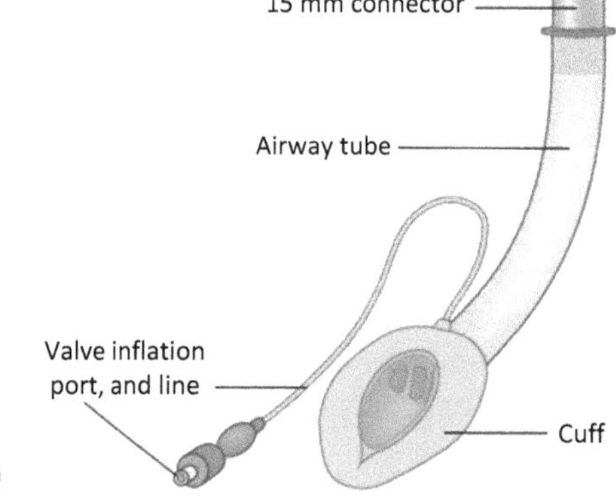

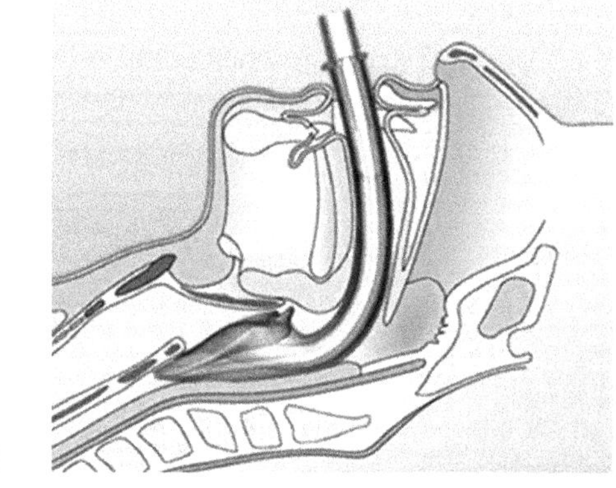

Figure 7.7 a) Laryngeal mask, b) placement of I-Gel.

have been trained to do. However, there is a public and professional expectation that all clinical staff can carry out CPR and ensure that expert help and equipment is summoned immediately. This basic requirement is the minimum expected of student nurses and newly qualified staff nurses.

When a patient suffers a cardiac arrest, there are four priorities needed to provide the best chance of a successful outcome. These are:

1 Early recognition of cardiac arrest and call for help; in all UK hospitals, there is now a standard number to use in the event of a cardiac arrest: 2222.
2 Early **basic life support (BLS)**, also termed **cardiopulmonary resuscitation (CPR)**.
3 Early **defibrillation**, if appropriate.
4 Post-resuscitation care, aimed at restoring quality of life.

These are often conceptualised as the chain of survival (see Figure 7.8).

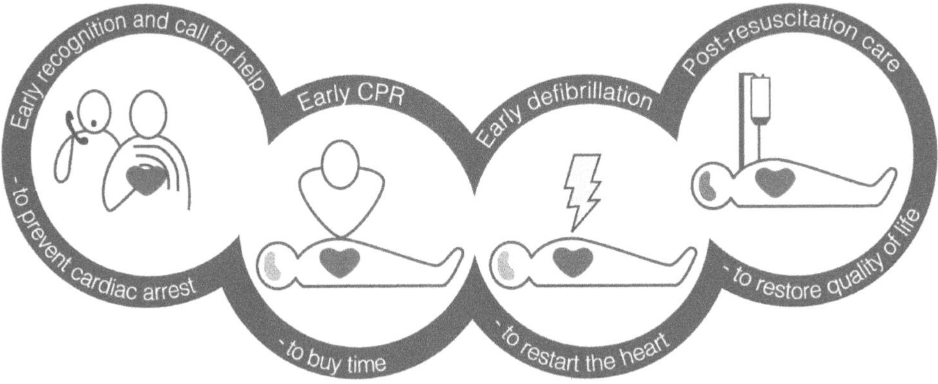

Figure 7.8 The chain of survival. *Source*: Resuscitation Council UK (2015) *2015 Resuscitation Guidelines*. Reproduced with the kind permission of Resuscitation Council (UK).

Each of the four links in the chain is essential – if any one of them is weak, the whole chain is weakened. Basic life support (BLS) is integral to advanced life support (ALS), and the transition between the two should be seamless.

Cardiac arrests are relatively rare events. It is therefore essential that clinical staff have the opportunity to rehearse and practice the algorithms on a regular basis, to ensure that the response is effective.

To help ensure that the collapsed patient receives the best chances of survival, it is necessary that clinical staff are familiar with the procedures to follow and the techniques to use. The Resuscitation Council UK (RCUK) sets the standards in relation to these procedures and techniques. The Council was established in 1981, with the objective of ensuring that health care professionals and the general public are educated in the most effective methods of resuscitation, appropriate to their needs. The guidance is reviewed every two to three years to ensure that it is in line with the latest evidence. The RCUK has produced a series of algorithms. These are diagrammatic representations of the steps to follow in the event of a cardiac arrest (see Figure 7.9). Emergency situations require a coordinated team response to achieve the best outcome. This is most likely to occur if everyone is following the same agreed process.

The chain of survival underpins the in-hospital resuscitation algorithm.

The sequence of events to follow for a collapsed person can be easily remembered by the acronym DRS ABC.

D = Danger

Check that the area around the patient is safe. Although there are relatively few documented cases of first responders to a cardiac arrest suffering adverse effects, your safety and that of the other members of the team is always the first priority.

Use appropriate personal protective clothing as soon as possible. In most cases, this will be non-sterile gloves and aprons, although masks and eye protection may be required in some circumstances, such as a major trauma.

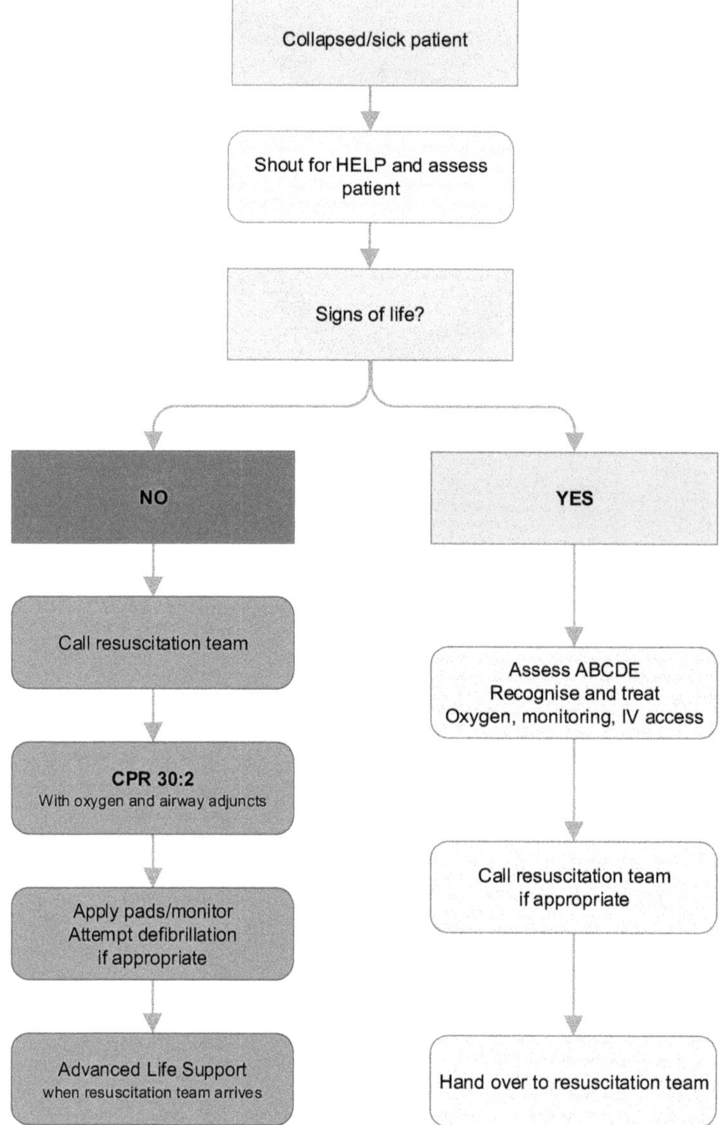

Figure 7.9 In-hospital resuscitation algorithm. *Source*: Resuscitation Council UK (2015) *2015 Resuscitation Guidelines*. Reproduced with the kind permission of Resuscitation Council (UK).

R = Response

Gently shake the shoulders and shout the name of the person who has collapsed to assess if there is a response.

S = Shout

Or summon help. In reality, checking for a response and getting help will usually occur simultaneously as, in most cases, if a patient appears to have collapsed, additional help of some kind will be required. As soon as it is apparent that a cardiac arrest has occurred, the resuscitation or medical emergency team (MET) *must* be called.

A = Airway

The airway should be opened by tilting the head back and lifting the chin up. This will cause the tongue to move away from the back of the pharynx, creating a patent airway (see Figure 7.10).

If necessary, the patient may need to be moved to enable opening of the airway, but, if other injuries are suspected, movement should be minimised until further help arrives. Despite the presence of other injuries, opening the airway is the priority in a collapsed unconscious casualty, because, if the airway remains closed, there is no chance of survival, regardless of the cause of collapse. It may be easier for you to open the airway without moving the casualty too much by employing the jaw-thrust manoeuvre (see Figure 7.11).

B = Breathing

With the airway open, the unconscious casualty may breathe spontaneously. To check if this is the case, it is necessary to:

- *Look* – at the chest for movement, coughing or other signs of life.
- *Listen* – for breath sounds with your face close to the casualty's.
- *Feel* – for movement of air against your face.

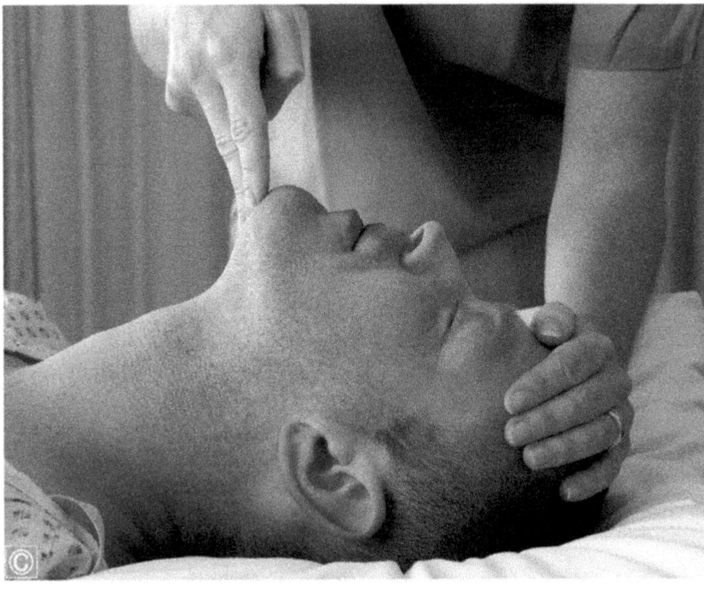

Figure 7.10 Head-tilt/chin-lift manoeuvre. *Source*: Resuscitation Council UK (2016) *Advanced Life Support*. Photographs reproduced with kind permission of Michael Scott and the Resuscitation Council (UK).

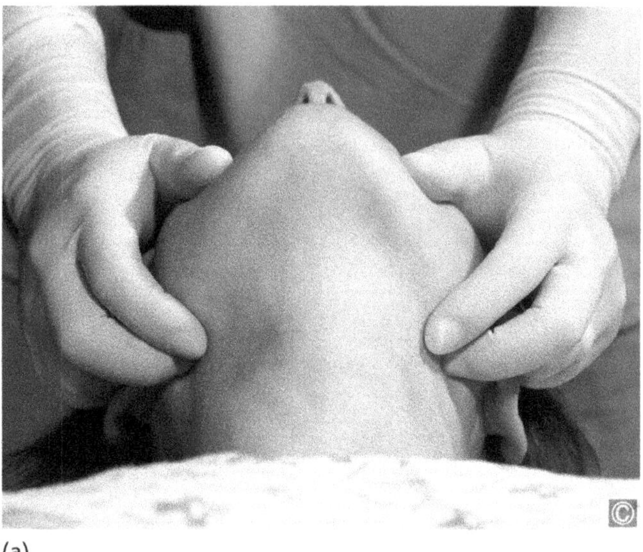

(a)

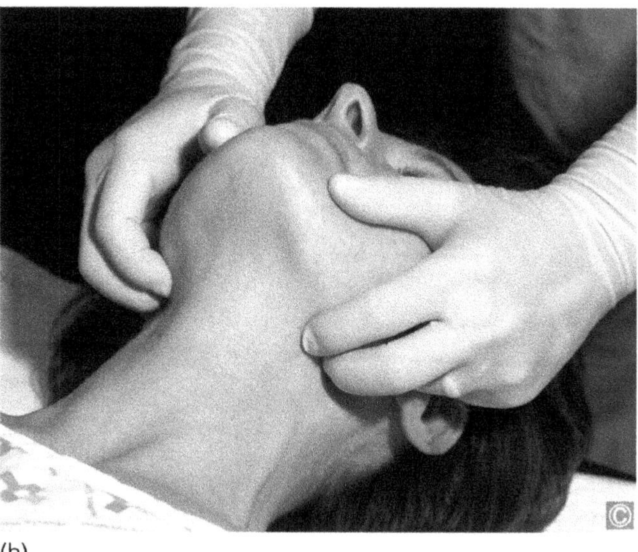

(b)

Figure 7.11 Jaw-thrust manoeuvre. *Source*: Resuscitation Council UK (2016) *Advanced Life Support*. Photographs reproduced with kind permission of Michael Scott and the Resuscitation Council (UK).

Occasional gasps, slow, laboured or noisy breathing, known as **agonal breathing,** is common in the immediate stage following cardiac arrest. This must not be confused with normal breathing.

If the casualty remains unconscious and there is no normal breathing, assume that a cardiac arrest has occurred and commence chest compressions.

If there are signs of life, assess the patient using the ABCDE approach, while waiting for assistance.

C = Compressions

Ensure help has been summoned and commence CPR (see Figure 7.12). This is achieved by:

- Locating the sternum.
- Interlocking your fingers.
- Applying downward pressure to the lower half of the sternum (centre of the chest) with straight arms (see Figure 7.12).
- 30 compressions should be performed.
- The pressure applied to the sternum should compress the chest by one-third of its depth (approximately 5–6cm).
- The rate of compression should be 100–120 compressions per minute.

> To avoid fatigue on the part of the person providing chest compressions, CPR providers should ideally change every two minutes to avoid a reduction in the quality of compressions. This change over should occur without long pauses in compressions as even minor delays have been shown to adversely affect the outcome of resuscitation.
>
> (Resuscitation Council UK 2015)

There should be minimal delay between cycles of compressions. Compressions generate a pressure in the arterial system, which enables the flow of oxygenated blood. Delays result in the pressure falling, reducing the oxygen supply to vital organs and tissues.

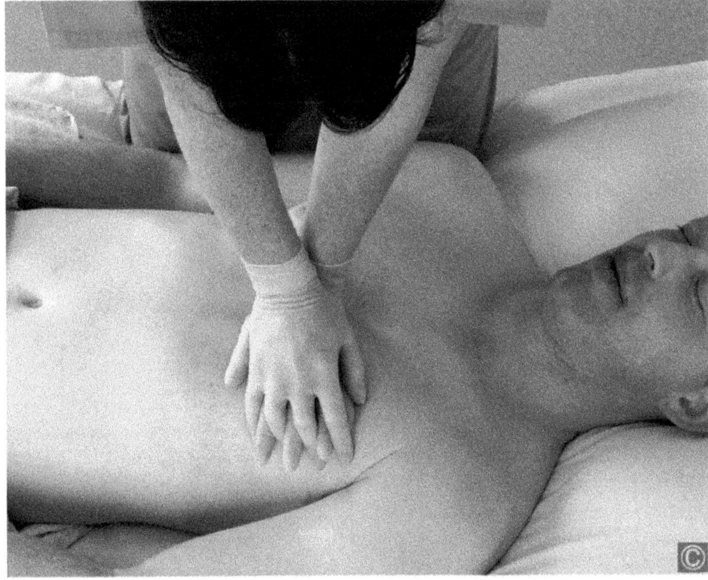

Figure 7.12 Chest compressions. *Source*: Resuscitation Council UK (2016) *Advanced Life Support*. Photograph reproduced with kind permission by Michael Scott and the Resuscitation Council (UK).

Two rescue breaths then immediately follow the 30 chest compressions.

Remember your safety. In a clinical setting, rescue breaths should never be attempted without using a pocket mask (Figure 7.13) at the very least. This is to protect the first responder from contamination from exhaled air and body fluids. These masks should be readily available in all areas and the time taken to complete the 30 compressions gives someone else time to get one for you. You should deliver the breath over one second and ensure you see the chest rise. If it does not, you may need to adjust the head position to ensure the airway is fully open.

Adjuncts to aid ventilation

A pocket mask (Figure 7.13) is used to safely deliver rescue breaths during a cardiac arrest. It can easily be used by one person as both hands are free to hold the mask firmly to the face, maintaining an airtight seal. It should be used in conjunction with an appropriately sized Guedel airway. Pocket masks are often situated in key areas and, as such, are often available before the crash trolley arrives. They have the benefit of ease-of-use.

Using only your expired air for rescue breaths is much better than nothing but this should be enriched with oxygen as soon as it is available. Set the oxygen flow to 15L

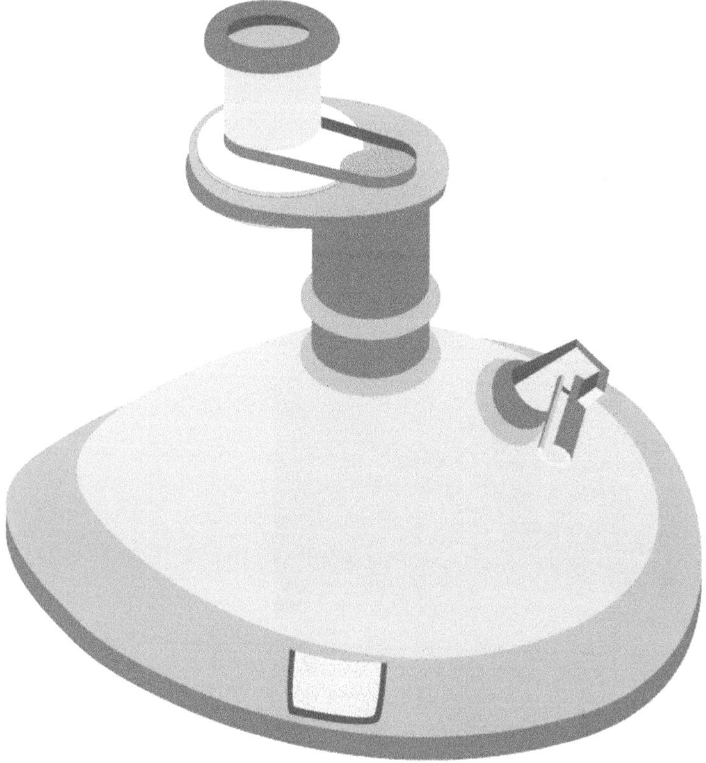

Figure 7.13 Pocket mask.

per minute and either attach to the port on the pocket mask or place the oxygen tubing under the mask.

A bag valve mask (see Figure 7.14) is a hand-held device designed to provide rescue breaths for a casualty who is not breathing or is breathing inadequately. The device consists of an air chamber, which can be attached to a reservoir bag, oxygen supply and a face mask. It can be used with air, but oxygen supply should be attached as soon as it is possible to do so at a flow rate of 15L/ minute. The device then has the benefit of giving high percentages of oxygen, without the rescuer using his/her own breaths. However, normally two people are required to operate this effectively: one to hold the mask to maintain an airtight seal, and the other to squeeze the bag in between the cardiac compressions. The ratio of 30 compressions to two rescue breaths is continued, until a request to stop is made by the resuscitation team.

Remember

The priority here is to ensure that effective rescue breaths are given.

If you find this easier to do with a pocket mask, then stick with that, rather than trying to use the bag valve mask device.

Don't forget to use an OPA if possible and add supplemental oxygen.

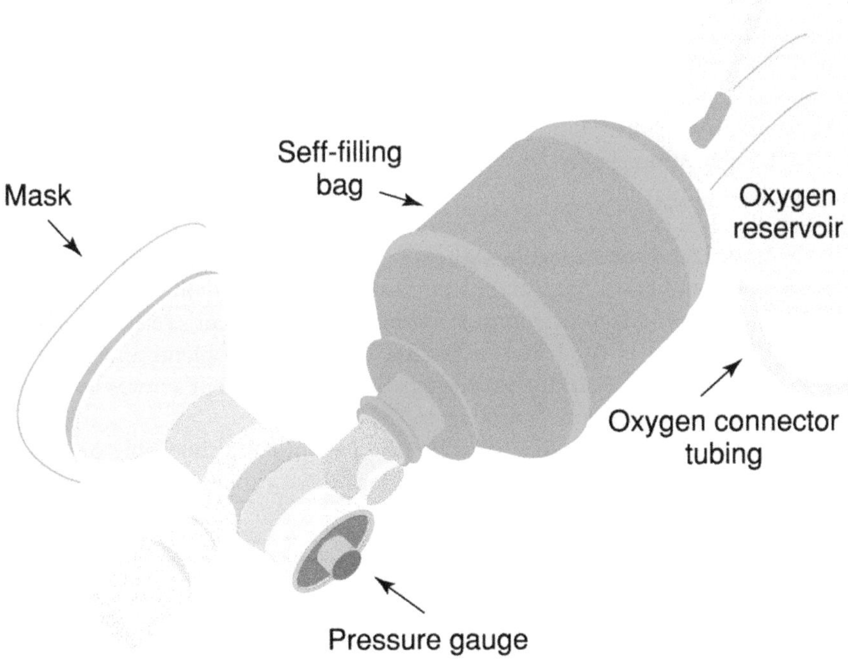

Figure 7.14 Bag valve mask.

Having followed these steps, you have ensured the first two links of the chain of survival have occurred: early recognition, calling for help and commencement of CPR. *You have already given the patient a significantly improved chance of survival.*

Defibrillation

The next link in the chain is early defibrillation, the purpose of which is to re-establish a rhythm capable of producing an adequate cardiac output.

Defibrillation consists of delivering a controlled amount of electrical energy to the heart, using a **defibrillator**. The aim is to depolarise the myocardium and terminate the arrhythmia. This allows normal sinus rhythm to be re-established by the sinoatrial node.

When a cardiac arrest occurs, the heart rhythm will be in one of two categories:

- Those that are amenable to reversal by defibrillation: shockable – **ventricular fibrillation (VF)** or pulseless **ventricular tachycardia (VT)**.
- Those that aren't amenable to reversal by defibrillation: non-shockable – **asystole** or **pulseless electrical activity** (PEA).

Asystole and PEA are the most common presentations in hospital arrests and are linked to hypoxaemia and hypotension, which have been unrecognised and/or inadequately treated.

As soon as the defibrillator arrives, the pads should be attached in order that the rhythm can be assessed. Chest compressions should continue whilst the pads are applied. As soon as the pads are applied, the rhythm must be assessed and chest compressions will need to stop whilst this occurs. It is at this point that we move from the in-hospital resuscitation algorithm to the ALS algorithm (Figure 7.15).

For rhythms that are amenable to defibrillation, the best chance of survival will be achieved if the first shock is delivered within three minutes of collapse.

It is essential to understand the probable sequence of events in advanced life support (ALS) as nurses are key members of the resuscitation team. This may involve drawing up, checking and recording drugs given, or communicating with the patient's relatives as the process continues. Knowledge of the patient's history, immediate problems and laboratory results are crucial to decision making during this stage. The patient's notes need to be available to the resuscitation team.

Rhythm assessment is vital to determine whether the patient has a shockable or non-shockable rhythm. If shockable, this needs to be performed without delay. Shockable rhythms include:

- VT (without a pulse) (see Figure 7.16)
- VF (see Figure 7.17).

Shocking a patient with asystole or PEA is of no value and could reduce the chances of survival by prolonging the pause in chest compressions.

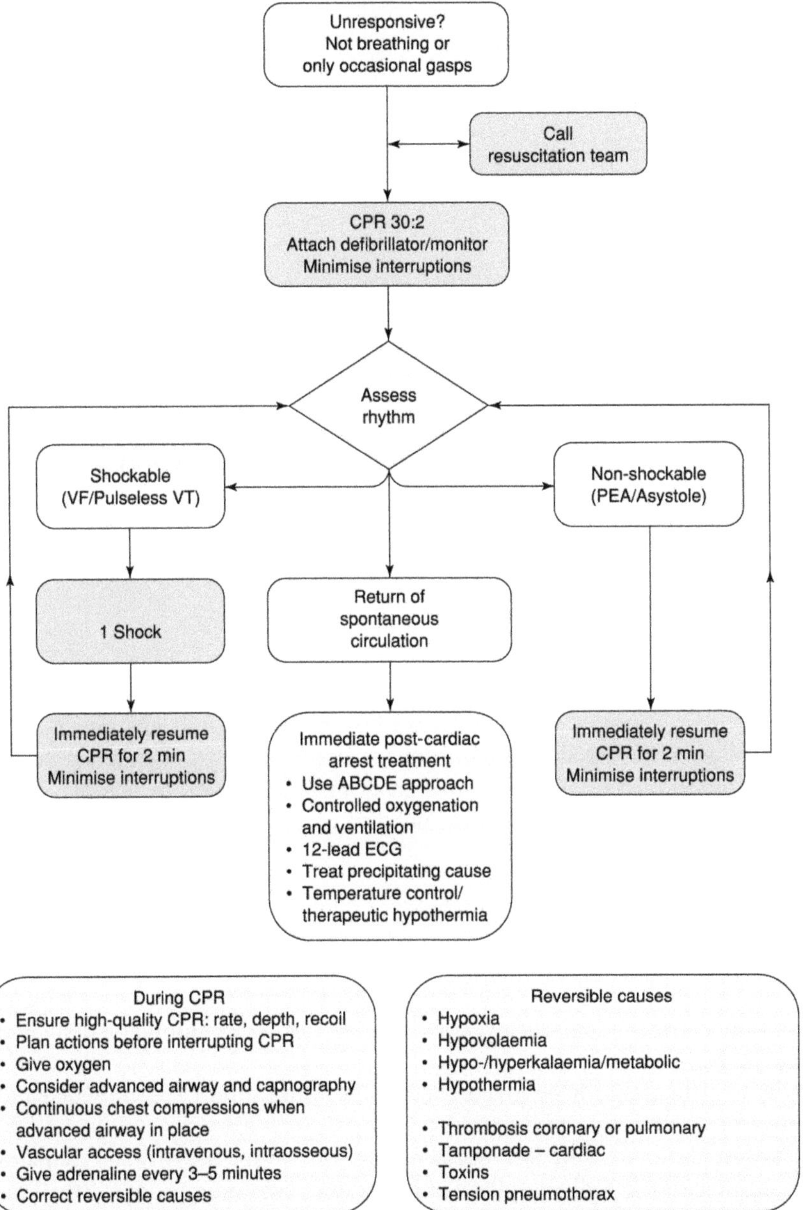

Figure 7.15 Adult advanced life support algorithm. *Source*: Resuscitation Council UK (2015) *2015 Resuscitation Guidelines*. Reproduced with the kind permission of Resuscitation Council (UK).

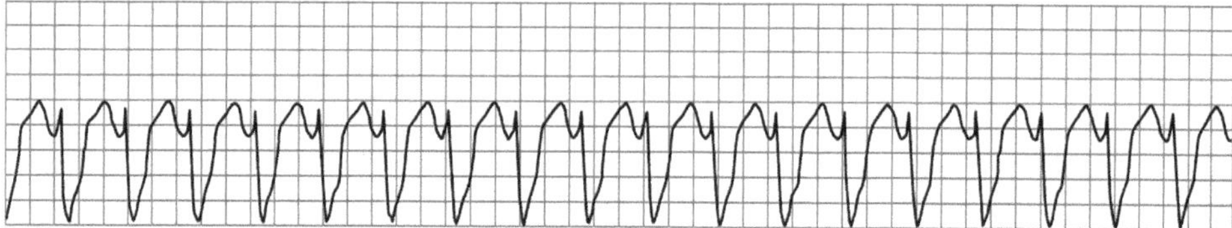

Figure 7.16 Ventricular tachycardia (VT) (without a pulse).

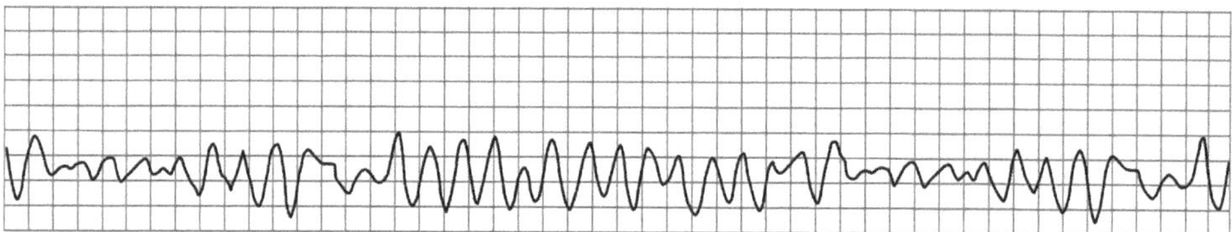

Figure 7.17 Ventricular fibrillation (VF).

Remember

Stopping compressions to assess the rhythm should be for the shortest time possible, no longer than five seconds. Prolonged interruptions to chest compressions reduce the chance of a defibrillation being successful in restoring a rhythm which can support an adequate cardiac output. Chest compressions need to be resumed immediately after delivering a shock.

Shockable rhythms

- Once the rhythm has been identified as shockable, the first shock should be delivered as soon as possible.
- As soon as the first shock has been given chest compressions must recommence and CPR resumed for another two minutes.
- After two minutes, the rhythm is reassessed and, providing the rhythm remains shockable, a further shock is given followed by another two minutes of CPR. This cycle continues unless the rhythm changes.
- Before the third shock is delivered, 1mg of **adrenaline** is given **intravenously** (IV).
- After this, further doses of adrenaline at the same dose are given before each alternate shock.

CPR commences immediately after defibrillation without checking for a pulse. This is because, even if a perfusing rhythm has been restored, it is unlikely that a pulse will be felt immediately, and the delay will be harmful if the defibrillation has not been successful.

CASE STUDY 7.1 STAFF NURSE AYAH: PART 1

SITUATION AND BACKGROUND

Ayah, a staff nurse returning from her break, passes a visitor waiting area and sees a lady collapsed on the floor.

ASSESSMENT

She checks the area is safe and approaches the lady, calling for assistance from John, a porter at the other end of the corridor, as she does so. The lady appears to be unconscious. Ayah kneels beside her and gently shakes her shoulders and asks her in a loud voice 'are you alright?' There is no response **(DRS).** There are no signs of any injury, so Ayah turns the lady onto her back and opens the airway using a head-tilt/chin-lift manoeuvre **(A)**.

Ayah checks for breathing by looking, listening and feeling, **(B)** while also checking for any signs of , such as movement or coughing. She tries to feel for a carotid pulse but is unable to find one. After 10 seconds, there is no breathing noted or any signs of life.

John, the porter, asks Ayah if he can help. Ayah asks him to phone 2222 and call the resuscitation team.

RESPONSE

Daniel, a second-year student nurse on Ayah's ward, has heard her call and she asks him to go to the nearest ward at the end of the corridor and to bring the emergency trolley and defibrillator. Ayah commences 30 chest compressions and continues until Daniel returns with the emergency trolley and pocket mask **(C)**.

Ayah confirms that Daniel knows how to do basic life support. Ayah asks Daniel to put on gloves and to prepare to continue with 30 more chest compressions, following two rescue breaths. She uses the pocket mask to administer two breaths. While Daniel takes over compressions, Ayah takes a size 3 Guedel airway from the trolley, places it in the patient's airway and adds oxygen at 15L/min to the pocket mask, ready for administration of the next two breaths.

Ayah is trained in defibrillation, so attaches the defibrillator pads onto the patient's chest and switches on the machine. The voice prompt requests that compressions are stopped while the rhythm is analysed.

The next voice prompt tells them the rhythm is shockable and to step away whilst the machine charges. Once the machine is charged, a further prompt reminds them to stand clear as the shock is delivered. They are then prompted to commence two minutes CPR.

Ayah, now wearing gloves, takes over the compressions and asks Daniel to continue the ventilation, using the pocket mask and oxygen at 15L/minute, and attach a pulse oximeter probe. At this point, the resuscitation team arrives.

Remember

The use of any defibrillator should **never** be attempted unless you have been trained in its use.

Types of defibrillator

There are different types of defibrillator available in clinical practice:

- Manual defibrillators: these require a high level of rhythm recognition skills on the part of the operator but have the advantage, when used in expert hands, of reducing the delay in compressions to less than five seconds.
- Automated external defibrillators (AEDs): these are sophisticated computerised devices that can reliably analyse the heart rhythm and, through voice and visual prompts, guide you through safe defibrillation. In areas where staff may not have skills in rhythm recognition and/or do not use defibrillators regularly, training in the use of AEDs is achieved much more easily and quickly than in the use of manual defibrillators, and offers a way of achieving the goal of delivering the first shock within three minutes of collapse.

Energy levels

The amount of electrical energy delivered is measured in joules (J). The number of joules delivered will depend on the type of defibrillator; most defibrillators in clinical practice are biphasic and the recommended energy level for the first shock is 150J. Subsequent shocks may be delivered at 150J or be escalated up to a maximum of 360J. This will depend on the device used and local protocols.

Defibrillators in clinical use are biphasic. This means the energy travels from one pad through the chest to the other pad and back again, therefore two 'jolts' of energy are delivered. This means the energy level set on the machine can be lower.

AEDs automatically select the energy level and guide you through the delivery of the shock.

- When using an AED, the voice prompts will tell you when to stand clear.
- When a manual defibrillator is being used, compressions must stop only during rhythm analysis and actual shock delivery. While the machine is charging, compressions must continue, although everyone else is asked to step away.
- If you are the person doing the compressions, you may feel quite vulnerable as everyone else has been asked to step away and you continue to have contact with the patient while the defibrillator is charging. It is important that you have confidence in the person operating the defibrillator and that you can see what that person is doing at all times.

Safety considerations

Defibrillation uses live electricity that is an obvious hazard and can pose risks. The use of AEDs does reduce some of these risks but there are still important safety considerations to take into account when using any defibrillator.

- Ensure the area around the patient and the patient's chest are dry – this could be an issue if, for example, the patient has collapsed in the bathroom.
- No one should touch the patient whilst the shock is being delivered – this includes indirect contact, such as touching the bed or IV stand.
- Always use self-adhesive pad electrodes.
- The combination of an oxygen-rich environment and a spark from a poorly applied pad could cause a fire. To minimise this risk, oxygen should be removed to at least one metre away from the patient during delivery of a shock. Once an endotracheal tube is *in situ*, the oxygen may be left connected, as this is a closed system.

It is recommended that each member of the team wears gloves. This not only protects them from body fluid contamination but may also provide limited protection from electrical current in the event of inadvertent contact during defibrillation.

Non-shockable rhythms

Non-shockable rhythms are asystole (see Figure 7.18) and pulseless electrical activity (PEA).

Early data from the National Cardiac Arrest Audit (NCAA) indicate that, of those people who suffer a cardiac arrest in hospital, approximately 20% of these will present with a shockable rhythm, of whom 44% survive, whereas, of those who present with a non-shockable rhythm, only 7% survive to discharge (Nolan et al. 2014).

Asystole is when there is no electrical activity detected on the monitor. Always ensure the pads/electrodes are securely attached and that the correct monitoring mode and gain are selected.

Pulseless electrical activity occurs when some organised electrical activity within the myocardium is detected on the monitor (this could even look like a normal ECG trace) but does not result in a cardiac output sufficient to produce a pulse. Unless a treatable cause can be found quickly, survival from asystole or PEA is unlikely. Because these rhythms are not amenable to defibrillation, the focus is on high-quality CPR and early identification of a possible cause.

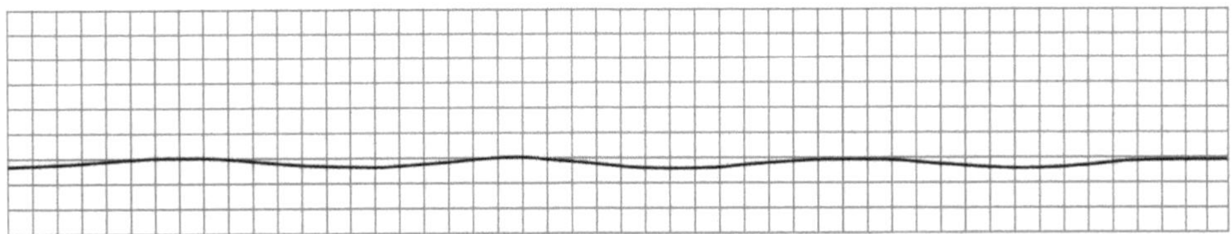

Figure 7.18 Asystole.

The sequence of events is therefore:

- Commencement of CPR at a ratio of 30:2.
- Administration of 1mg of adrenaline IV as soon as access is established.
- Recheck the rhythm every two minutes; if it becomes shockable (VF or VT), then move to the shockable side of the algorithm.
- If the rhythm remains non-shockable, continue with CPR and repeat the adrenaline dose on alternate cycles of CPR (every 3–5 minutes).

The purpose of giving adrenaline repeatedly during a cardiac arrest is that it increases coronary and cerebral blood flow, and may therefore improve the effectiveness of CPR.

During CPR

In both shockable and non-shockable sides of the algorithm, there is much to be done to improve the patient's chances of survival.

Remember

Ventilation must be supplemented with high-flow oxygen as soon as possible and monitored, using a pulse oximeter, aiming for saturations of 94–98%. Avoid over-inflation as this may result in gastric regurgitation.

- The most important task is maintenance of high-quality CPR.
- The gold standard for protecting the airway is tracheal intubation but this can only be performed by someone expert in the technique. Until this point, ensure ventilation is achieved by whichever means you are competent to perform.
- Once tracheal intubation is achieved, ventilations can be administered at a rate of 10 per minute without stopping compressions.
- Once tracheal intubation has been undertaken, waveform capnography should be used.
- Intravenous access should be obtained as soon as possible.
- If it is not possible to achieve intravenous access, **intraosseous** access may be considered, using either the tibia or the humerus. Either drugs or fluids can be administered *via* this route.

Benefits of waveform capnography during CPR include:

Ensuring correct placement of the endotracheal tube.

Monitoring the rate of ventilation and avoidance of hyperinflation.

Monitoring the quality of compression; end-tidal CO_2 values increase with optimal compression depth and ventilation rate.

Identifying a return of spontaneous circulation (ROSC) – an increased end-tidal CO_2 value can indicate ROSC and avoid unnecessary adrenaline administration.

Prognostication – low end-tidal CO_2 values during CPR have been associated with lower ROSC rates and increased mortality, and high values have been associated with better ROSC and survival (Grmec et al. 2007; Kolar et al. 2008; Sheak et al. 2015). However, this should not be used on its own as an indicator to stop CPR, although it might contribute to decision making (RCUK 2015)

Whereas you may not be able to perform some of the tasks during an arrest, you still have an important part to play once the resuscitation team arrives:

- Helping to keep effective CPR going, which is vital.
- Assisting with tracheal intubation.
- Preparing drugs, such as adrenaline.
- The team leader may designate someone to document events and the drugs that were given.
- There may be relatives or other patients, who need support.

Reversible causes

In all cases of cardiac arrest, it is important to consider the factors that could be the primary cause or be aggravating factors and which may be reversible.

To make these easier to remember, it is helpful to think of them as the four Hs and the four Ts.

Four Hs

1. **Hypoxia**: this is minimised by:
    - Ventilating during the arrest with 100% oxygen. Oxygen saturation should be monitored, aiming for an SpO_2 reading of 94%–98%.
    - Ensuring adequate chest movement with each breath.
    - Ensuring patency and correct placement of any artificial airway.
2. **Hypovolaemia**: this may be a primary cause of PEA, often due to severe bleeding:
    - Bleeding may be obvious, as in severe trauma, or hidden, as in the case of a gastrointestinal bleed.
    - Hypovolaemia may also be caused by severe dehydration, for example, as a result of prolonged or excessive diarrhoea and vomiting.
    - Circulating volume should be restored rapidly with delivery of blood and/or fluids and, if necessary, surgery to stop the haemorrhage.
3. **Hyperkalaemia** may be present as a result of renal insufficiency and can be treated immediately with an infusion of dextrose and insulin, but it may require renal replacement therapy in the longer term.

    Other metabolic abnormalities that should also be considered are:
    - **Hypokalaemia**: this may happen following aggressive diuretic therapy and is treated by administering a potassium chloride infusion.
    - Hypoglycaemia, treated with a bolus of 50% dextrose.
    - Hypocalcaemia, treated with calcium chloride.

    These disturbances may be detected by biochemical tests or from the patient's history, for example, renal impairment.

    Either hyper- or hypoglycaemia post-arrest is not uncommon and either is associated with poor outcome. The aim is to keep the blood sugar between 4 and 6mmol/L.
4. **Hypothermia**: this should be suspected in any cases of near-drowning or exposure. Attempts should be made to rewarm the patient using warmed IV fluids and warming blankets.

Four Ts

1. **Tension pneumothorax**: this could be the primary cause of PEA and is initially relieved by needle decompression and then by insertion of a chest drain.
2. **Cardiac tamponade**: this is a build-up of fluid in the pericardial sac, restricting myocardial contraction and resulting in PEA. It can be difficult to diagnose as the clinical signs of low blood pressure and distended neck veins are difficult to observe during an arrest, but penetrating chest injury or arrest immediately post-cardiac surgery should raise suspicions.
3. **Toxic**: this may be difficult to detect unless there is history of intentional or accidental overdose or ingestion of toxic substances.
4. **Thromboembolic**: massive **pulmonary embolism** (PE) is the commonest cause of mechanical circulatory obstruction. If a PE is thought to be the cause, thrombolytic drug therapy should be considered.

Post-resuscitation care

Following a successful resuscitation, as determined by a return of spontaneous circulation (ROSC), the patient will need to be transferred to an intensive care unit or high-dependency facility for close monitoring and further management. This process usually takes some time and, while awaiting transfer, the patient should be monitored and managed, using the ABCDE approach. The aim of this is to optimise oxygenation and tissue perfusion while looking for, identifying and treating any complications, such as hypoglycaemia or convulsions. During this time, a member of the medical team will usually remain with the patient.

Patients admitted to Intensive Care Units (ICUs) following cardiac arrest, who are comatose but with a ROSC, have a survival-to-discharge rate of 40–50%, the majority of whom will have a good neurological outcome (Moulaert et al. 2009; Cronberg et al. 2015; Lilja et al. 2015; Sulzgruber et al. 2015). The key interventions in post-resuscitation care, that will guide immediate and ongoing management, are detailed in Figure 7.19.

Decisions to stop resuscitation

Remember

It is unfortunately more likely that the person will die rather than survive as a result of a cardiac arrest, however prompt and well-co-ordinated the response.

Despite the improvement in survival rates, the majority of people who suffer an in-hospital cardiac arrest, sadly, do not survive, and, therefore, there will come a point during the resuscitation process where a decision to stop needs to be made. This is a difficult situation for all concerned. The most senior doctor present has the legal responsibility to take the decision to stop, but, in reality, when this occurs, there is a need to take into account the views of the whole team and, in some cases, the family. As time elapses, the chances of a

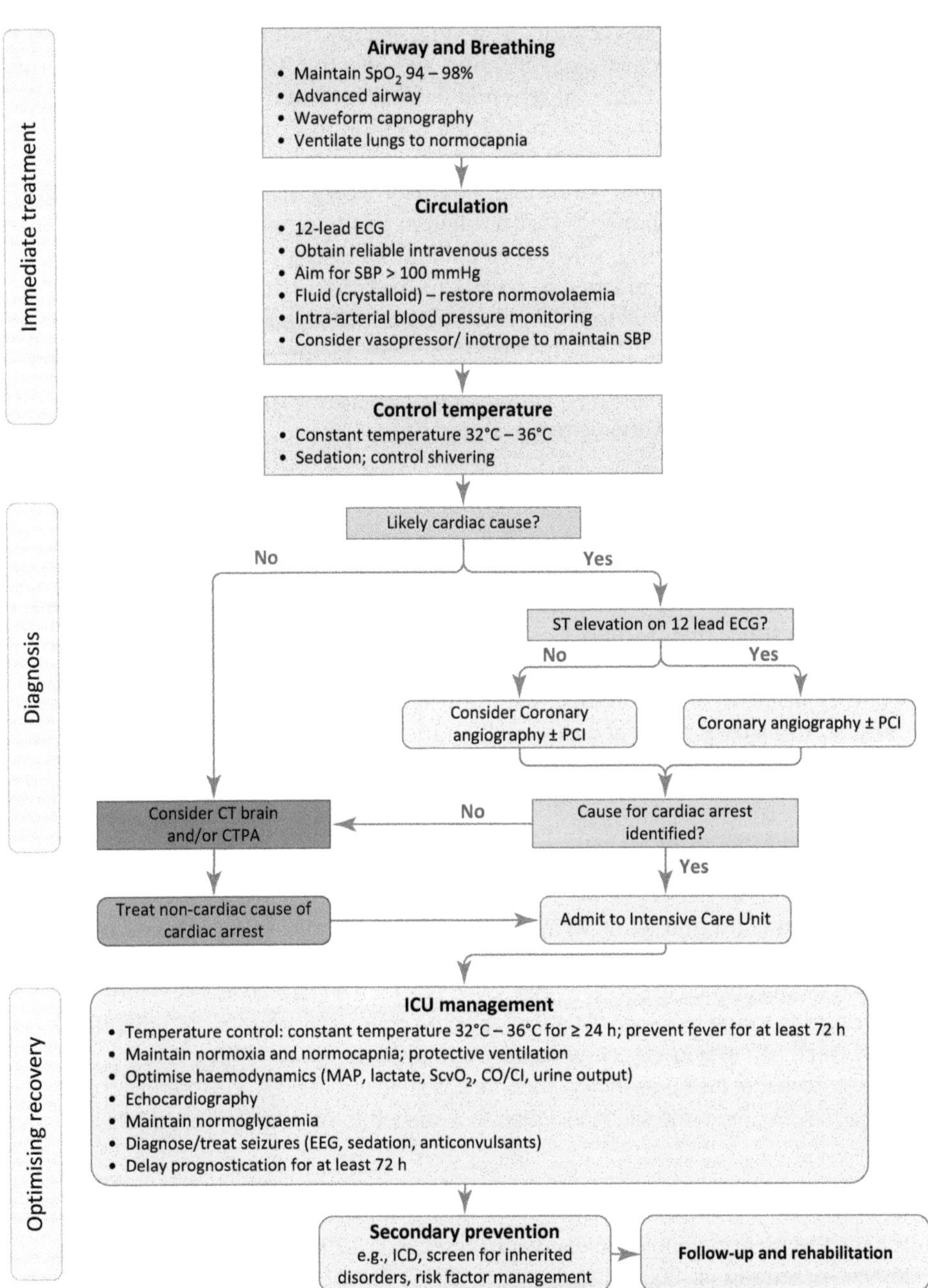

Figure 7.19 Post resuscitation care. *Source*: Resuscitation Council UK (2015) *2015 Resuscitation Guidelines*. Reproduced with the kind permission of Resuscitation Council (UK).

successful outcome decrease, although recovery can occur even after prolonged resuscitation attempts, particularly in cases of near-drowning, electrocution, hypothermia or some drug overdoses. Assuming adequate oxygenation and effective CPR and the absence of an untreated reversible cause, failure of repeated defibrillation and drug treatment usually signals that the point has been reached to take the decision to stop.

Following a period of intense activity focused on saving the patient's life, this outcome is often emotional and sometimes confusing. You may worry that, as the first responder, it was something you did or didn't do that resulted in this outcome. If you adhere to the principles of the chain of survival, this is very unlikely to be the case.

It is now considered good practice to have a team debrief after the event. This does not need to be very long but will focus on constructive feedback and learning rather than the apportioning of any blame.

Presence of relatives at resuscitation attempts

It is becoming increasingly common for relatives to be present during the resuscitation. It has been recognised for the past two decades that many relatives would choose to remain during resuscitation, if given the option (Hansen and Strawser 1992; Adams et al. 1994; McLaughlan et al. 1996). In 1996, the Resuscitation Council UK published the findings of a working party which favoured relatives' attendance, provided that that was their wish and that they received support and information (Resuscitation Council UK 1996). Work by Grice et al. (2003) indicated that 56% of medical staff and 66% of nurses working in an adult intensive care unit felt that relatives should be given the option to stay. If relatives requested to stay, 70% of medical staff and 82% of nurses said they would allow this.

Benefits to relatives of being present during a resuscitation attempt

- It helps with coming to terms with the death and enables a healthier bereavement process.
- They have the chance to speak to their loved one for the last time.
- It is possible to see that everything that could be done was done.
- They can touch their loved one while the body is still warm.
- They believe that their presence is important, both to themselves and their loved one.
- To be removed from the situation, when they wished to be present, would be highly distressing.

Authors have also identified possible disadvantages (Crisci 1994; Schilling 1994; Compton et al. 2009; Guzzetta et al. 2007; Doolin et al. 2011; Twibell et al. 2018). Some of the identified benefits and disadvantages of relatives being present at a resuscitation attempt are summarised in the boxes below.

Interestingly, the rationale for decision making for nurses and medical staff was found, by Twibell et al. (2018), to have a slightly different focus. Whereas both disciplines had much in common, the family's potential to interrupt life-saving efforts and possibly compromise patient care, weighed more heavily with the medical staff than with the nurses.

The nurses focused on the potential for the family to be traumatised *versus* the potential of family benefit.

Disadvantages of relatives being present during a resuscitation attempt

- Watching the resuscitation attempt could be distressing, particularly in the absence of support.
- Relatives may hinder the resuscitation attempt or may be offended by remarks made by the team.
- They may be disturbed by the memory of the events, although evidence suggests that people are disturbed less by facts than by what they imagine.

In any other end-of-life scenario, most health care practitioners would accept that the presence of family and loved ones is both desirable and entirely normal. Given that the majority of resuscitation attempts will result in the person's death, we must ask ourselves, why should this be different?

Each situation, though, must be judged individually, taking into account the circumstances, the wishes of the relatives and any known wishes of the patient. Perceptions vary in different cultural settings, and both positive and negative effects need to be considered (Sak-Dankosky et al. 2014).

The UK and European Resuscitation Guidelines (RCUK 2016; Lippert et al. 2010) advocate allowing families to remain during resuscitation attempts, should they wish to. In line with the Nursing and Midwifery Council Code (2018), nurses should support the decision of relatives, whatever that may be.

The person who stays and supports relatives should be appropriately qualified. You may be allocated this task, particularly if you know the family already. There is no script to follow but there are a few principles that could help you to manage this emotional situation:

- Acknowledge how difficult this is for them.
- Make it clear that the choice to stay or go is entirely theirs and that either choice is fine.
- Let them know that they will be looked after, whatever their choice. If the family decides to leave, then go with them, if possible.
- Give clear explanations about what has happened, for example, 'John's heart has stopped beating and we are doing everything we can to re-start it' and also what to expect, 'we are giving John oxygen through a special mask and pressing down on his chest to pump the oxygen around the body while his heart is not beating.'
- Offer them the chance to touch the patient when this is appropriate and be clear about when and why it is not appropriate, for example, during defibrillation.
- Answer any questions honestly. Some questions may be asked which you can't answer such as 'Is he going to live?' 'Will he be brain damaged?' It is OK to say you can't answer those questions at present as the situation is too uncertain but offer reassurance that they will be kept informed at all stages.
- Don't be afraid of silences; in these situations, people often need time to take in what is happening and may not wish to, or need to, talk.

'Do Not Attempt Cardiopulmonary Resuscitation' (DNACPR) orders

Successful resuscitation has led to many people experiencing extended and useful lives, precious to them and their loved ones. Unfortunately, these success stories remain in the minority, and it must be recognised that resuscitation carries the risk of causing morbidity and suffering by prolonging the process of dying.

It is essential to differentiate between the natural process of death and a reversible cardiac arrest.

It is not always appropriate to attempt resuscitation, for example:

- Where the chances of success are very slight.
- If a successful outcome would result in a reduced quality of life. This is often the most common reason given and the most difficult area to make decisions about.
- If there is a known wish expressed by the patient not to be resuscitated. This may be written or verbal but must be valid – made by a patient competent to make the decision and in full possession of the facts. It is important to bear in mind that situations change, which could affect the validity of the previous decision.

In-depth guidance and advice on this topic has been produced by the British Medical Association, Resuscitation Council (UK) and the Royal College of Nursing (2016). This is a complex area, and, for detailed information, this document is recommended reading. There are, however, some key points:

- Decisions related to DNACPR should be made carefully and on an individual basis, in consultation with the patient, wherever possible, and including the family, unless the patient does not wish this to be the case. In the case of a patient who lacks capacity, the discussion should involve the family to explore the patient's likely feelings, wishes and beliefs.
- Whereas the final decision rests with the senior doctor in charge of the case, there should be consultation with the multi-professional team involved.
- Advance care planning, including making decisions about CPR, is part of high-quality clinical care for persons who may be at risk of cardiac arrest, such as people with chronic heart or lung disease.
- It is not necessary to have these discussions with patients for whom there is no reason to believe that they are at risk of a cardiac arrest.
- Once made, decisions should be accurately documented, communicated and reviewed.
- Any patient, with the capacity to do so, who refuses CPR or those who lack capacity but have made a valid advance decision refusing CPR, should have their wishes respected.
- A DNACPR order should not override clinical judgement. For example, in the unlikely event of a patient with a DNACPR order developing a sudden reversible cause of cardiac arrest, unrelated to the underlying condition, such as choking or anaphylaxis, the decision may be taken to attempt CPR.
- Where there is no explicit advance decision or in circumstances where this is unclear or unknown, then CPR should always be attempted.
- DNACPR orders only refer to CPR and not to other forms of treatment.

This final point is important. The presence of a DNACPR does not preclude other treatments, that may include oxygen therapy, ventilation, pain relief, antibiotics and nutritional support, among others. High-quality, safe and effective nursing care remains paramount.

CASE STUDY 7.2 STAFF NURSE AYAH: PART 2

Ayah, with the assistance of John and Daniel, has ensured the first three links of the chain of survival have been implemented before the medical emergency team (MET) arrived:

- She assessed the situation, recognised a cardiac arrest had occurred and ensured the MET was called.
- CPR was started quickly, and the emergency equipment was brought to the scene as soon as possible. This enabled rescue breaths to be delivered *via* a pocket mask, with a Guedel airway *in situ*, supplemented with high-flow oxygen.
- Pads were applied and the rhythm analysed. By the time the MET arrived, one shock had been delivered and two minutes of further CPR were underway.

Both Ayah and Daniel put on gloves as soon as it was practical to do so, in order to protect themselves from any bodily fluids.

As the MET arrives, a second lady comes into the room, carrying two cups of coffee, and becomes very distressed as the lady on the floor is, apparently, her mother.

A member of the MET advises Ayah and Daniel to continue with CPR and helps the daughter, whose name is Laura, to a chair and asks her if she wishes to leave the room or stay. The daughter is reassured that her presence will not be a problem if she wishes to stay.

Two minutes of CPR are complete and the voice prompt on the defibrillator advises stopping compressions in order to analyse the rhythm.

The next voice prompt tells them the rhythm is shockable and to step away whilst the machine charges. Once charged, a further prompt reminds them to stand clear as the shock is delivered. They are then prompted to commence two minutes CPR.

- Daniel continues with chest compressions and the anaesthetist takes over the management of the airway and prepares to intubate the patient.

The team leader asks Ayah to relate the events so far, then requests that she remain with Laura and explain what has happened and what is going on now. Ayah finds out that Laura and her mother Mary were visiting her (Laura's) father, who is an in-patient following a knee replacement. Mary has had 'heart problems' for years.

Two minutes of CPR are completed and the anaesthetist has secured the airway with an endotracheal tube. A peripheral IV cannula has been inserted and a dose of adrenaline 1mg IV is given and flushed with 20mL saline. The team leader has switched the defibrillator to manual mode and requests Daniel to stop compressions to permit analysis of the rhythm. A second member of the team is designated to operate the defibrillator. The rhythm is confirmed as VT and the operator requests Daniel to recommence compressions as the machine charges. Everyone else is asked to step away. The anaesthetist leaves the oxygen connected to the re-inflatable bag and the ET tube as a closed circuit. As soon as the defibrillator is charged, Daniel is asked to step away and the operator discharges the shock. Once the shock is delivered a third member of the team takes over compressions for another two minutes of CPR.

Ayah explains to Laura that she had found her mother collapsed on the floor and that her heart had stopped. She says she realises that this is a huge shock and a lot to take in but that all efforts were now being made to restart Mary's heart. She offered Laura the option to stay or to wait in another area, reassuring her that she (Ayah) would stay with her throughout.

After another two minutes of CPR, compressions were stopped, and the rhythm was analysed again. Atrial fibrillation now showed on the monitor. This is a rhythm that could be consistent with an output. The anaesthetist confirmed the presence of a weak carotid pulse.

A full ABCDE assessment was commenced, and the ICU was contacted to arrange a bed for post-resuscitation care. Laura was able to come and sit next to her mother and hold her hand.

At the point of transfer to ICU:

Airway and breathing

Mary remained intubated but was making some respiratory effort. Oxygen saturations 97%.

Circulation

Her heart rate was 112 in AF with a blood pressure of 110/85, she was cool peripherally, with a capillary refill time of > 3 second.

Disability

Her blood glucose level was 5.3 mmol/L and she responded to painful stimuli.

Exposure

No obvious wounds or abnormalities were noted, although she had been incontinent of urine.

Ayah accompanied Laura to ICU and assisted in the handover to ICU staff.

Following the transfer to ICU, Ayah and Daniel were commended for their efforts during the team brief for acting so promptly. It was likely that Mary had suffered a myocardial infarction. She had a shockable rhythm that reverted, after three shocks, to atrial fibrillation which, due to Mary's cardiac history, could be her normal heart rhythm.

Caring for the bereaved

In the case study, Mary is transferred to intensive care, following a successful resuscitation. Sadly, however, as mentioned at the beginning of this chapter, most people who experience a cardiopulmonary arrest will die (Resuscitation Council UK 2015). Whereas the focus of care is very different following the death of the person concerned, it is imperative that a high level of sensitive and practical support continues to be provided to the suddenly bereaved (Kent and McDowell 2004), some of whom may have witnessed the resuscitation attempt. This is of significance, both in terms of your role in helping to facilitate a positive grieving process and also when doing so after having only just met the bereaved and then under very traumatic circumstances.

Whereas some may wish to be involved in the last offices of the deceased, this needs to be dealt with on an individual basis. The bereaved may request to have a spiritual leader contacted or would be comforted to receive one of the hospital chaplaincy members as key support at this time.

Breaking bad news

When the resuscitation has been unsuccessful, news of the patient's death needs to be delivered (preferably face-to-face, although this may not always be possible) and it is generally done by a senior member of staff, preferably in a quiet and private area. You may, however, be on hand to support this process. This news can be devastating for the bereaved, although a sudden and unexpected death may carry different meanings to different families, and the responses to such news can be very diverse. This makes it very stressful for the clinicians involved, who may never have met the relative before (Walker 2010).

How the bad news is broken can have a major impact on the bereaved (Edwards and Shaw 1998; Kent and McDowell 2004; Walker 2010), and, if not handled well, can become a traumatic memory seared into their consciousness. The language used needs to be simple, clear and unambiguous, avoiding all euphemisms, and delivered at a gentle pace, outlining exactly what was done during the resuscitation. It needs to be made clear that all attempts to prevent the person's death were made and that the deceased was not left to die alone (DH 2005). Explaining how the patient may now look and small details, such as why the deceased's clothes were removed or cut, can go a long way to avoiding unnecessary distress on the part of the bereaved. Such difficult discussions require significant empathy and competence in communication skills (Wilson and White 2011).

Giving the bereaved the opportunity to view and be with the deceased in a quiet and private space is an important part of the aftercare, especially if the relatives or next-of-kin were not present when the patient died. The evidence shows that this can minimise any later difficulties in the grieving process experienced by the bereaved (Raphael 1984; Wright 1996).

Spiritual and cultural care

The aftercare you provide needs to be sensitive and supportive, with regard to any particular cultural or religious rituals that are important to the bereaved family you are caring for.

Information provision

There are a number of important practical responsibilities that need to be undertaken following the death of a patient, and these also need to be dealt with sensitively and in a timely manner. For example, all necessary paperwork, e.g., the registration of death and the death certificate, should ideally be dealt with quickly and efficiently, and given to the bereaved with appropriate explanations. They should also be informed of the process that will be followed, regarding a post-mortem, if appropriate, and when and how they might obtain the results and from whom (DH 2005). If the deceased is not known to the hospital, the death may be referred to the coroner, then the issuing of documentation, such as the death certificate, may be delayed, and this can be very stressful for the bereaved. The bereaved may also require information regarding funerals or cremation and also helpful external contacts, who may be able to give information regarding support, both in the immediate term and in the longer term (Murray Parkes 1998; Pattison 2008). These may be specific local services that are available in the trust (DH 2005; Walker 2010) or through other national organisations, some of which are listed in the text box. Providing informative leaflets to the bereaved (ideally translated into other languages) about support services may be helpful (Walker 2010).

National bereavement support

CRUSE BEREAVEMENT CARE

A nationwide service that provides bereavement counselling advice, information and social contact.

Website: www.https://www.cruse.org.uk/
Helpline: 0808 808 1677

THE COMPASSIONATE FRIENDS

An organisation that offers grief support to parents and bereaved families after the death of a son or daughter.

Website: www.tcf.org.uk
Helpline: 0345 120 3785 email: helpline@tcf.org.uk

Conclusion

For many patients who experience a cardiac arrest, the efforts made do not result in survival and, of those who do survive, some will suffer long-term effects. However, at the outset it is often impossible to judge who will survive and make a full recovery. Following the guidance set out in this chapter will enable you to provide the best possible chances of a happy outcome. Adherence to the Resuscitation Council UK (2015) algorithms ensures that all those attending the cardiac arrest will be following the same procedures, enabling a coordinated and uniform response.

In addition to the care of the patient, the support of relatives, regardless of the outcome, has been discussed. A cardiac arrest may present you not only with many challenges but also the opportunity to provide high-quality care to patients and families at a

very difficult time. Because of the challenges and difficulties involved in this situation, it is important that, following the event, whatever the outcome, you are involved in some sort of debrief. This does not need to be very time consuming, but it is important to help you to put things into perspective. If you have followed the guidance given here, it is very unlikely that anything you did or didn't do will have negatively affected the outcome. However, if you are left with feelings of worry and uncertainty, you must seek guidance from a practice assessor or supervisor, preceptor or more senior colleague.

Glossary 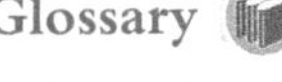

Adrenaline Naturally occurring hormone, also known as epinephrine, given during cardiac arrest to increase coronary and cerebral perfusion.

Agonal breathing Deep sighing, irregular gasping breathing, also known as Cheyne–Stokes breathing, which occurs at the end of life.

Algorithm Step-by-step procedure for problem-solving, often expressed as a diagram or flow chart.

Asystole Complete absence of electrical and mechanical activity in the heart.

Bag valve mask A device used to provide artificial ventilation, which consists of a manual compressible chamber with an oxygen reservoir at one end and a one-way valve and mask at the other.

Basic life support See **Cardiopulmonary resuscitation**.

Cardiopulmonary arrest The sudden cessation of breathing and effective cardiac output.

Cardiopulmonary resuscitation (CPR) Emergency procedures to be undertaken in the event of cardiopulmonary arrest, aimed at preventing irreversible brain damage caused by lack of oxygen. CPR consists of rescue breathing and cardiac compressions. CPR is also known as basic life support (BLS).

Defibrillation The reversal of fibrillation (inefficient and non-rhythmic contraction) by the delivery of a controlled electric shock.

Embolism Circulating foreign object such as air, fat or a blood clot, which can lodge in and block a vessel.

Hyperkalaemia High level of potassium in the blood.

Hypokalaemia Low level of potassium in the blood.

Hypothermia Abnormally low temperature.

Hypovolaemia Low circulating blood volume.

Hypoxia Low levels of cellular oxygen.

Intraosseous The inside of a bone.

Intravenous The inside of a vein.

Pulmonary embolism The blockage of a pulmonary artery by a blood clot, fat or air.

Pulseless electrical activity (PEA) Organised electrical cardiac activity in the absence of a pulse.

Tamponade Compression of the heart by the accumulation of fluid in the pericardial space.

Tension pneumothorax Presence of air in the pleural space that occurs when air escapes into the pleural cavity from a bronchus but cannot regain entry into the bronchus. As a result, continuously increasing air pressure in the pleural cavity causes progressive collapse of the lung tissue.

Ventricular fibrillation Disorganised electrical activity in the ventricular myocardium, resulting in an absence of effective cardiac output.

Ventricular tachycardia Cardiac arrhythmia originating from within the ventricles, characterised by rapid ventricular complexes at a rate greater than 100/min. It may or may not be associated with a pulse.

Waveform capnography Continuous monitoring of end-tidal CO_2 in expired air *via* a device attached to an endotracheal tube.

TEST YOURSELF 

1 On discovery of a collapsed unresponsive casualty who is not breathing, the sequence of events you should follow is:
   a. assess for danger, assess for response, shout for help, open the airway, assess breathing, commence compressions.
   b. shout for help, open the airway, assess for response, assess breathing, assess for danger, commence compressions.
   c. check for response, commence compressions, shout for help, assess for danger, open the airway, assess breathing.
   d. assess for danger, open the airway, assess for response, assess breathing, commence compressions, shout for help.

2 In *partial* airway obstruction:
   a. there will be no sound.
   b. there will be paradoxical chest movement.
   c. the casualty may be talking, breathing may be noisy.
   d. there will be tracheal tug with intercostal and subcostal recession.

3 The interventions that contribute to a successful outcome following a cardiac arrest are known as:
   a. the weakest link.
   b. the chain reaction.
   c. the chain of survival.
   d. the chain of resuscitation.

4 Which of the following rhythms would you shock in a cardiac arrest situation?
   a. pulseless electrical activity (PEA).
   b. pulseless ventricular tachycardia.
   c. atrial fibrillation.
   d. asystole.

5 During a cardiac arrest, adrenaline is given to:
   a. restart the heart.
   b. slow the heart rate.
   c. prevent further arrythmias.
   d. increase cerebral and coronary perfusion.

6 When using a defibrillator, you should:
   a. be trained in its use.
   b. ensure oxygen is removed at least one metre away from the patient.
   c. ensure everyone is clear of the immediate area before delivering a shock.
   d. all of the above.

7 During a cardiac arrest, chest compressions:
   a. should continue without any interruptions at all times.
   b. should only stop during defibrillation.
   c. should be continuous once the trachea is intubated.
   d. should be delivered at a rate of 150 per minute.

8 A *reversible* cause of a cardiac arrest is:
   a. hypovolaemia.
   b. deep vein thrombosis.
   c. angina.
   d. pyrexia.

9 A reason to abandon a resuscitation attempt could be:
   a. the cardiac arrest team is called to another arrest.
   b. discovery of cardiac tamponade.
   c. asystole for more than 20 minutes without a reversible cause.
   d. the casualty is over 80 years of age.

10 A 'Do not attempt cardiopulmonary resuscitation' (DNACPR) order may be considered / put in place when:
   a. the patient has a terminal illness.
   b. there is a documented request from a competent patient not to resuscitate.
   c. the quality of life following a successful outcome is predicted to be very poor.
   d. all of the above.

Answers

1 a
2 c
3 c
4 b
5 d
6 d
7 c
8 a
9 c
10 d

References

Adams S, Whitlock M, Bloomfield P, Baskett PJF. (1994). Should relatives watch resuscitation? *BMJ*, 308, 1687–1689.

Aiken LH, et al. (2014). Nurse staffing and education and hospital mortality in nine European countries: a retrospective observational study. *Lancet*, 383, 1824–1830.

Benoit JL, Gerecht RB, Steuerwald MT, McMullan JT. (2015). Endotracheal intubation versus supraglottic airway placement in out-of-hospital cardiac arrest: a meta-analysis. *Resuscitation*, 93, 20–26.

Chan PS, McNally B, Tang F, Kellermann A, Group CS. (2014). Recent trends in survival from out-of-hospital cardiac arrest in the United States. *Circulation*, 2, 130, 1876–1882.

Compton S, et al. (2009). Post-traumatic stress disorder symptomology associated with witnessing unsuccessful out-of-hospital cardiopulmonary resuscitation. *Academic Emergency Medicine*, 16(3), 226–229.

Crisci C. (1994). Local factors may influence decision (Letters). *BMJ*, 309, 406.

Cronberg T, et al. (2015). Neurologic function and health-related quality of life in patients following targeted temperature management at 33 degrees C vs 36 degrees C after out-of-hospital cardiac arrest: a randomized clinical trial. *JAMA Neurology*, 72, 634–641.

DH (Department of Health). (2005). *When a Patient Dies. Advice on Developing Bereavement Services in the NHS*. London: DH.

Doolin CT, et al. (2011). Family presence during cardiopulmonary resuscitation: using evidence-based knowledge to guide the advanced practice nurse in developing formal policy and practice guidelines. *Journal of the American Academy of Nurse Practitioners*, 23(1), 8–14.

Edwards L, Shaw D. (1998). Care of the suddenly bereaved in cardiac care units: a review of the literature. *Intensive and Critical Care Nursing*, 14, 144–152.

Findlay G, Shotton H, Kelly K, Mason M. (2012). *Time to Intervene? A Review of Patients who Underwent Cardiopulmonary Resuscitation as a Result of an in-Hospital Cardiorespiratory Arrest*. A Report by the National Confidential Enquiry into Patient Outcome and Death. Accessed from: http://www.ncepod.org.uk/2012report1/downloads/CAP_fullreport.pdf.

Girotra S, et al. (2012). Trends in survival after in-hospital cardiac arrest. *New England Journal of Medicine*, 367, 1912–1920.

Grice AS, Picton P, Deakin CDS. (2003). Study examining attitudes of staff, patients and relatives to witnessed resuscitation in adult intensive care units. *British Journal of Anaesthesia*, 91(6), 820–824.

Grmec S, Krizmaric M, Mally S, Kozelj A, Spindler M, Lesnik B. (2007). Utstein style analysis of out-of-hospital cardiac arrest – bystander CPR and end expired carbon dioxide. *Resuscitation*, 72, 404–414.

Guzzetta CE, et al. (2007). *Presenting the Option for Family Presence*. Des Plaines, IL: Emergency Nurses Association.

Hansen C, Strawser D. (1992). Family presence during CPR: Foote hospital 9-year perspective. *Journal of Emergency Nursing*, 18, 104–106.

Kause J, Smith G, Prytherch D, Parr M, Flabouris A, Hillman K. (2004). A comparison of antecedents to cardiac arrests, deaths and emergency intensive care admissions in Australia and New Zealand, and the United Kingdom – the ACADEMIA study. *Resuscitation*, 62, 275–282.

Kent H, McDowell J. (2004). Sudden bereavement in acute care settings. *Nursing Standard*, 19(6), 38–42.

Kolar M, Krizmaric M, Klemen P, Grmec S. (2008). Partial pressure of end-tidal carbon dioxide successful predicts cardiopulmonary resuscitation in the field: a prospective observational study. *Critical Care*, 12, R11.

Lilja G, et al. (2015). Cognitive function in survivors of out-of-hospital cardiac arrest after target temperature management at 33 degrees C versus 36 degrees C. *Circulation*, 131, 1340–1349.

Lippert FK, et al. (2010). European resuscitation council guidelines for resuscitation 2010 section 10. The ethics of resuscitation and end-of-life decisions. *Resuscitation*, 81(10), 1445–1451.

Lyon RM, Ferris JD, Young DM, McKeown DW, Oglesby AJ, Robertson C. (2010). Field intubation of cardiac arrest patients: a dying art? *Emergency Medicine Journal*, 27, 321–323.

McLaughlan C, et al. (1996). *Should Relatives Witness Resuscitation?* London: Resuscitation Council (UK).

Moulaert VRMP, Verbunt JA, van Heugten CM, Wade DT. (2009). Cognitive impairments in survivors of out-of-hospital cardiac arrest: a systematic review. *Resuscitation*, 80, 297–305.

Murray Parkes C. (1998). *Bereavement. Studies of Grief in Adult Life*. Harmondsworth: Penguin.

NCEPOD. (2005). *A Report of the National Confidential Enquiry into Patient Outcome and Death 2005 an Acute Problem?* London: NCEPOD. Available from: https://www.ncepod.org.uk/2005report/summary.pdf.

Needleman J, Buerhaus P, Mattke S, Stewart M, Zelevinsky K. (2002). Nurse-staffing levels and the quality of care in hospitals. *New England Journal of Medicine*, 346, 1715–1722.

Nolan JP, Soar J. (2008). Airway techniques and ventilation strategies. *Current Opinion in Critical Care*, 14, 279–286.

Nolan JP, Soar J, Smith GB, Jerry P, Gwinnutt C, Parrott F, Power S, Harrison D, Nixon E, Rowane K, On behalf of the National Cardiac Arrest Audit. (2014). Incidence and outcome of in-hospital cardiac arrest in the United Kingdom national cardiac arrest audit. *Resuscitation*, 85, 987–992. doi:10.1016/j.resuscitation.2014.04.002.

Nursing & Midwifery Council. (2018). *The Code: Professional Standards of Practice and Behaviour for Nurses, Midwives and Nursing Associates.* Retrieved from: http://www.nmc.org.uk/globalassets/sitedocuments/nmc-publications/revised-new-nmc-code.pdf.

Pattison N. (2008). Caring for patients after death. *Nursing Standard*, 22(51), 48–56.

Raphael B. (1984). *The Anatomy of Bereavement. A Handbook for the Caring Professionals.* London: Hutchinson.

Resuscitation Council UK. (1996). *Should Relatives Witness Resuscitation? A Report from a Project Team of the Resuscitation Council (UK).* London: Resuscitation Council UK.

Resuscitation Council (UK). (2015). *Resuscitation Guidelines.* London: Resuscitation Council UK. Available from: https://www.resus.org.uk/resuscitation-guidelines/.

Resuscitation Council (UK). (2016). *Advanced Life Support*, 7th Edition. London: RCUK.

Royal College of Nursing, British Medical Association and the Resuscitation Council UK. (2016). *Decisions Relating to Cardiopulmonary Resuscitation*, 3rd Edition, 1st Revision. London: BMA, RCUK, RCN.

Sak-Dankosky N, Andruszkiewicz P, Sherwood P, Kvist T. (2014). Integrative review: nurses' and physicians' experiences and attitudes towards inpatient-witnessed resuscitation of an adult patient. *Journal of Advanced Nursing*, 70(5), 957–954. doi:10.1111/jan.12276.

Schilling RJ. (1994). No room for spectators (Letters). *BMJ*, 309, 406–412.

Sheak KR, et al. (2015). Quantitative relationship between end-tidal carbon dioxide and CPR quality during both in-hospital and out-of-hospital cardiac arrest. *Resuscitation*, 89, 149–154.

Soar J, Nolan JP, Bottiger BW, et al. (2015). European resuscitation council guidelines for resuscitation 2015, section 3: Adult advanced life support. *Resuscitation*, 95, 99–146.

Sulzgruber P, et al. (2015). Survivors of cardiac arrest with good neurological outcome show considerable impairments of memory functioning. *Resuscitation*, 88, 120–125.

Twibell R, Siela D, Riwitis C, Neal N, Waters N. (2018). A qualitative study of factors in nurses' and physicians' decision making related to family presence during resuscitation. *Journal of Clinical Nursing*, 27(1–2), e320–e334. doi:10.1111/jocn.13948.

Walker WM. (2010). Sudden cardiac death in adults: causes, incidence and interventions. *Nursing Standard*, 24(38), 50–56.

Wilson J, White C. (2011). *Guidance for Staff Responsible for Care After Death (Last Offices).* London: The Stationery Office.

Wissenberg M, et al. (2013). Association of national initiatives to improve cardiac arrest management with rates of bystander intervention and patient survival after out-of-hospital cardiac arrest. *JAMA*, 310, 1377–1384.

Wright B. (1996). *Sudden Death. A Research Base for Practice*, 2nd Edition. New York, NY: Churchill Livingstone.

8 The patient with acute renal problems

Ian Naldrett

AIM

The aim of this chapter is to familiarise you with the functions of the kidney and the presentation and management of acute renal problems.

OBJECTIVES

After reading this chapter you will be able to:

- Identify the major anatomical structures of the renal system.
- Identify the anatomical components of the nephron and describe the physiological properties of each component.
- Differentiate, from a physiological perspective, the three phases of urine production: tubular filtration, tubular reabsorption and tubular secretion.
- Distinguish between objective and subjective assessment data and the nurse's role in collecting this information.
- Critically discuss the nursing care and medical interventions that might be implemented in order to optimise renal status.

Introduction

The renal system has a crucial role to play in maintaining homoeostasis. The primary function of the kidneys is to produce urine as a waste product that can then be excreted from the body by the accessory renal organs, the ureters, the urinary bladder and the urethra. This is a complex physiological process, because, as the blood plasma is filtered through the kidneys, many adjustments are made to the water and solute levels in order to maintain a dynamic equilibrium within the body. Renal impairment, from a primary or secondary cause, or a systemic illness, such as sepsis, can quickly lead to life-threatening complications. Nurses have a key role to play in the prevention of acute renal injury in all patients (but particularly those most at risk) and in the early recognition and assessment of renal problems. Nurses must also effectively plan, implement and evaluate all interventions for those individuals with established renal dysfunction, liaising effectively with other members of the multidisciplinary team in the provision of quality care.

In this chapter, we will discuss four key areas: the applied anatomy and physiology of the renal system, common acute renal problems affecting patients, renal assessment and, finally, the ways in which renal status can be optimised through nursing care and multidisciplinary management.

Gross anatomy of the kidney

The kidneys are situated on the posterior abdominal wall, outside the peritoneal cavity. Located on either side of the vertebral column, they are approximately 11cm in length, 5 to 6cm in width and 3–4cm thick. They are partially protected by the eleventh and twelfth pairs of ribs and they are capped by the adrenal glands. Each kidney is surrounded by three layers: a tough fibrous covering, the 'renal capsule', a layer of protective fat and a layer of connective tissue, the 'renal fascia', which attaches the kidney to the posterior abdominal wall (see Figure 8.1).

Each kidney has a hilum where the nerves, blood vessels, lymphatics and the ureter enter and exit. The renal artery, from the abdominal aorta, branches into interlobar, arcuate and interlobular arteries and finally into the afferent arterioles, which eventually form tufts of capillaries called glomeruli. Venous return is *via* a single efferent arteriole, which

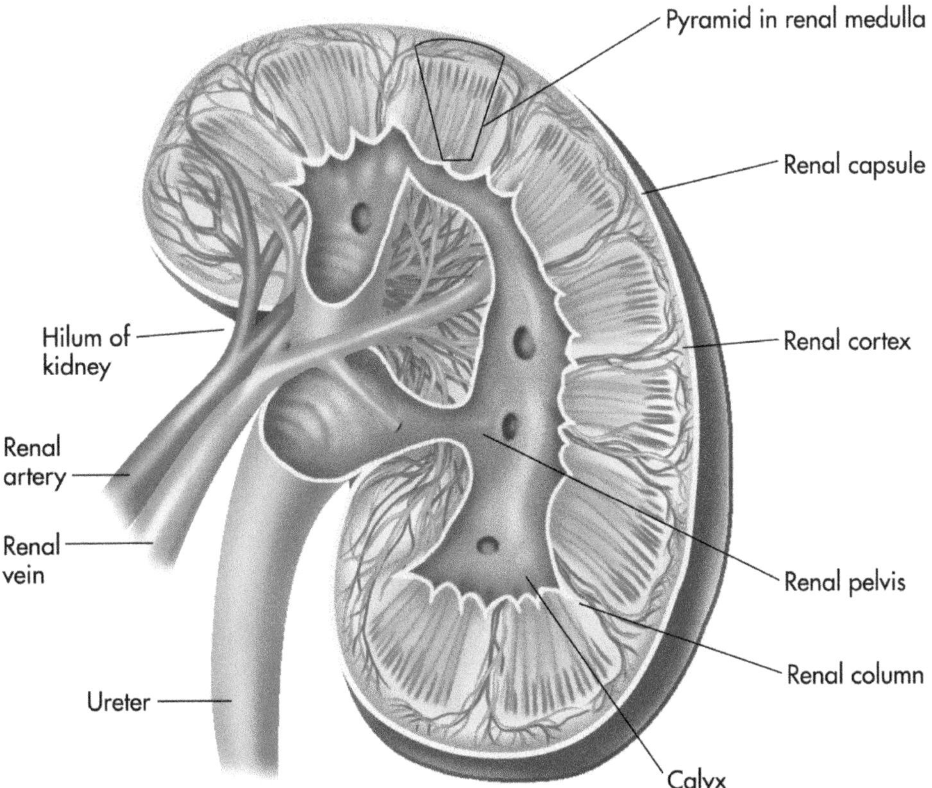

Figure 8.1 Internal and external anatomy of the kidney.

branches to form a second capillary bed, the 'peritubular capillaries', and then interlobular, arcuate and interlobar veins leading to the renal vein and, ultimately, the inferior vena cava (see Figure 8.2). Lymphatic vessels follow the larger renal blood vessels and drain into the lateral aortic lymph nodes. The nerve supply to the kidney is *via* the sympathetic branch of the autonomic nervous system, with afferent fibres entering the spinal cord at T10, T11 and T12. Blood flow is regulated by vasodilation and vasoconstriction, thereby controlling blood pressure in the glomerulus.

The *nephron* is the functional unit of the renal system. There are approximately one million of them per kidney and, put together, they would have a combined length of about 80 kilometres. Each nephron consists of two sections. Firstly, a tubular area consisting of the glomerulus, the proximal convoluted tubule, the loop of Henle, the distal convoluted tubule and the collecting duct, and secondly, a vascular area called the **vasa recta** (see Figure 8.3).

There are three specific areas in the kidney. There is an outer section called the *renal cortex*, which contains all of the glomeruli and portions of the tubule. The inner section is known as the *renal medulla*, and this contains the straight segments of the proximal and distal tubules and the collecting ducts. Renal pyramids are found here, and these cone-shaped areas have their apices ending in the papillae, which open into the minor calyx. Urine passes from the collecting ducts in the pyramid to two small cavities, the minor calyces and the

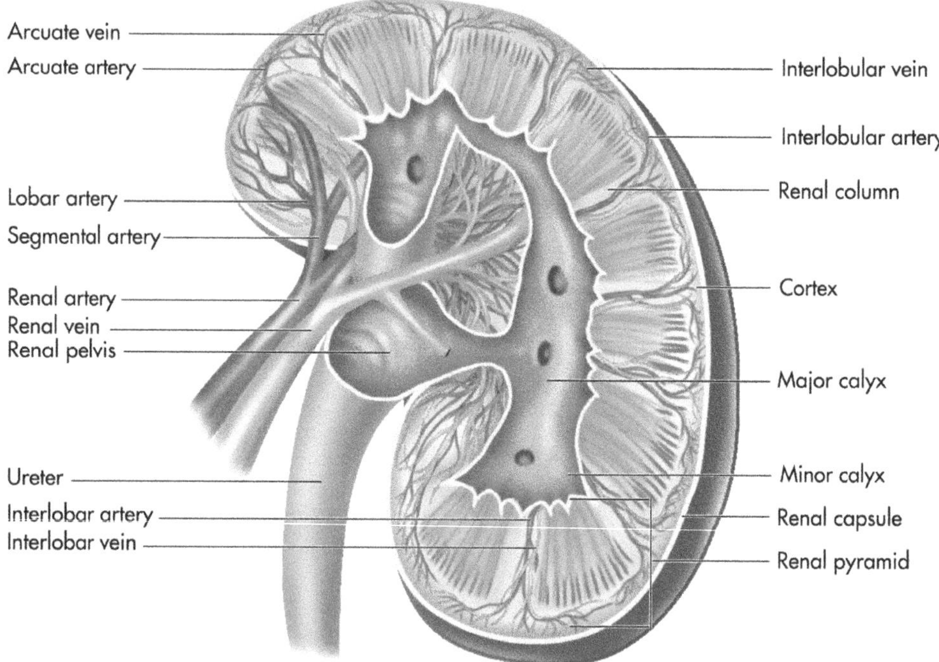

Figure 8.2 Renal blood vessels and the pathway of blood through the renal system.

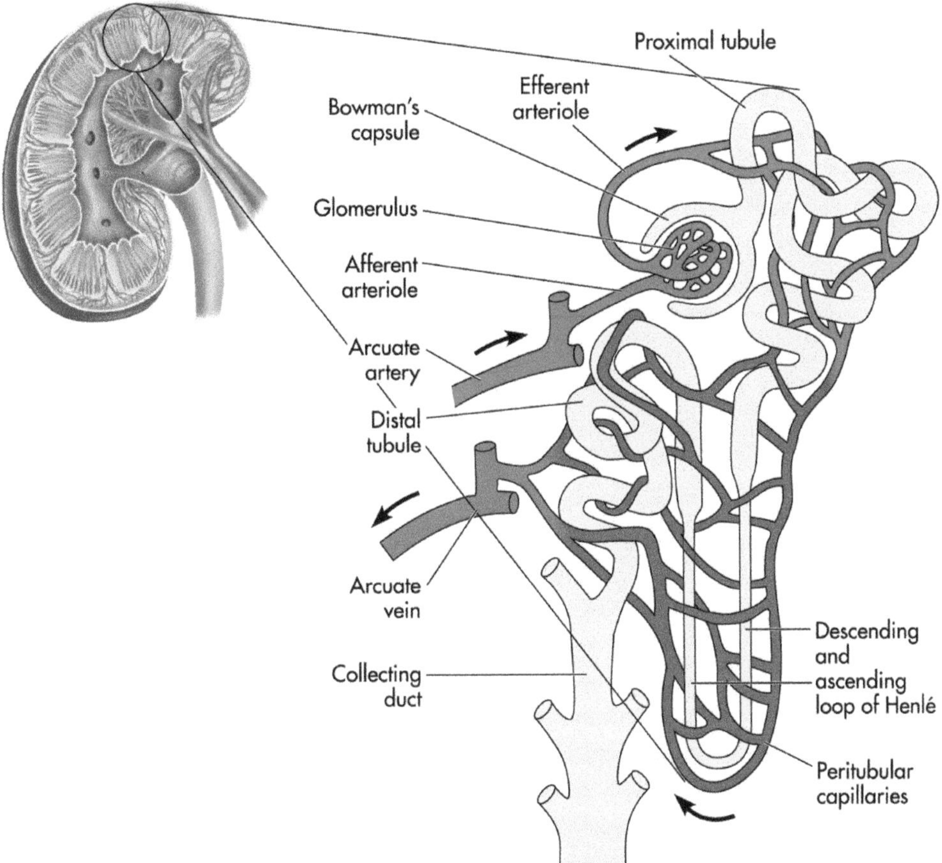

Figure 8.3 The nephron.

major calyces, and, from here, it enters the renal pelvis. Finally, the *renal pelvis* is formed from the expanded upper section of the ureter and it acts as a collecting space.

Accessory structures of excretion

There are several accessory structures of excretion in the renal tract (see Figure 8.4).

The ureters

These two tubes, approximately 28–34cm in length, convey urine from the renal pelvis to the bladder. In cross section, each ureter has a star shape and is composed of three layers:

- The tunica mucosa, an inner mucous lining.
- The tunica muscularis, a muscular middle layer (which propels urine by peristalsis along the ureters).
- The tunica adventitia, an outer fibrous layer.

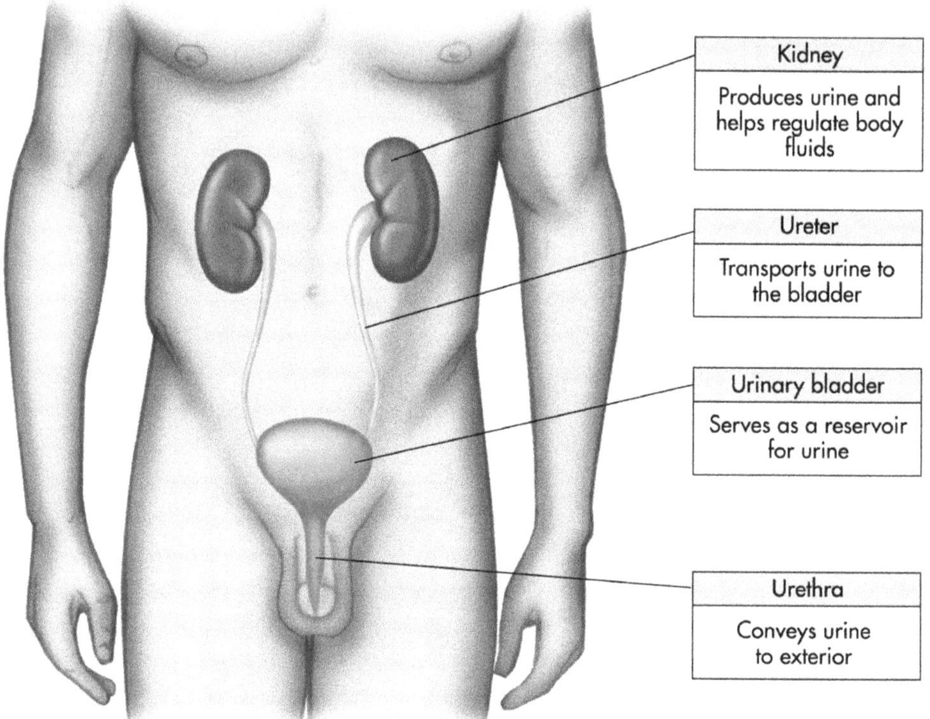

Figure 8.4 Anatomy of the urinary system.

The ureters run obliquely for a short distance within the bladder wall, and this enables them to act as valves, preventing back flow of urine from the bladder into the ureters. In the female, the ureters are close to the cervix and the ovaries, whereas, in the male, they are adjacent to the seminal vesicles and the prostate gland.

The bladder

The bladder is a hollow, muscular bag, located behind the symphysis pubis and in front of the rectum. In females, it rests on the anterior vagina and in front of the uterus, whereas, in males, it is situated above the prostate gland. The wall of the bladder is made up of three different layers:

- The tunica mucosa: this has folds, called rugae, in it and they allow the bladder to distend, while acting as a reservoir for urine before it is excreted from the body.
- The tunica muscularis: this consists of three layers of meshed smooth muscle. In this area, a network of muscle fibres cross over one another in different directions and these are known collectively as the detrusor muscle.
- The tunica serosa or adventitia: this outer layer moistens the tissues and lubricates surfaces so that, when the bladder is full, it does not compress other organs.

The average bladder can hold up to 300mL of urine before the desire to void is noted. Passing urine begins with voluntary relaxation of the external sphincter muscle of the bladder and then different regions of the detrusor muscle contract, forcing urine out of the bladder and through the urethra. Parasympathetic fibres from the autonomic nervous system transmit impulses that cause bladder contraction; injury to the central nervous system can result in problems with passing urine.

Urethra

This is a small tube lined with mucous membrane, leading from the floor of the bladder (trigone) to the outside of the body. In the female, it lies behind the symphysis pubis and in front of the vagina, extending down for approximately 3cm. In the male, the urethra is about 20cm long and it passes through the centre of the prostate gland, where it is joined by two ejaculatory ducts, thus also serving as a pathway for semen. From there, it extends downwards and forwards into the penis and ends as the urinary meatus at the tip of this organ. Urine is prevented from mixing with semen during ejaculation by a reflex closure of sphincter muscles at the bladder's opening.

Applied physiology

Functions of the kidney

The kidneys have a major role in maintaining homoeostasis and, when their function is impaired through disease or injury, physiological effects can be seen throughout the body, affecting all organs. Through the regulation of body fluid volume, composition and pH, the subsequent production of urine to excrete waste products, and the production and secretion of various hormones (e.g., erythropoietin), the kidneys maintain equilibrium within the body (see Figure 8.5).

The regulation of body fluids and the production of urine

The tubular components of the nephron have a specific role to play in the formation of urine, which occurs in three stages: **filtration**, **tubular reabsorption** and **tubular secretion**.

Glomerular (Bowman's) capsule

This is where the first stage of urine production, filtration, takes place. Filtration is defined as the passage of a fluid and the substances in that fluid through a membrane under pressure. So, in this case, the blood and all of the constituents in the blood are pushed, by the arterial blood pressure (at around 60–70mmHg), through the glomerular capillaries and then into the Bowman's capsule, *via* the glomerular-capsular membrane. This membrane has three special filtration layers in it, with different-sized pores, and the purpose of these is to retain key substances that are required in the blood and to select others to be excreted *via* the renal tubules. Firstly, the endothelial layer prevents the passage of blood cells, secondly, the basement membrane prevents the passage of large proteins, and, thirdly, the visceral layer prevents the passage of medium-sized proteins. Apart from the varying size of the pores in these different layers, there is another reason that blood and

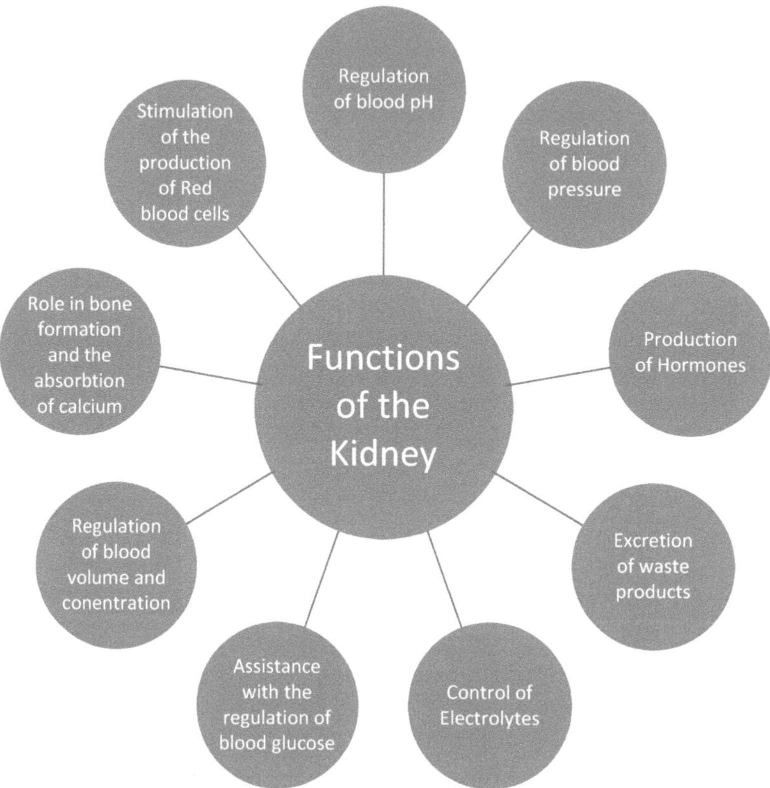

Figure 8.5 The functions of the kidney.

proteins cannot pass through from the blood into the filtrate and that is because these glycoproteins are carrying a negative electrical charge. The filtration membrane also carries a negative electrical charge and therefore repels them. Therefore, in health, blood cells and proteins should not be filtered out of the blood because they are needed in order to maintain normal blood function and to maintain the integrity of the intravascular space. Remember, also, that the kidney has an important role in regulating blood components through the production of **erythropoietin**.

> The hormone erythropoietin stimulates red blood cell production (erythrogenesis) in the bone marrow.

In contrast, whereas larger molecules cannot pass through, substances of lower molecular weight, like water, electrolytes, **urea** and amino acids, can. Ultimately, therefore, this means that the kidneys are able to excrete certain amounts of these substances from the body. On average, 180 litres of plasma are filtered per day by the kidneys. Significant factors in this filtration process are, firstly, the arterial blood pressure and the degree of renal perfusion (especially if this is lowered), secondly, the presence of proteins in the blood, such as albumin, globulins and fibrinogen, which may be impaired by conditions such as hypoalbuminaemia, and thirdly, the pressure exerted by the Bowman's capsule itself, which might be altered in disease processes such as **glomerulonephritis**. In good health, the kidneys have the ability to regulate filtration by adjusting blood flow into and out of the glomerulus through vasoconstriction or vasodilation of the afferent arteriole. On the other hand, if any of the aforementioned parameters are disturbed, such as by hypovolaemia, for example, this can affect the filtration pressure and, in turn, can lead to an abnormal **glomerular filtration rate** (GFR). The average GFR for an adult male is about 125mL per minute and for an adult female, 105mL per minute, but these parameters would be much reduced under conditions where poor renal perfusion occurs, such as in the case of dehydration (see Figure 8.6).

Significant factors in filtration, therefore, are the arterial blood pressure, the presence of plasma proteins in the blood and the pressure exerted by the Bowman's capsule itself.

The kidney secretes an enzyme called **renin** from cells in the juxtaglomerulus apparatus, and this plays a significant role in regulating fluid balance and subsequently in controlling

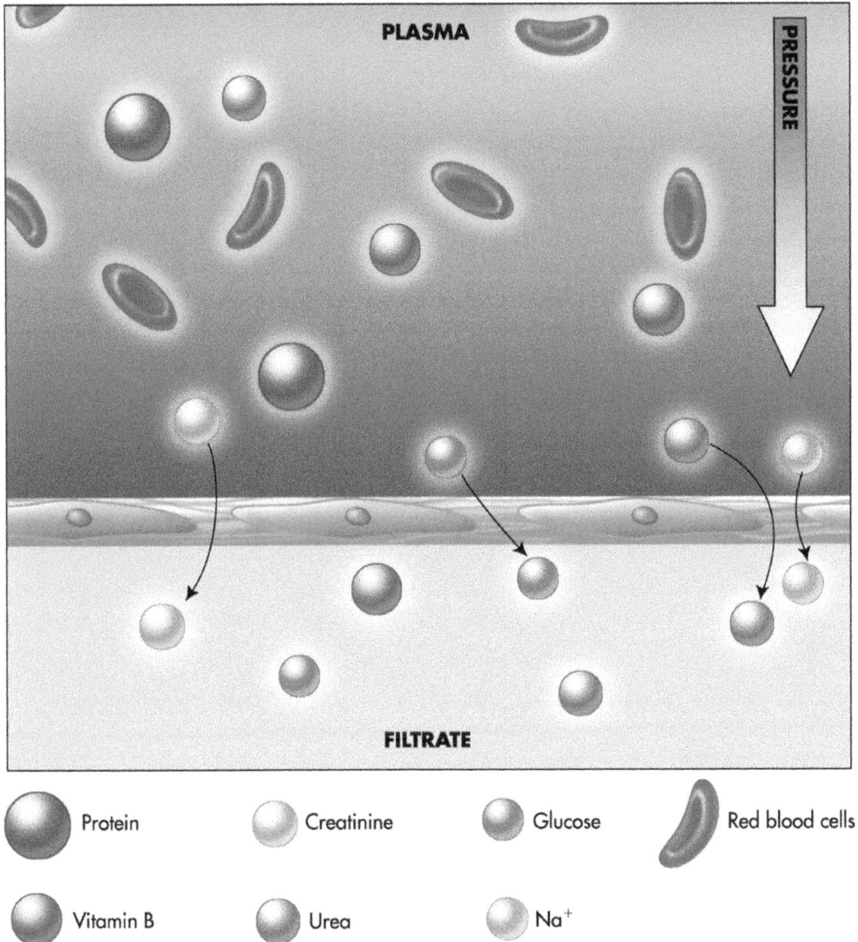

Figure 8.6 Filter selectivity.

blood pressure. Renin is a vasoconstrictor and it leads to the release of other substances with similar properties. The chain of events that it initiates is collectively known as the renin–angiotensin–aldosterone system. Renin leads to the release of angiotensinogen, produced by hepatocytes, and converted in the plasma into angiotensin 1. This is then converted in the lungs into angiotensin 2, a very powerful vasopressor. The latter has two main functions:

- Vasoconstriction of the afferent arterioles, leading to a reduced glomerular filtration rate.
- Activation of aldosterone from the adrenal cortex, which leads to the reabsorption of sodium into the extracellular space, with chloride and water following it.

The overall effect of these measures is to increase the circulating blood volume by fluid replenishment and, ultimately, to increase the arterial blood pressure. Should the perfusion to the kidney continue to decrease, however, more drastic physiological responses are called for. In this case, the sympathetic autonomic nervous system will be activated, and the release of norepinephrine will lead to increased vasoconstriction of the renal vasculature and a further reduction in the glomerular filtration rate.

Proximal convoluted tubule

The second stage of urine production, tubular reabsorption, begins in this section of the nephron. The filtrate coming from the glomerulus passes over the epithelial microvilli found here and is then reabsorbed back into the peritubular capillaries. In fact, 99% of the plasma being filtered per day will be reabsorbed back into the blood via **active transport** mechanisms (using energy, namely ATP, adenosine triphosphate) and passive electrochemical gradients, such as **osmosis** and **diffusion**. Two-thirds of this plasma will have been reabsorbed by the time the filtrate reaches the end of the proximal convoluted tubule. A key substance to be reabsorbed is sodium, and glucose and amino acids are co-transported with it. Other substances, such as potassium, calcium, phosphate, bicarbonate, magnesium, uric acid, amino acids, small polypeptides, lactic acid and water-soluble vitamins, will also be reabsorbed under the influence of sodium in this part of the nephron. Reabsorption of all of these solutes increases the **osmolality** (concentration) of, firstly, the tubule cells, and, secondly, the interstitial fluid and, finally, the blood. This, in turn, attracts water by osmosis and thereby ensures that the blood is osmotically balanced. In fact, 65% of the filtered water is reabsorbed into the proximal convoluted tubule, at a rate of about 80mL per minute.

Remember

The kidneys can perform gluconeogenesis ('the production of new glucose', from non-carbohydrate precursors). This provides more glucose for energy production.

The kidney has an important role in calcium homeostasis, with 95% of filtered calcium being reabsorbed in the distal convoluted tubule. Calcium is needed for muscle contraction and, together with phosphate, builds the extracellular bone matrix.

In this section of the nephron, some tubular secretion, the third stage of urine production, also takes place. Hydrogen ions are actively exchanged for sodium ions, to maintain electrochemical balance, and ammonia, a toxic waste product derived from various amino acids, is filtered out into the tubular fluid in the form of urea, most of which is secreted. Other agents, like **creatinine**, and some drugs, such as penicillin, are also secreted here.

Loop of Henle

The loop of Henle reabsorbs about 20–30% of the filtered sodium, potassium and calcium, and there is also some bicarbonate, chloride and water reabsorption taking place here. This part of the nephron is composed of ascending and descending limbs; filtrate flows in one direction down the descending limb and then in the other direction up the ascending limb, therefore flowing in opposing directions in parallel tubes. For this reason, this is often referred to as 'the counter-current mechanism'. Ultimately, the purpose of these limbs is to concentrate the filtrate and form an osmotically concentrated urine for excretion. This is achieved by the descending and ascending limbs having varying degrees of permeability to water and other solutes, and also by having differences in their capacity to transport substances, such as sodium and urea. Key factors influencing how concentrated urine becomes are active transport mechanisms and hormonal influences, such as the action of the anti**diuretic** hormone (ADH), called **vasopressin**. This is made in the hypothalamus and secreted from the posterior lobe of the pituitary gland. Its role is to control the level of water reabsorption or excretion by the kidney.

Distal convoluted tubule

This structure begins with a convoluted section, which is virtually impermeable to water; because the water is retained in the lumen, it is able to contribute to the dilution of the tubular fluid. The second, straighter segment is more permeable to water and is regulated by the antidiuretic hormone. Sodium can also be reabsorbed here and potassium actively secreted, both under the influence of the hormone aldosterone, secreted by the adrenal cortex.

The kidneys and the lungs together control the acid-base balance. In the kidney, the distal convoluted tubule contributes to this process by secreting hydrogen ions. Hydrogen is very important because it maintains the integrity of cellular membranes and it facilitates enzyme action. The body produces about 50 to 100mEq of body acids per day through the metabolism of proteins, fats and carbohydrates, but the concentration of this acid in the body (in the form of hydrogen ions) must be kept within a fairly narrow range with a pH of 7.35–7.45. Even slight changes in the level of body acids can lead to cellular instability and altered biological processes in tissues. In acute and critical illness, a disturbance of the acid-base balance often occurs, and this can lead to organ damage.

pH changes in the blood can lead to problems with perfusion and oxygenation.

In summary, when the blood pH decreases (plasma becomes more acidic, 'acidaemia'; for example, pH 7.23), the kidneys secrete more hydrogen ions (acidic) and simultaneously reabsorb more bicarbonate ions (basic), with the net effect being to increase the blood pH back to normal. In contrast, if the blood pH increases (plasma becomes more alkalotic, 'alkalaemia'; for example, pH 7.51), the kidneys will secrete less hydrogen ions and decrease bicarbonate reabsorption. This lowers the pH back to normal.

The collecting duct

This is a large straight tubule that extends down from the cortex of the kidney into the medullary section. On its route through the kidney, it is joined by the distal tubules of several nephrons. The collecting duct then joins larger ducts and eventually forms a renal pyramid, and these structures finally converge to form a tube that enters into the small calyces. From here, the filtrate, now called urine, drains into the renal pelvis and then into the bladder.

In summary, each of the components of the renal tubule plays a key role in the production and finally excretion of the filtrate as urine (see Figure 8.7).

Normal urine composition

In good health, urine is composed of water (approximately 95%) and various solutes, with a normal pH of 5.0–6.5 (although this may vary, and become more alkaline after eating). It has a distinctive odour (which should not be offensive) and a characteristic yellow colour, the latter being due to the presence of yellow pigments called urochromes, which are produced by the breakdown of red blood cells in the liver. Bilirubin and its by-product, urobilinogen, also found in urine, are generated by the breakdown of old red blood cells.

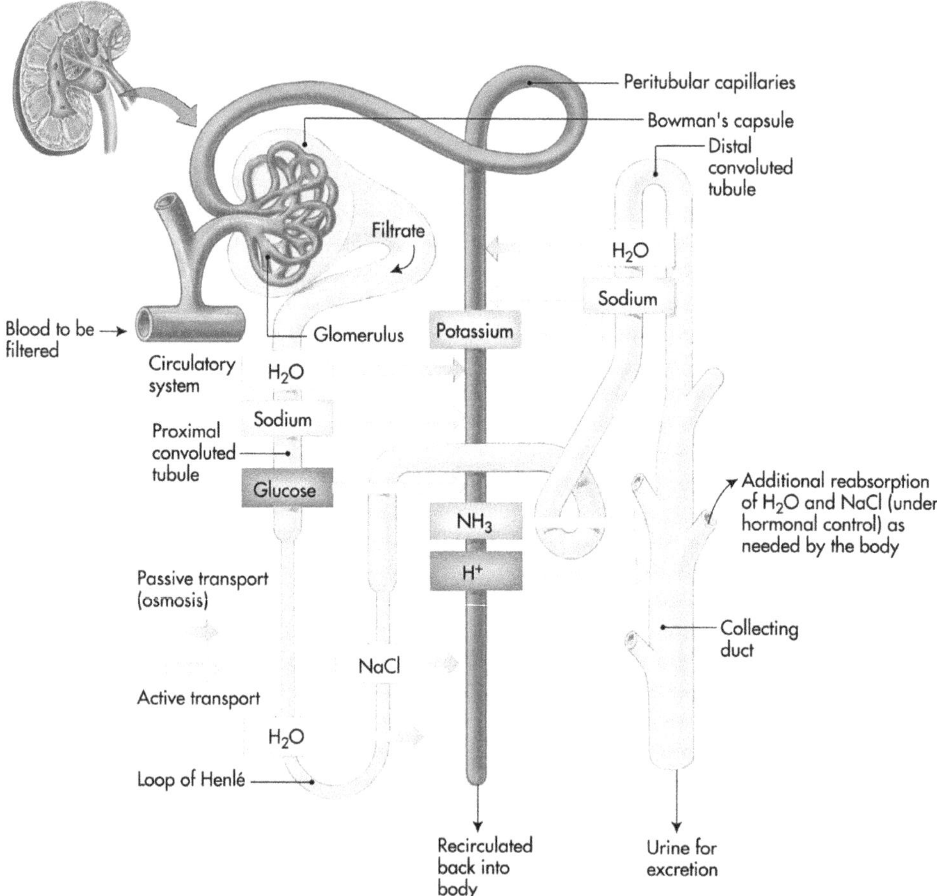

Figure 8.7 Sites of tubular reabsorption and secretion.

Urinalysis is a vital tool in management of the acutely ill adult in determining aspects of urine composition and the detection of abnormalities; this should be undertaken as soon as acute kidney injury (AKI) is suspected (NICE 2013a).

Specific gravity is the estimated level of solutes in the urine and the normal range is between 1.016 and 1.022; the greater the solute concentration in relation to water, the greater the specific gravity. To illustrate this, during dehydration, the reading might be high, for example 1.030, owing to reduced levels of water in the blood in comparison to solutes. Urea constitutes the bulk of the solute in urine and this, together with other substances produced by protein catabolism, such as uric acid, urea and creatinine, form the nitrogenous waste products. There are also a number of electrolytes present, such as sodium, potassium, ammonium, chloride, bicarbonate, phosphate and sulphate. In health, the amounts of these substances will vary slightly with diet. Hormones can also sometimes be found in urine (if levels of these substances are high in the blood) and Toxins, such as bacteria, may also be present in the event of ill health (Tortora et al. 2017).

When things go wrong – common acute renal problems

Glomerular disorders

Many disorders of the glomerulus are related to immunologic factors, but toxins, such as drugs, and some systemic diseases, like diabetes mellitus, can all contribute to the development of glomerular dysfunction. They may present initially as acute problems and, whereas most people recover quite well, they can lead to a chronic disorder in some individuals, requiring haemodialysis, or even renal transplantation.

One common complaint is glomerulonephritis, which is the collective name for all disorders that lead to inflammation of the glomerulus. Some patients presenting with this disease have what is known as a **nephrotic syndrome**. McCance and Huether (2018) outlined the characteristic symptoms of this disorder:

- A reduced glomerular filtration rate.
- **Haematuria** and **proteinuria**. These abnormalities occur because the filtration membrane has been damaged. This leads to increased permeability and loss of the normal negative electrical charge, thus allowing these substances to pass into the urine when they would not usually be able to do so.
- Oedema secondary to loss of plasma proteins in the urine such as albumin.
- Hypertension secondary to excess fluid retention.
- Hyperlipidaemia secondary to increased triglyceride and cholesterol production by the liver.

Depending on the cause, people with this problem often require pharmacological intervention, in the form of **diuretic** or antihypertensive therapy, to relieve oedema and hypertension, antibiotic administration to counteract infection, steroid administration to reduce inflammation, or lipid-lowering drugs to reduce elevated blood fat levels (McCance and Huether 2018). Specialist dietary advice should also be sought in order to reduce fat and replace lost proteins.

Infection

In health, urine is naturally acidic, the bladder empties completely, flushing the urethra and there is no back flow of urine into the renal tract; this means that, above the urethra, the urine is sterile. If, however, any part of the urinary tract becomes infected, a large number of bacteria, usually Gram-negative in nature, will be found in the urine, (Tortora et al. 2017). These infections may affect the lower urinary tract, resulting in conditions such as urethritis (inflammation of the urethra) or cystitis (inflammation of the bladder), or they may colonise the upper urinary tract, involving the ureters and kidneys. One very common reason for bacterial colonisation of the urinary tract is urinary catheterisation (O'Callaghan 2017). The catheter can introduce bacteria into the bladder on insertion, it can cause damage to the urethra, creating a portal for bacterial entry, and it bypasses the normal voiding process. When caring for a patient with an indwelling urinary catheter, the nurse must ensure that a sterile closed system is used, drainage bags are changed in line with manufacturer's instructions, and that effective hand-decontamination practices are observed pre- and post-handling of the catheter and drainage system (Loveday et al. 2013). The need for a urinary catheter should be assessed daily for each patient and it should be removed when no longer clinically indicated. Where infection is suspected, samples of urine should be aseptically obtained and sent to the microbiology department for microscopy, culture and sensitivity testing, as ascending infection is easily introduced into the urinary tract and any infection that has occurred needs to be identified early, so that appropriate treatment can be instigated.

The insertion of a urinary catheter is a common cause of urinary tract infection.

One of the most common kidney infections is pyelonephritis. In many cases, this is caused by the spread of bacteria such as *Escherichia coli* from the gut and, as with most urinary tract infection, it is more commonly seen in females, due to the short urethra and the close proximity of the rectal and urethral openings. With pyelonephritis, the infection ascends into the bladder and then progresses to the ureters and eventually the kidneys, affecting the renal tubules and blood vessels. The symptoms are similar to those of all urinary tract infections, in that they may include increased urgency and frequency of urination, pyrexia, back pain, increased leucocytes in the blood, dysuria and cloudy urine, with bacteria present. If the infection becomes a chronic problem, scar tissue can form on the kidneys and lead to impaired function (McCance and Huether 2018). Once infection is established, treatment is required in order to prevent long-term renal damage. This includes increased fluid intake to 'flush' the system (instigated for most patients, unless there are specific reasons not to do so, such as fluid overload), antibiotic therapy and the prescription of antispasmodic drugs.

Signs and symptoms of a urinary tract infection include:

- Frequent, painful urination.
- Pyrexia.
- Back pain.
- Increased white cell count.
- Cloudy urine.

Renal calculi ('kidney stones')

These kidney stones are made up of calcium and other minerals found in urine and they can accumulate in the renal pelvis and calyces, leading to renal obstruction. Factors that predispose individuals to this problem include dehydration, excessive intake of vitamin D or calcium, high levels of uric acid and renal infection (Tortora et al. 2017). Small stones can pass through the ureters and urethra and be excreted in the urine, but larger stones can lead to obstruction of the ureters, especially as they may sometimes have jagged edges. When this happens, it leads to intense, stabbing pain called 'renal colic', where the muscles of the affected ureter rhythmically contract in an attempt to dislodge the stone. The pain often starts in the flank of the affected side and radiates into the groin, and it may be accompanied by other urinary tract symptoms, such as frequent urination or urge incontinence. If the stone cannot be moved, hydronephrosis may occur, which is when the kidney swells due to the obstructed flow of urine (Tortora et al. 2017).

Renal calculi cause severe pain as the muscles of the ureters try to pass the stones.

Renal calculi are usually diagnosed by a combination of history taking, clinical assessment and investigative procedures, such as abdominal X-ray (90% of renal stones are radio-opaque), **intravenous pyelogram (IVP)** or a **computerised tomography (CT) scan**. Once diagnosed, treatment includes analgesia for the pain, an increase in water intake to help flush the stones out, an increase in dietary fibre because this binds calcium in the bowel and reduces its absorption and excretion in the urine, and, finally, antibiotic therapy to treat any infection. Historically, surgical intervention was always required for the removal of stones that could not be passed. Whereas this method of treatment may still be an option for very large stones, more recently shock wave lithotripsy has been used to remove most calculi. In this radiological procedure, high-energy shock waves are used to reduce the stone to smaller fragments which can then be excreted in the urine (Tortora et al. 2017.)

Acute urinary obstruction

Patients may present with difficulties in voiding urine, owing to lower urinary tract obstruction. They can present with acute urinary retention, requiring immediate catheterisation (possibly suprapubic) and then diagnosis of the cause. The common reasons for this problem include:

- In men, prostatic hypertrophy of benign or malignant origin. The passage of urine is impaired as the urethra passes through an inflamed or enlarged prostate gland.
- In women, organ prolapse. The uterus can herniate through the vaginal canal, so severely in some cases that it is visible on inspection of the external genitalia. A cystocele (when a portion of the bladder wall descends into the vaginal canal) or a rectocele (where the rectum bulges into the vaginal canal) can also develop and these disorders nearly always occur secondary to childbirth, although it is not usually until the menopause that they become evident.
- In men or women, urethral stricture may occur secondary to infection or trauma.
- In men and women, tumours of the renal tract may occur and these tend to affect individuals in the fifth and sixth decades of life. Common symptoms include haematuria,

pain in the affected area and sometimes a swelling of tissue. Kidney tumours are usually malignant in origin, metastasise early and often lead to urinary obstruction, with hydronephrosis. Bladder cancers are also common, but, with early intervention, the prognosis is better than for kidney tumours. The development of bladder carcinoma is strongly linked to smoking and exposure to industrial chemicals. Aromatic amines, found in paints, dyes and other substances of a similar nature, have all been linked with the occurrence of the disease (Tortora et al. 2017).

Treatment for these disorders depends on the severity and the progression of the problem, but often surgical intervention is required to rectify the anatomical injury or disease.

Acute kidney injury

Acute kidney injury occurs when there is a sudden impairment of renal function, leading to the accumulation of waste products in the blood. It is often a reversible condition, but, if left untreated, can lead to chronic renal failure. There are many susceptibilities to AKI, including advanced age, female gender, black race and hypertension (KDIGO 2012).

Risk factors for acute kidney injury:

- Advanced age.
- Female gender.
- Black race.
- Hypertension.

Acute kidney injury is classified according to the degree of blood chemistry impairment and the extent to which the urinary output is abnormal. In 2012, the Kidney Disease: Improving Global Outcomes AKI working group devised the current KDIGO staging system (KDIGO 2012). This is outlined in Table 8.1. This system of staging was devised from two previous AKI staging systems, the RIFLE and AKIN criteria.

Table 8.1 The KDIGO criteria

Stage 1	Increased serum creatinine to 1.5–1.9 times baseline OR increase in serum creatinine to ≤0.3 mg/dL (≤ 26.5 μmol/L) Urine output < 0.5mL/kg/hour for 6–12 hours
Stage 2	Increased serum creatinine to 2.0–2.9 times baseline. Urine output < 0.5mL/kg/hour for ≥ 12 hours
Stage 3	Increased serum creatinine to 3.0 times baseline OR increase in serum creatinine to ≥4.0 mg/dl (≥353.6 μmol/l) Urine output < 0.3mL/kg/hour for ≥ 24 hours or anuria ≥12 hours OR Initiation of renal replacement therapy OR in patients <18 years, decrease in eGFR to <35 mL/minute per 1.73 m^2

With this classification system (KDIGO), there are two defining features: serum creatinine concentration and the degree of **oliguria**. If either or both these are increasingly abnormal, the AKI is worsening and increasing levels of intervention are required. The risks of mortality increase as AKI worsens (Thomas et al. 2015).

The causes of acute kidney injury fall into three main categories

- Pre-renal.
- Acute intrinsic.
- Post-renal.

Pre-renal

- This volume-responsive injury occurs when there is a significant reduction in perfusion to the kidneys. It may happen as a result of a variety of conditions, but commonly loss of circulating volume caused by dehydration, hemorrhage or burns.
- Cardiac impairment, leading to low cardiac output state.
- Dilation of peripheral blood vessels, reducing the peripheral vascular resistance and therefore affecting the blood pressure (this occurs in sepsis).
- Obstruction of renal blood vessels, for example, renal artery stenosis.

Remember

A lack of circulating volume leads to poor renal perfusion and a poor urine output of less than 0.5mL/kg/hour.

In all cases, the sympathetic autonomic nervous system and the renin–angiotensin–aldosterone system, once activated as part of a normal homoeostatic response to changes in blood volume, contribute to the vasoconstriction and a further reduction in blood supply to the kidneys.

Acute intrinsic

This is when actual structural damage to the nephrons has occurred and it may lead to acute tubular necrosis, where tubular cells die and are shed into the tubule lumen, resulting in tubular blockages. The most common causes for this are as follows:

- Prolonged hypoperfusion.
- Nephrotoxic drug therapy, especially the aminoglycoside antibiotics and the non-steroidal anti-inflammatory agents.
- Exposure to radiocontrast agents.
- Infections, for example unresolved glomerulonephritis.
- Other diseases that can affect tubular function, such as sickle-cell disease and certain malignancies.

All nephrotoxic drugs should be stopped if the patient has renal impairment, in order to avoid further renal injury.

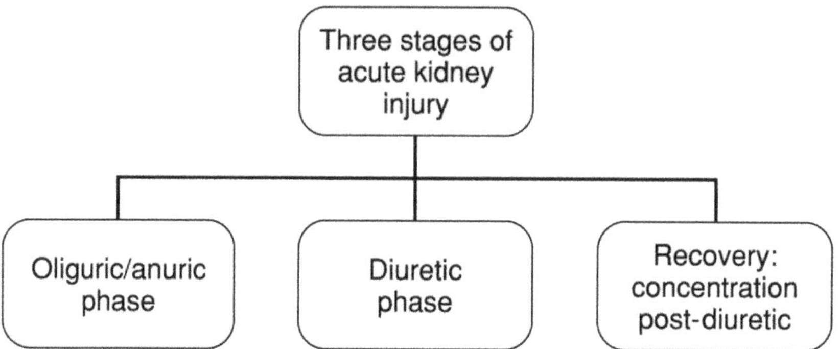

Figure 8.8 The stages of renal failure.

Post-renal

This is where an obstruction anywhere in the renal tract is unresolved and eventually leads to kidney damage.

Stages of acute kidney injury

There are said to be three distinct phases to acute kidney injury, whatever the original cause (Donald 2011). These are illustrated in Figure 8.8.

The patient's initial clinical presentation depends on the progression and severity of the disease, but commonly includes the following signs and symptoms:

- Urine output of less than 0.5mL/kg/hour.
- Metabolic acidosis, which may or may not be compensated.
- Raised serum creatinine level above 111umol/L.
- Raised serum potassium level above 5.1mmol/L.
- Raised serum urea level above 7.0mmol/L.
- Serum sodium levels may be high or low, depending on the kidney's ability to reabsorb the sodium into the blood.

Renal assessment

Historically, there have been problems with the late recognition and treatment of renal impairment amongst ward patients. Significantly, poor fluid balance management and unsatisfactory record keeping by the multidisciplinary team have been contributing factors. In such cases, the signs and symptoms of renal dysfunction have not been identified early enough and this has sometimes been followed by poor investigation and poor treatment of the patients' problems (NICE 2013a). In 2009, a report from the National Confidential Enquiry into Patient Outcome and Death (NCEPOD 2009) noted that the substandard management of individuals with a diagnosis of acute kidney injury had led to increased mortality for this patient group. This led to the development of the National Institute for Health and Care Excellence (NICE) guidelines, Acute Kidney Injury: Prevention, Detection and Management (NICE 2013a).

Clinical presentations and laboratory findings associated with AKI include:

- Urine output of less than 0.5mL/kg/hour.
- Metabolic acidosis on blood gas analysis (pH< 7.35).
- Raised serum creatinine, urea and potassium.
- High or low serum sodium.

In order to address these issues from a nursing perspective, a systematic approach to patient assessment must be adopted. The use of the ABCDE format and effective implementation of physiological track and trigger systems will monitor clinical parameters, identifying any significant changes. All **early warning scoring systems,** most notably NEWS 2, enable recognition of deterioration risk from the onset and facilitate optimal intervention.

In previous chapters, the importance of recording subjective and objective data during the assessment process has been highlighted. A considerable amount of valuable information can be gathered from the patient's general medical history, any medication they are taking, the history of the current problem, the patient's perception of what is troubling them, their physical appearance and, finally, a physical examination. We also have a range of tests and investigations that can be used to determine renal status.

Subjective data

If any part of the renal tract is not working normally, the patient will probably be aware of it and report a range of unpleasant symptoms. In addition, such is the importance of the kidney to health that, when problems do occur, all of the body's systems can be affected. A range of complaints may arise if there are any abnormalities with the production and/or excretion of urine. These include, among others, lethargy and drowsiness, feelings of breathlessness, dizziness, palpitations, difficulties with urination, weight gain, pruritus, feeling hot or cold, nausea and vomiting and sometimes severe pain.

Objective data

Monitoring of vital signs is crucial in renal impairment. Patients with acute renal problems may exhibit changes in respiratory rate, heart rate and pattern, blood pressure, temperature and oxygen saturation, all owing to a number of physiological factors including pain, pyrexia, dehydration or fluid overload, electrolyte disorders and acid-base imbalance. Frequent monitoring of these parameters, calculating deterioration risk, using NEWS, and the perceived severity of the patient's condition will alert nursing staff to any deterioration.

Obtaining the patient's weight gives useful information regarding fluid status.

One important issue is fluid balance. As discussed earlier, urine output should be at least 0.5mL/kg/hour, but, if this volume is abnormal, the patient may become dehydrated or overloaded. For this reason, the patient's weight should be recorded, as this will reveal important information about their fluid status. It is very helpful to have access to an accurate weight, that reflects the normal weight for the patient *before* they became unwell. The patient may have become fluid depleted or, alternatively, fluid accumulation (oedema) may have significantly increased their normal 'dry' weight. If the severity of the patient's condition prevents them from being weighed, an estimate should be made from their physical appearance (height and body mass). Following this, accurate measurement and charting of fluid gains and losses must be undertaken. The balance is calculated every 24 hours, with the fluid deficit or fluid accumulation being reported to medical staff immediately. Nurses should also be aware of insensible losses, for example, fluid lost through profuse sweating. All of this information needs to be taken into account when reporting fluid balance. Nurses must also always ensure that a urinary catheter is patent before assuming that the patient is oliguric or anuric. Bladder ultrasonography may be requested in order to establish if there is urine in the bladder (Serlin et al. 2018). A bladder washout may be required if the catheter becomes blocked, although this must be risk assessed, due to the high risk of infection associated with breaking the sterile catheter circuit (RCN 2019).

Always maintain an accurate fluid balance chart and take into account insensible losses.

Any urine that is passed is tested for specific gravity, pH and the presence of abnormal constituents, such as blood and protein, both of which can indicate malfunctioning kidneys. Remember, though, that it is important when testing urine to ensure that other causes of abnormal findings have been excluded, such as haematuria secondary to menstruation or urethral trauma following catheterisation. Similarly, there may be proteinuria following contamination of a collecting receptacle. The appearance and smell of urine is also significant; for example, cloudy urine with an offensive odour is likely to indicate that a urinary tract infection is present.

A number of investigations into renal function may also be ordered by the medical staff. Nursing staff require knowledge of all invasive and non-invasive procedures so that they can work collaboratively with medical colleagues in treating the patient and act as a resource should the patient seek further information. Common renal investigations are outlined in Table 8.2.

Table 8.2 Renal investigations

Blood biochemistry	Looking at serum values of sodium, potassium, creatinine, urea and albumin amongst others
Full blood count	To diagnose whether or not the patient is anaemic, has an abnormal white cell count or low platelets – all common findings as renal function deteriorates
Arterial blood gas analysis	To measure the pH of the blood and identify metabolic acidosis consistent with renal failure
Microbiology	Cultures of blood and urine may be required in order to identify specific infections
Histology	A percutaneous renal biopsy may be needed to diagnose tumours and other causes of renal disease
Ultrasound	This test is performed so that the size of the kidneys can be ascertained and so that any obstruction can be located
Angiography	A variety of techniques can be employed to inject contrast media into the renal tract so that its different structures can be visualised more closely. It should be noted that the radio-contrast agent that is used for this investigation can be nephrotoxic and sometimes protective pharmacology, in the form of N-acetylcysteine, is administered prior to the procedure being carried out

Physical examination

In order to identify patients at risk, nurses have a professional responsibility to conduct a thorough holistic assessment, using appropriate diagnostic and decision-making skills (Nursing and Midwifery Council 2018). It is important to remember, however, that, whereas technology may be very useful in assisting this process, it can fail. The nurse must therefore not become complacent and rely exclusively on information gathered in this way, but instead use an array of assessment strategies to recognise and monitor the patient's condition (Browne and Cook 2011). As we have seen in earlier chapters, the ABCDE approach is a comprehensive assessment strategy to employ. This tool, together with the key skills of looking, feeling and listening, can reveal vital information about a patient's condition.

Remember

- Look.
- Feel.
- Listen.

Inspect ('look')

Observing a patient with renal problems can give the nurse vital information, for example, when assessing the patient's ability to maintain their own airway, visual inspection and listening for abnormal airway sounds are important. Immediate action is required with airway compromise. The nurse should take into account the recorded levels of urea and electrolytes in the blood. As we have seen earlier, these can be grossly disturbed in acute renal dysfunction, and particular problems, like a rising urea concentration or a sodium imbalance, can affect the level of consciousness and, subsequently, airway maintenance.

Even if the patient is able to maintain an airway, their breathing may be affected by the renal impairment for several reasons. As a result of metabolic acidosis, the patient may increase their respiratory rate in an attempt to excrete more carbon dioxide *via* the lungs and ultimately increase the pH of the blood.

An increased respiratory rate may be due to metabolic acidosis
For example, the arterial blood gas analysis may reveal

- pH: 7.35 (within range of 7.35–7.45)
- $PaCO_2$: 3.0kPa (reduced, normal range 4–6kPa)
- PaO_2: 11.0kPa
- HCO_3^-: 16mmol/L (reduced, normal range 22–26mmol/L)
- base deficit: -8 mmol/L (reduced, normal range -/+ 2)

This is a compensated metabolic acidosis, as the $PaC0_2$ has moved below its normal range (through hyperventilation) and restored the pH to within normal range.

It is essential to maintain an accurate fluid balance chart because some patients may also be fluid overloaded and this can lead to the development of pulmonary oedema, where fluid fills the alveoli and prevents normal gas exchange.

Observe for respiratory distress, falling oxygen saturations and frothy sputum – a sign of pulmonary oedema.

Hypoxaemia and, eventually, retention of carbon dioxide will occur, and these will be evident on clinical presentation and arterial blood gas analysis. The work of breathing is greatly increased, and the respiratory rate increases but may become shallow; changes to the pattern of breathing and use of the accessory muscles of respiration will be seen, and SpO_2 may fall precipitously. The nurse may also see frothy, pink-tinged secretions expectorated by the patient and these are very characteristic of pulmonary oedema. The patient will be in distress and urgent action is required to maximize SpO_2 with supplemental oxygen in line with the British Thoracic Society emergency oxygen guidelines (2017), with care escalation. On further examination, the patient might appear oedematous, with fluid retention in the face and limbs (the latter particularly in dependent areas, due to gravity). There may also be a noticeable weight gain and as the problem progresses, changes to the vital signs may be evident in the form of hypertension and tachycardia as the workload of the heart is increased. A more detailed discussion on this is included in Chapter 6.

Observe for signs of anaemia, such as pallor, dyspnoea and lethargy.

Although it is more common in chronic renal impairment, the patient with AKI may be pale in appearance and very tired, due to anaemia; as discussed earlier in this chapter, the kidney produces the hormone erythropoietin and the production of this hormone, and consequently red blood cells, may be impaired. A blood sample should be sent for full blood count analysis to confirm suspected anaemia and appropriate treatment started, if necessary. This is a significant clinical issue, because anaemia will further increase the work of breathing for the patient, due to the lack of haemoglobin available for oxygen transport.

Whereas some patients with renal impairment may be fluid overloaded, some, in contrast, will present with fluid depletion owing to a loss of circulating volume, as a result, for example, of severe haemorrhage. When assessing the circulatory function, it might be noted on inspection that the patient's skin is dry with a loss of elasticity. They may have a furred tongue, cracked lips and sometimes sunken eyes. In this case, if there is any urine output, it will be diminished in volume (less than 0.5mL/kg/hour) and appear very dark and concentrated, with a high specific gravity noted on urinalysis. This patient may also present with hypotension and tachycardia, due to hypovolaemia.

Observe for signs of dehydration, such as dry skin, furred tongue, cracked lips and sunken eyes.

A problem common to all patients with renal insufficiency is electrolyte imbalance and this may lead to the development of cardiac arrhythmias (the existing metabolic acidosis will further contribute to cardiac instability because of cellular disruption). If a cardiac monitor is *in situ* or a 12-lead electrocardiograph (ECG) recording is taken, specific changes may be noted, such as arrhythmias or damage to one particular area of the heart. All ECG changes need to be recognised and acted upon quickly, in order to prevent life-threatening arrhythmias, such as ventricular tachycardia, ventricular fibrillation and asystole, from occurring. A more detailed discussion on electrolyte imbalance can be found in Chapter 4 and in Chapter 6 on cardiac electrophysiology.

Monitor the patient for cardiac arrhythmias and record a 12-lead ECG.

Holistic assessment of the patient is important when renal impairment is suspected as the inability of the body to excrete waste products can affect all organs. We have already noted how the patient's level of consciousness may be impaired by the accumulation of urea; the higher the concentration of this substance in the blood, the more likely the patient will become comatose. Individuals with deteriorating renal function can develop uraemic encephalopathy, which occurs when high levels of urea in the blood impair neurotransmission. Similarly, visual inspection of the skin is important, not just for an estimate of the patient's fluid status, but to determine whether or not the uraemia is worsening. The skin can take on a yellow tinge, as can the mucous membranes, as the urea accumulates. The patient may subsequently complain of intense pruritus and this may lead to an increased risk of infection through skin trauma. As the gut is also affected by rising urea levels in the blood, the patient may have signs of gastrointestinal illness such as persistent hiccupping, vomiting and diarrhoea (O'Callaghan 2017).

Palpation and percussion ('feel')

In renal dysfunction, the nurse can gather important assessment data from touching the patient. Feeling the patient's pulse can identify if it is weak, as occurs with volume depletion, bounding, as in volume overload, or irregular, as in the presence of arrhythmias. Touching the skin can detect pyrexia, hypothermia or poor perfusion; the latter can be further assessed by testing capillary refill. Oedema and swelling can also be noted from palpation and percussion.

Always take a patient's pulse manually so that its strength and regularity can be assessed.

It is also important to remember that, from a psychological perspective, touch can be therapeutic for the patient, creating a means of non-verbal reassurance and comfort (Anderson et al. 2016). Touching the patient's hand during the assessment process may relieve anxiety and instill a sense of peace, although the nurse should always be sensitive to the appropriateness of physical contact and explain all actions. From a cultural perspective, touch may be deemed inappropriate by some patients, especially if there is a difference in gender between patient and nurse (Giger 2016).

Auscultation ('listen')

Listening is an important skill for the nurse to acquire and perfect. In the first instance, we need to listen carefully to our patients and note what they are actually saying. Unless a patient is unconscious, they can often report significant symptoms that will facilitate nursing care and assist medical diagnosis and treatment. Patients with renal colic, for example, can inform us of the location, duration and intensity of their pain; similarly, patients with urinary tract infections can recall the unpleasant sensations of the frequency and urgency of micturition. They can also directly evaluate therapeutic interventions and, although some patients are better historians than others, chart the progress of a disorder from onset to resolution.

Listen for:

- Sounds of a partially obstructed airway, such as stridor, snoring, crowing.
- Abnormal breath sounds on auscultation, such as crackles or wheezing

The way in which a patient speaks is also significant, as there may be evidence of confusion or the patient may be very breathless and unable to complete sentences. Even if patients are unable to verbalise, nurses can still gather valuable information through listening to physiological sounds. A patient with a compromised airway, due to uraemic encephalopathy, may start to make a snoring noise as the muscular tone in the oropharynx is reduced. Other noises, indicative of impaired airway patency, include stridor, caused by occlusion, or the high-pitched crowing noise characteristic of laryngeal spasm (Jevon et al. 2012). These problems require the nurse to initiate emergency airway management, an issue discussed in more detail in Chapters 5 and 7.

Auscultating a patient's chest can also reveal useful information. The frothy secretions that occur in pulmonary oedema create adventitious breath sounds, and coarse crackles can be heard when a stethoscope is placed appropriately on the chest wall. Wheezing may also be heard if there is a degree of bronchoconstriction present.

CASE STUDY 8.1 MR HEIDEN WITH AN ACUTE KIDNEY INJURY SECONDARY TO VOLUME DEPLETION 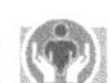

PATIENT HISTORY AND INITIAL ASSESSMENT

Mr Heiden, a 65-year-old Human Resources manager, has been admitted to the acute assessment ward (AMU) from the emergency department, accompanied by his wife. He has been admitted with confusion secondary to a suspected urinary tract infection.

10:00

On his transfer to the ward, you are told his vital signs and NEWS (4) (RCP 2017); as soon as he is settled, you perform an ABCDE assessment.

10:15

Airway: His airway is clear, with no added sounds that would suggest partial patency. He is able to talk and cough but is complaining that he wants to 'get out of this place'. You explain that you are doing your best to help, which seems to settle him a little, as he allows you to continue your assessment.

Breathing: His breathing does not appear laboured, with no evidence of accessory muscle use. His respiratory rate, though, is raised at 22 per min with his SpO_2 of 96% on room air. His target oxygen saturation is 94–98%, and Scale 1 is being used to record his respiratory observations on NEWS.

Breathing NEWS: (2+0+0) = 2

Circulation: He looks flushed, and feels warm peripherally, but is not sweaty. You offer to remove his blankets as he says he feels warm. You take his pulse manually to assess rate and rhythm, and find it to be strong, regular but a little fast at 105 bpm.

His blood pressure is recorded at 98/60mmHg with a MAP of 73mmHg. He has a past medical history of hypertension, so this is lower than expected.

He has not been able to eat and drink normally. His wife tells the nurse caring for him that he has only had sips of water due to nausea for the past three days. He is confused and now refuses to drink; he has not passed any urine for about eight hours, but, on being offered a bottle, he produces 50 mL of concentrated urine. You check his weight; at 80kg, you would have expected 40mL of urine for each hour. You ask the HCA to perform urinalysis and discover a specific gravity of 1.020, +ve for nitrates, protein and leucocytes. The urine smells offensive, and a sample is sent for microscopy. This is all consistent with his initial diagnosis of urinary tract infection. An IV cannula was inserted in the emergency department and a stat dose of IV Co-amoxiclav, a broad-spectrum antibiotic, was given about 20 minutes ago. He has been prescribed for a fluid challenge of 500mL Plama-Lyte, but this has not yet been given, so you prioritise this on completion of your assessment.

Circulation NEWS: (2+1) = 3

Disability: Mr Heiden is unable to tell you where he is, but he does know that he is not at home. He is confused about the time of day but is reassured that his wife is present. He does not seem to understand where he is, or why he is there. After consulting with his wife, you ascertain that this level of confusion has only been present for a few hours, so you assess him as having new confusion. His blood sugar was checked in the emergency department and was within normal range

Disability NEWS = 3

Exposure: His temperature is 37.7°C, slightly higher than the normal range. You check his skin from head to toes and ask if he has any other problems. Nothing significant is seen.

Exposure NEWS=0

TOTAL NEWS** = 2+3+3=0=**8

This is an increase of 4 from his NEWS in the emergency department. This is due to an increase in his respiratory rate and a drop in BP. The SpR walks onto the ward just as you are looking up his admission blood results, before calling her. NEWS of 8 requires an **emergency response**. They tell you that the chest X-ray taken previously has no abnormalities reported and together you review the blood results. You ask a colleague to prepare the Plasma-Lyte for commencement of the fluid challenge.

Blood results reveal:

Haemoglobin: 14.5g/dL (range: 13.0–17.5g/dL)
White cell count: 12.5×10^9/L (range: 4.5–11.0 ×10^9/L) **raised,** consistent with infection.
Platelets: 325 ×10^9/L (range: 140–450 ×10^9/L)
Sodium: 142mmol/L (range: 135–145mmol/L)
Potassium: 5.0mmol/L (range 3.5–5.1mmol/L)
Urea: 17.9 (range: 3.2–7.0mmol/L) **raised**, consistent with dehydration and possibly poor renal function
Creatinine: 189 (range: 63–111μmol/L) **raised** (?x1.5–2), but no baseline value is available for comparison. This value is consistent with AKI

Glucose: 7mmol/L (range: 4–8mmol/L)
Inflammatory marker C-reactive protein: 100 (range 0–8mg/L) **raised**, consistent with a bacterial infection

These blood results, together with the history and the initial physical examination, confirm that the problem is probably of an infective origin. They also confirm that there is renal impairment, with the development of borderline elevated serum potassium, and increased urea and creatinine levels. Given the history and the blood analysis, dehydration is the most likely cause of his AKI. Mr Heiden has lost body fluids through the borderline pyrexia, and lack of oral fluids.

The SpR is keen for the fluid challenge to be given as soon as possible. An influx of patients from a recent traffic collision had maybe influenced this early transfer to AMU. The SpR asks you to raise the end of his bed to 45^0, in a passive leg raise manoeuvre, and a quick assessment of BP saw a rise to 110mmg systolic, and a reduction in his HR to 100, suggesting a positive response. The Plasma-Lyte is given, 500mL over 15 minutes. The SpR explains that they are concerned about his risk of sepsis and takes an arterial blood sample. You note that the NEWS>5 means that sepsis should be considered and, with the existing evidence of infection, required action. You were pleased that the antibiotics and fluids were already being acted upon and made a note to check whether blood cultures had been taken, before the antibiotics were given.

10:30

Assessment after fluid challenge

A: clear
B: respiratory rate 21, SpO_2 96% on air: NEWS (2+0+0) =2
C: HR 82bpm, BP 105/68mmHg, no further urine passed: NEWS (1+0) =1
D: remains confused: NEWS =3
E: no change

Total NEWS=6

The SpR has stayed on the ward to review the response to fluid challenge and his ABGs.

Arterial blood gas analysis reveals

pH: 7.32 (range: 7.35–7.45)
$PaCO_2$: 4.5 (range: 4.5–6.1kPa)
PaO_2: 10.5 (range: 11–13kPa)
HCO_3-: 19 (range: 22–26mmol/L)
BE: -4 (range: -2 to +2mmol/L)
Lactate: 1.3mol/L

10:35

The ABG analysis show an acidosis (pH: 7.34), which, as the $HC0_3^-$ and BE are lowered, demonstrates a metabolic acidosis. The lactate is within the normal range and so sepsis is discounted for now. The metabolic acidosis, though, is consistent with dehydration. The positive response, with the NEWS falling by 2 in response to the first fluid challenge, is noted.

Mr Heiden is moved to the monitored area of the ward and continuous vital sign monitoring continues throughout this period. He is then given a further 1 litre of the same crystalloid solution, in two fluid boluses over the next hour. The critical care outreach team have been alerted due to the elevated NEWS score. They recommend a urinary catheter is placed to observe his urine output hourly and that he remains continually monitored, under their review, until his NEWS score decreases below 4.

11:35

Following further fluid administration, his vital signs are as follows:

- SpO_2: 97% on room air, RR 19 (NEWS 0).
- Heart rate: 82 beats per minute, sinus rhythm.
- Blood pressure: 112/75mmHg, no urine output (NEWS 0) (but no urine is a cause for concern)
- Remains mildly confused, but more settled (NEWS 3).

NEWS Score = 3

There is, however, no improvement in his urinary output. Caution is required with further IV fluid therapy, due to his anuria. A bladder scan confirms an empty bladder, and, after some discussion, the urinary catheter is inserted, and a further 20mL drained. A decision is made that no other immediate treatment be instigated at this time and the plan is to refer him to the renal consultant for further assessment and management of the oligo/anuria.

The nurse documents all findings and prepares to inform colleagues, at the nursing handover, that Mr Heiden has been diagnosed with acute kidney injury secondary to hypovolaemia. The initial plan is to cautiously continue with the administration of intravenous fluids to fully rehydrate him and to closely monitor his renal function over the next 24–48 hours. If this does not improve, with the target goal of a urine output of at least 0.5mL/kg/hour, further medical management of his renal dysfunction will be required.

17:30

Mr Heiden has a significant increase in his urine output over the next 6 hours, exceeding the 0.5mL/kg/hour target. His NEWS score decreases to 0, with a resolution of his acute confusion. He is discharged from the critical care outreach team review list and de-escalated to a level 0 bed with ward level monitoring. His serum urea has normalised, and the creatinine is falling towards the normal range. He is now drinking oral fluids and has asked his wife to bring in his favourite snacks. The blood cultures came back negative, but his urine showed growth of *Proteus mirabilis* sensitive to Co-amoxiclav.

Mr Heiden is discharged home 48 hours later, on a continuing course of oral antibiotics, with patient education regarding hydration and nutrition. A discharge letter is sent to his General Practitioner, detailing the events of his in-patient stay, with instructions for ongoing monitoring for any long-term renal deterioration.

Optimising renal status

The aims of treating a patient with acute renal impairment are the early recognition of the problem and the restoration of normal fluid and electrolyte status. All therapeutic interventions are focused on rectifying the kidneys' inability to excrete the waste products of metabolism and on preventing further kidney injury from developing. For some patients, this will not be possible and they will go on to develop chronic renal dysfunction, but, for a large number of individuals who have sustained a perfusion injury in acute illness, early effective medical intervention and good nursing care can prevent further deterioration and ultimately preserve renal function.

Fluid replacement

There has been some debate in recent years as to which type of intravenous fluid a hypovolaemic patient should be given to increase their circulating volume, namely **colloid** or **crystalloid** solutions (NICE 2013b). Blood products and other colloid infusions, like gelofusine, contain larger molecules and are therefore able to increase blood pressure without the administration of large volumes of fluid. They do this by expanding the plasma compartment and increasing the plasma osmolality; their large molecules generate an oncotic pressure and pull water from the interstitial compartment and subsequently increase the circulating volume (Lewis et al. 2018). Colloids are now seldom used initially in acute practice for this purpose, due to the risks of:

- Allergic reaction for some patients.
- Clotting impairment.
- Reduction of haemoglobin levels through haemodilution.

Recent guidance by NICE (2013b, updated in 2017) recommends the use of balanced crystalloid fluids for fluid resuscitation and fluid maintenance.

Crystalloid solutions include normal saline 0.9%, Compound Sodium Lactate (Hartmann's), Plasma-Lyte and Dextrose Saline. These are isotonic in nature, that is, they have a concentration of solutes very similar to plasma. Crystalloids increase the circulating volume, but, as the molecules are small, they move through the capillary wall into the interstitial fluid. It has been suggested that larger volumes of these solutions are required to have the same circulatory effect as colloids. They contain similar sodium concentrations to the extracellular fluid and are distributed to all body compartments, their plasma expansion effects being quite short lived. Balanced crystalloid solutions, such as Compound Sodium Lactate and Plasma-Lyte, have been recommended for fluid replacement due to the risk of hyperchloraemia and hypernatraemia in patients treated with large volumes of 0.9% saline (NICE 2013b). As with all fluid administration, the risk of fluid overload is present, and this should be assessed during IV fluid administration, with an accurate record kept of fluid balance.

A 24-hour urine collection may be requested to identify creatinine clearance.

Which then is better – colloid or crystalloid? In fact, there is little clinical evidence to suggest that either is superior, although, in recent years, crystalloid fluid has prevailed as the preferred intravenous fluid replacement. Both have advantages and disadvantages that nursing staff need to be aware of when administering.

One useful guide to fluid restoration is to replace what has been lost from the body. For example, if haemorrhage has occurred, then blood will be required due to the loss of blood components and clotting factors. In contrast, if a patient has severe dehydration through persistent diarrhoea and vomiting (as with Mr Heiden in the case study), then crystalloid fluid replacement is required.

Remember

Pyrexia increases fluid loss through sweating and increased respiratory rate.

Whatever is prescribed, the nurse must ensure that strict monitoring and charting of all fluids lost (including any wound, nasogastric drainage or diarrhoea) and all fluids administered is carried out in order to avoid further physiological complications. Twenty-four-hour urine collections are often requested in order to gain additional information about fluid and electrolyte balance, especially creatinine clearance. The nurse should also be aware of insensible fluid losses, particularly in the presence of pyrexia, when assessing a patient's fluid status. Historically, a patient receiving fluid resuscitation will have had a central venous catheter sited so that accurate assessment of central venous pressure and fluid status can be determined. In recent years, however, research has disputed the accuracy of this monitoring and it has been removed from many international guidelines as a recommended measure of fluid status (De Backer and Vincent 2018). Fluid challenges (for example, 500mL of balanced crystalloids, given over 15–30 minutes intravenously) are often administered in the first instance, so that cardiac and renal response to volume loading can be safely assessed prior to the administration of larger volumes of fluid (NICE 2013b). If a patient is known to have a compromised cardiac status, smaller volumes of fluid, such as 250mL, would be given as a fluid challenge (NICE 2013b). More recently, the use of passive leg raising as a measure of fluid responsiveness has been suggested as an accurate and low-risk approach to fluid status monitoring. This is where the legs are raised to 45° while the patient is in a semi-recumbent position, and monitoring of the blood pressure over the next 30–90 seconds determines fluid responsiveness, by looking for an increase in blood pressure during this time (Rameau et al. 2017).

A fluid challenge or passive leg raise (PLR) may be requested to determine response to volume loading.

Correction of abnormal electrolyte levels

In the fluid and electrolyte chapter (Chapter 4), we learned of the significance of maintaining optimal electrolyte levels in the body. Abnormal levels, whether they are too high or too low, can be life threatening for the patient. Sodium, potassium, calcium and magnesium, in particular, are required for cellular stability, and levels that are out of the normal range can lead to severe problems with cardiac, renal and neuromuscular function. The nurse will need to be vigilant for any signs of electrolyte imbalance, such as lethargy, muscle weakness, paraesthesia, gastrointestinal symptoms and, most significantly, hypotension and arrhythmias. Together with careful observation of fluid balance, cardiac monitoring should be in process and regular 12-lead ECG readings taken.

In acute renal impairment, the following may be seen:

- Sodium levels may be high or low, depending on whether or not the kidney is able to reabsorb sodium back into the blood, a process that should naturally occur in health. In advancing states of renal dysfunction, the kidney is often unable to reabsorb the sodium and the patient develops a polyuria, the ability of the body to conserve water being lost. In all cases, careful fluid management is required.

Some patients with renal dysfunction can present with polyuria as their condition worsens.

- Potassium reabsorption and secretion should be regulated by the kidney, but, when function is impaired, levels will start to rise in the blood and this can lead to fatal arrhythmias, among other problems. A significantly high potassium level (greater than 5.5mmols/L) needs to be treated urgently, usually by the administration of one of the following pharmacological interventions. Firstly, intravenous dextrose and insulin in combination or, secondly, administration of the beta 2 agonist salbutamol (nebulised or intravenous). Either therapy can be used in prescribed doses to lower the serum potassium level. These agents will work by promoting potassium transport from the serum into the intracellular space. Calcium (10mL of calcium gluconate 10% by slow intravenous injection) may also be given, where ECG changes are present, because this has cardioprotective properties. It will prolong the plateau phase of the action potential and therefore prevent any tachyarrhythmias from occurring. Any of these drugs will have a temporary effect but will allow time for the underlying cause to be identified and specific treatment commenced (Deprèt et al. 2019).

Abnormal electrolyte levels can be life threatening and require immediate correction.

- Serum calcium levels are usually normal in patients with acute kidney injury, but patients who are developing a chronic renal impairment often present with low levels of this cation in their blood, due to inadequate vitamin D production by the kidneys. Calcium replacements will then be required. This problem is often accompanied by rising levels of phosphate in the blood.
- Magnesium levels may be low in patients with renal disease, especially those who consume excessive amounts of alcohol.

Other pharmacological interventions

Drugs are metabolised in different ways, according to their molecular properties; some are protein bound, some lipid soluble and some water soluble. Many of them are excreted by the kidney and, if there is renal impairment, toxic levels of the agent can accumulate in the blood. Impaired glomerular filtration and ineffectual tubular secretion can lead to certain drugs reaching harmful levels, in addition to which patients with renal problems can often develop increased sensitivity to drugs, with poor tolerance of their side effects.

Two key issues to address, then, are, firstly, what is being prescribed and whether or not adjustments need to be made to the drug dosage in the interests of patient safety? Secondly, are any known nephrotoxic agents currently being taken by or given to the patient? Drugs such as ampicillin, gentamicin and digoxin can all reach toxic levels and need to be monitored closely. Others, like non-steroidal anti-inflammatory drugs, can lead to direct kidney injury and would need to be stopped immediately (Jevon et al. 2012).

The nurse should check that nephrotoxic drugs have been stopped or are being monitored very closely.

Some pharmacological agents are used in the treatment of renal impairment, the choice of which depends on the type of kidney injury and the severity of the problem:

- *Oxygen therapy*, previously discussed in Chapter 5, may be prescribed for some patients in order to optimise gas exchange, where fluid overload has impaired oxygenation. Careful monitoring of the patient's colour, perfusion and SpO_2 readings must be carried out and arterial blood gas analysis, where required, adhering to the BTS guidelines on emergency oxygen therapy (O'Driscoll et al. 2017).
- *Diuretic therapy*, in the form of furosemide, is often prescribed if patients are deemed to be fluid overloaded, especially if there is a degree of pulmonary oedema secondary to heart failure. This drug is classified as a loop diuretic and it works by inhibiting reabsorption from the ascending limb of the loop of Henle in the renal tubule. It has several side effects, most significantly hypokalaemia (because it is not a potassium-sparing diuretic), hyponatraemia, hypocalcaemia, hypomagnesaemia and hypotension, all as a result of excessive diuresis. Another side effect of furosemide, if given in large enough doses, is ototoxicity, which may damage hearing. When diuretic therapy is prescribed, the nurse should be aware of the possibility of hypotension and excessive electrolyte loss in the urine.

There are many reasons diuretics are prescribed for patients in renal insufficiency. Patients with chronic kidney disease (CKD) and/or congestive heart failure may require diuretics to maintain circulatory function; these are often taken daily and monitored through fluctuations in the patient's daily weight and symptom management. Traditionally, a loop diuretic, given in response to low urine output, was a standard treatment in acute hospitals. This practice is now disputed and the use of loop diuretics to prevent or treat AKI is not recommended unless the patient is in acute fluid overload or awaiting the start of renal replacement therapy (NICE 2013a; KDIGO 2012)

- *Correction of metabolic acidosis* may be necessary. This problem is common to all types of renal impairment and cannot be left untreated, because it will impair tissue perfusion and have a depressant effect on the myocardium. In the first instance, it can often be remedied by fluid therapy, as this will restore tissue and renal perfusion. However, if the patient is fluid overloaded, then diuretic therapy may be required to promote the

excretion of metabolic acids. Of more concern, though, is the severe acidosis (pH less than 7.10) that is resistant to these preliminary interventions; in such cases, intravenous sodium bicarbonate may be administered, and transfer to a higher level of care may be required. This solution will buffer the excess hydrogen ions that have accumulated and therefore increase the pH of the blood. Caution must be taken, however, as side effects include metabolic alkalosis, with respiratory compensation, and an increased serum sodium level, which may ultimately affect fluid balance in the body (Leach 2014).
- *Vasopressor therapy* is occasionally used to manage renal impairment under higher levels of care, although it is not widely recommended. There is sometimes a need to increase the mean arterial pressure to improve renal perfusion; in such cases, noradrenaline may be prescribed (Leach 2014). The use of dopamine at a 'renal dose' (2–5 μg/kg/minute) is not recommended and should not be offered to patients to prevent or treat any stage of acute kidney injury (NICE 2013a).

Remember

For accurate and safe administration of inotropic drugs, the dose must be calculated in μg/kg/minute. Patients with vasoactive/inotropic drug therapy require a higher level of care, such as high dependency or ITU.

Renal replacement therapy

Renal replacement therapy will be required if the acute kidney injury fails to respond to fluid therapy and pharmacological interventions. With this treatment, fluid and solutes are removed from the patient's blood as it passes through a membrane or filter, and the filtered blood is then returned into the systemic circulation. It may take the form of peritoneal dialysis, haemofiltration or haemodialysis, although haemofiltration is the mode of choice for acutely ill patients as this removes substances in a slower, continuous way, which is better tolerated if there is any haemodynamic instability (O'Callaghan 2017; Leach 2014). Transfer to a higher level of care will be required for many of these therapies.

Renal replacement therapy should be considered when the following symptoms of AKI do not respond to medical therapy (NICE 2013b):

- Hyperkalaemia.
- Metabolic acidosis.
- Symptoms or complications of uraemia (for example, pericarditis or encephalopathy).
- Fluid overload.
- Pulmonary oedema.

Holistic nursing care for patients with renal dysfunction

Patients with a diagnosis of renal dysfunction require skilled nursing care. Continual assessment of the patient's condition and careful planning, implementation and evaluation of nursing interventions is essential if actual and potential problems are to be addressed and the patient's safety ensured. Accurate documentation and record keeping are also part of this process, as is effective communication with all members of the multidisciplinary team (Nursing and Midwifery Council 2018).

Physically, renal patients present with many signs and symptoms which may lead, not only to systemic instability and a risk of further deterioration, but will leave them feeling very weak, tired and generally unwell. Full nursing care is required, with particular attention being paid to the skin, which may easily break down or become infected, and oral care is needed, especially if the patient has impaired consciousness, is dehydrated or receiving oxygen therapy. In most cases the patients will also have a degree of anorexia and malnutrition, requiring the nurse to encourage oral intake (if oral diet is permitted) or to provide enteral or parenteral nutrition. Specialist advice should be sought from the dietician when addressing the dietary needs of renal patients, especially with regard to the protein, potassium and sodium content of food and drinks, as these need to be carefully calculated on an individual basis, according to the patient's renal function. Once the diet has been reviewed, the nurse then has an important role in health education and health promotion, as the patient may find it difficult to adhere to the regime (Nursing and Midwifery Council 2018).

To effectively address the dietary needs of renal patients, specialist advice must be sought from the dietician, as specific guidelines exist for different renal conditions (KDIGO 2012).

Psychosocially, the patient may have other needs. They may be very concerned about the diagnosis of renal dysfunction because, unless a good response to initial treatment is seen, long-term dialysis may be required with the introduction of strict dietary and fluid restrictions. These treatments will have a considerable impact on the patient's lifestyle, in some cases raising difficulties with personal relationships or with their employment status, and possibly leading to financial hardship. In addition, the patient may ultimately undergo renal transplantation if a suitable donor can be found and will then have further treatment modalities to adhere to post-operatively. If the patient (and their family) wishes to discuss any concerns, the nurse needs to spend time listening and, where appropriate, to offer advice and guidance, with appropriate referral to colleagues, such as the social worker, where necessary. It is important that, as a health care provider, the nurse works across professional boundaries and acts as a change agent within the multidisciplinary team, providing leadership and direction to care delivery (Nursing and Midwifery Council 2018).

A diagnosis of renal failure can have a profound psychological effect on the patient, especially if long-term dialysis is required.

Conclusion

In this chapter, we have reviewed the anatomy and physiology of the renal system and explored the ways in which acute dysfunction may manifest itself. Investigations into renal function and how the patient's clinical condition might be improved by nursing and medical intervention has also been addressed.

In summary, the kidneys play a key role in maintaining fluid, electrolyte and acid-base balance, as well as in producing and regulating several hormones within the body. When problems occur with any of these functions, patients often become acutely unwell and they are at an increased risk of further deterioration. Nurses must therefore have the requisite skills and knowledge to conduct a thorough assessment of each patient, collecting and recording subjective and objective data that will contribute towards accurate diagnosis, optimal management and effective evaluation of care. Through constant liaison and communication with other members of the multidisciplinary team, a holistic, cohesive approach can be adopted that will ultimately enhance the delivery of quality care.

Glossary 

Active transport Using energy in the form of adenosine triphosphate (ATP) to move fluid and solutes between cellular compartments.

Acute kidney injury An abrupt reduction in kidney function, characterised by a rising serum creatinine level and a reduction in the urine output.

Anuria Less than 100mL of urine in 24 hours.

Colloid A solution with large insoluble molecules that can generate an osmotic pressure and expand the plasma compartment.

Computerised tomography (CT) scan A specialised X-ray where pictures are taken from a multidimensional perspective.

Creatinine A waste product of muscle metabolism secreted by the kidney.

Crystalloid An aqueous solution that contains mineral salts and other water-soluble molecules.

Diffusion The movement of solutes from a state of higher concentration to one of lower concentration.

Diuretic A drug that increases urine output.

Erythropoietin A hormone, produced in the kidney, that promotes erythrogenesis in the bone marrow.

Filtration (renal) The forcing of blood and the substances in it through the glomerular-capsular membrane under arterial pressure.

Glomerular filtration rate (GFR) The rate at which substances pass through the filtration membrane and enter the proximal convoluted tubule.

Glomerulonephritis Inflammation of the glomerulus.

Haematuria The presence of blood in the urine.

Inotropic therapy Drugs that work on the contractility of the myocardium, ultimately improving cardiac performance.

Intravenous pyelogram (IVP) Investigation of the kidney and ureters for obstructive lesions (using contrast media).

National Early Warning System (NEWS) A scoring system that detects early deterioration in a patient's condition.

Nephrotic syndrome An inflammatory disease of the glomerulus characterised by proteinuria, hypoalbuminaemia, oedema and hyperlipidaemia.

Oligoanuria Less than 100mL of urine in 24 hours.

Oliguria 100–400mL of urine in 24 hours.

Osmolality The concentration of solutes in a kilogram of water.

Osmosis The distribution of water from a lesser area of solute concentration to an area of higher concentration.

Proteinuria The presence of protein in the urine.

Renal calculi Stones made up of calcium and other minerals that can obstruct the ureters.

Renal replacement therapy An extra-corporeal circuit used to filter excess fluid and waste products from the blood.

Renin A protein produced by the juxtaglomerular apparatus that leads to the formation of angiotensin 2.

Specific gravity A measurement of urine osmolality.

Tubular reabsorption Reabsorption of the filtrate back into the peritubular capillaries.

Tubular secretion Substances are filtered out of the blood into the tubular fluid for secretion.

Ultrasound The production of an image from ultrasound waves that are created by structures within the body.

Urea A waste product of protein metabolism.

Vasa recta A network of blood vessels found in the cortex and medullary regions of the kidney.

Vasopressin Also known as the antidiuretic hormone, this polypeptide controls water reabsorption and secretion

TEST YOURSELF 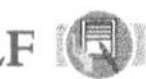

1 The nephron is the functional unit of the kidney. Which of the following structures is not part of the tubular area?
   a. glomerulus
   b. proximal convoluted tubule
   c. loop of Henle
   d. vasa recta
   e. distal convoluted tubule
   f. collecting duct

2 The ureters and bladder have three layers, name them.

3 Name the three stages of urine production.

4 During urine production, which of the following substances are filtered out into the tubular fluid?
   a. blood
   b. albumin
   c. creatinine

5 What is the average glomerular filtration rate for an adult male?
   a. 125mL per minute
   b. 160mL per minute
   c. 180mL per minute

6 Which substance regulates water reabsorption or excretion in the body?
   a. Renin
   b. Erythropoietin
   c. vasopressin

7 Which of the following is not a usual symptom of a urinary tract infection?
   a. pyrexia
   b. oliguria
   c. back pain
   d. increased leucocytes in the blood

8 When diagnosing acute kidney injury, which blood test result is the most significant?
   a. urea
   b. creatinine
   c. sodium
   d. albumin

9 When conducting a nursing assessment of a patient with renal dysfunction, which of the following is not a sign of a volume responsive injury?
   a. urine output less than 0.5mL/kg/hour
   b. raised serum potassium

c. weak dilute urine
d. metabolic acidosis

10 Which of the following drugs could be used *directly to* lower high serum potassium levels?
a. intravenous dextrose and insulin in combination
b. intravenous delivery of nebulised salbutamol
c. intravenous calcium gluconate

Answers

1 d
2 the tunica mucosa; the tunica muscularis; the tunica adventitia
3 tubular filtration; tubular reabsorption; tubular secretion
4 c
5 a
6 c
7 c
8 b
9 c
10 a

References

Anderson, J., Friesen, M. A., Swengros, D., Herbst, A., Mangione, L. (2016). Examination of the use of healing touch by registered nurses in the acute care setting. *Journal of Holistic Nursing*, 35(1), 97–107.

British Thoracic Society. (2017). BTS guidelines for oxygen use in adults in healthcare and emergency settings. *Thorax*, 72(Suppl. 1), i1–i90.

Browne, M., Cook, P. (2011). Inappropriate trust in technology: implications for critical care nurses. *Nursing in Critical Care*, 16(2), 92–98.

De Backer, D., Vincent, J. L. (2018). Should we measure the central venous pressure to guide fluid management? Ten answers to 10 questions. *Critical Care*, 22, 43.

Deprèt, F., Peacock, F., Liu, K., Rafique, Z., Rossignol, P., Legrand, M. (2019). Management of hyperkalemia in the acutely ill patient. *Annals of Intensive Care*, 9, 32.

Donald, R. (2011). Caring for the renal system. In Macintosh, M., Moore, T., (Eds.), *Caring for the Seriously Ill Patient*, 2nd Edition. London: Hodder Arnold, p. 80.

Giger, J. (2016). *Transcultural Nursing Assessment and Intervention*, 7th Edition. St Louis, MO, USA: Mosby.

Jevon, P., Ewens, B., Singh Pooni, J. (2012). *Monitoring the Critically Ill Patient*, 3rd Edition. Oxford: Blackwell Publishing.

Kidney Disease Improving Global Outcomes (KDIGO). (2012). KDIGO clinical practice guidelines for acute kidney injury. *Kidney International*, 2, 1–124. Available from https://kdigo.org/wp-content/uploads/2016/10/KDIGO-2012-AKI-Guideline-English.pdf.

Leach, R. (2014). *Acute and Critical Care Medicine at a Glance*, 3rd Edition. Oxford: Wiley.

Lewis, S. R., Pritchard, M. W., Evans, D. J. W., Butler, A. R., Alderson, P., Smith, A. F., Roberts, I. (2018). Colloids versus crystalloids for fluid resuscitation in critically ill people. *Cochrane Database of Systematic Reviews*. Available from https://www.cochranelibrary.com/cdsr/doi/10.1002/14651858.CD000567.pub7/full.

Loveday, H., Wilson, J., Pratt, R., Golsorkhi, M., Tingle, A., Bak, A., Browne, J., Prieto, J., Wilcox, M. (2013). Epic3: national evidence-based guidelines for preventing healthcare-associated infections in NHS hospitals in England. *Journal of Hospital Infection*, 8651 Supplement 1, S1–S70.

McCance, K. L., Huether, S. E. (2018). *Pathophysiology: The Biologic Basis for Disease in Adults and Children*, 8th Edition. St Louis, MO, USA: Mosby.

NCEPOD. (2009). *Adding Insult to Injury: A Review of He Care Of Patients Who Died in Hospital with a Primary Diagnosis of Acute Kidney Injury (Acute Renal Failure)*. Available form https://www.ncepod.org.uk/2009report1/Downloads/AKI_summary.pdf.

NICE. (2013a). *Acute Kidney Injury: Prevention, Detection and Management*. Available from https://www.nice.org.uk/guidance/cg169/resources/acute-kidney-injury-prevention-detection-and-management-pdf-35109700165573.

NICE. (2013b). *Intravenous Fluid Therapy in Adults in Hospital*. Available from https://www.nice.org.uk/guidance/cg174/resources/intravenous-fluid-therapy-in-adults-in-hospital-pdf-35109752233669.

Nursing and Midwifery Council. (2018). *Future Nurse: Standards of Proficiency for Registered Nurses*. Available from https://www.nmc.org.uk/globalassets/sitedocuments/education-standards/future-nurse-proficiencies.pdf.

O'Callaghan, C. (2017). *The Renal System at a Glance*, 4th Edition. Oxford: Blackwell.

O'Driscoll, R., Howard, L., Earis, J., Mak, V., Bajwah, S., Beasley, R., Curtis, K., Davison, A., Dorward, A., Dyer, C., Evans, A., Falconer, L., Fitzpatrick, C., Gibbs, S., Hinshaw, K., Howard, R., Kane, B., Keep, J., Kelly, C., Khachi, H., Asad, M., Khan, I., Kishen, R., Mansfield, L., Martin, B., Moore, F., Powrie, D., Restrick, L., Roffe, C., Singer, M., Soar, J., Small, I., Ward, L., Whitmore, D., Wedzicha, W., Wijesinghe, M., BTS Emergency Oxygen Guideline Development Group On behalf of the British Thoracic Society. (2017). BTS guideline for oxygen use in adults in healthcare an emergency settings. *Thorax*, 72(S1), i1–i20.

Rameau, A., De With, E., Boerma, E. C. (2017). Passive leg raise testing effectively reduces fluid administration in septic shock after correction of non-compliance to test results. *Annals of Intensive Care*, 7, 2.

RCN. (2019). *Catheter Care, RCN Guidance for Health Care Professionals*. Available from https://www.rcn.org.uk/professional-development/publications/PUB-007313.

Royal College of Physicians. (2017). *National Early Warning Score (NEWS) 2 Standardising the Assessment of Acute-Illness Severity in the NHS*. Available from http://www.rcplondon.ac.uk/resources/national-early-warning-score-news. Accessed on 14 January 2019.

Serlin, D., Heidelbaugh, J., Stoffel, J. (2018). Urinary retention in adults: evaluation and initial management. *American Family Physician*, 98(8), 596–503.

Thomas, M., Blaine, C., Dawnay, A., Devonald, M., Fthou, S., Laing, C., Latchem, S., Lewington, A., Milford, D., Ostermann, M. (2015). The definition of acute kidney injury and its use in practice. *Kidney International*, 87(1), 62–73.

Tortora, G., Gerard, J., Derrickson, B. (2017). *Principles of Anatomy and Physiology*, 15th Edition. Chichester: Wiley.

Further reading

Himmelfarb, J., Alp Ikizler, T. (2019). *Chronic Kidney Disease, Dialysis, and Transplantation*, 4th Edition. Amsterdam: Elsevier.

Reneke, H. G., Denker, B. M. (2019). *Renal Pathology. The Essentials*, 5th Edition. Philadelphia, PA: Lippincott.

Thomas, N. (2019). *Renal Nursing: Care and Management of People with Kidney Disease*, 5th Edition. Oxford: Wiley-Blackwell.

9 The patient with acute neurological problems

Kit Tong

AIM

This chapter aims to provide you with improved knowledge of the structure and function of the nervous system, allowing you to relate normal physiology to the pathophysiology of neurological disease or injury and understand the nurse's role in the assessment and management of patients with deteriorating neurological status.

OBJECTIVES

After reading this chapter you will be able to:

- Describe the anatomy of the nervous system.
- Describe the structure of a neurone and the physiology of nerve impulses, and relate this to the pathophysiology of neuromuscular disease.
- Explain the normal function of the autonomic nervous system and relate this to the **stress response** seen in acute illness.
- Describe the techniques used in neurological assessment.
- Explain the pathophysiology and clinical management of neurological emergencies.
- Identify clinical interventions to optimise neurological function.

Introduction

The nervous system communicates with and controls all other body systems. It is essential for consciousness, cognitive thought and memory, movement and manual dexterity, perception and behaviour. Together with the endocrine system, it is responsible for homeostasis, the maintenance of a stable internal environment irrespective of external conditions. It is a rapid response system that responds to a crisis without hesitation, yet is also essential for relaxation and sleep. This chapter focuses on the cells that make up the nervous system and the way in which the nervous system is organised. The structure and function of the central and peripheral nervous system are discussed, and an overview of the autonomic nervous system is presented. Common neurological diseases and injuries are reviewed, and neurological assessment described. Competence in neurological assessment is an important nursing skill and is essential for the early detection and management of neurological and medical emergencies.

Applied anatomy and physiology of the nervous system

The nervous system has two main subdivisions; the **central nervous system (CNS)** and the **peripheral nervous system (PNS)**. The brain and spinal cord form the CNS and the cranial nerves, **spinal nerves** and their branches form the PNS. The PNS is subdivided into the autonomic and **somatic nervous systems**.

The function of the nervous system can be considered under three main headings: sensory, integrative and motor.

- *Sensory*: **sensory receptors** detect information internally and externally. For example, sensory receptors in the brain detect body temperature while sensory receptors in the skin detect environmental temperature. Sensory information is transmitted to the brain by cranial and spinal nerves.
- *Integrative*: sensory information received by the brain is analysed, some information is stored, and decisions are made about the type of response that is required. This process is called integration. Perception is essential for cognitive thought and is an important integrative function.
- *Motor*: having received and integrated the sensory information, the brain decides whether a motor response is necessary, and appropriate muscles or glands are stimulated via cranial and spinal nerves.

These three key activities provide a continuous mechanism of feedback and regulation to maintain **homeostasis** and manage emergencies.

Cells of the nervous system

There are two main cell types within the nervous system: **neurones** and **glial cells**.

Neurones

It is estimated that the central nervous system (CNS) contains 100 billion neurones. Neurones vary in shape and size depending on their location and function. All neurones have the same structure: a **cell body**, which is the main part of the neurone, **dendrites** that bring information to the cell body and an **axon** that carries **nerve** impulses away from the cell body. There are two types of neurons, motor and sensory (see Figure 9.1).

The neurone *cell body* is similar to other cells and contains a nucleus with a prominent nucleolus, mitochondria, Golgi apparatus, free ribosomes and rough and smooth endoplasmic reticulum and lysosomes, all surrounded by cytoplasm and contained by a cell membrane. Neurones synthesise vast amounts of protein to maintain cell membrane proteins, intracellular organelles and **neurotransmitters** and to support the neural processes that extend from the cell body. Protein is synthesised by large numbers of free ribosomes and rough endoplasmic reticulum called **Nissl bodies** or granules.

Dendrites increase the surface area of the cell membrane and connect with other neurones. This function is maximised by the presence of **dendritic spines**, small hair-like projections on the dendrites. Dendrites bring information to the cell body.

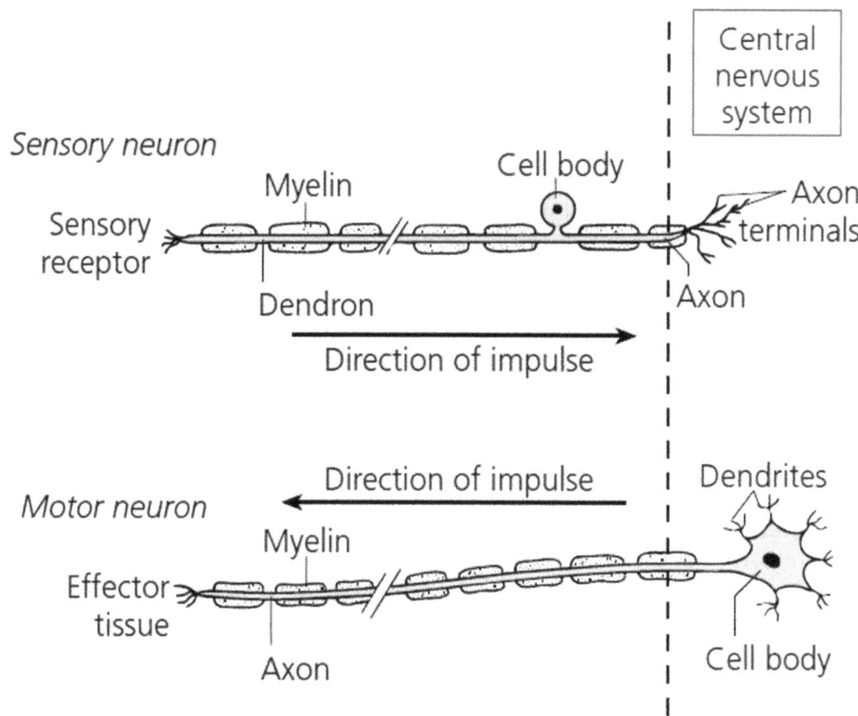

Figure 9.1 Sensory and motor neurons within the nervous system. Source: Clancy, John and Andrew J. McVicar (2009), Physiology and Anatomy for Nurses and Healthcare Professionals: A Homeostatic Approach Clancy and McVicar, 3rd ed. Taylor Francis, p. 163. Figure 8.2, Copyright © 2009. Reproduced by permission of Taylor Francis.

Dendrite: from the Greek word for *tree*, dendrites often look like little trees extending from the cell body.

Axons transmit information away from the cell body. Axons vary in length from less than 1mm to over a metre. The proximal portion of the axon is called the **initial segment** and is the origin of the **action potential** required for nerve transmission. Action potentials are electrical signals that travel along the surface of a neurone. The signal is maintained (or propagated) by the movement of ions (electrolytes) across the membrane of the neurone.

When touching something hot, sensory nerves rapidly transmit information to the brain, which responds immediately by sending a motor signal to withdraw from the source of heat. This takes a fraction of a second

Axons divide to form branches with button-like endings called **terminal boutons**, where neurotransmitters are stored in synaptic vesicles.

The connection between a terminal bouton and another tissue structure is called the **synapse**. Terminal boutons form the presynaptic component of the synapse and the structure it connects to forms the post-synaptic component. Neurotransmitters released from synaptic vesicles inhibit (suppress) or excite (stimulate) the post-synaptic component. When a neurone connects with a muscle fibre, the synapse is termed a **neuromuscular junction** and the post-synaptic component is termed the **motor end plate** (see Figure 9.2).

Most axons are wrapped in a lipid-based substance called **myelin**, which insulates the axon and increases the speed of conduction along the axon. Neurones wrapped in myelin are classified as **myelinated neurones**; those not wrapped in myelin are classified as **unmyelinated**.

Neurones are classified as sensory or motor neurones according to their function. Sensory neurones detect or sense internal or external stimuli and transmit sensory information to the brain. The brain receives and integrates sensory information and produces an appropriate motor response. Sensory neurones are also known as **afferent neurones** (afferent means carried towards), whilst **motor neurones** are termed **efferent neurones** (efferent means away from).

A nerve is a bundle of many hundreds of axons together with their blood vessels and connective tissue. They only occur within the PNS. Bundles of axons within the CNS are called tracts.

A **ganglion** is the term used to describe a cluster of neurone cell bodies within the PNS. Clusters of neurone cell bodies within the CNS are called **nuclei**.

Neuroglia

Neuroglia, or glial cells, are the dominant cell structure making up 90% of all cells within the CNS. Glial cells are structural cells providing support, nutrition and protection for neurones. They do not generate or conduct **nerve impulses** and do not form synapses, but they can divide by mitosis to create new cells. Glial cells are the main cause of primary tumours within the nervous system, because of their ability to reproduce.

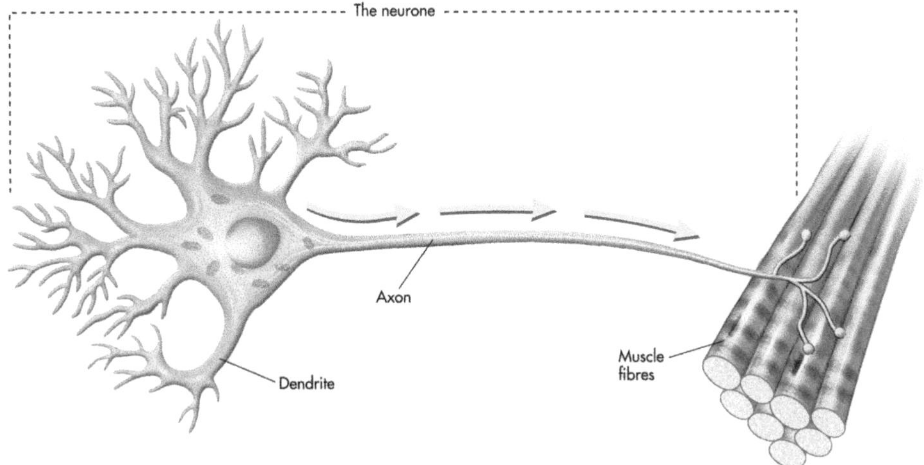

Figure 9.2 A neurone connecting to skeletal muscle fibres.

Glial cells are classified as **macroglia** or **microglia** – big and small glial cells. There are several types of macroglia within the CNS: **astrocytes**, **oligodendrocytes** and ependymal cells. Microglia are the macrophages of the CNS, removing cell debris and microorganisms by phagocytosis.

Glia: from the Greek meaning *glue*; also translates as 'holding together'.

Astrocytes are so named because of their star-like appearance. Multiple processes extend from the cell body, some of which end in foot processes that interface with cerebral blood vessels. Astrocytes are important for the movement of molecules from the blood to the brain, and they form part of the blood–brain barrier.

Ependymal cells form a single layer of cells lining the ventricles of the brain and the central canal of the **spinal cord**. They contain microvilli and cilia and are involved with the circulation of **cerebrospinal fluid**.

Oligodendrocytes generate myelin within the CNS (see Figure 9.3). **Schwann cells**, also a type of glial cell, generate myelin in the PNS. Schwann cells wrap around axons, forming a myelin sheath. The outer layer includes the Schwann cell's cytoplasm and nucleus and is called the **neurolemma**. The neurolemma is thought to promote axon regeneration in the PNS. When a myelinated axon is examined microscopically, there appear to be gaps in the myelin called **nodes of Ranvier**. One Schwann cell myelinates the segment of axon between two nodes of Ranvier; myelinated nerves will therefore have several Schwann cells (see Figures 9.3 and 9.4).

Myelination is different within the CNS. A single oligodendrocyte can myelinate up to 50 adjacent axons. Oligodendrocytes project multiple processes that wrap around the axons, but because the cell body and nucleus are not wrapped around the axon, there is no neurolemma. This may contribute to the lack of axonal regeneration within the CNS. Myelinated neurones within the CNS have fewer nodes of Ranvier than neurones in the PNS.

Demyelination describes the loss or destruction of myelin. Rapid shifts in serum sodium can cause CNS demyelination and neurological injury with symptoms similar to hypoxic brain injury. Abnormal serum sodium levels must be corrected slowly, at a rate not exceeding 5mmol/L per day. CNS demyelination is a side effect of some chemotherapy regimens. Inflammatory demyelinating diseases also occur and form part of a group of diseases called polyneuropathies, for example **multiple sclerosis (MS)** and **Guillain-Barré syndrome (GBS)**.

MS, a chronic demyelinating disease of the CNS, is an autoimmune disease characterised by degeneration of the myelin sheath. The name comes from the pathophysiology of the disease. The myelin sheaths degenerate in *multiple* areas, until they form hardened plaques called *scleroses*. Plaques are found in the brain and spinal cord of MS sufferers. Demyelination prevents **saltatory conduction** and reduces nerve transmission. Symptoms include muscle weakness, altered sensation and blurred vision. Acute episodes are followed by periods of remission, but frequency and severity of the attacks increases with time.

Autoimmune: describes a disease in which the body is attacked by the patient's own immune system.

GBS, an acute demyelinating disease of the PNS, often presents after a bacterial illness. It is a rare neurological condition in which the body's immune system attacks its peripheral

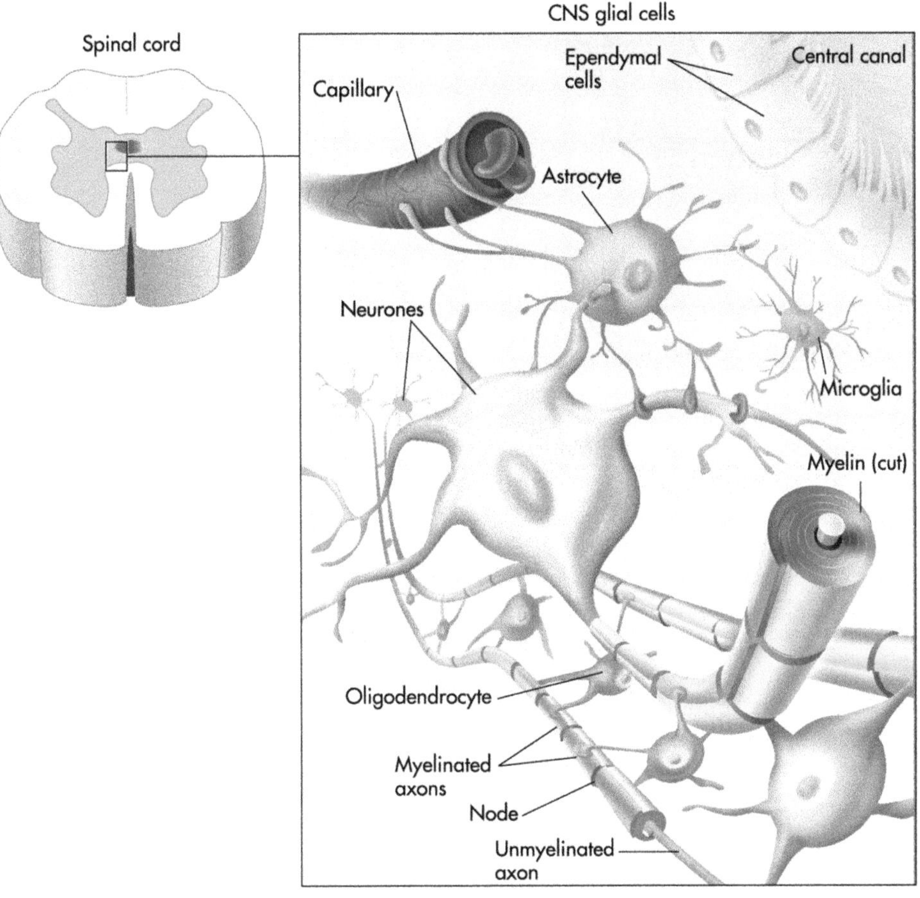

CNS glial cells	**PNS glial cells**
Astrocyte – metabolic and structural support	Schwann cells – produce myelin
Microglia – remove debris	
Oligodendrocytes – make lipid insulation (myelin)	
Ependymal cells – cover and line cavities	

Figure 9.3 Glial cells and their functions.

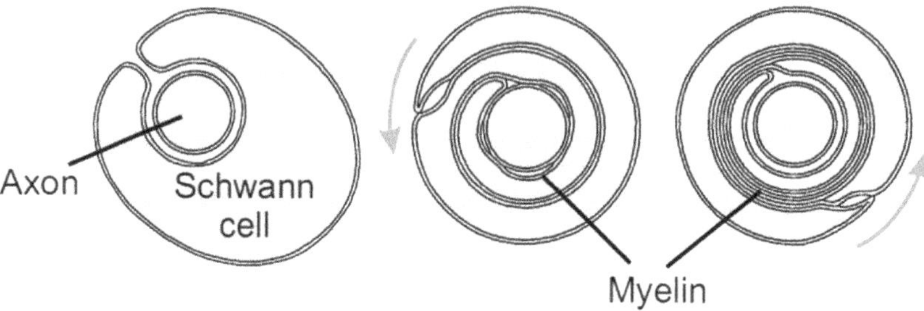

Figure 9.4 Schwann cells and peripheral axons. *Source*: Carpenter, R., and Reddi, B. (2013) *Neurophysiology: A Conceptual Approach*, 5th ed. Florida: CRC Press, p.9.

nervous system. Macrophages attack myelinated axons, stripping away the myelin sheath. Its symptoms can range from a mild condition, tingling sensation or weakness at the periphery, to severe condition, paralysis in which the respiratory muscles could be affected. GBS can progress rapidly over a few days and up to four weeks, and the severity of the muscle weakness or paralysis is different in each individual. When the patient's respiratory muscle is affected or become totally paralysed, this is a life-threatening condition, as the breathing can be affected and even the blood pressure and heart rate could be compromised (National Institute of Neurological Disorders and Stroke 2019). If respiratory muscles are affected, patients may require intubation and ventilation. Treatment is directed towards the immune system using plasmapheresis (plasma exchange) and intravenous immunoglobulin therapy.

Nerve impulses

A nerve impulse, or action potential, is a series of electrical events that take place sequentially along the length of an axon. An action potential has two phases: **depolarisation** and **repolarisation**. When a neurone is stimulated, sodium ions (Na^+) flow rapidly across the initial segment and into the cytoplasm of the axon: this is depolarisation. Depolarisation changes the electrical charge of that section of the axon causing potassium ions (K^+) to flow rapidly out of the axon and into the interstitial space: this is repolarisation. The sequential depolarisation and repolarisation of the axon cell membrane is like a row of dominoes; once the first action potential has occurred it causes neighbouring sections of the membrane to depolarise. The Na^+/K^+ pump on the axon cell membrane ensures the Na^+ and K^+ ions are restored to their normal positions, ready for the next action potential to occur (see Figure 9.5).

Nerve transmission requires a series of action potentials to be generated in sequence along the length of the axon, from the initial segment all the way to the terminal boutons. Nerve impulses are transmitted more rapidly by myelinated axons. The impulse jumps between the nodes of Ranvier in a process known as **saltatory conduction**.

Saltatory: from the Latin for *leap or jump*.

The diameter of the axon affects nerve transmission: the bigger the neurone, the faster it will transmit. Pain is one of example of this: local anaesthetic agents such as lidocaine

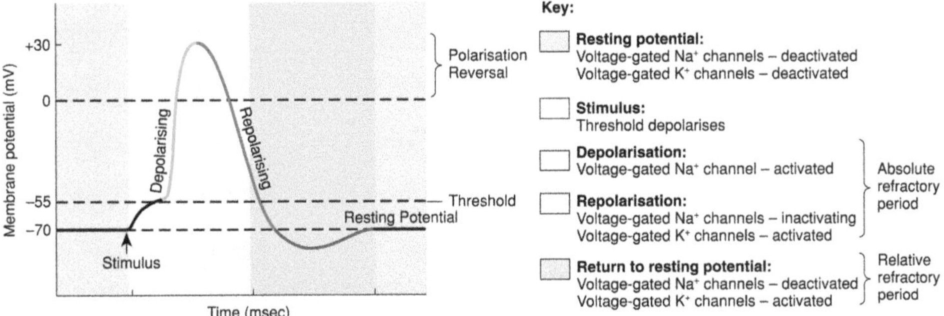

Figure 9.5 Action potential.

work by blocking the influx of Na^+ and preventing the action potential from being generated. If the action potential cannot be generated, the impulse cannot pass along the axon, preventing transmission of pain signals to the brain.

Ice can also be used to reduce the sensation of pain by locally cooling the nerve supplying the injured tissue. Cooling slows the transmission of nerve impulses, reducing the number of pain signals transmitted to the brain.

Action potentials can be affected by electrolyte imbalances. Disturbance of action potentials within the CNS may result in altered cerebral function, with symptoms ranging from irritability to seizures and coma. Disturbance of action potentials in the PNS can result in muscle weakness or excessive muscle contraction, known as tetany.

Hyponatraemia, **hypernatraemia**, **hypocalcaemia**, **hypomagnesaemia** and uraemia can all affect cerebral function. Hypo- and hypernatraemia are common causes of seizures. Hypocalcaemia and hypomagnesaemia can cause tingling of the hands and feet and in extreme cases, **tetany**. Hypocalcaemia can be identified by the Chvostek's sign. This is a twitching of the facial muscles in response to tapping on the cheek (Mohebbi, Rosenkrans and Jung 2013). Please see Chapter 4 for further consequences of electrolyte imbalance.

The synapse

The synapse is a collective term describing the interface between a terminal bouton and another tissue structure, which may be another nerve but could be a blood vessel, a muscle, an organ or a gland.

Synapses can be electrical or chemical. Electrical synapses are found in cardiac muscle and the smooth muscle of the gastrointestinal (GI) tract, they also occur in the CNS. Electrical synapses are special channels directly connecting the cytoplasm of neighbouring cells. This allows the flow of ions between cells and accounts for the 'wavelike' muscular activity seen in cardiac contraction and gut motility. The rapid spread of electrical information ensures the entire muscle is synchronised and produces a coordinated contraction. Electrical synapses are faster than chemical synapses.

Most synapses are chemical; neurotransmitters are used to bridge the gap between the terminal bouton and the post-synaptic structure (see Figure 9.6). Neurotransmitters released from the presynaptic terminal diffuse across the synaptic cleft and bind to the

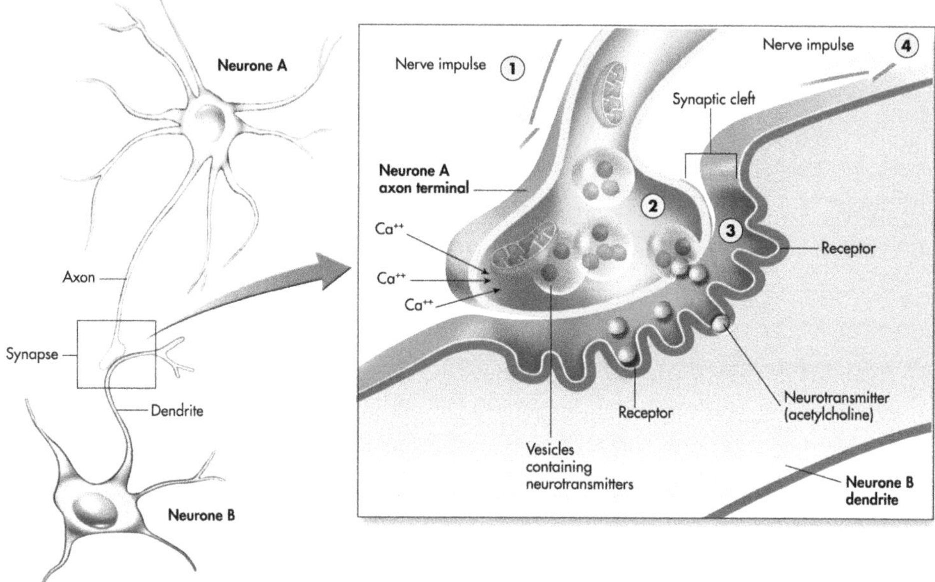

Figure 9.6 The chemical synapse: step 1, the impulse travels down the axon; step 2, vesicles are stimulated to release neurotransmitter (exocytosis); step 3, the neurotransmitter travels across the synapse and binds with the receptor site of the post-synaptic cell; step 4, the impulse continues down the dendrite.

post-synaptic terminal, where they inhibit or excite the post-synaptic structure. Inhibition blocks the post-synaptic structure, and excitation stimulates the post-synaptic structure.

Calcium is important in chemical synapses. As the electrical impulse arrives at the terminal bouton, the action potential causes calcium to flow into the terminal bouton from the interstitial space, triggering the synaptic vesicles to release the neurotransmitter into the synaptic cleft. The neurotransmitter diffuses across the **synaptic cleft** and binds with the receptors on the post-synaptic structure, generating an action potential in the post-synaptic cell.

Chemical synapse requires the following steps:

1. Step 1: neurotransmitter synthesised by neurone cell body and transported to axon terminal.
2. Step 2: neurotransmitter stored in synaptic vesicles within the terminal boutons, ready for release.
3. Step 3: nerve impulse reaches the axon terminal and triggers the influx of Ca^{++} from the interstitial space.
4. Step 4: increase in Ca^{++} triggers the release of the neurotransmitter into the synaptic cleft.
5. Step 5: neurotransmitter diffuses across the synaptic cleft and binds to a specific receptor, causing ion channels to open.

6. Step 6: an influx of ions from the synaptic cleft generates an action potential at the post-synaptic component, stimulating or inhibiting the post-synaptic cell.
7. Step 7: neurotransmitter is removed from synaptic cleft by enzyme inactivation, reuptake or by diffusing away from the synapse.

In summary, the impulse begins as an electrical signal transmitted along the axon of a neurone. When the signal reaches the terminal bouton, it is converted into a chemical signal that diffuses across the synaptic cleft and binds to the post-synaptic cell. The post-synaptic cell converts the chemical signal back into an electrical signal.

Once the synapse has occurred, the neurotransmitter must be cleared from the synaptic cleft. Otherwise, the post-synaptic cell will be stimulated repeatedly. Neurotransmitters can be cleared in three ways:

- Enzyme inactivation: enzymes break down the molecular structure of the neurotransmitter, e.g., **acetylcholine** is inactivated by **acetylcholinesterase**.
- Cellular uptake: neurotransmitters are transported back to the neurone that released them and are reused, e.g., norepinephrine (noradrenaline), or taken up by glial cells.
- Diffusion: neurotransmitters diffuse away from the synaptic cleft, preventing contact with their receptor sites.
- Neurones receive thousands of synapses. Weak synapses do not generate action potentials: if the signal is strong enough, an action potential will occur, and an impulse will be transmitted. This is described as an 'all or nothing' event.

Neurotransmitters

Neurotransmitters are chemicals that excite, inhibit or modify the response of another cell. They are classified by their molecular size into small-molecule neurotransmitters and neuropeptides (Tortora and Derrickson 2017). Small molecule neurotransmitters include acetylcholine, norepinephrine, **epinephrine** and **dopamine**. Acetylcholine (ACh), an important neurotransmitter in both the PNS and the CNS, is inactivated by the enzyme acetylcholinesterase (AChE).

Myasthenia gravis is caused by the autoimmune destruction of ACh receptors. ACh produced at the synapse is broken down by AChE before the patient's muscles have contracted. By blocking AChE, the breakdown of ACh is prevented, and the muscle is stimulated until it contracts. Drugs that block AChE are called **acetylcholinesterase inhibitors**, for example, pyridostigmine, and are the mainstay of myasthenia gravis management.

Norepinephrine and epinephrine are classified as catecholamines because of their chemical structure and are both neurotransmitters and hormones. As well as being released at synapses, norepinephrine and epinephrine are released directly into the bloodstream by the adrenal medulla. Norepinephrine and epinephrine are inactivated by reuptake from presynaptic neurones and are recycled or destroyed by enzymes.

Dopamine, also a catecholamine, is active in both the CNS and the PNS. In the CNS, dopamine is involved in emotion and pleasure and may be associated with addictive behaviours. In the PNS, dopamine helps to regulate muscle tone: it is deactivated by reuptake in presynaptic neurones.

Parkinson's disease is caused by inadequate levels of dopamine creating an imbalance in the ratio of dopamine to ACh, resulting in involuntary muscle contractions and producing the characteristic clinical feature of tremor. Involuntary movements interfere with voluntary movements, for example buttoning a shirt is difficult because the hands shake. Dopamine cannot be administered orally or by injection, as it cannot cross the **blood–brain** barrier. Levodopa (L-dopa) does cross the blood–brain barrier, and once inside the CNS, is converted to dopamine, restoring dopamine levels and controlling symptoms. However, L-dopa does not slow down the progression of Parkinson's disease.

Interestingly, an excess of dopamine has been linked to schizophrenia. Therefore, most effective antipsychotic treatments are targeted at dopamine and its neurochemical pathways (Brisch et al. 2014).

Neuropeptide neurotransmitters: chains of amino acids linked by peptide bonds, examples include **endorphins** and **substance P**. Neuropeptides are synthesised in neurone cell bodies, formed into vesicles and transported to the terminal boutons; they are active in the CNS and the PNS.

Endorphins, described as opioid peptides, function as natural analgesics by binding to opiate receptors in the CNS. Endorphins can be triggered by acupuncture and acupressure, providing pain-relieving effects.

Substance P is released in the PNS by neurones responsible for the transmission of pain information to the CNS. Substance P is also found in spinal cord pathways and in parts of the brain associated with pain. Substance P increases the perception of pain. Endorphins inhibit the release of substance P and reduce the perception of pain.

The brain

The brain is surrounded and protected by the skull and the **meninges**. The section of skull enclosing the brain is called the **cranium** and is made up of eight bones. Swelling of the brain causes **intracranial pressure** to rise because the adult skull is unable to expand to accommodate the swelling. Swelling of the brain is termed **cerebral oedema**, and if not treated, may lead to fatal brain herniation.

The meninges is a collective term describing the three membranes that cover and protect the brain and spinal cord. The acronym *PAD* may help you to remember the names of the meninges. Starting from the surface of the brain and working outwards, the membranes are the **pia mater**, the **arachnoid mater** and the **dura mater**. Inflammation of the meninges is called meningitis (see Figure 9.7).

Cerebrospinal fluid (CSF) protects the brain and spinal cord from injury. Adults have 80150mL of CSF circulating continuously around the brain and spinal cord (Tortora and Derrickson 2017). CSF transports oxygen, glucose and electrolytes from the blood to the neurones and neuroglia of the CNS and removes waste from neural tissues. CSF makes the brain buoyant, effectively floating within the skull, ensuring the brain is not damaged from resting against the skull.

CSF is a colourless, clear liquid produced by a network of capillaries called the **choroid plexus** in the walls of all four ventricles within the brain. The choroid plexus is surrounded by ependymal cells (glial cells) that continuously generate CSF from the plasma of the blood by a process of filtration and secretion. As well as a blood–brain barrier, the brain also has a blood–CSF barrier, protecting it from harmful substances that may be carried in the plasma of the blood. Ependymal cells form the blood–CSF barrier, controlling the substances that are allowed to enter the CSF.

CSF flows from the two lateral ventricles into the third ventricle, where another choroid plexus generates more CSF. CSF then flows through the cerebral aqueduct, or

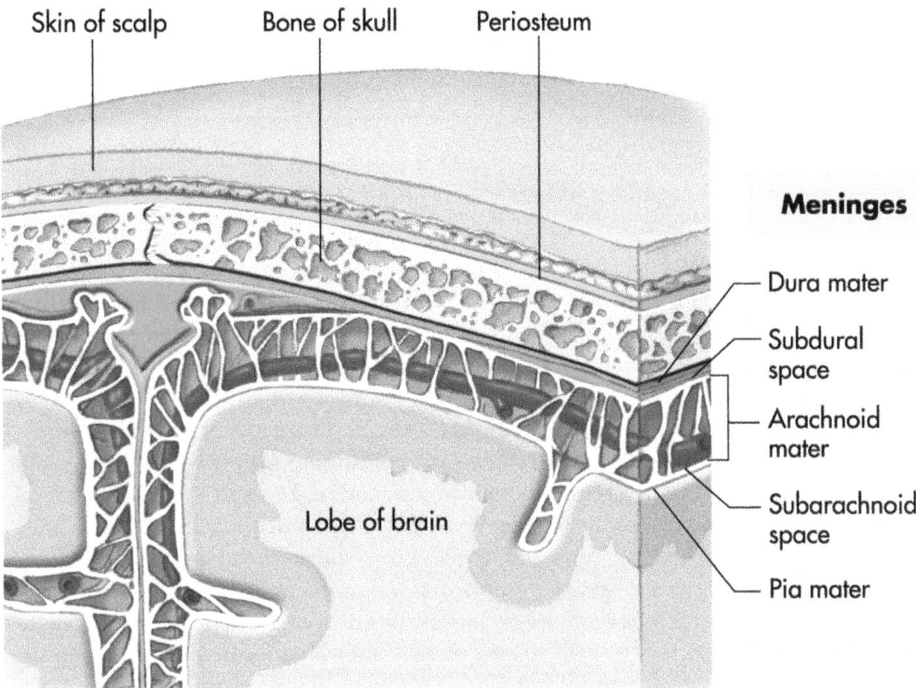

Figure 9.7 The meninges.

aqueduct of Sylvius, into the fourth ventricle, where further CSF is generated. The CSF then enters the **subarachnoid space**, the space between the arachnoid mater and the pia mater, through openings in the ceiling of the fourth ventricle. CSF circulates in the subarachnoid space around the brain and spinal cord and also in the central canal of the spinal cord. CSF is absorbed back into the blood by arachnoid villi, finger-like projections of the arachnoid mater. If the volume of the CSF is to remain constant, then the CSF must be produced and reabsorbed at the same rate. Once generated, the CSF should flow unobstructed from the ventricles through the arachnoid space and into the spinal canal. The flow of CSF can be affected by tumours, inflammatory conditions like **ventriculitis** and by intraventricular or **subarachnoid haemorrhage**, which can cause CSF flow to become obstructed by thrombus. If this happens, CSF continues to be produced, but cannot drain adequately, and the pressure of the CSF increases: this clinical condition is termed **hydrocephalus**. Hydrocephalus can be controlled temporarily by the insertion of an extra-ventricular drain (EVD), or permanently by the insertion of a ventriculoperitoneal (VP) shunt. Any increase in CSF pressure will result in an increase in intracranial pressure (ICP, normal range 3–15mmHg) because adult skull bones are fused. This may be a clinical emergency if left unattended.

Blood supply to the brain

The internal carotid and vertebral arteries provide most of the blood supply to the brain. The internal carotids branch to form the anterior cerebral artery and the middle cerebral artery. Anastomoses of the right and left internal carotid arteries and the basilar artery form a special cerebral circulation at the base of the brain called the **circle of Willis**. Most of the brain is supplied by arteries arising from the circle of Willis. The circle of Willis equalises blood pressure across the brain and provides an alternative blood supply if an artery within the brain becomes blocked or diseased.

The internal carotid artery supplies the eyeball, ear, most of the cerebrum, pituitary and nose.

Neurones reply on a constant supply of glucose and oxygen for normal brain function. Brief interruptions in blood flow can cause **unconsciousness**, for example, standing up too fast and fainting, or **transient ischaemic attacks (TIAs)** caused by temporary obstruction of an artery by thrombus or atherosclerosis. Loss of blood flow (and therefore oxygen) for four minutes or more, for example, during cardiac arrest, causes irreversible brain injury.

The brain stores very little glucose and relies on a continuous supply of glucose via the bloodstream. Hypoglycaemia can result in confusion, seizures and altered **consciousness**.

Patients who are unexpectedly drowsy, confused or unconscious should have their blood glucose checked, as hypo/hyperglycaemia affects level of consciousness. Hypoglycaemia can be corrected by the use of oral or intravenous glucose preparations and by the administration of glucagon. Alert patients with hypoglycaemia can be given a sugary drink and carbohydrates to eat. Sugar quickly raises blood glucose, and carbohydrates provide a slow release supply of glucose to prevent recurrence of hypoglycaemia. Patients who are less alert can be given an oral preparation of glucose that can be rubbed on the gums. Unconscious patients are treated with intravenous glucose or intramuscular glucagon (JBDS-IP 2018; NICE 2019b). For further discussion on glycaemic management, please see Chapter 11.

The blood–brain barrier

The **blood–brain barrier** is an important structure that prevents harmful substances in the bloodstream from entering brain tissue. The blood–brain barrier has two main components: a thick capillary basement membrane and tight junctions between the endothelial cells of the capillaries. Capillaries in other parts of the body have gaps between the endothelial cells that allow substances to diffuse across the capillary wall and enter the interstitial space. Tight junctions in brain capillaries and the thick basement membrane prevents diffusion, the brain relies on astrocytes to control the movement of substances from blood to brain. The foot processes of astrocytes press tightly against the endothelial wall of brain capillaries, secreting chemicals that control the permeability of the capillary. This structure is semipermeable to some water-soluble substances like glucose, but not others, for example, proteins and antibiotics. However, it is permeable to fat-soluble substances, e.g., oxygen, carbon dioxide, alcohol and most anaesthetic agents (Tortora and Derrickson 2017). The blood–brain barrier is affected by trauma and inflammation and can malfunction.

The brain is primarily divided into four parts: the **cerebrum**, the **diencephalon**, the **cerebellum** and the **brainstem** (see Figure 9.8).

The *cerebrum* is the largest part of the brain and is subdivided by the *great longitudinal fissure*: each half is called a **cerebral hemisphere**. In cross-section, the hemispheres consist

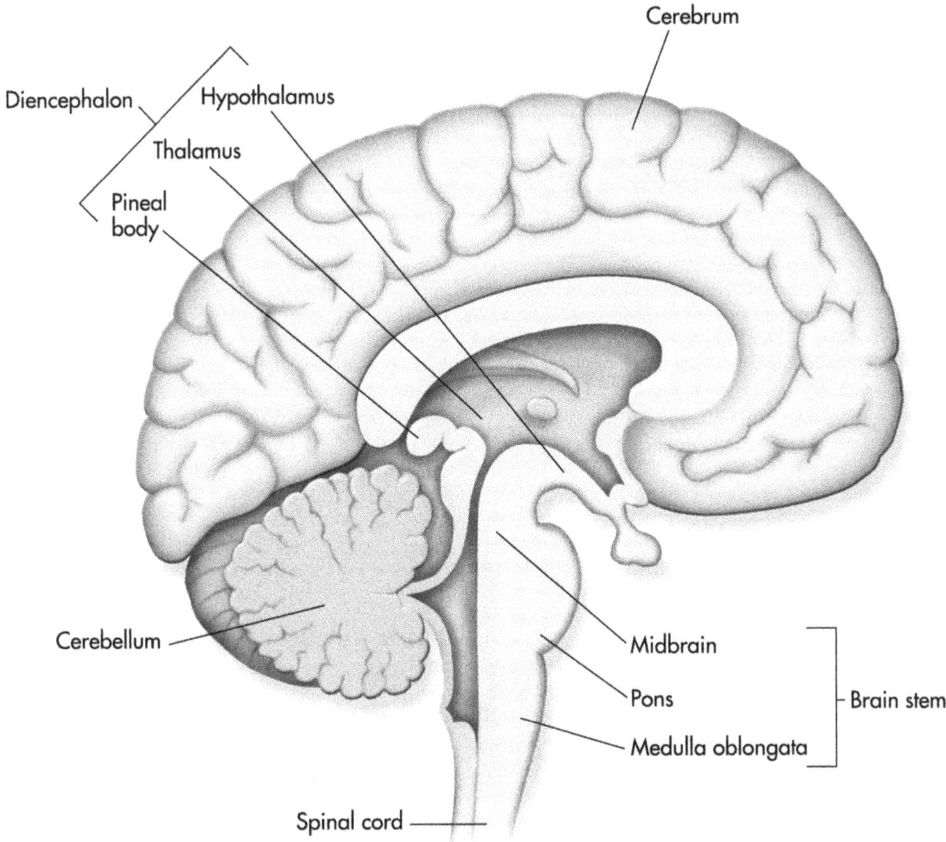

Figure 9.8 Internal anatomy of the brain.

of an outer layer of **grey matter** and an internal area of **white matter**. White matter is made up mainly of myelinated axons; grey matter is mainly made of neurone cell bodies, dendrites, unmyelinated axons and neuroglia. The outer layer of grey matter is approximately 3mm thick, contains billions of neurones and is called the **cerebral cortex**.

The surface of each hemisphere has multiple folds called **gyri**, which increase the surface area of the brain (see Figure 9.9). The deep grooves between the gyri are called **fissures**. The shallower grooves are called **sulci**. The two hemispheres are connected by the **corpus callosum**, which is a band of white matter filled with axons running between the hemispheres.

Sulci: the plural of sulcus.
Gyri: the plural of **gyrus**.

The hemispheres are subdivided into paired lobes named after the skull bones that cover them: frontal lobe, parietal lobe, occipital lobe, temporal lobe. Each lobe is separated by

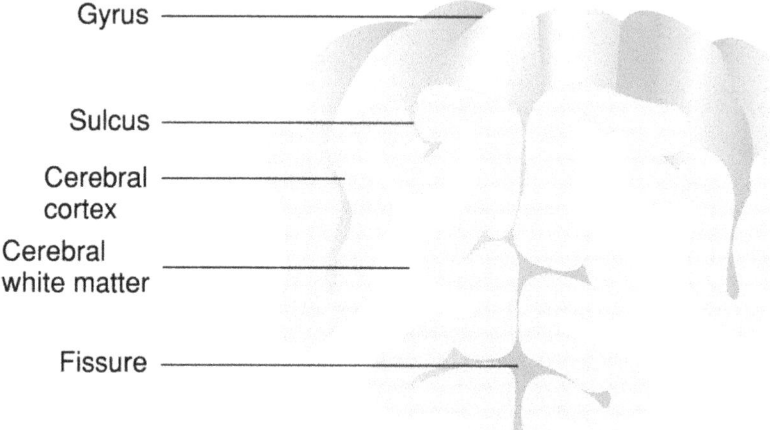

Figure 9.9 Detail of a gyrus, sulcus and fissure.

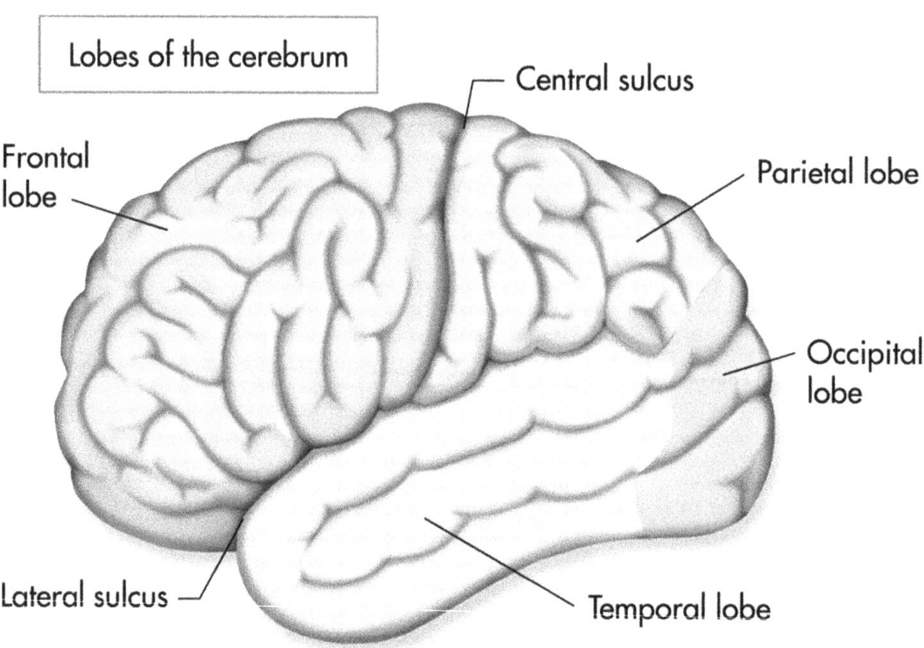

Figure 9.10 External brain anatomy.

a **sulcus** (see Figure 9.10). One hemisphere is usually more highly developed than the other; this is known as **cerebral dominance**: 90% of the population have a dominant left hemisphere, which results in right-handedness, an important consideration when dealing with unilateral brain injuries such as acute stroke. Motor control of speech is usually located within the dominant hemisphere.

Function of the cerebral cortex

The cerebral cortex processes sensory, motor and integrated signals. The central sulcus is an important area of the cerebral cortex, because it separates the primary somatosensory area from the **primary motor area** in each hemisphere (see Figure 9.11).

The primary somatosensory area is a highly specialised area of the cerebral cortex containing a 'map' of the body: each point on the body surface can be mapped to a specific part of the primary somatosensory area (see Figure 9.12). The amount of cortex receiving signals from a particular part of the body depends on the number of receptors in that body part, not the size of the body part. For example, the tongue is relatively small, but a relatively large part of the primary somatosensory area receives signals from the tongue because the tongue contains large numbers of sensory nerve endings.

The **primary somatosensory area** is important for perception of sensation including touch, tickle, itch, pain, temperature and joint posture. Other senses are interpreted in different parts of the cortex:

- *Sight and visual perception*: posterior portion of the occipital lobe.
- *Taste*: parietal cortex.
- *Smell*: temporal cortex.
- *Hearing*: temporal cortex.

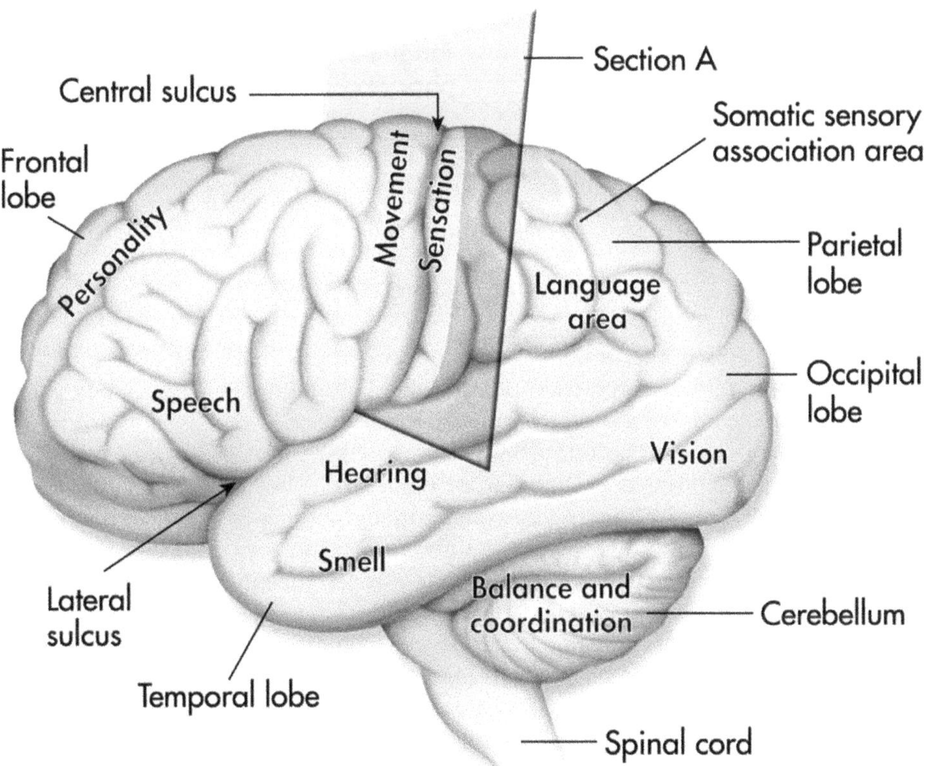

Figure 9.11 Primary somatosensory area.

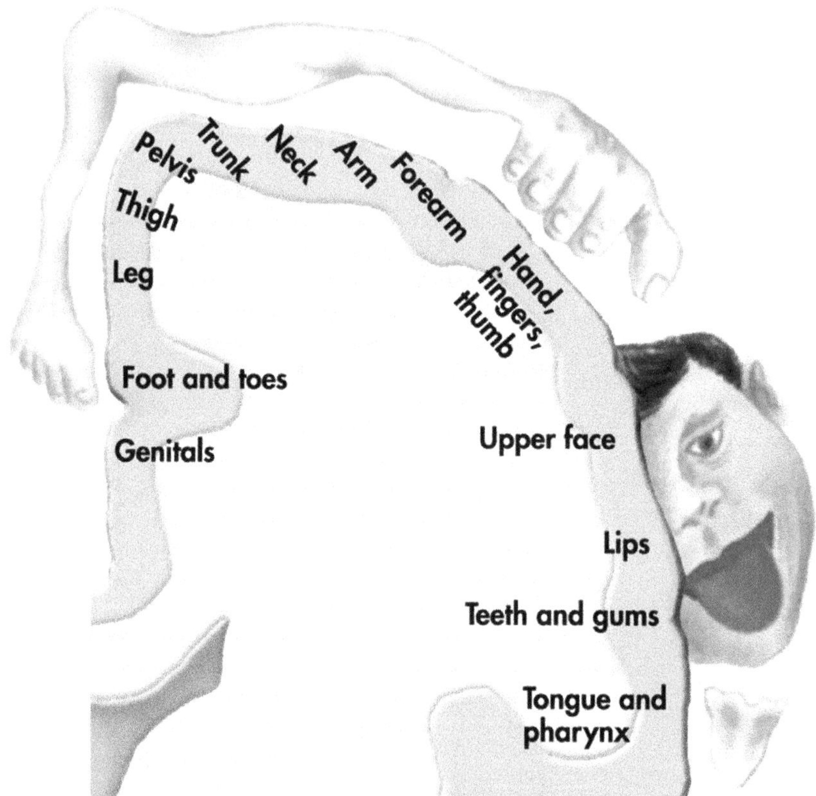

Figure 9.12 Primary somatosensory area, cross-sectional view of section A in Figure 9.11, showing how different parts of the body map to different areas of the sensory cortex.

The *primary motor area* of the cerebral cortex is located immediately anterior to the primary somatosensory area in the posterior section of the frontal lobe. Stimulation of the primary motor area results in contraction of a specific skeletal muscle. Again, body parts do not map in proportion to their size, but in proportion to the number of motor neurones present in that particular part of the body. Large parts of the cortex relate to muscles that are required for complex, skilled or delicate movements. For example, highly dextrous parts of the body, such as the fingers, contain more motor neurones than the toes.

Speech is an important motor function and is controlled in a specialised zone of the motor cortex called **Broca's speech area** in the left frontal lobe. Motor neurones connect Broca's speech area with the larynx, pharynx, mouth and the respiratory muscles. Speech is the result of high-level coordination between talking, breathing and swallowing.

Wernicke's area, located broadly within the left temporal and parietal lobes, interprets speech by recognising spoken words and translating them into thoughts.

The areas in the right hemisphere corresponding to Broca's area and Wernicke's area are responsible for the emotional elements of speech.

Conversation requires integrated sensory functions; speech must be heard (auditory function), interpreted (cognitive function) and translated into speech (verbal function).

Brain injuries such as acute stroke can cause a range of communication problems. Damage to Broca's area results in **expressive aphasia**, where the patient is capable of thought but incapable of speech. Damage to Wernicke's area results in **receptive aphasia**, the inability to put words together coherently. The patient may be capable of a diverse range of words, but cannot create a meaningful sentence. This is usually due to left-sided brain injuries, irrespective of hemisphere dominance.

Aphasia: from the Greek *aphatos*, meaning *speechless*.

The *diencephalon* is located below the cerebrum and includes the **thalamus**, **hypothalamus**, **subthalamus** and **epithalamus**.

The *thalamus* is a pair of oval-shaped structures made of grey matter; in most individuals, the right and left halves are joined by a bridge of grey matter. The thalamus acts as a relay station between the cerebral cortex and the spinal cord, between different areas of the cerebrum and between the cerebrum and the cerebellum. It is involved with consciousness.

The hypothalamus is beneath the thalamus and controls temperature, water metabolism, autonomic function, physical emotion and pituitary secretions such as growth hormone. The hypothalamus contains a feeding centre which contributes to the sense of hunger and a satiety centre that causes a sense of fullness and triggers individuals to stop eating. The thirst centre is also located within the hypothalamus. **Osmoreceptors** in the hypothalamus are stimulated by an increase in blood osmotic pressure, triggering the sensation of thirst. The hypothalamus influences the circadian rhythm of the body – the sleep/wake cycle.

The subthalamus is the most ventral part of the diencephalon and is wedged between the thalamus and the midbrain. It forms part of the basal ganglia and has a role in movement modulation. This is the target for deep brain stimulation (DBS), which is one of the treatments for Parkinson's Disease (Alkemade 2013).

The epithalamus consists of the **pineal gland** and the **habenular nuclei**. The pineal gland secretes melatonin and is considered an endocrine gland. The habenular nuclei have an integrative role, linking smell and emotion. For example, a particular smell may evoke a specific memory.

Beneath the diencephalon are the cerebellum and the brainstem. The cerebellum lies posterior to the brainstem. The surface of the cerebellum is similar to the surface of the cerebrum, has multiple sulci and gyri and contains a rim of grey matter. The cerebellum regulates posture and balance and is important for the coordinated contraction of skeletal muscle. Damage to the cerebellum affects muscle coordination and causes ataxia. Ataxia is most noticeable when walking, as individuals appear to stagger or have an abnormal gait. Similar signs of ataxia can be seen after excessive alcohol consumption; alcohol inhibits cerebellar function.

The brainstem contains the **midbrain**, the **pons** and the **medulla oblongata**. The spinal cord is an extension of the brainstem descending into the vertebral column (see Figure 9.11).

The midbrain contains sensory and motor pathways controlling movement of the eyes, head and trunk in response to visual and auditory stimuli. The midbrain is the origin of **cranial nerves** III–V.

The pons also contains sensory and motor pathways and is a relay station between the cerebral cortex and the cerebellum. Together with the medulla, the **apneustic** and

pneumotaxic areas of the pons control breathing. The pons is the origin of cranial nerves V–VIII.

The medulla oblongata contains the **vasomotor centre**, also called the cardiovascular centre. This regulates the heartbeat and controls the diameter of blood vessels, thereby controlling blood pressure. The medulla is also responsible for the rhythmical pattern of breathing. The medulla contains ascending sensory pathways and descending motor pathways connecting the spinal cord with other parts of the brain. The area where the medulla joins the spinal cord is where most of the ascending and descending pathways (tracts of axons within the CNS) cross over; as a result, each cerebral hemisphere is responsible for sensation and voluntary movement on the opposite side of the body.

Nuclei (clusters of cell bodies within the CNS) within the medulla control important protective reflexes including swallowing, coughing, vomiting, sneezing and hiccoughing. The medulla also contains sensory nuclei involved in sensations of touch, pressure, vibration, taste, balance and hearing. The medulla is the origin of cranial nerves V, VII, VIII–XII.

Cranial nerves

There are 12 pairs of cranial nerves, and they form part of the PNS. Each nerve is named according to its function and is identified numerically by Roman numerals.

Brainstem injuries have the potential to affect several cranial nerves because most of them originate within the brainstem. Cranial nerves I and II are the only cranial nerves whose origins are not in the brainstem; they originate from the cerebral hemispheres.

Cranial nerves can be tested by asking the patient to perform an action that the cranial nerve usually controls.

Cranial nerves

I. **Olfactory** (sensory – smell).
II. **Optic** (sensory – sight).
III. **Oculomotor** (motor – eye movement, upper eyelid control and pupil constriction).
IV. **Trochlear** (motor – eye movement).
V. **Trigeminal** (sensory and motor – face, scalp, nose and mouth).
VI. **Abducens** (motor – eye movement).
VII. **Facial** (motor and sensory – closing eyes, crying, smiling, grimacing, taste, salivation).
VIII. **Vestibulocochlear** (sensory – hearing and balance).
IX. **Glossopharyngeal** (sensory and motor – sensation and taste, tongue and pharynx).
X. **Vagus** (motor and sensory – pharynx, larynx, heart, lungs, gut, viscera).
XI. **Spinal accessory** (motor – shoulder and head movement).
XII. **Hypoglossal** (motor – speech, swallowing).

The spinal cord and spinal nerves

The spinal cord lies within the spinal canal inside the vertebral column and is protected by the meninges and cushioned by CSF. The spinal cord is an extension of the brainstem running from the medulla oblongata to the top of the second lumbar vertebra, approximately 45cm long and 1cm wide.

In cross-section, the spinal cord has areas of white and grey matter (see Figure 9.13). Grey matter is arranged in an H shape and divided into regions called horns. Horns are classified as anterior (ventral) or posterior (dorsal) depending upon location. The **posterior horns** contain sensory axons, the **anterior horns** contain motor axons. The white matter is divided into regions called columns: anterior, posterior and lateral white columns. The amount of grey and white matter varies in different sections of the cord.

Spinal nerves are part of the PNS, and together with the cranial nerves, they connect the CNS with the rest of the body. 31 pairs of spinal nerves exit the spinal column between each vertebra and are named according to the section of the vertebral column they emerge from (see Figure 9.14).

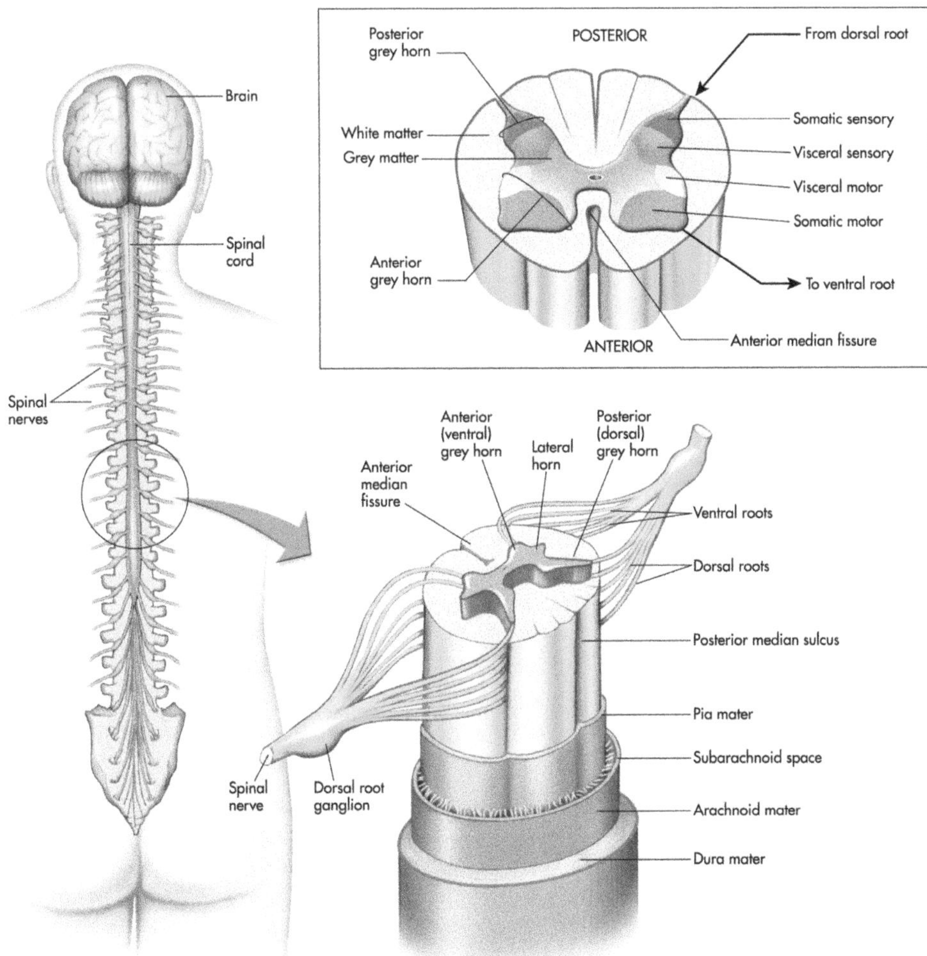

Figure 9.13 Internal anatomy of the spinal cord.

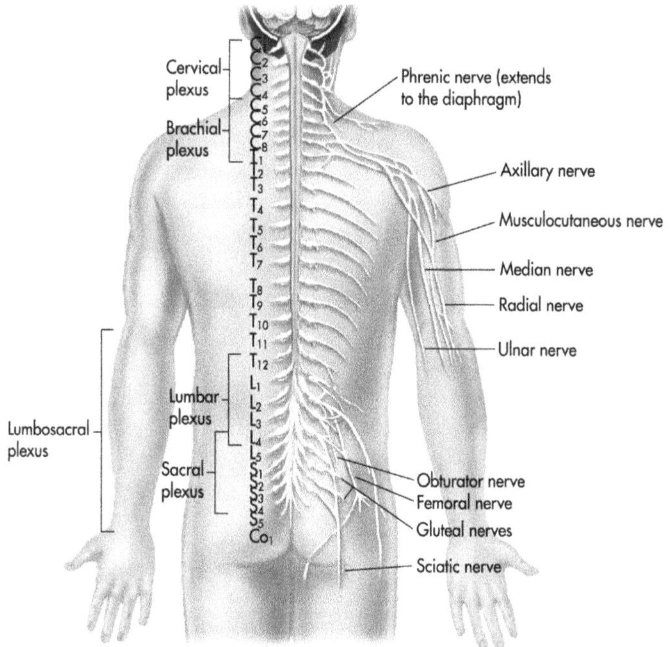

SPINAL NERVE PLEXUSES

PLEXUS	LOCATION	SPINAL NERVES INVOLVED	REGION SUPPLIED	MAJOR NERVES LEAVING PLEXUS
Cervical	Deep in the neck, under the sternocleidomastoid muscle	C_1–C_4	Skin and muscles of neck and shoulder; diaphragm	Phrenic (diaphragm)
Brachial	Deep to the clavicle, between the neck and the axilla	C_5–C_8, T_1	Skin and muscles of upper extremity	Musculocutaneous Ulnar Median Radial Axillary
Lumbosacral	Lumbar region of the back	T_{12}, L_1–L_5, S_1–S_4	Skin and muscles of lower abdominal wall, lower extremity, buttocks, external genitalia	Obturator Femoral Sciatic Pudendal

Figure 9.14 Spinal cord plexuses.

Spinal nerves are arranged as follows:

- 8 pairs of **cervical nerves** (C1–C8).
- 12 pairs of **thoracic nerves** (T1–T12).
- 5 pairs of **lumbar nerves** (L1–L5).
- 5 pairs of **sacral nerves** (S1–S5).
- 1 pair of **coccygeal nerves** (Co1).

Spinal nerves have two connections to the spinal cord: an anterior and a posterior root containing sensory and motor axons. Classified as mixed nerves, spinal nerves branch many times and directly innervate many peripheral structures.

Motor neurone disease (MND) is a degenerative disease affecting the ventral horns of the spinal cord and the ventral nerve roots that connect with skeletal muscle. Loss of nerve stimulation leads to muscle-wasting and weakness. Because the ventral horns contain motor neurones, MND affects voluntary muscle, causing progressive weakness and finally, inability to walk, talk, swallow and breathe ensues.

The spinal cord does not extend below the second lumbar vertebra. Beneath L2, the spinal canal is filled with the lumbar, sacral and coccygeal nerve roots that continue down the spinal canal exiting at their appropriate level. This collection of nerve roots is called the **cauda equina**.

Cauda equina: Latin for 'horse's tail' – the nerve roots in the spinal canal look like a horse's tail.

Figure 9.14 shows the parts of the body supplied by spinal nerves. These areas have been mapped out, and the resulting map is called a **dermatome**.

Spinal cord injury (SCI) describes damage to the spinal cord resulting in loss of mobility or sensation. SCI is a lifelong condition affecting over 40,000 people in the UK (NICE 2016). The spinal cord does not have to be severed for loss of function to occur; bruising and tearing can cause long-term injury. Fractured vertebrae do not necessarily cause spinal cord injury.

Traumatic causes of SCI include:

- Falls.
- Sports injuries.
- Stabbings.
- Shootings.
- Road traffic accidents (RTA).

Diseases that can cause SCI include:

- Spina bifida.
- Polio.
- Primary or metastatic tumours.
- Severe disc prolapse.
- Inflammatory diseases, such as rheumatoid and osteoarthritis.
- Infective diseases, such as TB of the spine, osteomyelitis and epidural abscess.
- Haematoma.
- Ageing.

Spinal cord injuries can have several phases:

- Primary injury, i.e. trauma.
- Secondary injury, i.e. cord ischaemia.
- Subsequent injury, i.e. additional injury from manual handling.

Primary injury is usually traumatic, and damage begins at the moment of injury. The primary trauma causes vascular and chemical changes leading to secondary injury, such as cord ischaemia, hypoxia and oedema. Secondary injuries may also be caused by arterial insufficiency, thrombosis or hypotension.

SCI is classified by the clinical effects of the injury:

- **Quadriplegia** (also called tetraplegia).
- **Paraplegia**.

Both types of injury may be complete or incomplete.

In incomplete SCI, the ability of the brain and spinal cord to convey messages is not entirely lost; some degree of motor or sensory function is present below the level of the injury. Patients with complete SCI have no function below the level of the injury, no sensation and no voluntary movement; both sides of the body are equally affected. Understanding the anatomy of the spinal nerves helps predict how the patient will be affected.

Cervical injuries usually cause quadriplegia and affect diaphragm control and breathing. Patients with complete high cervical injuries (C1–3) lose diaphragm function and cannot cough or breathe effectively, usually requiring a tracheostomy, and are often ventilator-dependent. All function below the level of the injury is lost.

Injuries at thoracic level usually cause paraplegia; breathing is not as badly affected, and patients usually retain the use of their arms and hands. Spinal cord injury, though, can result in neurogenic bowel dysfunction. Patients may depend on routine interventional bowel care, including the digital (manual) removal of faeces (DRF). Lesions above T6 predispose patients to **autonomic dysreflexia** – an excessive autonomic response to a stimulus below the level of the SCI, for example, a blocked catheter or constipation. A patient safety alert (NHS Improvement 2018) was issued following the identification of 61 reports of significant delays in providing DRF, which resulted in 3 cases of autonomic dysreflexia. The extreme rise in blood pressure could lead to some types of stroke or even death (Nazarko 2018) and is a medical emergency which requires prompt treatment to prevent complications.

Signs of autonomic dysreflexia

- Severe, uncontrolled hypertension, 200/100mmHg.
- Blood pressure greater than 20mmHg above baseline for both systolic and diastolic.
- Bradycardia at onset, tachycardia may follow.
- Respiratory distress or bronchospasm.
- Severe headaches.
- Sweating or shivering.
- Anxiety.
- Blurred vision.
- Flushing of the skin above the injury.
- Coolness of the skin below the injury.

Lumbar injuries affect leg muscles and walking. Sacral injuries affect bowel, bladder and sexual function.

Initial SCI management focuses on stabilising the spine, reducing oedema, maintaining cord blood flow and preventing further injury.

Staff caring for patients with SCI must be trained in the safe handling of SCI patients.

The autonomic nervous system

The **autonomic nervous system** (ANS) is regulated by centres within the brainstem and the hypothalamus; it is subdivided into the **sympathetic** and **parasympathetic nervous systems**.

The sympathetic nervous system is involuntary and maintains the body in a state of readiness to deal with any problems that arise. It is active during times of stress and generates the body's 'fight or flight' response. Sympathetic fibres arise from the thoracic section of the spinal cord, T1–T12. One of the neurotransmitters released by the sympathetic nervous system is norepinephrine, also known as noradrenaline; consequently, the **sympathetic nervous system** is described as *adrenergic*. Noradrenaline binds to adrenergic receptors and creates a physiological effect. Adrenergic receptors are divided into different subtypes: α_1, α_2, β_1, β_2.

The parasympathetic nervous system is also involuntary and, in general, counteracts the action of the sympathetic nervous system, restoring the body to its resting state; it is needed for relaxation and sleep. Parasympathetic fibres arise from cranial nerves III, VII, IX and X and also from the sacral section of the spinal cord, S2–S4. The neurotransmitter released by the parasympathetic nervous system is acetylcholine; the parasympathetic nervous system is described as *cholinergic*. Acetylcholine binds to **cholinergic receptors** to produce a physiological effect.

Cholinergic receptors are divided into two subtypes: **nicotinic receptors** and **muscarinic receptors**. Most organs are innervated by sympathetic and parasympathetic fibres. The major exception is the vascular system, which is generally under sympathetic control. The systemic effects of the sympathetic and parasympathetic nervous system can be seen in Table 9.1.

Table 9.1 Systemic effects of the sympathetic and parasympathetic nervous system

Location	*Sympathetic*	*Parasympathetic*
Heart muscle	Increases heart rate and contractility (β_1)	Decreases heart rate and contractility (mAChR)
Coronary arterioles	Vasodilation (β_2)	Vasoconstriction (mAChR)
Bronchial smooth muscle	Bronchodilation (β_2)	Bronchoconstriction (mAChR)
Skeletal muscle arterioles	Vasodilation (β_2)	No known effect
Pupils	Dilation (α_1)	No known effect
Liver	Glycogenolysis and gluconeogenesis	Glycogen synthesis
Kidney	Secretion of renin (β_1)	No known effect
Bladder	Relaxation of bladder (β_2) Constriction of sphincter (α_1)	Contraction of bladder and relaxation of sphincter (mAChR)
GI tract	Reduced motility (α_1, α_2, β_2) Contraction of sphincters (α_1)	Increased motility Relaxation of sphincters (mAChR)
Skin arterioles	Vasoconstriction (α_1)	No known effect
Arrector pili muscle (hair follicles)	Contraction, hairs stand up (α_1)	No known effect
Sweating	Increased sweating on the palms of the hand (α_1)	No known effect

Imagine walking home one evening and hearing footsteps in the dark. An instant decision is made either to turn to confront the person or to run away. This is the 'fight or flight' response of the sympathetic nervous system. Whichever action is taken requires the release of **adrenaline**, and an important series of physiological events automatically occur:

- *Pupils dilate*: improving environmental awareness.
- *Heart rate and contractility increases*: sending more blood to the muscles, facilitating the physical response.
- *Coronary arteries dilate*: delivering more oxygen to the myocardium whilst it works harder.
- *Bronchi dilate*: increasing airflow and improving oxygenation.
- *Arterioles supplying blood to skeletal muscle dilate*: delivering more oxygen to the muscles.
- *Arterioles supplying the skin vasoconstrict*: diverting blood to essential organs, causing the peripheries to cool.
- *Kidneys releases renin*: a vasoconstrictor that increases blood pressure.
- *Liver breaks down stored glycogen to form glucose, which is released into the bloodstream*: maintaining the supply of glucose to the brain and the muscles.
- *Adipose tissue is broken down*: to provide more energy.
- *Gut motility is reduced, sphincters constrict*: the gut is not essential in a crisis.
- *The trigone of the bladder relaxes, allowing the bladder to fill*: reducing the urge to urinate.
- *Arrector pili muscles contract*: the hairs on the skin stand on end.
- Palms of the hands may begin to sweat.

The sympathetic nervous system has instantly prepared the body to deal with the crisis. When the crisis is over, the parasympathetic system takes over and reverses the sympathetic effects. Parasympathetic effects can be quite noticeable. The acronym SLUDD helps to remember the five key parasympathetic responses (Tortora and Derrickson 2017):

S – salivation
L – lacrimation (tears)
U – urination
D – digestion
D – defaecation.

The parasympathetic system decreases the heart rate and constricts the bronchi and the pupils.

Stress is physiological as well as environmental. Acute and critical illness creates physiological stress, and a sympathetic response occurs. Patients become tachycardic, hypertensive, tachypnoeic, peripherally cool, clammy, hyperglycaemic and if conscious, may become anxious. Acutely ill patients may experience these symptoms for days or weeks and may exhibit all the effects listed in Table 9.2, including constipation and urinary retention.

Neurological emergencies

The unconscious patient

Consciousness refers to a state of awareness of oneself and one's surroundings. An acute episode of unconsciousness is a medical emergency, irrespective of the cause.

Table 9.2 Common causes of acute unconsciousness

• Hypotension	• Seizures
• Hypoglycaemia	• Head injury
• Diabetic ketoacidosis	• Raised intracranial pressure
• Hyponatraemia	• Hypoxia
• Uraemia	• CO_2 narcosis
• Sensitivity to narcotics	• Alcohol excess
• Overdose and poisoning	• Anaphylaxis
• Hepatic encephalopathy	• Hypothermia
• Acute stroke	• Dysrhythmias
• Cerebral haemorrhage	• Cardiac arrest
• Meningitis	
• Encephalitis	

Unconsciousness has many potential causes, not all of which are neurological, but the treatment of the patient will be the same until the diagnosis has been made. Common causes of acute unconsciousness can be found in Table 9.2.

If the patient is unresponsive, call for expert help immediately; in hospital, it is appropriate to make peri-arrest, cardiac arrest or medical emergency calls; in the community, dial 999 for an ambulance.

The first-line management of all medical emergencies is the same – ABCDE – airway, breathing, circulation, disability, exposure. For the management of cardiac arrest, see Chapter 7.

Having established that the patient is not in cardiac arrest (i.e. they are breathing), place the patient in the recovery position to optimise the airway. Reduced consciousness is potentially life-threatening and may result in postural airway obstruction and loss of airway reflexes such as cough, gag and swallow reflexes. Without these reflexes, the patient is at risk of aspirating secretions or vomit. A nasopharyngeal airway may be required if positioning alone does not maintain the airway.

Administer oxygen initially at 15L/min via non-rebreathing face mask; when stable, the inspired oxygen can be titrated to maintain oxygen saturations within the normal range of 94–98% (unless a target of 88–92% has been directed). A full set of vital signs should be recorded.

The cause of reduced consciousness requires formal medical diagnosis; the blood glucose should be checked to detect hyper- or hypoglycaemia. Hypoglycaemia should be treated immediately with intravenous glucose or glucagon injection (NICE 2019b).

Unconscious patients are unable to give consent to treatment, but it is a professional expectation that nurses will act in the best interests of the patient and provide all necessary care until the patient regains consciousness and competence (Nursing and Midwifery Council 2018b).

Care of the unconscious patient includes:

- *Psychological support*: explaining all nursing actions prior to carrying them out, not talking over patients, actively orientating patients to time and place.
- *Hydration*: intravenous or enteral fluids to meet hydration requirements, including insensible losses. Maintain accurate intake and output records, calculating fluid balance at least 12-hourly (NMC 2018a).

- *Nutrition*: nasogastric (NG) feeding to meet calorie requirements as advised by dietetics, checking and recording NG position prior to use and supplementing electrolytes as indicated by blood results.
- *Oral hygiene*: oral suction if needed, and toothbrush and paste to maintain oral hygiene.
- *Eye care*: if unable to blink, eyes should be kept closed, if possible, and the corneas lubricated with eye drops or eye ointment.
- *Positioning*: to promote airway maintenance, normal limb posture and to prevent pressure injury. Pressure-relieving mattresses as indicated by regular assessment, using a pressure risk-assessment tool.
- *Bowel management*: laxatives as required to prevent constipation; record bowel actions on a bowel chart and follow local policy for diarrhoea management.
- *Urinary management*: catheterisation or urinary sheath (Conveen) to monitor urine output and to prevent skin breakdown.
- *Skin care*: control of secretions, use of barrier creams to prevent skin excoriation, prompt incontinence management, avoidance of incontinence pads, regular washes if diaphoretic. Men should be shaved if this is their normal practice. Fingernails should be kept clean and trimmed, toenails should be kept clean and trimmed (refer to podiatry or chiropody if patient is diabetic).
- *Observations*: frequency appropriate to the patient's condition and agreed with the nurse in charge, report abnormal observations immediately assessing deterioration risk using NEWS. For those with altered consciousness use the Glasgow Coma Scale (GCS) assessment if applicable, to assesses neurological status, to promote consistency of scoring and detection of subtle changes.
- *Thromboprophylaxis*: administer anticoagulants and apply anti-emboli stockings or compression devices in accordance with local policy, regular reassessment of risk.
- *Vascular access*: regular assessment of all vascular access insertion sites utilising a phlebitis scoring tool; document findings. To prevent infection of the vascular access site, both timely removal of devices when no longer required, and timely replacement of devices that have reached maximum dwell time are recommended (Loveday et al. 2014).
- *Medications*: administer as prescribed, monitor drug levels, electrolytes and vital signs as indicated for each particular medication (NMC 2018a).
- *Support family and friends*: provide support and information appropriately whilst maintaining an appropriate level of patient confidentiality (NMC 2018a, b).

Assessing change in level of consciousness

An acutely ill patient may present with an altered mental status, manifesting as a new acute confusion or delirium. This altered mental status may have stemmed from one or a combination of the following causes: hypoxia, hypotension, sepsis or metabolic disturbances (Royal College of Physician [RCP] 2017). Altered mental status is associated with deterioration, requiring an immediate clinical assessment and response. The ACVPU scale is embedded in the National Early Warning Score (NEWS) 2. The ACVPU scale is simple to use and can rapidly record a change in conscious level. 'A' is used to record alert, 'C' records *new onset* of confusion or delirium and adds a score of 3 to NEWS, 'V' records responding to verbal stimuli, 'P' records response to painful stimuli only and 'U' records unresponsiveness. Only 'A' scores 0, and each of CVPU scores 3, reflecting the risk of deterioration associated with altered mental status. If it is unclear whether the altered mentation is new, it is recommended that it should be regarded as new onset until proven otherwise (RCP 2017). Further information regarding patient confusion can be gleaned from relatives, who will be able to explain what normal confusion (as with dementia) might be for their loved one, or confirm that the current level of confusion is not normal/worse that their normal state. If the patient is unconscious, or if there are suspicions of underlying neurological pathology, e.g., stroke or fall, a full neurological assessment using the **Glasgow Coma Scale (GCS)** gives a more consistent and detailed approach.

Neurological assessment

Neurological assessment is performed for the following reasons:

- To establish baseline neurology.
- To identify change in relation to an earlier neurological assessment.
- To identify neurological abnormalities or deficits.
- To identify the impact of a neurological deficit on the activities of living (AL).

Specific elements of neurological assessment vary, depending upon the patient's level of consciousness, their ability to follow simple commands and their clinical situation. The frequency of neurological assessment is dictated by the patient's clinical condition. Acutely unstable neurological patients may require observation every 5–15 minutes; the stable neurological patient may require observation every 4–8 hours. Clinical judgment is required when performing neurological assessment; if the patient's condition is deteriorating, frequency of assessment should increase. Neurological assessment is recorded on a neurological observation chart, which includes the Glasgow Coma Scale and may incorporate NEWS.

A neurological observation chart includes:

- Assessment of consciousness, (eye opening, best verbal response).
- Limbs assessment (best motor response, power and type of response).
- Pupil size, shape, equality and reaction to light.
- Respiratory rate and pattern.
- Blood pressure, pulse and temperature.

Assessing consciousness using the Glasgow Coma Scale

The **Glasgow Coma Scale (GCS)** is probably the most widely used neurological assessment tool in the world (Teasdale et al. 2014). GCS is designed to be used in the acute phase of head injury, to monitor any fluctuations in level of consciousness, when the condition might change rapidly.

GCS assessment has three elements:

- Best eye-opening response.
- Best verbal response.
- Best motor response.

Each element contains subcategories with a score (see Table 9.3).

Table 9.3 Glasgow coma scale

Best eye-opening response	Eyes open spontaneously	4
	Eyes open to sound	3
	Eyes open to pressure	2
	No eye opening	1
Best verbal response	Orientated to person, time and place	5
	Confused	4
	Words	3
	Sounds	2
	None	1
Best motor response	Obeys commands	6
	Localising	5
	Normal flexion/withdrawal	4
	Abnormal flexion	3
	Extension	2
	None	1

(Teasdale 2015).

4 steps for GCS assessment

- Step 1: check.
- Step 2: observe.
- Step 3: stimulate.
- Step 4: rate.

The four steps to assessment are used for assessing three components:

- Eye opening.
- Verbal response.
- Best motor response.

Briefly, firstly the nurse must *check* for any factors that might interfere with the patient's response, for example, is the patient deaf or is their eye swollen? What language is understood best by the patient? Then, the nurse will *observe* for any spontaneous movement or communication, for example, are the eyes opening spontaneously? Can they talk clearly and coherently; are they moving normally? Observations are recorded on the chart.

2 types of *stimuli* may be used; initially, verbal requests are made, with the voice raised if no initial response seen. If required, a physical stimulus such as the trapezius squeeze is used to illicit a response. The *rating* is then scored for each component and a total score obtained. If it has not been possible to test an area, then not tested (NT) it recorded. The score is reported at a total GCS and with each separate component, for example, E4 V5 M6 (Teasdale et al. 2014).

The maximum possible score is 15/15; the lowest score is 3/15. A drop of 2 or more is significant, and a score of eight or less indicates a medical emergency. This low score is associated with severe brain injury and must be escalated for immediate airway management (National Institute for Health and Care Excellence 2017).

GCS is intended to be an objective assessment of the patient's level of consciousness, however, as individual judgement for rating the patient's responses is required, a certain amount of subjectivity is inevitable. For this reason, it is considered good practice for nurses to jointly assess GCS at handover to ensure both agree on the GCS. If the GCS deteriorates, a second competent nurse can immediately check the GCS, confirming the deterioration prior to alerting the medical team. However, referral to the medical team should not be delayed, should the second competent nurse not be available (NICE 2017).

In a busy ward environment, in daylight or when the lights are on, most patients will be awake. The fact that a patient is sleeping in a noisy environment may be the first indication that the GCS is not 15/15, even if there is no primary neurological problem. If the patient wakes and opens their eyes as the nurse approaches, the eye-opening score will be 4 for spontaneous eye opening (see Table 9.3). If the patient's eyes do not open spontaneously as the nurse approaches the bed space, it will be necessary to use a stimulus to assess the patient. As discussed, there are two types of stimulus – verbal and pressure stimuli.

Verbal stimuli refers to use of voice to stimulate a response. Begin by greeting the patient in a normal tone to see if their eyes open: 'Hello, Mr Smith'. If unsuccessful, repeat the greeting with a raised voice. If the patient opens their eyes, continue the GCS assessment. If the patient does not open their eyes, speak loudly into both ears, ensuring hearing aids are present if the patient is deaf. If the patient opens their eyes, it will be a score of 3. While talking, observe for spontaneous limb movement. If verbal stimulus is unsuccessful, tactile stimulus is needed.

Pressure stimuli: neurological patients often sleep very deeply; it may be necessary to ensure the patient is fully awake before proceeding with GCS assessment. If the patient does not open their eyes to sound, pressure is applied to the fingertips using a pen or pencil, with increasing intensity for 10 seconds, until the maximum pressure is obtained (see Figure 9.15). If the patient opens their eyes, this scores 2 for eye opening. If there is no response, despite pressure being applied, this will scores as 1. However, if the patient's eyes are closed due to local swelling or other factors, it should be written as 'not testable' (NT).

The patient's verbal response is elicited through compulsory questions to establish whether the patient is orientated to person, time and place. The nurse must ask the patient their name and where they are. If the patient knows they are in hospital, the nurse should

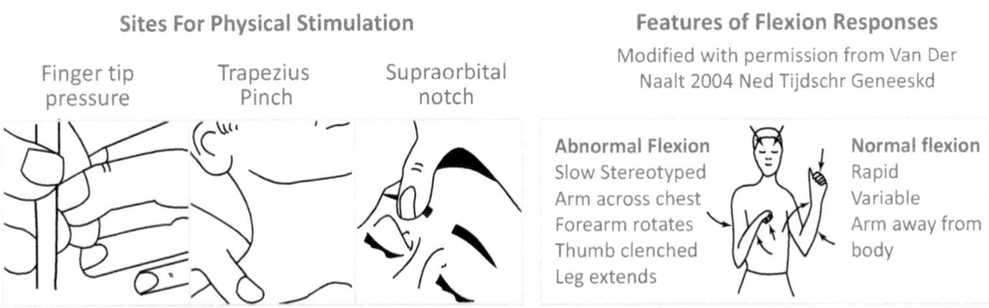

Figure 9.15 The new standard to perform neurological observation and Glasgow Coma Scale chart (Teasdale 2015). For further information and video demonstration please see www.glasgowcomascale.org.

be more specific and ask the patient to name the hospital. Next, ask the patient to state the month; if the patient answers correctly, this indicates orientation to person, time and place and scores 5 for the verbal response (see Table 9.3). If the patient answers incorrectly to any of the three questions, they should be scored as confused, even if they are able to speak coherently. For example, the patient may be in hospital, but might think they are at home; the answer is relevant to the question but incorrect, so they will score 4 for confusion. If the patient answers with words and lacks sentence structure or phrases, it is classified as 'words' and scores 3 points. Unintelligible speech, making sounds, not words, classifies the response as 'sounds', scoring 2 points. If there is no verbal response at all, the patient scores 1 point (Teasdale et al. 2014). Patients may be unable to speak because of intubation or a cuffed tracheostomy tube; these patients have no air flow through their vocal cords. In this situation, the nurse annotates the score as 'not testable' (NT).

After assessing verbal response, the motor response is assessed. As seen in Table 9.3, motor response has six possible results. The nurse asks the patient to perform two specific actions to determine whether the patient is capable of obeying commands (Teasdale et al. 2014). It is important to choose an action that the patient is unlikely to perform by coincidence. A hand squeeze can be used to assess motor function. For this command, the nurse places their fingers on the ventral side of the patient's fingers, not across the palm of the patient's hand. This avoids triggering the grasp reflex, which may occur without cognitive intention. For the second command, either ask the patient to raise their arms or, if they are unable to move their arms, to stick out their tongue.

Dorsal: upper, back or posterior surface.
Ventral: lower, under or anterior surface.

There are several ways to apply a central pain stimulus, and not all are clinically appropriate. The application of supraorbital pressure is a type of central pain stimulus, but is contraindicated in patients with facial fractures and should not be attempted unless trained to do so (see Figure 9.15). A sternal rub can easily bruise the soft tissue over the sternum, and is strongly not recommended (Teasdale et al. 2014). The easiest and most common method of applying a central pain stimulus is to squeeze the trapezius muscle between the neck and the shoulder joint. If the trapezius squeeze is contraindicated, for example, if the collar bones are fractured, mandibular pressure may be applied by using the index and middle finger to press upwards and inwards at the hinge of the mandible.

Prior to applying a pain stimulus, the nurse should ensure that the patient is positioned appropriately and that the arms and the feet have been uncovered in order to observe limb responses. Arms should be placed away from the body, allowing enough space for the limbs to move freely. If the arms are too close to the patient's body, it may be difficult to interpret the motor response of the upper limbs.

A central pain stimulus should be used for motor response; peripheral pain stimuli can invoke spinal reflexes and may result in an incorrect GCS assessment. A spinal reflex is a signal that travels via a sensory nerve to the spinal cord, producing a motor response from the spinal cord back to the periphery. The impulse does not travel via the brain and is not an indicator of motor function.

Nurses may be hesitant to apply a pain stimulus, concerned about hurting the patient. This misplaced concern may result in an incorrect GCS assessment, which may be detrimental to the patient. Nurses caring for patients with altered consciousness have a professional obligation to assess the patient accurately in order to ensure the patient receives the most appropriate treatment. Nurses must overcome their anxiety and learn to apply a central pain stimulus correctly.

A trapezius squeeze is performed using the thumb and index finger to grasp about 5cm of trapezius muscle at the base of the neck, squeeze and twist the muscle while observing carefully for eye opening and for motor response of all four limbs. Pain stimulus should be maintained for about 10 seconds, until the nurse is certain of the patient's response.

Having applied a pain stimulus, the motor response must be interpreted, and a score awarded (see Table 9.3). To achieve a motor score of five, the patient must localise to pain. If the brain is intact, the normal response to pain is to move away from the pain or to remove the source of the pain. Having applied a trapezius squeeze, if the patient moves their arm purposely towards the source of the pain, attempting to remove the assessor's hand, they are said to be localising to pain. The patient's hand must be raised to the height of the chin to award a motor score of 5. This is a positive sign, suggesting a relatively intact brain.

If the patient is unable to raise their arm to chin height, but has rapidly flexed their arm, they may be awarded a score of 4, for 'withdrawal or normal flexion'. **Flexion/**withdrawal suggests that the patient is unable to make a purposeful attempt to remove the source of the pain. It should be noted that this flexion is a brisk movement. If the patient is flexing the arm, bringing the hand towards the body by bending the elbow and wrist slowly in an abnormal manner, they are scored 3 for abnormal flexion.

When the pain stimulus is applied, the shoulders appear to move upwards, the elbows appear to flex and, as the pain stimulus continues, arms internally rotate, fingers flex to form a fist and the arms push down and extend away from the source of pain, legs extend and toes point. This is extension and will score 2 points (see Table 9.3). If there is no response to central pain, try to apply supraorbital pressure (this is contraindicated in patients with facial fracture). One point is awarded for motor function if no response is elicited. If different responses are observed, for example, normal flexion is seen over the right arm (scoring 4) while the left arm is abnormal flexion (scoring 3), the best response should be recorded, which is a score of 4.

By now, a score will have been generated for all three sections of the GCS. The scores are recorded and communicated to identify each section of the score as well as giving a total score. For example, E2 V3 M4 gives a GCS of 9/15.

The motor section of the GCS carries the most weight. A GCS of 7/15 that is achieved by E1 V1 M5 is viewed more positively than a GCS of 7/15 that is achieved by E4 V1 M2. By presenting the information for each section, it becomes clear where the patient has lost points.

When patients are unable to obey commands, it is difficult to assess limb power. Muscle tone can be assessed by moving each limb through the normal range of passive movement. This reveals whether the limb is normal, flaccid or has increased tone.

When patients are able to obey commands, limb power is graded from 0–5 (see Table 9.4).

It is important to note that GCS only forms part of the assessment about a patient's neurological status. It is vital that other assessments, for example, pupillary assessment and vital signs, are included to provide a more complete picture.

Assessing pupils

This element of neurological assessment is performed on conscious and unconscious patients, unless the eyes are closed by oedema, in which case a 'NT' is marked on the

Table 9.4 Grading limb power

Grade	*Indicator of limb power*
5	Active movement against gravity; full resistance; normal strength
4	Active movement against gravity; some resistance that can be overcome by the examiner
3	Active movement against gravity; unable to resist the examiner
2	Active movement when gravity is eliminated
1	No active movement; weak muscle contraction can be palpated
0	No muscle contraction detected

neurological observation chart. Assessment of the pupils is not a part of GCS assessment, however, it is usually assessed when performing a neurological assessment, as the pupillary reaction provides additional information about the brain, for example, brain stem function and increased intracranial pressure.

Pupil size, pupil shape, reactivity to light and equality of pupil size should be assessed and recorded on the neurological observation chart.

A pupil gauge, printed on the neurological observation chart, is used to measure pupil size. Normal pupil size ranges from 2–6mm, but abnormal pupils may be as large as 9mm. Extremely small pupils are described as pinpoint and may result from opiate administration. Pupils that are large, dilated and unreactive to light are described as 'fixed and dilated'. This is a severe sign of raised intracranial pressure and may indicate that death is imminent.

Pupils are normally round, but pupil abnormalities do occur. An oval-shaped pupil indicates raised intracranial pressure and must be reported immediately. A keyhole pupil is the result of eye surgery and is not a neurological sign.

To assess the pupils, both eyelids should be elevated simultaneously, and pupil size compared. Bright overhead light should be switched off, as it will be more difficult to observe response in a bright room. Using a pen torch, shine light into the eye; observe the pupil, it should constrict immediately as light is applied and should dilate when the light is withdrawn – this is the direct light reflex. The application of light to one pupil should cause a simultaneous response in both pupils – this is the consensual light reaction. Reactions of the pupils to light can be described as brisk, sluggish or fixed.

A plus sign (+) indicates pupil reactivity on the neurological observation chart, and a minus sign (-) indicates no reaction. A reduction in pupil reactivity is an important sign of neurological compromise and should be reported immediately.

GCS PUPIL SCORE

The GCS gives a good indication of the overall change in brain function, or conscious level. The addition of information regarding pupil reaction and age has been suggested to give a clearer prognostic indicator of outcome than GCS alone (Murray et al. 2018). The GCS pupil score (GPS-P) can be calculated by subtracting a score of 2 (for two unreactive pupils), 1 (for one unreactive pupil) or 0 (for both pupils reacting normally) from the GSC Score. GPS-P can be derived from the information recorded on a neurological assessment chart encompassing the GSC score and pupil response. The GPS-P score in combination with CT scans and patient age may guide the medical team in their decision-making, and improve their information sharing with the patient, relatives and health care team (Brennan et al. 2018).

Respiratory assessment

Respiration may be affected by conscious level and brain pathology. Respiration is controlled by the pons and the medulla in the brainstem. Abnormal respiratory patterns suggest brainstem pathology. Brainstem injury is associated with tachypnoea, bradypnoea and **apnoea**.

Cheyne–Stokes breathing: a cyclical pattern of rapid breathing becoming progressively slower and shallower until apnoea occurs. The patient usually starts breathing again spontaneously, but may be stimulated to breathe by tactile stimulation if apnoea is prolonged. This respiratory pattern is associated with widespread cortical lesions and thalamic dysfunction. Apnoea is an important observation and should be reported. Non-invasive respiratory monitoring and support is indicated if apnoea is frequent or prolonged.

Vital signs assessment

Thermoregulation may be affected by neurological disease or injury. Hyperthermia is more common than hypothermia; it may be central in origin and is associated with subarachnoid haemorrhage, blood in the CSF and in patients with posterior fossa surgery. It is important to remember that fever may not be neurological in origin; it is also seen in acute MI, PE, sepsis and local infection.

Hyperthermia increases cell metabolism, which increases oxygen demand, CO_2 production and lactic acid. CO_2 is a potent vasodilator within the systemic circulation and has the potential to increase intracranial pressure (ICP) by increasing blood flow. Hyperthermia in neurological patients has been shown to independently contribute to increased length of stay and poorer neurological outcomes in neuro-critical care units (Bonds et al. 2015). Attempts should be made to control temperature, but it is important to prevent shivering in acute or unstable patients, as shivering increases ICP. Antipyretics, tepid sponging, removing blankets and increasing skin exposure all help to reduce fever. Induced hypothermia, where the patient was cooled to 33–35°C, has been practiced in neurological units as it was considered to be neuroprotective, improving long-term neurological outcomes. However, this practice is not currently recommended, as a recent study highlights that cooling did not improve neurological outcomes at six months. Cooling may actually increase additional risks, for example, pneumonia, that affect outcome (Cooper et al. 2018). The Prophylactic Hypothermia Trial to Lessen Traumatic Brain Injury-Randomized Clinical Trial (POLAR-RCT) recommends the maintenance of normothermia in patients with traumatic brain injury (Cooper et al. 2018).

Maximising neurological status

Raised ICP is damaging to brain tissue and must be prevented or managed urgently. The skull contains brain tissue, CSF and blood vessels, and strategies to reduce ICP focus on one or more of these elements.

Removal of brain tissue is not desirable unless clinically indicated, and strategies to control brain tissue generally focus on the control of cerebral oedema or the relief of pressure. Cerebral oedema is managed by administration of osmotic diuretics and steroids and the restriction of fluids. Raised ICP is relieved by the creation of burr holes (holes drilled in the skull) or by craniectomy (a surgical procedure to remove a flap of bone).

Position

Patients with reduced or fluctuating levels of consciousness are at risk of aspiration if protective airway reflexes are lost. Elevating the head of the bed to 30° reduces this risk. Head elevation also increases venous drainage from the head, helping to control cerebral blood volume and reduce ICP. For patients with acute elevations in ICP, extreme flexion of the hips and knees is contraindicated, as this may increase intra-abdominal pressure with a resulting increase in thoracic pressure and intracranial pressure. It is important to ensure the head is maintained in a neutral position, avoiding rotation of the head or hyperextension and flexion of the neck, as this will affect the venous drainage from the head, resulting in increased ICP.

Optimising cerebral blood flow

The cerebral blood vessels and the blood contained within them take up approximately 10 per cent of the space within the skull. Blood vessel diameter affects the amount of space that the blood vessels occupy within the brain. Blood vessels may dilate due to increased blood volume or because of metabolic factors influencing blood vessel tone, for example, pH, PaO_2, and $PaCO_2$. Hypoxia, hypercapnia and acidosis cause vasodilation of blood vessels, increasing ICP. The reverse is also true: hypocapnia and alkalosis cause vasoconstriction, reducing cerebral blood flow. As a result of these effects on the cerebral blood vessels, the partial pressure of carbon dioxide in arterial blood gas ($PaCO_2$) is monitored closely and maintained within normal limits between 4.6–6kPa for optimal cerebral blood flow (Carney et al. 2016).

Oxygen is administered to maintain PaO_2 greater than 11kPa or oxygen saturation >95% (Carney et al. 2016). This high target PaO_2 is important in order to help optimise vessel tone and ICP control. Intubation and ventilation may be needed to control $PaCO_2$ and to optimise oxygenation. By preventing hypoxia and hypercapnia, the blood vessels remain in a state of partial tone and will occupy less space within the brain.

A good cerebral blood flow and oxygen delivery is essential for normal cerebral function. Although the brain only weighs about 1.5kg, or 2% of body weight, it receives approximately 20% of the cardiac output and 20% of available oxygen. The brain is able to autoregulate to control cerebral blood flow. Autoregulation describes the brain's ability to maintain a constant blood flow irrespective of changes to blood pressure. This phenomenon only functions correctly when mean arterial pressure (MAP) is between 60 and 150mmHg. Below 60mmHg, cerebral blood flow diminishes, and above 150mmHg, it increases. Hypotension causes cerebral ischaemia and brain injury. Neurological management focuses on the maintenance of MAP by the administration of fluids and vasopressors.

Calculating cerebral perfusion pressure: MAP – ICP = CPP
For example:

80mmHg (MAP) – 13mmHg (ICP) = 67mmHg (CPP) [normal range 60–70mmHg]

In health, little notice is taken of **cerebral perfusion pressure (CPP)** because the brain autoregulates. However, for patients with acute neurological problems, CPP is considered to be important, as it has implications for cerebral blood flow. CPP is calculated by subtracting the ICP from the mean arterial blood pressure, with an aim of maintenance between 60–70mmHg to prevent cerebral ischaemia (Carney et al. 2016). From the formula, it can be concluded that if MAP were to fall and ICP were to rise, CPP would be significantly affected. Trauma to the vasomotor centre, located in the medulla of the brain, may cause autoregulation to fail. Hypotension from failure of the vasomotor centre is termed neurogenic shock.

Meningitis

Meningitis is the term used to describe inflammation of the meninges surrounding the brain and spinal cord. Inflammation can be caused by bacteria, viruses, fungi, protozoa, cancer cells or by irritant drugs. The most serious form of meningitis is bacterial meningitis. Bacterial meningitis affects the subarachnoid space and the meninges either side of the space, the pia and arachnoid mater as well as the CSF. It can be fatal, even when medical treatment is started promptly, as the bacterial infection progresses rapidly, which could lead to sepsis/septic shock (Meningitis Research Foundation 2019). Therefore, regardless of whether or not the patient has meningitis, once the patient presents with signs of sepsis, early recognition and intervention are vital to improving the patient's prognosis.

Bacterial meningitis is common in immunocompromised groups, for example, children, particularly new-borns, adolescents, those over 65 and certain disease groups. Meningococcal meningitis is the most common type of bacterial meningitis and is particularly dangerous, often associated with outbreaks, or small epidemics (Meningitis Research Foundation 2019). There are 6 identified serogroups of meningococcal infection: A, B, C, W, X and Y. Meningococcal B (MenB) and Meningococcal C (MenC) were once the most prevalent, but these have been significantly reduced with the introduction of the MenB and MenC vaccination (Public Health England 2016). However, since 2009, Meningococcal W (MenW) has increased across all age groups. Therefore, the Joint Committee on Vaccination and Immunisation (JCVI) recommend that the Men ACWY vaccine should replace the teenage MenC dose in the school-based programme for those aged 14–18 years old (Public Health England 2016).

The people most at risk are those living in close quarters, such as student halls of residence, hostels, nursing homes, overcrowded households or military barracks. Hence, the vaccination programme further recommends that those who are under 25 years old and who have missed the Men ACWY vaccines should be immunised before they start attending University (PHE 2016). There are other strains of bacteria causing meningitis, and vaccines are developed for a specific strain. These vaccines are mostly offered to babies at 2 months and children from 1–15 years old. Some vaccines are offered to those at risk, e.g., the elderly and those who had long term serious condition. However, not all vaccines are available, as some are still being researched, e.g., Group B Streptococcal bacteria.

Bacterial meningitis can also occur following neuro-surgery, lumbar puncture, skull fracture or penetrating head injury. This type of meningitis is not contagious and is caused by bacteria entering the meninges when the CNS is opened.

Severe headache, fever, nausea, vomiting and feeling unwell are early symptoms of meningitis; hyperpyrexia is common. Neck stiffness is also an early sign and may be associated with lethargy and confusion. Lethargy can quickly progress to unconsciousness. **Photophobia** and non-blanching rash are also common. Other signs may also include physical signs such as Brudzinski's sign (pain when the neck, hips and knees flex simultaneously) and Kernig's sign (with the patient supine, the knee is flexed and then straightened; straightening causes acute pain).

The immune system responds to the bacterial invasion of the meninges and inflammation develops. Inflammation may affect blood vessels, causing thrombus or haemorrhage. Inflammation also damages brain tissue and may cause seizures, stroke and cerebral oedema. Cerebral oedema can obstruct CSF drainage, leading to hydrocephaly and raised ICP. Meningococcal meningitis can lead to life-threatening sepsis and multi-organ failure.

Clinical symptoms are often poor predictors of meningitis; therefore, diagnosis is confirmed by mainly by lumbar puncture (LP). However, CT scan should be urgently performed if there are clinical signs of brain shift presented as focal neurological signs or deterioration in GCS score (Griffiths, McGill and Solomon 2018). Due to the potential mortality from meningitis, treatment should start immediately. Intravenous empirical antibiotics, as according to guidelines for meningitis, are given until culture results are known. If bacterial meningitis is suspected, corticosteroids like dexamethasone should be given (Griffiths, McGill and Solomon 2018). Corticosteroids are also used to suppress the inflammatory response and reduce cerebral oedema. There is no specific treatment for viral meningitis, and antivirals such as Acyclovir (an anti-viral medication) should only be considered if there are signs of encephalic involvement, such as impairment of consciousness, focal neurological signs and inflammation of the brain parenchyma in the temporal lobe.

Intravenous fluids are given to maintain hydration, intravascular volume and MAP. Insensible losses from sweating and measurable losses from vomiting must be replaced. The risk of seizures means that usually, **anticonvulsants** such as intravenous phenytoin are prescribed.

If ICP is dangerously high, (above 22mmHg) intravenous mannitol, an osmotic diuretic, may be given (Carney et al. 2016). Mannitol is a large-molecule sugar solution that rapidly increases the osmotic pressure of the blood. The increased osmotic pressure draws water from the interstitial space into the blood compartment, reducing interstitial cerebral oedema. Increases in blood volume are detected by the aortic and carotid baroreceptors and the atrial diastolic stretch receptors. Increased signals are sent to the vasomotor centre, indicating that the circulating volume is too high. Antidiuretic hormone is inhibited, and reabsorption of water by the kidneys ceases, causing an immediate diuresis. Mannitol is a potent osmotic diuretic, and patients may pass several litres of urine per hour. It is essential to maintain the patient's electrolytes within normal range, particularly potassium, to prevent cardiac dysrhythmias as a complication of diuresis.

Another widely used hyperosmolar agent is hypertonic saline (Shah and Kimberly 2016). This can effectively reduce ICP rapidly, with no rebound increase. Caution is required, though, due to risks of electrolyte imbalance and possible heart failure, so it should be administered with close monitoring in a higher level of care.

Acute stroke

Acute stroke is a common condition – someone suffers an acute stroke every five minutes in England. In the developed world, approximately 15 per cent of strokes are haemorrhagic and 85 per cent are ischaemic (Stroke Association 2018).

Ischaemic strokes can occur due to:

- A blot clot obstructing a cerebral blood vessel.
- An embolus from elsewhere in the body travelling to block a cerebral vessel.
- Low blood pressure or shock.

A haemorrhagic stroke may be cause by:

- An intracerebral haemorrhage (bleeding within the brain).
- Subarachnoid haemorrhage – bleeding occurring outside the brain tissue, but within the skull, usually within the meninges that surround the brain

A number of risk factors for stroke exist; some are modifiable, some are not. Non-modifiable risk factors for stroke include:

- Age: the risk of stroke increases exponentially with age.
- Gender: men are at increased risk when compared to women.
- Ethnicity: individuals of black and Asian origin have a greater risk of stroke when compared to white people.
- Genetics: a family of history of stroke in individuals under 65 years of age is a risk factor for stroke.

(Boehme, Esenwa and Elkind 2017)

Modifiable risk factors (factors which the individual can influence) include:

- Smoking.
- Obesity.
- Socio-economic class.
- Sedentary lifestyle.
- Alcohol excess.
- Hypertension.
- Diabetes.
- Hypercholesterolaemia.
- Metabolic syndrome.
- The oral contraceptive pill.
- Diet.

Problems such as atrial fibrillation (AF) can increase the incidence of stroke by an embolus from thrombus formation in the atria impeding cerebral blood flow. Anticoagulation is used to reduce this risk in those with known AF, but many who may have this problem (AF) are unaware of its existence.

The first sign of stroke may be collapse, but patients may also be aware of the following symptoms and may know that a stroke is occurring:

- Facial weakness or numbness.
- Difficulty walking.
- Difficulty speaking.
- Paralysis or numbness of one side of the body.
- Visual disturbance.
- Headache.

Immediate medical review is indicated: the more quickly a stroke is treated, the better the outcome. Patients with an acute stroke should receive brain imaging within one hour and be admitted to a specialist acute stroke unit where they can be assessed for thrombolysis and receive the appropriate therapy (NICE 2019c).

FAST, for stroke recognition:

Face: has the face fallen on one side, can they smile?
Arms: can they raise both arms and keep them there?
Speech: is their speech slurred?
Time: time to call 999 if you see any one of the signs.

The FAST campaign was first launched in 2009, by the UK government, to introduce the FAST tool to enable the public to recognise the early signs of stroke in the community. Although there was an improvement in the response to major stroke, the response to Transient Ischaemic Attack (TIA) and minor stroke had not improved, which could be attributed to the transient or less severe signs of the two conditions (Wolters et al. 2018). The Act FAST campaign was relaunched in 2018 to identify the symptoms of stroke as quickly as possible, ensuring emergency medical management is provided (PHE 2018).

A patient admitted with a suspected stroke or TIA may benefit from the use of ROSIER (recognition of stroke in the emergency room) (Nor et al. 2005), supported by NICE (2019c). This tool may be superior to FAST in identifying stroke (Jian et al. 2014), but is a little more complex.

ROSIER: Recognition of stroke in the emergency room (Nor et al., 2005)

• Has there been LOC or syncope?	Yes -1	No 0
• Has there been a seizure?	Yes -1	No 0

Is there a new acute onset of:

• Asymmetrical arm weakness.	Yes +1	No 0
• Asymmetrical leg weakness.	Yes +1	No 0
• Speech disturbance.	Yes +1	No 0
• Visual field defect.	Yes +1	No 0

Total Score between -2 to +6

If score >0 stroke is likely.
If score is </=0, stroke is less likely but not totally excluded.

It is imperative to determine that hypoglycaemia is not a cause of the neurological deterioration. A patient with suspected stroke should be admitted to a specialist stroke unit as soon as possible.

Patients with haemorrhagic stroke are transferred to a neurosurgical unit for monitoring. Any deterioration of neurological function requires urgent imaging (NICE 2019c), so frequent and accurate neurological observations are essential. Craniotomy may be indicated to evacuate the haematoma and control intracranial pressure in those who are deteriorating. Those with a thrombotic stroke may require clot removal.

Whatever the setting, patients experiencing an acute stroke require neurological assessment, vital signs assessment and support for ABCDE. Patients are nursed in a semi recumbent position, with the head elevated at a 30° angle to help prevent aspiration pneumonia. It is recommended that patients with acute stroke have their swallowing assessed by a specially trained health care professional prior to being given fluid or medication (NICE 2019c). Nutrition and hydration needs may need to be supported by the nurse until they recover their independence.

CASE STUDY 9.1 ROBERT WITH DROWSINESS, ACUTE ONSET OF CONFUSION AND WEAKNESS IN THE RIGHT ARM: PART 1

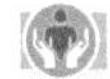

Robert, aged 65, was admitted to the medical unit for pneumonia 4 days ago. He was commenced on antibiotics and seemed to be making a good recovery. He had a past medical history of hypertension with a blood pressure of 150/80mmHg and irregular heart rate due to atrial fibrillation. He was on Amlodipine, 5mg once a day for treatment of his hypertension and Apixaban, 2.5mg twice daily for his atrial fibrillation. He was recovering well and was expected to be discharged home today. The nurse who took over from the night shift went into the room to check on Robert.

Initial assessment

On examination, Robert was lying on his back in a semi-recumbent position. His eyes were closed and he was not moving.

Airway: Robert did not speak when spoken to, but when the nurse spoke more loudly, then gently shook his shoulder, he was able to vocalise indistinctly, indicating the airway was patent and Robert was conscious. However, his speech was slurred, and he appeared anxious. There was no evidence of stridor or paradoxical breathing. However, the nurse noticed that the right side of his mouth was drooping. The nurse suspected that Robert may have had a stroke or transient ischaemic attack, and this may be a medical emergency. A rapid ABCDE assessment was completed to fully evaluate clinical status, and NEWS was completed to evaluate deteriorating risk. Robert's airway may need closer observation, as it might be compromised if his condition deteriorates.

Breathing: Robert looked short of breath, using accessory muscles of breathing. His colour was pink, and there was no sign of sweat. His chest appeared be moving equally. On auscultation, his breath sounds were clear on both the left and the right. No adventitious sound was heard.

Robert's respiratory rate was 20bpm, his respiratory pattern was regular and oxygen saturation was 95% on room air. His target saturation was 94–98%, recorded on the prescription chart. Even though Robert's respiratory rate was 20, within the normal range, the fact that he looked short of breath and that his oxygen saturation was slightly on the lower end of the normal range could be a cause for concern. This could be due to the fact that he was recovering from his pneumonia or it could be an indication that there might be another problem.

Breathing: NEWS (0 + 1 + 0) = 1

Circulation: Robert looked anxious and verbalised that he felt palpitations in his chest. Robert's pulse rate was 106bpm on palpation; the pulse was irregular, and the pulse volume was reduced. Robert felt centrally and peripherally warm with no peripheral oedema. His blood pressure was 140/70mmHg with a MAP of 93mmHg, and the CRT was two seconds.

Robert is known to have hypertension, therefore, the nurse was not too worried about his BP. However, the nurse suspected that Robert might have a worsening of his known cardiac dysrhythmia, atrial fibrillation, as his pulse felt fast and irregular. A colleague was asked to take a 12 lead electrocardiogram (ECG). Whilst not totally confident in ECG interpretation, the irregular heart rate was easy to see. There was no sign of the normal p wave that signifies atrial depolarisation, and a wavy line connected the irregular fast and narrow QRS complexes. It was noted that the ECG rate was 120, faster than the palpated pulse of 106, which is not unusual in fast AF. Not all ventricular contractions deliver an effective stroke volume due to poor atrial filling, therefore, not all heart beats are felt at the radial artery. This fast AF, though, increases myocardial oxygen use and can feel very uncomfortable for the patient.

Circulation: NEWS (0 + 1) = 1

Disability: Robert did not wake when approached and did not speak until a light tactile stimulus was applied. He opened his eyes when he spoke, but tended to mumble. The nurse noticed a slight downturn on the right side of his mouth. On questioning, Robert replied that he was at home, and he didn't know what year it was, indicating he was confused. He was able to obey commands when asked to squeeze the nurse's hand, but his right-hand grip was weaker than his left. He could raise both arms, but his right arm only partially. He was able to stick out his tongue, but it was slightly deviated to the side. The nurse was aware that the facial droop, weaker right arm and the deviated tongue could be signs of stroke.

The blood sugar had previously been stable, and as Robert was not clammy, the nurse did not think that the new onset of confusion could be due to glucose level. The nurse decided to measure this after talking to the doctor.

The nurse used the FAST pneumonic to confirm their suspicions:

F: facial drooping was present.
A: both arms were raised but the right not to the same extent as the right.
S: speech was slurred.
T: time for help to be summoned!

Disability: NEWS = 3

Exposure: Robert was apyrexial at 36.5°C. He did not have abdominal or calf pain. His abdomen was soft and non-tender on palpation. He had scanty bowel sounds, and his calves were soft and non-tender. His skin appeared intact, and he was continent.

Exposure: NEWS = 0
TOTAL NEWS 1 + 1 + 3 = 5

As Robert had developed new confusion, the concern with the FAST finding is that he may have been having an acute onset of stroke. GCS was performed on him as a baseline neurological assessment. His GCS was E3V4 M6 = 13/15. Pupils were size 2, equal and reactive to light. The nurse recorded the pupil responses as '+' on the neurological observation chart. Blood glucose was 10.1mmol/L.

The nurse realised that the elevated blood glucose level may be due to physiological stress, activating the sympathetic nervous system, thereby causing glycogenolysis and gluconeogenesis. The sympathetic nervous system may also have been responsible for the quiet and infrequent bowel sounds heard. Robert then required regular blood glucose monitoring.

Care escalation

In view of the NEWS of 5 presentation and clinical findings, which include slurred speech, drooping right side of mouth, deviated tongue, weaker right side and tachycardia, a provisional diagnosis of stroke is made. This required urgent escalation. The NEWS of 5 with the addition of new confusion and history of chest infection also meant that sepsis must be considered.

The doctor arrived promptly, concerned by the change in NEWS and neurological status.

The doctor prescribed the O_2 to be titrated to maintain the oxygen saturation greater than 95%, according to NICE guidelines NG 128 (2019).

A large-bore peripheral cannula was inserted and 500mL of 0.9% NaCl was given over 15 minutes, in light of his raised heart rate. Blood was taken for full blood count, electrolytes, C-reactive protein, liver function tests and a clotting screen at the time of cannulation. Robert was cannulated using aseptic technique. An arterial blood gas was taken as well to check his respiratory status and his serum lactate.

A quick calculation by the doctor revealed the **ROSIER** score to be +2, as there was right-sided arm weakness and speech disturbance, further suggesting stroke as a likely diagnosis.

Robert's nurse recorded the GCS and the vital signs, and it was agreed that Robert would remain on continuous monitoring with hourly recording of observations. An urgent referral to the neurologist and a CT scan of the head is requested. It was explained to Robert that he would remain nil by mouth for the moment, and that a scan would confirm his diagnosis and indicate the treatment required. The nurse asked if he would like his wife to be called, to let her know what was happening.

Seizures and epilepsy and status epilepticus

Seizures and epilepsy

A seizure is as brief and transient occurrence of signs and/or symptoms such as temporary confusion, loss of awareness and uncontrollable movements of arms or legs due to abnormal excessive neuronal activity in the brain (Fisher et al. 2017). A seizure refers to a *single episode* of abnormal cerebral activity resulting in a temporary state of altered consciousness, whereas epilepsy is the disease condition describing the high probability of recurrent epileptic episodes (Falco-Walter, Scheffer and Fisher 2018). People who have two or more seizures without other cause are likely to be diagnosed with epilepsy. Epilepsy is, in effect, recurrent seizures, and is one of the most common neurological disorders.

It is important to note that not all seizures are due to epilepsy, as other conditions may cause seizures, such as:

- Low blood sugar.
- Stroke.
- Hypoxia.
- Meningitis.

It is vital that the healthcare professional exclude these causes during their patient assessment.

Over the years, there have been many attempts to classify seizure and epilepsy types, as they may present in many ways. This classification will assist clinicians in selecting treatment of the condition. The International League Against Epilepsy (ILAE) has set up a new task force to develop and publish a new definition of epilepsy as well as a new classification of seizures and epilepsies (Falco-Walter, Scheffer and Fisher 2018).

Basic classification of seizure is based on the onset, which are defined as:

- Focal.
- Generalized.
- Unclassifiable.

Focal seizure refers to onset of the seizure activity in one hemisphere of the brain, and the person experiencing this may be aware or have impaired awareness. There may not be motor involvement, such as jerking or stiffening of the limbs, but movement may be isolated to a muscle group such as the arm or face.

Generalised onset seizure is when both hemispheres of the brain are involved, while unknown onset is when there are manifestations of seizure present, but onset is unknown.

Unclassifiable refers to where there is clearly a seizure event, but it is unclassifiable

Seizure triggers and patterns

Seizures may be triggered by particular risk factors such as trauma, alcohol, brain tumour, electrolyte imbalance, Alzheimer's disease and neurodegenerative diseases. For some individuals, triggers can be specific, such as flashing lights, a specific smell or a particular type of music. General triggers include tiredness, lack of sleep, fever, menstruation, constipation and emotional stress.

Seizures may follow a predictable pattern:

- *Aura*: a warning sign that a seizure is imminent. Auras may be visual, auditory or gustatory (taste) and are usually consistent in their presentation.
- *Automatisms*: coordinated involuntary activities that precede the seizure, such as pacing about or lip smacking.
- *Autonomic symptoms*: physical symptoms resulting from stimulation of the ANS, such as sweating, flushing and pupil dilation.
- *Tonus*: major contraction of voluntary muscles, resulting in generalised stiffness and extension of the arms and legs; the jaw is clamped shut (the tongue may be bitten), and apnoea and incontinence may occur.
- *Clonus*: muscular spasms with a violent rhythmic pattern of muscular rigidity and relaxation; the *clonic phase* of seizure may be accompanied by hyperventilation, eye rolling, frothing at the mouth and tachycardia.
- *Postictal*: the after phase, when patients may be deeply asleep and difficult to rouse, but the muscle spasms have ceased. This may last several hours, and on waking, patients may be disorientated or amnesic.

Due to the unpredictable nature of seizures, patients may sustain secondary injuries, such as falls, burns or head injuries. Recurrent seizures are usually recorded on a seizure or fit chart, allowing objective assessment of the frequency and duration of seizures and evaluation of management strategies.

Treatment focuses on the epilepsy aetiology and underlying cause, such as correction of electrolyte imbalance or removal of brain tumour. For chronic sufferers, avoidance of triggers is important.

Management of seizures

Seizures are transient and are unlikely to cause long-term harm unless injury is sustained during the seizure.

- Ensure sharp objects are out of the way.
- Do not try and stop movements.
- Keep calm and be reassuring; preserve dignity where possible, as patient may be incontinent.
- Time the seizure length.
- Place the patient on their side to protect the airway, when it is safe to do so.
- Do not place anything in the patient's mouth.
- Stay with the patient until the seizure ends.
- Reassure and stay with the patient immediately post-seizure; they may feel lethargic, drowsy and confused.
- Consider normal seizure medication.

Pharmacological management includes the use of traditional anti-epileptic medications such as phenytoin, or more modern agents, such as levetiracetam (Keppra), lamotrigine, sodium valproate and topiramate, which have proven to be effective in generalised epilepsy. However, safety advice should be considered when using sodium valproate in young women and girls of childbearing age (Medicines and Healthcare products Regulatory Authority [MHRA] 2018).

Status epilepticus or prolonged seizures

Status epilepticus refers to a seizure lasting 5 minutes or longer, or several recurrent seizures (more than 3 seizures in an hour), where the patient does not regain consciousness between seizures (Galizia and Faulkner 2018; NICE 2019a). This emergency condition is sometimes referred to as simply 'status'. Status is associated with significant morbidity and mortality if treatment is delayed; help needs to be sought immediately. The Scottish Intercollegiate Guidelines Network (SIGN) have issued guidelines on the management of acute and prolonged seizures (SIGN 2018). The healthcare team should consider the following when supporting a patient with prolonged seizures:

- Prevent environmental harm by removing sharp objects; raise bed sides using pillows to protect from injury.
- Secure/protect the patient's airway (do not place objects in mouth whilst patient is having a seizure). Place the patient on their side, if possible; make sure their airway is not obstructed by the pillows used to protect them from injury.
- Give oxygen, 15L via non-rebreathe bag.
- Assess cardiac and respiratory function.
- Secure intravenous access in large veins; check for and treat hypoglycaemia.
- Aim for termination of the seizure with medications:
  - Buccal midazolam (first line in community).
  - Intravenous lorazepam, 4mg (if intravenous access available) should be given as soon as possible (NICE 2019a).
  - Diazepam, 10mg rectal or IV, if midazolam or lorazepam are unavailable.
- EEG can be used for both diagnosis and for monitoring the effect of treatment.
- *After 10 minutes*, if benzodiazepines (such as midazolam) fail, then repeat dose.
- *After 30 minutes*, consider IV sodium valproate (20–30mg/min) (balance risk with benefits for young women of child bearing age).
- *After 60 minute, admit to ITU and administer general anaesthetic, intubation and ventilation.*

It is important to identify the cause of the prolonged seizure, so abnormal serum electrolytes should be managed; a toxicology screen may be appropriate where drug problems are suspected; malignant hypertension and possible brain trauma should be explored along with the possibility of a brain tumour.

CASE STUDY 9.2 ROBERT WITH ACUTE ONSET OF STROKE AND WEAKNESS IN THE RIGHT ARM: PART 2

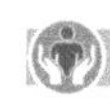

It is important that a CT scan is done without delay to ensure that treatment, such as thrombolysis or thrombectomy, can be started as soon as possible, within 4.5 to 6 hours from onset of the stroke symptoms (NICE 2019). Robert required a thrombectomy and was transferred to the neurology high-dependency unit for neurological and neurovascular monitoring (Nakamura and Serondo 2019). The nurse in the neurology HDU assessed him after his return from the procedure, just as the ward nurse was bringing his belongings to the unit. The ward nurse was keen to see how he was post procedure.

Airway: Robert was still slightly drowsy after his thrombectomy, but he answered the nurse, indicating a patent airway. In addition, the nurse did not hear any partial upper airway obstruction, e.g., stridor or snoring sounds. If Robert had been drowsy, or there was any evidence that he could not maintain a patent airway, the nurse would have selected an appropriately sized nasopharyngeal airway from the emergency bedside equipment.

Breathing: Robert looked pink, with no signs of central or peripheral cyanosis. His breathing was quiet, and the respiratory rate was 16 bpm. Oxygen saturations were 98% on room air. Chest movements were symmetrical. On auscultation, the nurse could hear bilateral air entry, and both lungs were clear. The neuro HDU did not use NEWS to escalate care, but the ward nurse wanted to check his score compared to prior to his procedure.

Respiratory: NEWS (0 + 0 + 0) = 0

Circulation

The cardiac monitor displayed atrial fibrillation, with a rate of 92/min; the radial pulse was counted at 90bpm, and the blood pressure was 130/70mmHg. CRT was 2 seconds, and Robert's hands and feet were slightly cool. This was probably due to the effects of the cold environment in the angiogram room causing vasoconstriction. Monitoring of the blood pressure post-procedure is vital, as the blood pressure must be sufficient to ensure an adequate cerebral perfusion pressure (NICE 2019).

Circulation: NEWS (0 + 1) = 1

Disability

Robert was still a little drowsy from the effects of the anaesthesia post-thrombectomy, but he could speak more clearly. The ward nurse was able to confirm that his mouth looked to be a better shape, which was encouraging. It was vital to closely monitor his GCS post-procedure, as 37% of patients may deteriorate within 24 hours post-thrombectomy (Nakamura and Serondo 2019). Any changes in GCS would need to be reported to the neurologist. His E3 V5 M6 = 14/15. His pupils were size 2 and reactive to light. The nurse also monitored his blood sugar, which had returned to a normal range, at 6mmol/L. It is important to prevent hyperglycaemia, as it is a predictor of 30-day increase of mortality and parenchymal damage in the first 7 days post-procedure (Nakamura and Serondo 2019).

Disability: NEWS = 0

Exposure: Robert looked comfortable, and he did not complain of pain. The nurse ensured that the pressure bandage on the wound site at the groin was intact, and the dressing was dry and clean. The nurse also needs to frequently monitor the patient's pedal pulse on the site of the procedure to detect arterial occlusion neuropathy; the pulse is strong at present. Robert's temperature is 36.5°C. It is vital to monitor the patient for hyperthermia and determine its source. Hyperthermia needs to be treated aggressively, with antipyretics and cooling measures to achieve normothermia to protect the brain. Other complications post-procedure that the HDU nurse is alert to include retroperitoneal haemorrhage and pseudoaneurysm.

Exposure: NEWS = 0

Total NEWS = 0 + 1 + 0 + 0 = 1

Robert was stable following the procedure, and his neurological signs much improved. Whilst he will stay on HDU overnight for close monitoring, he should return to the ward soon. It is hoped that the prompt recognition and treatment of his stroke has minimized long-term problems for the future, and a full recovery is possible.

Conclusion

The nervous system is a highly integrated system that ensures an appropriate response to changes in the internal or external environment. Diseases of the nervous system may be acute or chronic. Nurses must understand the anatomy and physiology of the nervous system in order to understand neurological disease processes and to anticipate the clinical implications of neurological dysfunction. Competence in neurological assessment is a key clinical skill for nurses faced with a medical emergency in any clinical setting, and is an essential skill within a neuroscience setting. Neurological emergencies have the potential to be life-threatening if normal control of airway, breathing or circulation is lost. Ability to assess patients using an ABCDE approach is essential for the management of neurological emergencies.

Glossary

Abducens VIth cranial nerve, motor control of eye movements.

Acetylcholine A neurotransmitter of the parasympathetic nervous system released by many neurones within the peripheral nervous system and by a few neurones in the central nervous system.

Acetylcholinesterase The enzyme that destroys the neurotransmitter acetylcholine.

Acetylcholinesterase inhibitors Drugs that block the production of the enzyme acetylcholinesterase, e.g., pyridostigmine.

Action potential An electrical signal that travels along the surface of a neurone; the signal is propagated by the movement of ions across the cell membrane of the neurone.

Adrenaline Now called epinephrine; neurotransmitter of the sympathetic nervous system.

Afferent neurone An alternative name for a sensory neurone; carries information towards the brain.

$\alpha_1$receptor Receptor within the sympathetic nervous system located on the post-synaptic surface; responds to epinephrine creating a physiological effect, e.g., vasoconstriction.

$\alpha_2$receptor Receptor within the sympathetic nervous system located on the pre-synaptic surface; detects unused or surplus epinephrine and inhibits further epinephrine secretion.

Anterior horns Section of the spinal cord; comprised of grey matter and containing motor axons.

Anticonvulsants Drugs used to control seizures.

Aphasia Absence of speech.

Apneustic centre Located within the pons; controls breathing in conjunction with the pneumotaxic centre and the medulla.

Apnoea Temporary cessation of breathing, usually self-terminating; more prevalent following brainstem injury.

Arachnoid mater Middle layer of the meninges.

Astrocyte A type of glial cell within the central nervous system; star-like in appearance, with multiple processes extending from the cell body, some of which end in foot processes that interface with cerebral blood vessels forming part of the blood–brain barrier.

Autonomic dysreflexia Extreme autonomic response that can occur in patients with spinal cord injury above the level of T6.

Autonomic nervous system Branch of the peripheral nervous system containing two major subdivisions: the sympathetic and parasympathetic nervous systems.

Axon The section of the neurone that extends away from the cell body.

β_1 receptors Part of the sympathetic nervous system; adrenergic receptors located within the heart muscle; stimulation causes increase in heart rate and contractility.

$\beta_2$receptors Part of the sympathetic nervous system; adrenergic receptors with widespread activity, including vasodilation and bronchodilation.

Blood–brain barrier An important structure that prevents harmful substances from entering the brain tissue. The blood–brain barrier has two main components: a thick capillary basement membrane and tight junctions between the endothelial cells of the capillaries.

Brainstem An essential structure within the brain containing the *midbrain*, the *pons* and the *medulla oblongata.*

Broca's speech area Motor control of speech within the cerebral cortex; motor neurones connect Broca's speech area with the larynx, pharynx, mouth and respiratory muscles to enable coordination of talking, breathing and swallowing.

Cauda equina A collection of lumbar, sacral and coccygeal nerve roots within the spinal canal below the height of L2.

Cell body The main part of the neurone containing cytoplasm and organelles.

Central nervous system A subdivision of the nervous system comprising the brain and spinal cord; often referred to as the CNS.

Cerebellum Part of the brain that lies beneath the cerebral hemispheres and posterior to the brainstem; regulates posture and balance; important for the coordinated contraction of skeletal muscle.

Cerebral cortex Outer rim of grey matter that forms part of the cerebral hemispheres.

Cerebral dominance The development of one cerebral hemisphere more than the other.

Cerebral hemispheres The two halves of the cerebrum.

Cerebral oedema Swelling of the brain.

Cerebral perfusion pressure Or CPP; calculated from the mean arterial blood pressure minus the ICP; the pressure of the blood perfusing the brain.

Cerebrospinal fluid Also called CSF; a colourless, clear liquid that circulates around the brain and spinal cord, produced by a network of capillaries in the cerebral ventricles called the choroid plexus.

Cerebrum The largest part of the brain, divided into two parts by the *great longitudinal fissure*; each half is called a *cerebral hemisphere.*

Cervical nerves A group of eight spinal nerves that arise from the cervical section of the spinal column and are annotated C1–C8.

Cholinergic receptors Receptors within the sympathetic nervous system, divided into two subtypes: nicotinic receptors and muscarinic receptors.

Choroid plexus A network of capillaries in the walls of all four ventricles of the brain.

Circle of Willis Anastomoses of the right and left internal carotid arteries and the basilar artery which form a special cerebral circulation at the base of the brain.

Coccygeal nerves A pair of spinal nerves that arise from the coccygeal section of the spinal column and are annotated Co1.

Consciousness A state of awareness of oneself and one's surroundings.

Corpus callosum A band of white matter that connects the two cerebral hemispheres.

Cranial nerves A set of 12 nerves arising from within the brain and forming part of the peripheral nervous system; each nerve is named in accordance with its function and is identified numerically by the use of Roman numerals.

Cranium The section of the skull that encloses the brain.

CSF Cerebrospinal fluid.

Decerebrate One of two types of extensor motor response.

Decorticate One of two types of extensor motor response.

Demyelination The loss or destruction of myelin.

Dendrites Projections from the cell body of the neurone that increase the surface area of the cell membrane, making it easier to connect with other neurones and bringing information to the cell body.

Dendritic spines Small hair-like projections on the dendrites that maximise the surface area of the dendrites.

Depolarisation The first phase of an action potential, where the membrane potential changes from negative to positive due to the influx of sodium ions.

Dermatome A map of the parts of the body that are innervated by spinal nerves.

Diencephalon Located below the cerebrum; made up of the *thalamus*, *hypothalamus* and *epithalamus.*

Dopamine A neurotransmitter within the central and peripheral nervous systems.

Dorsal horns Section of the spinal cord; comprised of grey matter and containing sensory axons; also called the posterior horns.

Dura mater Outer layer of the meninges.

Efferent neurone An alternative name for a motor neurone; information is transmitted from the brain towards the periphery.

Endorphins A neuropeptide neurotransmitter; also described as an opioid-peptide; functions as a natural analgesic by binding to opiate receptors within the central nervous system.

Ependymal cells A single layer of cells that line the ventricles of the brain and the central canal of the spinal cord, they form the blood–CSF barrier to control substances entering the CSF.

Epinephrine A neurotransmitter of the sympathetic nervous system; also a catecholamine and a hormone; used to be called adrenaline.

Epithalamus Region of the diencephalon comprising the pineal gland and the habenular nuclei.

Expressive aphasia Patients are capable of thought but incapable of speech.

Facial nerve VIIth cranial nerve; sensory and motor control for closing eyes, crying, smiling, grimacing, taste and salivation.

Fissures Deep grooves between the gyri of the cerebral hemispheres.

Flexion A motor response where the limbs move towards the body in response to a pain stimulus.

Ganglion A cluster of neurone cell bodies within the peripheral nervous system.

Glasgow Coma Scale An assessment tool for assessing consciousness.

Glial cells Also known as neuroglia; the dominant cell structure within the central nervous system; cells that support neurones.

Glossopharyngeal nerve IXth cranial nerve; sensory and motor control of tongue and pharynx.

Grey matter Outer layer of the cerebral hemispheres; mainly made of neurone cell bodies, dendrites, unmyelinated axons and neuroglia; also found within the spinal cord, where it is arranged in an H shape and divided into regions called horns.

Guillain–Barré syndrome An acute demyelinating disease of the peripheral nervous system, also called acute inflammatory demyelinating polyradiculoneuropathy (AIDP).

Gyri The pleural of gyrus.

Gyrus Folds on the surface of the cerebral hemispheres that increase the surface area of the brain.

Habenular nuclei Located within the epithalamus; have an integrative role linking smell and emotion, for example, a particular smell may evoke a specific memory.

Homeostasis The maintenance of a stable internal environment irrespective of external conditions.

Hydrocephaly Increase in CSF caused by obstruction of CSF drainage.

Hypernatraemia High-serum sodium.

Hypocalcaemia Low-serum calcium.

Hypoglossal nerve XIIth cranial nerve; motor function for speech and swallowing.

Hypomagnesaemia Low-serum magnesium.

Hyponatraemia Low-serum sodium.

Hypothalamus Part of the diencephalon; situated under the thalamus; controls temperature, water metabolism, autonomic function, physical symptoms of emotion and pituitary secretions such as growth hormone. Also contains a feeding centre, a satiety centre and a thirst centre.

Initial segment The proximal portion of the axon where the action potential is generated.

Intracranial pressure The pressure within the skull.

Lumbar nerves A group of five paired spinal nerves that arise from the lumbar section of the spinal column and are annotated L1–L5.

Macroglia Large glial cells.

Medulla oblongata Part of the brainstem; contains the vasomotor centre, which regulates the heartbeat and controls the diameter of blood vessels, thereby controlling blood pressure. Responsible for the rhythmical pattern of breathing. Contains ascending sensory pathways and descending motor pathways that connect the spinal cord with other parts of the brain. Contains important protective reflexes: swallowing, coughing, vomiting, sneezing and hiccoughing as well as sensory nuclei for sensations of touch, pressure and vibration, taste, balance and hearing. It is the origin of cranial nerves VIII–XII.

Meninges A collective term describing the three membranes that enclose the brain and spinal cord.

Meningitis Inflammation of the meninges.

Microglia Small glial cells.

Midbrain Part of the brainstem; contains sensory and motor pathways, involved in the movement of eyes, head and trunk in response to visual and auditory stimuli; also the origin of cranial nerves III–IV.

Motor end plate The post-synaptic surface of a synapse between a nerve and a muscle fibre.

Motor neurone An alternative name for an efferent neurone; information is carried from the brain towards the periphery.

Multiple sclerosis A chronic demyelinating disease of the central nervous system; also known as MS.

Muscarinic receptor A type of receptor within the parasympathetic nervous system that responds to the neurotransmitter acetylcholine.

Myasthenia gravis An autoimmune degenerative disease in which acetylcholine receptors are destroyed, resulting in muscle weakness.

Myelin A lipid-based substance that is secreted by Schwann cells within the peripheral nervous system and by oligodendrocytes within the central nervous system. Myelin insulates axons and increases the speed of conduction along the axon.

Myelin sheath Up to 100 layers of myelin wrapped around an axon.

Myelinated neurone A neurone whose axon is wrapped in myelin.

Nerve A bundle of many hundreds of axons together with their blood vessels and connective tissue. They only occur within the peripheral nervous system.

Nerve impulse The transmission of an electrical signal along a bundle of axons within the peripheral nervous system.

Neuroglia Cells that support neurones, the dominant cell structure within the central nervous system.

Neurolemma The outer layer of a myelin sheath containing the nucleus of the Schwann cell, only found in the peripheral nervous system.

Neuromuscular junction A synapse between a neurone and a muscle fibre.

Neurones Cells within the nervous system that are capable of generating an action potential.

Neurotransmitters Chemicals within the nervous system that are released from terminal boutons and diffuse across the synapse to excite or inhibit post-synaptic structures.

Nicotinic receptor A type of receptor within the parasympathetic nervous system that responds to the neurotransmitter acetylcholine.

Nissl bodies Rough endoplasmic reticulum within the cell body of the neurone, also called Nissl granules.

Nodes of Ranvier Gaps between sections of myelin where action potentials can jump along the axon in a process known as saltatory conduction. Nodes of Ranvier are more prevalent within the peripheral nervous system.

Nuclei Clusters of neurone cell bodies within the central nervous system.

Oculomotor nerve IIIrd cranial nerve; motor control of eye movement, upper eyelid control and pupil constriction.

Olfactory nerve Ist cranial nerve; sensory function for sense of smell.

Oligodendrocytes A type of glial cell which produces myelin within the CNS.

Optic nerve IInd cranial nerve; sensory interpretation of sight.

Osmoreceptors Sensory neurones in the hypothalamus that are stimulated by a change in the osmotic pressure of the blood and trigger the sensation of thirst.

Paraplegia Partial or complete loss of motor and sensory function from the thoracic region downwards.

Parasympathetic nervous system A branch of the autonomic nervous system; involuntary and, as a generalisation, counteracts the action of the sympathetic nervous system, it restores the body to its resting state and is needed for relaxation and sleep.

Parkinson's disease A chronic disease caused by inadequate levels of dopamine with a consequent imbalance in the ratio of dopamine to acetylcholine.

Peripheral nervous system A subdivision of the nervous system comprising the cranial nerves, spinal nerves and their branches; often referred to as the PNS.

Photophobia Intolerance of light.

Pia mater Innermost layer of the meninges.

Pineal gland Part of the epithalamus; secretes the hormone melatonin, considered an endocrine gland.

Pneumotaxic area Located within the pons; influences breathing.

Pons Part of the brainstem; contains sensory and motor pathways, a relay station between the cerebral cortex and the cerebellum; contains the apneustic and pneumotaxic areas which influence breathing. The pons is the origin of cranial nerves V–VIII.

Posterior horns Section of the spinal cord; comprised of grey matter and containing sensory axons.

Primary motor area A highly specialised area of the cerebral cortex located immediately anterior to the primary somatosensory area in the posterior section of the frontal lobe, immediately anterior to the central sulcus; important motor control of complex, skilled or delicate movements.

Primary somatosensory area A highly specialised area of the cerebral cortex located in the anterior portion of each parietal lobe, immediately posterior to the central sulci; important for perception of sensations including touch, tickle, itch, pain, temperature and joint posture.

Quadriplegia Partial or complete loss of sensation and motor function from the neck down.

Receptive aphasia Inability to put words together coherently.

Repolarisation A phase within the action potential where the membrane potential changes from positive to negative by the efflux of potassium ions and returns to its resting state.

Sacral nerves A group of five paired spinal nerves which arise from the sacral section of the spinal column and are annotated S1–S5.

Saltatory conduction The term used to describe an action potential that jumps from one Node of Ranvier to another. This only occurs in myelinated axons.

Schwann cells A type of glial cell responsible for myelin production within the peripheral nervous system.

Sensory receptors Nerve endings that detect information internally and externally.

Somatic nervous system A subdivision of the peripheral nervous system.

Spinal accessory nerve XIth cranial nerve; motor control of shoulder and head movement.

Spinal cord An extension of the brainstem that runs from the medulla oblongata to the top of the second lumbar vertebra.

Spinal cord injury Damage to the spinal cord that results in loss of mobility or sensation; also known as SCI.

Spinal nerves Part of the peripheral nervous system; a group of 31 pairs of spinal nerves that exit the spinal column between each vertebra.

Stress response Activation of the sympathetic nervous system by an environmental or physiological stressor.

Subarachnoid haemorrhage Haemorrhage into the subarachnoid space.

Subarachnoid space The space between the arachnoid mater and the pia mater.

Substance P A neuropeptide neurotransmitter released by neurones in the peripheral nervous system that are responsible for the transmission of pain information to the central nervous system.

Sulci The pleural of sulcus.

Sulcus Shallow groove between the gyri of the cerebral hemispheres.

Sympathetic nervous system A division of the autonomic nervous system that is involuntary, controls the 'fight and flight' response and maintains the body in a state of alertness.

Synapse A collective term that describes the interface between a terminal bouton and another tissue structure, which may be another nerve but could also be a blood vessel, a muscle, an organ or a gland. Synapses can be electrical or chemical.

Synaptic cleft The space between the presynaptic surface and the post-synaptic surface.

Terminal boutons 'Button-like' terminals at the ends of the axon branches containing synaptic vesicles where neurotransmitters are stored.

Tetany Muscle spasms caused by low-serum calcium.

Thalamus A pair of oval-shaped structures within the diencephalon; comprised of grey matter and usually joined by a bridge of grey matter. A relay station between the cerebral cortex and the spinal cord; also relays information between different areas of the cerebrum and between the cerebrum and the cerebellum. The thalamus is involved with consciousness.

Thoracic nerves A group of 12 paired spinal nerves that arise from the thoracic section of the spinal column and are annotated T1–T12.

Transient ischaemic attacks Brief episodes of altered consciousness caused by temporary obstruction of the arterial blood supply to the brain; also known as a TIA.

Trigeminal nerve Vth cranial nerve; sensory and motor control of face, scalp, nose and mouth.

Trochlear nerve IVth cranial nerve; motor control of eye movement.

Unconsciousness Lack of awareness of oneself and one's surroundings.

Unmyelinated neurone A neurone whose axon is not wrapped in myelin.

Vagus nerve Xth cranial nerve, motor and sensory control of pharynx, larynx, heart, lungs, gut, viscera.

Vasomotor centre Located within the brainstem, regulates the heartbeat and controls the diameter of blood vessels, thereby controlling blood pressure; also called the cardiovascular centre.

Ventriculitis Inflammation of the ventricles within the brain.

Vestibulocochlear nerve VIIIth cranial nerve; sensory control of hearing and balance.

Wernicke's area Located within the left temporal and parietal lobes; interprets speech by recognising spoken words and translating them into thoughts.

White matter Inner area of the cerebral hemisphere; mainly comprised of myelinated axons; also found within the spinal cord, where it is divided into regions called columns: anterior, posterior and lateral white columns.

TEST YOURSELF 

1 The autonomic nervous system is a division of:
   a. The central nervous system
   b. The peripheral nervous system
2 A cluster of neurone cell bodies within the CNS is called:
   a. A ganglion
   b. A nucleus
3 Which type of glial cell forms part of the blood–brain barrier?
   a. Ependymal cells
   b. Oligodendrocytes
   c. Astrocytes
   d. Microglia
4 Guillain–Barré syndrome is a disease of the:
   a. Central nervous system
   b. Peripheral nervous system
5 Which of the following neurotransmitters are classified as catecholamines?
   a. Acetylcholine
   b. Norepinephrine
   c. Dopamine
   d. Substance P
6 CSF is produced from:
   a. The medulla oblongata
   b. The subarachnoid membrane
   c. The choroid plexus
   d. The cerebral cortex
7 The vasomotor centre is responsible for:
   a. Temperature regulation
   b. Respiratory rate regulation
   c. Blood pressure regulation
   d. Heart rate regulation
8 Cranial nerves are part of the:
   a. Central nervous system
   b. Peripheral nervous system

9 The neurotransmitter of the parasympathetic nervous system is:
   a. Acetylcholine
   b. Noradrenaline
   c. Dopamine
   d. Endorphins
10 Which type of sympathetic receptor is found in the heart?
   a. α_1
   b. β_1
   c. α_2
   d. β_2

Answers

1 b
2 b
3 c
4 b
5 b, c
6 c
7 c, d
8 b
9 a
10 b

References

Alkemade, A. (2013). Subdivisions and anatomical boundaries of the subthalamic nucleus. *Journal of Neuroscience*, 33(22), 9233–9234. doi:10.1523/JNEUROSCI.1266-13.2013.

Boehme, A. K., Esenwa, C. and Elkind, M. S. V. (2017). Stroke risk factors, genetics, and prevention. *Circulation Research*, 120, 472–495. doi:10.1161/CIRCRESAHA.116.308398.

Bonds, B. W., Hu, P., Li, Y., Yang, S., Colton, K., Gonchigar, A., Cheriyan, J., Grissom, T., Fang, R. and Stein, D. M. (2015). Predictive value of hyperthermia and intracranial hypertension on neurological outcomes in patients with severe traumatic brain injury. *Brain Injury*, 29(13–14), 1642–1647. doi:10.3109/02699052.2015.1075157.

Brennan, P. M., Murray, G. D. and Teasdale, G. M. (2018). Simplifying the use of prognostic information in traumatic brain injury. Part 1: the GCS-Pupils score: an extended index of clinical severity. *Journal of Neurosurgery*, 128, 1612–1620.

Brisch, R., Saniotis, A., Wolf, R., Bielau, H., Bernstein, H.-G., Steiner, J., Bogerts, B., Braun, K., Jankowski, Z., Kumaratilake, J., Henneberg, M. and Gos, T. (2014). The role of dopamine in schizophrenia from a neurobiological and evolutionary perspective: old fashioned, but still in vogue. *Frontiers in Psychiatry*, 5, 47. doi:10.3389/fpsyt.2014.00047.

Carney, N., Totten, A. M., O'Reilly, C., Ullman, J. S., Hawryluk, G. W. J., Bell, M. J., Bratton, S. L., Chesnut, R., Harris, O. A., Kissoon, N., Rubiano, A. M., Shutter, L., Tasker, R. C., Vavilala, M. S., Wilberger, J., Wright, D. W. and Ghajar, J. (2016). Guidelines for the management of severe traumatic brain injury, 4th ed. *Neurosurgery*, 80, 1–10. doi:10.1227/NEU.0000000000001432.

Cooper, D. J., Nichol, A. D., Bailey, M., Bernard, S., Cameron, P. A., Pili-Floury, S., Forbes, A., Gantner, D., Higgins, A. M., Huet, O., Kasza, J., Murray, L., Newby, L., Presneill, J. J., Rashford,

S., Rosenfeld, J. V., Stephenson, M., Vallance, S., Varma, D., Webb, S. A. R., Trapani, T. and McArthur, C. (2018). Effect of early sustained prophylactic hypothermia on neurologic outcomes among patients with severe traumatic brain injury: the POLAR randomized clinical trial. *JAMA*, 320(21), 2211–2220. doi:10.1001/jama.2018.17075.

Falco-Walter, J. J., Scheffer, I. E. and Fisher, R. S. (2018). The new definition and classification of seizures and epilepsy. *Epilepsy Research*, 139, 73–79. doi:10.1016/j.eplepsyres.2017.11.015.

Fisher, R. S., Cross, J. H., French, J. A., Higurashi, N., Hirsch, E., Jansen, F. E., Lagae, L., Moshe, S. L., Peltola, J., Perez, E. R., Scheffer, I. E. and Zuberi, S. M. (2017). Operational classification of seizure types by the international league against epilepsy: position paper of the ILAE commission for classification and terminology. *Epilepsia*, 58(4), 522–530. doi:10.1111/epi.13670.

Galizia, E. C. and Faulkner, H. J. (2018). Seizures and epilepsy in the acute medical setting: presentation and management. *Clinical Medicine*, 18, 409–413. doi:10.7861/clinmedicine.18-5-409.

Griffiths, M. J., McGill, F. and Solomon, T. (2018). Management of acute meningitis. *Clinical Medicine*, 18(2), 164–169. doi:10.7861/clinmedicine.18-2-164.

Jiang, H., Chan, C., Leung, Y., Li, Y., Graham, C. and Rainer, T. (2014). Evaluation of the recognition of stroke in the emergency room (ROSIER) scale in Chinese patients in Hong Kong. *PLoS One*. doi:10.1371/journal.pone.0109762.

Joint British Diabetes Societies for Inpatient Care (JBDS-IP). (2018). *The Hospital Management of Hypoglycaemia in Adults with Diabetes Mellitus*, 3rd Edition. JBDS 01. Available from https://www.diabetes.org.uk/professionals/position-statements-reports/specialist-care-for-children-and-adults-and-complications/the-hospital-management-of-hypoglycaemia-in-adults-with-diabetes-mellitus. Accessed 29 August 2019.

Loveday, H. P., Wilson, J. A., Pratt, R. J., Golsorkhi, M., Tingle, A., Bak, A., Browne, J., Prieto, J. and Wilcox, M. (2014). epic3: national evidence-based guidelines for preventing healthcare-associated infections in NHS hospitals in England. *Journal of Hospital Infection*, 86(S1), S1–S70.

Medicines and Healthcare Products Regulatory Authority (MHRA). (2018). *Drug Safety Update*, Vol. 12(2). MHRA, pp. 1–11. Available from https://assets.publishing.service.gov.uk/government/uploads/system/uploads/attachment_data/file/743094/Sept-2018-DSU-PDF.pdf. Accessed: 13 September 2019.

Meningitis Research Foundation. (2019). *Are You At Risk?* Available from https://www.meningitis.org/meningitis/are-you-at-risk. Accessed: 29 August 2019.

Mohebbi, M. R., Rosenkrans, K. A. and Jung, M. J. (2013). Chvostek's and Trousseau's signs in a case of hypoparathyroidism. *Journal of Clinical and Diagnostic Research*, 7(5), 970.

Murray, G. D., Brennan, P. M. and Teasdale, G. M. (2018). Simplifying the use of prognostic information in traumatic brain injury. Part 2: graphical presentation of probabilities. *Journal of Neurosurgery*, 128(6), 1621–1634.

Nakamura, C. and Serondo, D. (2019). *Caring for the Post Procedure Mechanical Thrombectomy Patient*. Available from https://currents.neurocriticalcare.org/blogs/currents-editor/2019/02/08/caring-for-the-post-procedure-mechanical-thrombect. Accessed 12 September 2019.

National Institute for Health and Care Excellence. (2016). *Spinal Injury: Assessment and Initial Management*. Clinical Guideline 41. Available from https://www.nice.org.uk/guidance/ng41/evidence/full-guideline-2358425776. Accessed 27 April 2019.

National Institute for Health and Care Excellence. (2017). *Head Injury: Assessment and Early Management*. Clinical Guideline *[CG176]*. Available from https://www.nice.org.uk/guidance/cg176/chapter/1-Recommendations. Accessed 30 April 2019.

National Institute for Health and Care Excellence. (2019a). *Epilepsy*. Available from https://cks.nice.org.uk/epilepsy#!management. Accessed 13 September 2019.

National Institute for Health and Care Excellence. (2019b). *Hypoglycaemia: Treatment of Hypoglycaemia*. Available from https://bnf.nice.org.uk/treatmentsummary/hypoglycaemia.html. Accessed 27 April 2019.

National Institute for Health and Care Excellence. (2019c). *Stroke and Transient Ischaemic Attack in the Over 16's: Diagnosis and Management*, ng 128. Available from www.nic.org.uk/guidance/ng128. Accessed 29 August 2019.

National Institute of Neurological Disorders and Stroke. (2019). *Guillain Barre Syndrome Fact Sheet.* Available from https://www.ninds.nih.gov/Disorders/Patient-Caregiver-Education/Fact-Sheets/Guillain-Barr%C3%A9-Syndrome-Fact-Sheet. Accessed 28 August 2019.

Nazarko, L. (2018). Safety alert for bowel care. *Nursing and Residential Care*, 20(10), 487. Available from https://www-magonlinelibrary-com.ezproxy.uwl.ac.uk/doi/pdfplus/10.12968/nrec.2018.20.10.487. Accessed August 2019.

NHS Improvement. (2018). *Patient Safety Alert: Resources to Support Safer Bowel Care for Patients at Risk of Autonomic Dysreflexia.* Available from https://improvement.nhs.uk/documents/3074/Patient_Safety_Alert_-_safer_care_for_patients_at_risk_of_AD.pdf. Accessed 25 July 2015.

Nor, A. M., Davis, J., Sen, B., Shipsey, D., Louw, S. J., et al. (2005). The recognition of stroke in the emergency room (ROSIER) scale: development and validation of a stroke recognition instrument. *Lancet Neurology*, 4, 727–734.

Nursing and Midwifery Council. (2018a). *Future Nurse: Standards of Proficiency for Registered Nurses.* Available from https://www.nmc.org.uk/globalassets/sitedocuments/education-standards/future-nurse-proficiencies.pdf. Accessed 28 April 2019.

Nursing and Midwifery Council. (2018b). *The Code.* London: NMC.

Office for National Statistics. (2011). Available from http://www.statistics.gov.uk/cci/nugget.asp?id=6. Accessed 6 May 2011.

Public Health England. (2016). *Guidance on the Prevention and Management of Meningococcal Meningitis and Septicaemia in Higher Education Institutions.* Available from https://assets.publishing.service.gov.uk/government/uploads/system/uploads/attachment_data/file/582511/MenACWY_HEI_Guidelines.pdf. Accessed 7 September 2019.

Public Health England. (2018). *New Figures Show Larger Proportion of Strokes in the Middle Aged.* Available from https://www.gov.uk/government/news/new-figures-show-larger-proportion-of-strokes-in-the-middle-aged. Accessed 29 August 2019.

Royal College of Physician. (2017). *National Early Warning Score (NEWS) 2: Standardising the Assessment of Acute-Illness Severity in the NHS. Updated Report of a Working Party.* London: RCP.

Scottish Intercollegiate Guidelines Network. (2018). *SIGN 143: Diagnosis and Management of Epilepsy in Adults.* Available from https://www.sign.ac.uk/assets/sign143_2018.pdf. Accessed 14 September 2019.

Shah, S. and Kimberly, W. T. (2016). The modern approach to treating brain swelling in the neuro ICU. *Seminars in Neurology*, 36(6), 502–507. doi:10.1055/s-0036-1592109.

Stroke Association. (2018). *State of the Nation: Stroke Statistics Feb 2018.* Available from https://www.stroke.org.uk/sites/default/files/state_of_the_nation_2018.pdf. Accessed 7 September 2019.

Teasdale, G., Maas, A., Lecky, F., Manley, G., Stocchetti, N. and Murray, G. (2014). The Glasgow coma scale at 40 years: standing the test of time. *Lancet Neurology*, 13, 844–854.

Tortora, G. J. and Derrickson, B. H. (2017). *Tortora's Principles of Anatomy and Physiology*, 15th Edition. Hoboken, NJ: Wiley.

Wolters, F. J., Li, L., Gutnikov, S. A., Mehta, Z. and Rothwell, P. M. (2018). Medical attention seeking after transient ischemic attack and minor stroke before and after the UK face, arm, speech, time (FAST) public education campaign: results from the Oxford vascular study. *JAMA Neurology*, 75(10), 1225–1233. doi:10.1001/jamaneurol.2018.1603.

10 The patient with acute gastrointestinal problems

Rebecca Maindonald and Adrian Jugdoyal

AIM

The aim of this chapter is to identify key functions of the gastrointestinal system. This includes providing insight into how disordered physiology can cause a medical emergency and the nurse's role in recognising and responding appropriately to patients with acute gastrointestinal problems.

OBJECTIVES

At the end of this chapter you will be able to:

- Describe the major structures of the gastrointestinal system.
- Identify the main roles of the stomach, pancreas, liver and bowel, relating this to problems arising from disordered pathophysiology.
- Identify the common gastrointestinal emergencies and differentiate between patient presentations.
- Describe the nurse's role in undertaking an assessment of the abdomen.
- Describe the nurse's role in undertaking an assessment of fluid balance in relation to gastrointestinal emergencies.
- Identify interventions which maximise gastrointestinal status.

Introduction

The GI system can be affected primarily by specific disorders and also secondarily as a consequence of pathology elsewhere in the body. Both types of disturbance can result in a medical emergency. The nurse has an important role in assessing and monitoring the patient with gastrointestinal signs and symptoms in order to identify the potential for the patient to deteriorate. Deterioration can occur either as a result of the altered pathophysiological processes or because of life threatening complications such as infection or hypovolaemia.

Applied physiology

Overview of gastrointestinal (GI) tract

The GI tract (alimentary canal) consists of a continuous tube commencing at the mouth and ending at the anus. The organs forming this system include the mouth, most of the pharynx, oesophagus, stomach, small intestine and large intestine. The accessory organs contributing to this tract are the teeth, tongue, salivary glands, liver, gallbladder and pancreas.

The GI tract processes food from the time it is eaten until it is digested, absorbed or eliminated and in summary performs six processes:

- Ingestion: taking food and liquids into the mouth by eating and drinking.
- Secretion: the cells within the GI tract and accessory organs secrete water, acid, buffers and enzymes (total approximately 8 litres/day) into the tract lumen.
- Mixing and propulsion: alternating contraction and relaxation of the smooth muscle in the walls of the GI tract mixes the food and secretions and this peristaltic action promotes forward movement through the system.
- Digestion: food is digested mechanically by the teeth whilst in the mouth, and is subsequently digested chemically, commencing within the stomach.
- Absorption: following chemical digestion, the resulting products composed of small molecules are absorbed by the epithelial cells lining the GI tract. These then pass into the blood to be circulated systemically.
- Defaecation: Material consisting of wastes, indigestible substances, bacteria and cells from the lining of the GI tract is excreted in the form of faeces.

The oesophagus

The oesophagus is a hollow muscular tube which secretes mucus and transports food into the stomach, but does not produce any digestive enzymes. The oesophagus joins the stomach at the oesophagogastric junction via a group of muscles referred to as the lower oesophageal sphincter. If this sphincter becomes ineffectual, the highly acidic contents of the stomach can reflux into the oesophagus causing inflammation, erosion and ulceration. Excessive pressure due to vomiting can also cause damage (e.g., Mallory-Weiss Syndrome). Both of these situations may present as **haematemesis**. Another common cause of haematemesis is related directly to the gastro-oesophageal junction in the form of a variceal bleed. Oesophageal and gastric **varices** form and eventually rupture as a result of high pressure in the venous circulation to the liver arising from chronic liver damage.

The stomach

The stomach sits in the left side of the abdominal cavity under the diaphragm. It is divided into four regions: the cardiac, the fundus, the body and the pylorus (see Figure 10.1). The pylorus has two parts, the pyloric antrum connecting to the body of the stomach and the pyloric canal leading into the duodenum. The pyloric sphincter is located at the junction of the stomach and duodenum. The stomach acts as a temporary holding area for food that arrives from the oesophagus.

The stomach forms **chyme** by churning food, hydrochloric acid, intrinsic factor, pepsinogen, mucus and bicarbonate together. These substances are secreted by parietal cells in the stomach.

The secretory actions of the parietal cells keep the stomach contents acidic (pH 1.5–2.0) which prevents the growth of harmful bacteria, initiates the digestion of proteins and facilitates the digestion of plant and meat tissue.

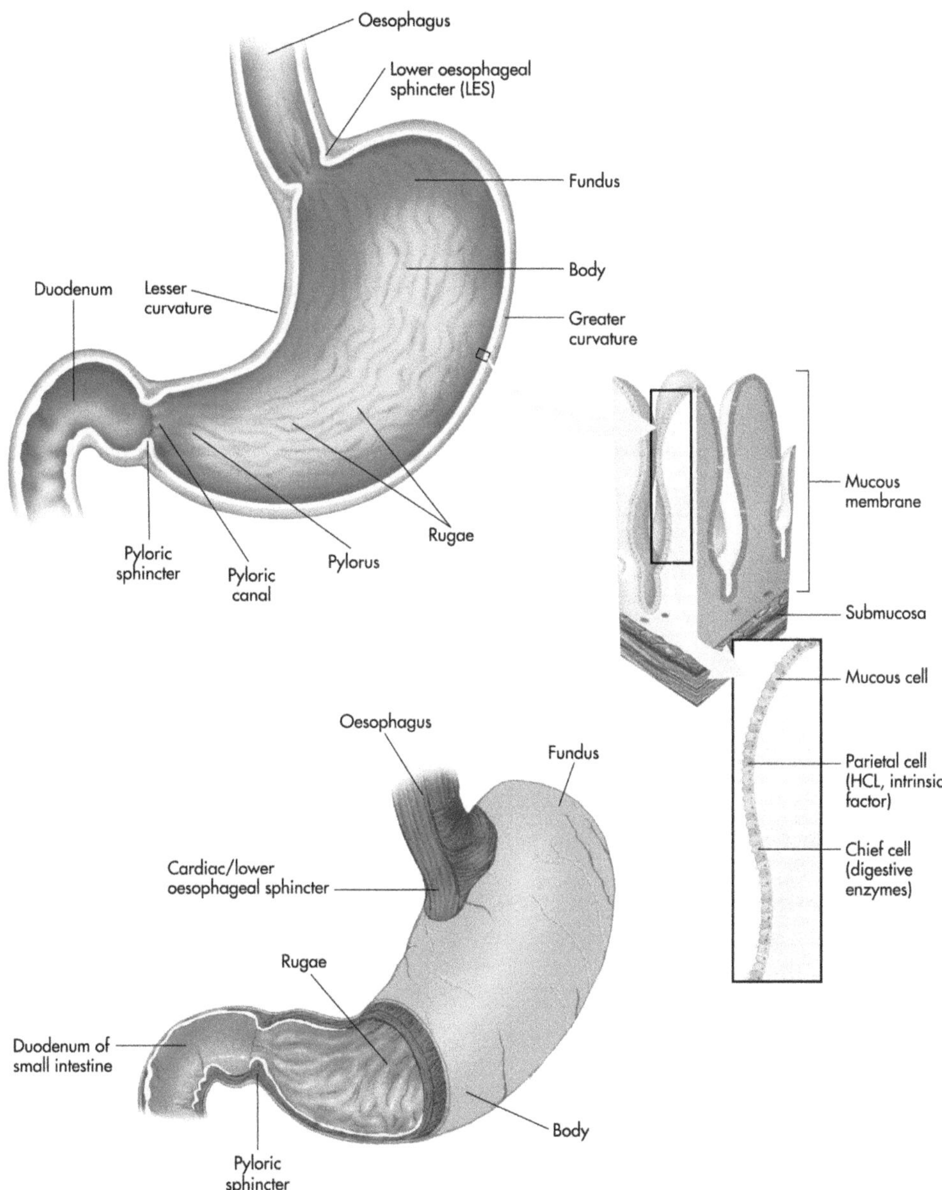

Figure 10.1 The stomach.

Vitamin B12, ingested mainly through dietary protein, is an essential component to maintain normal red blood cell function. Vitamin B12 cannot be absorbed without intrinsic factor, secreted by parietal cells. Conditions resulting in an absence of intrinsic factor will lead to Vitamin B12 deficiency, resulting in a condition known as pernicious anaemia. This anaemia occurs when the body's own immune system mistakenly attacks parietal cells, or a portion of the stomach is removed.

The pancreas

The pancreas is a retroperitoneal gland approximately 12–15cm long and 2.5cm thick. It is connected by the pancreatic duct to the common **bile** duct, which in turn empties into the duodenum. Structurally, the pancreas is composed of clustered epithelial cells, about 99% of which constitute the **exocrine** portion of the organ. They secrete approximately 1200–1500mL daily of pancreatic juice, consisting of water, salts, sodium bicarbonate and enzymes. Bicarbonate pancreatic juice mixes with acidic chyme in the duodenum to neutralise the substance. Pancreatic juices consist of several enzymes that aid in the digestion of carbohydrates, proteins and fats. The protein digesting enzymes are secreted initially within the pancreas in an inactive form (trypsinogen), as the active form would damage the pancreas itself. Trypsinogen is only activated when it reaches the duodenum and mixes with other enzymes. It is the premature activation of trypsinogen, when it is still in the pancreas, which causes serious problems (pancreatitis). The remaining 1% of the cells are organised into pancreatic islets (islets of Langerhans), which have an **endocrine** function. These cells secrete hormones such as glucagon, insulin, somatostatin and pancreatic polypeptide (see section on diabetic emergencies in Chapter 11).

The small intestine

The major processes of digestion and absorption of nutrients occur in the small intestine. Its length of approximately 3 metres provides a large surface area for these functions, which are further enhanced by the presence of circular folds, villi and microvilli. The circular folds aid absorption, not only by increasing surface area, but by causing the chyme to spiral, rather than move in a straight line as it passes through the small intestine (please see Figure 10.2).

The small intestine is divided into three regions: the duodenum (25cm) commencing at the pyloric sphincter of the stomach, the jejunum (100cm) and finally the ileum (200cm). The duodenum is a C-shaped tube which curves around the head of the pancreas and secretes bicarbonate to neutralise gastric acid. It can increase bicarbonate production in response to raised acidity. The close proximity of the duodenum to the stomach, however, makes it prone to ulceration as a result of the acidity of the stomach contents.

Intestinal juice is a clear yellow, alkaline fluid (1–2 litres/day) containing water and mucus. Pancreatic and intestinal juices together provide an environment that facilitates the absorption of the substances in chyme as they come into contact with the villi. The endothelial cells synthesise several digestive enzymes (brush border enzymes), which are inserted in the plasma membrane of the microvilli. This results in some of the enzymatic digestion occurring at the surface of the endothelial cells that line the villi, rather than in the lumen itself.

Following enzymatic digestion, the resulting nutrients are absorbed through the endothelial cells. These include: monosaccharides, amino acids, lipids, electrolytes and vitamins. In addition to these elemental nutrients, the small intestine absorbs water. Approximately 10 litres of water a day enters the small intestine (2 litres as ingested fluids and 8 litres as various gastrointestinal secretions), most of which is reabsorbed by osmosis. The remainder passes into the large intestine.

There are two types of movements in the small intestine: firstly, segmentations, which are localized contractions that occur in areas distended by chyme and mix the chyme and enzymes together. Secondly, this process is followed by **peristalsis**, whereby chyme is moved forward as a result of waves of muscular contractions. In total, the chyme is

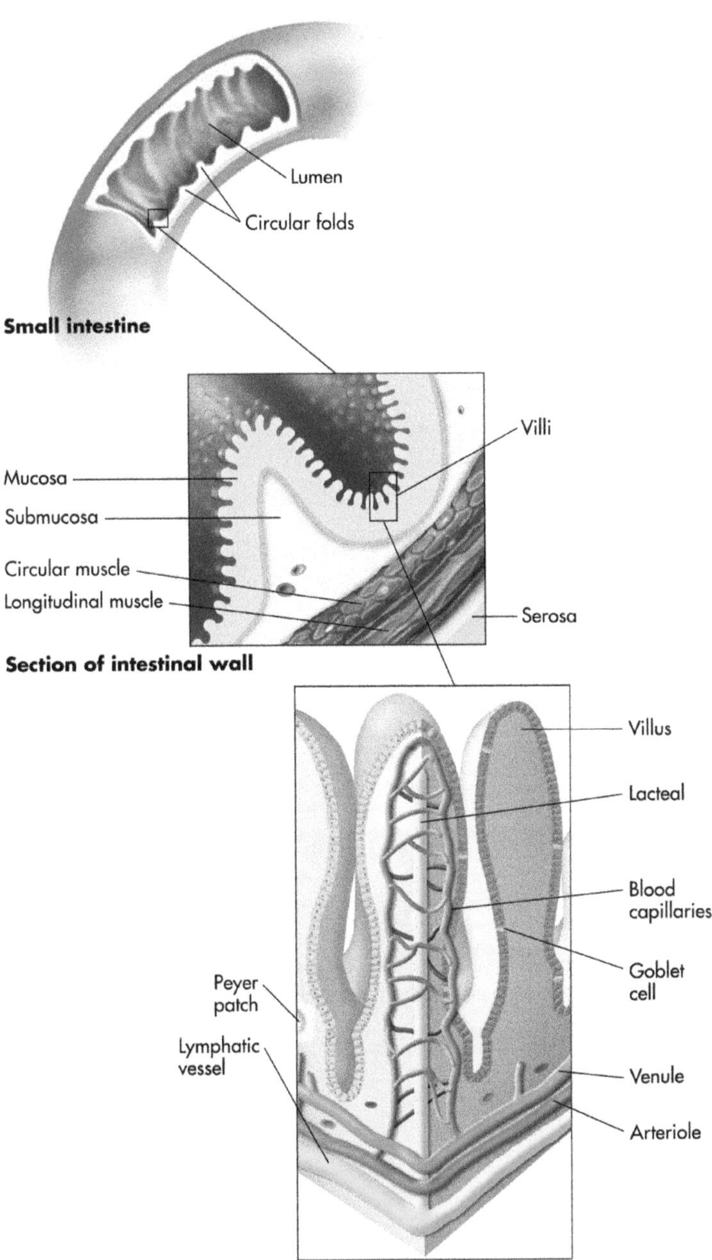

Figure 10.2 The small intestine and villi.

present in the small intestine for between 3 and 5 hours. The jejunum is the middle section of the small intestine. It has longer villi than the duodenum to provide an increased surface area from which to absorb nutrients such as glucose, amino acids and vitamins. The section following the jejunum is the ileum, whose function is to absorb Vitamin B12, bile salts and other substances not taken up by the jejunum.

The liver (and gallbladder)

The liver is the second largest organ in the body (after the skin). It weighs approximately 1.4kg and is positioned inferiorly to the diaphragm on the right side (please see Figure 10.3). The liver is the largest gland and the largest solid organ in the body. It holds approximately 13% (about one pint or 0.57 litres) of the total blood supply at any given time.

The liver is dark reddish-brown in colour and is divided into two main lobes (the larger right and the smaller left) which are further subdivided into approximately 100,000 small lobes, or lobules. About 60% of the liver is made up of liver cells called hepatocytes, which absorb nutrients and detoxify and remove harmful substances from the blood. A hepatocyte has an average lifespan of 150 days. There are approximately 202,000 hepatocytes in every milligram of liver tissue. The liver receives its blood supply via the hepatic artery and portal vein. Instead of capillaries, the liver has large endothelium lined spaces (sinusoids) through which blood passes. The sinusoids also contain fixed phagocytes called stellate reticuloendothelial (Kupffer) cells which perform several functions, including the breakdown of worn out red blood cells, bacteria and other foreign matter which can then pass into the venous circulation.

Bile (secreted by hepatocytes) enters into the small bile canaliculi and drains subsequently into the bile ductules and bile ducts, which eventually become the right and left hepatic ducts merging into the common hepatic duct. Having left the liver, the bile is stored in the gallbladder, which acts as a reservoir. This is a pear-shaped sac (7–10 cm) long, located in a depression of the posterior visceral surface of the liver. The gallbladder is divided into a fundus, body and neck. The cystic duct joins the common hepatic duct, which in turn merges into the common bile duct. Bile contains water, bile salts,

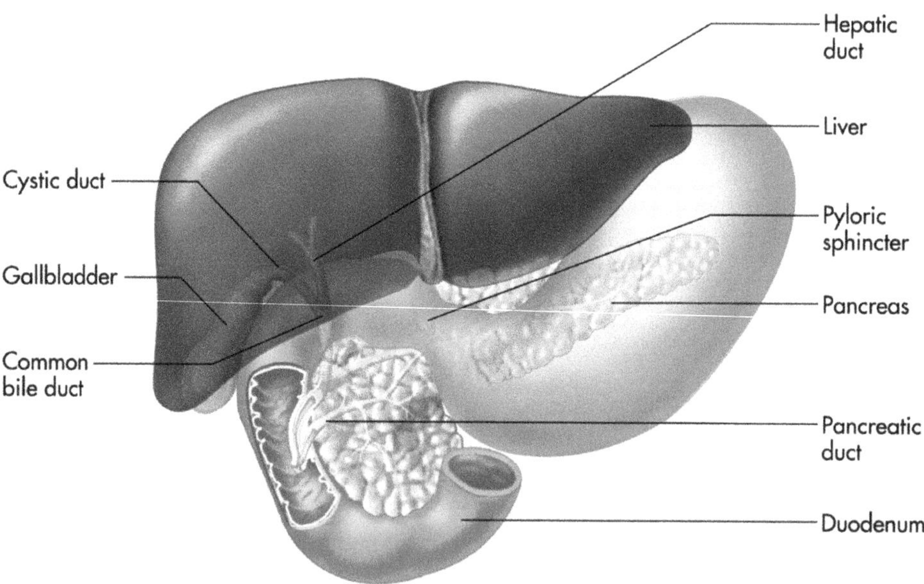

Figure 10.3 The liver.

bile pigments and electrolytes, and from the common bile duct, bile is emptied into the duodenum, where the bile salts emulsify fat.

The liver receives blood from two sources: the hepatic artery carries oxygenated blood (approximately 30% of liver blood flow), and the hepatic portal vein carries deoxygenated blood (approximately 70% of blood flow). The venous blood from the hepatic portal vein contains newly absorbed nutrients, drugs, microbes and toxins from the gastrointestinal tract. Branches of both of these blood vessels carry blood into the liver sinusoids where oxygen, most of the nutrients and some toxic substances are processed by the hepatocytes. The resulting venous blood drains into the hepatic vein to return to the systemic venous circulation.

The portal vein carries approximately 1500mL/min of blood from the intestines, spleen and stomach to the liver. Obstruction to this blood flow (whatever the aetiology) will result in elevated portal venous pressure. This, in turn, causes distension of the proximal veins and an increase in the intracapillary pressure in the organs drained by the obstructed veins. Particularly vulnerable to this increase in pressure is the gastro-oesophageal junction, where varices can develop and sometimes rupture, resulting in haemorrhage and haematemesis. Varices are portosystemic anastomoses, or a connection between the veins of the portal system and the systemic circulation. These communications between the two systems are formed when the direct drainage routes are blocked. The typical site of varices is the lower third of the oesophagus, between the lower oesophageal veins and the short gastric veins.

Functions of the liver

These are summarised in Figure 10.4.

STORAGE

- *Glucose*: the liver plays a major role in replenishing the blood's supply of glucose when the concentration falls below normal. Liver cells are highly permeable to glucose (digested carbohydrate) and will absorb 75% of the excess glucose in the circulation. This is accomplished by the enzyme glucokinase (regulated by blood insulin levels), which accelerates the rate of glucose uptake by the liver cell. The absorbed glucose is stored in the liver as glycogen.
- *Amino acids*: the amino acids derived from protein digestion travel to the liver by way of the portal vein. Intracellular enzymes in the parenchymal cells of the liver convert the excess amino acids into cellular proteins. These proteins are then stored in the liver and released as required to maintain equilibrium between the body's cellular and plasma proteins.
- *Fat-soluble vitamins (A, D, E + K):* Vitamin K is absorbed from the GI tract, and this is dependent, in turn, upon the liver's ability to secrete bile into the intestinal tract. More importantly, Vitamin K is a vital co-enzyme in the liver's ability to produce plasma proteins, prothrombin (Factor II) and some other clotting factors (e.g., VII, IX, X), and it activates enzymes in the clotting cascade. In addition to the Vitamin K-dependent clotting factors (II, VII, IX, X), the liver produces clotting factors I, V, XI, XII and XIII. Vitamin B12 is also stored by the liver, but is not fat-soluble.
- *The trace metals Iron (Fe) and Copper (Cu)*: are stored in the liver with an excess, resulting in Haemochromatosis and Wilson's Disease respectively.

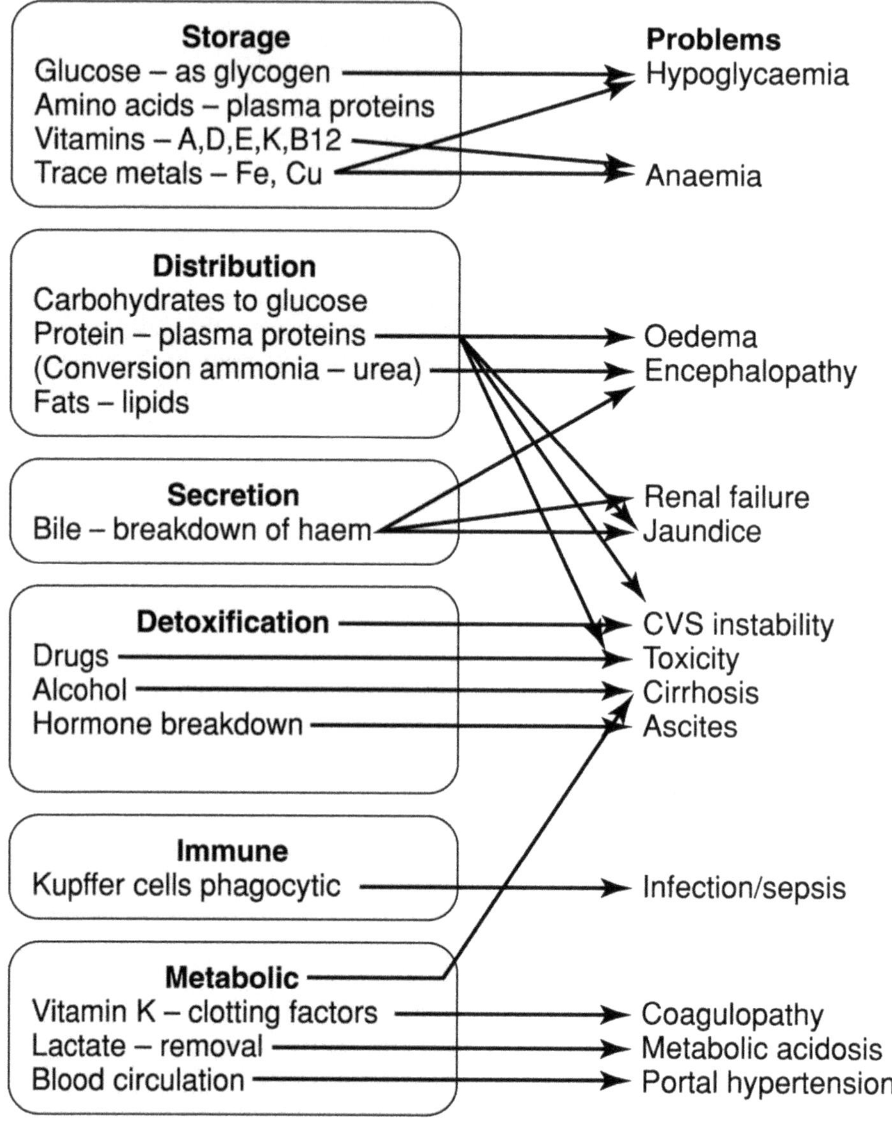

Figure 10.4 Summary of the Functions of the Liver.

CONVERSION

The liver plays an active role in the conversion of carbohydrates, proteins and fatty acids into the energy (in the form of ATP) which is required for all chemical reactions to occur at a cellular level.

- *Carbohydrates*: carbohydrates in the form of glucose are the primary source of energy for the body. The liver responds to low plasma glucose levels (and accompanying low plasma insulin levels) by both inhibiting the uptake of circulating glucose and by breaking down stored glycogen (glycogenolysis) to make more glucose available in the circulation.

- *Protein*: the end products of protein digestion circulate in the blood as amino acids, which are re-synthesised by the liver to form three plasma proteins (albumin, fibrinogen and globulins). Albumin is essential to maintain the colloid osmotic pressure, fibrinogen is vital for the coagulation process, and globulins are required for antibody formation. Of these, the liver produces all of the body's albumin and fibrinogen and 50% of the globulins. In addition, the liver, in conjunction with vitamin K, synthesises all of the body's prothrombin (Factor II) and Factors VII, IX and X essential for fibrinogen activation.
- Amino acids (from protein) are utilised also for gluconeogenesis, resulting in the formation of ammonia as a by-product. The liver converts this metabolically generated ammonia into urea. Ammonia produced by bacteria in the intestines is also removed from portal blood for urea synthesis. The liver therefore converts ammonia, a potential toxin, into urea, a compound that can be excreted in the urine.
- *Fatty acids*: triglycerides, phospholipids and cholesterol are the principle lipids which become the body's source of energy when glucose is not available. Triglycerides are broken down to fatty acids and glycerol, then to acetyl COA, then to ATP, CO_2 and H_2O for cellular energy. The additional processing of fatty acids into ketone bodies occurs primarily when the availability of glucose for metabolism is limited, such as during starvation or in uncontrolled diabetes. Under some conditions lipids may accumulate in the hepatocytes and result in a 'fatty liver', for example, in alcohol excess.

SECRETION

The only substance actually secreted by the liver is bile. Bile solution contains bile salts, cholesterol, bilirubin, fatty acids and plasma electrolytes. A litre a day is produced, but is concentrated in the gall bladder. 80% of bilirubin is derived from haem following the breakdown of haemoglobin in the liver, spleen and bone marrow. It is not water-soluble and is carried in the plasma bound to albumin. In the liver, it is transported into the hepatocytes, conjugated with glucuronic acid and excreted by active transport into the bile. In the terminal ileum and colon, bacteria reduce bilirubin to stercobilinogen, and thence further to stercobilin, which is excreted in the stool. A small amount is reabsorbed and excreted in the urine as urobilinogen.

DETOXIFICATION

- *Drugs*: the detoxification process that occurs in the liver protects the body from many harmful substances that enter the blood stream. The liver absorbs most drugs that enter the blood stream, usually modified and excreted. Most of these are fat-soluble, and their conversion by the liver into water-soluble substances facilitates excretion in bile or urine.
- *Alcohol*: ethanol is oxidised to acetaldehyde, but as this is unstable, it is further metabolised to acetic acid utilising the enzyme alcohol dehydrogenase. This, in turn, collaborates with a further enzyme (ACSS2) to form Acetyl-CoA, which is then available for cellular metabolism.
- *Hormone breakdown*: e.g., oestrogen.

IMMUNE FUNCTION

The Kupffer cells are phagocytic and are very efficient in digesting bacteria, viruses and other foreign matter. These cells are particularly important because they destroy bacteria that are constantly entering the portal blood flow directly from the GI tract. The main functions of Kupffer cells are:

- phagocytosis of bacteria, debris and other foreign matter in hepatic blood.
- a defence mechanism when **bacterial translocation** occurs.

OTHER

- *Acid-base balance*: the liver is metabolically active, both producing and consuming H+ ions. It consumes about 20% of the body's O_2 production and produces about 20% of the CO_2 excreted via the lungs. The liver normally removes 70% of lactate, and there can be decreased hepatic clearance in either poor perfusion of the liver (e.g., severe shock) or liver disease, resulting in a metabolic acidosis.
- *Heat Production*: the liver is second only to muscle tissue in the production of heat by its continuous cellular activity (thermogenesis). Under normal resting conditions, the liver is responsible for most of the body heat.

The liver acts also as a blood reservoir containing about 10% of the circulating blood volume. The liver is essential for life. A total hepatectomy would always be fatal, death occurring in less than 24 hours from hypoglycaemia.

The jejunum and ileum

The jejunum is the middle section of the small intestine. It has longer villi than the duodenum to provide an increased surface area from which to absorb nutrients such as glucose, amino acids and vitamins.

The large bowel

The large intestine is the final section of the GI tract and is approximately 1.5m long. The large bowel includes the appendix, a redundant structure situated near the junction of the ileum (small bowel) and the caecum (large bowel). The caecum merges with a long tube called the colon and this is divided anatomically into four areas (ascending colon, transverse colon, descending colon and sigmoid colon) before terminating in the rectum and anus.

The wall of the large intestine differs from that of the small intestine in that there are no circular folds or villi. Instead, the **mucosal lining** consists of simple columnar epithelium, connective tissue and smooth muscle. The cells absorb further water (approximately 700mL daily) and secrete mucus to lubricate the passage of the colonic contents.

Immune function of the gut

Protection against harmful organisms is a responsibility shared between several components of the gastrointestinal system. The epithelial cells lining the gut prevent migration of organisms and the mucosa itself acts as a physical barrier. The intestinal walls contain lymphocytes and macrophages, and regional lymph nodes can be found in the abdominal lining. Intraluminal Peyer's Patches secrete immunoglobulin A (IgA) to prevent adherence of bacteria to the mucosal cells. These gut actions supplement the activities of the Kupffer cells in the liver and the spleen's role in trapping and phagocytosing bacteria. These immune functions can become compromised in cases of acute illnesses such as hypovolaemia, ischemia and sepsis as well as immunosuppression or increased bacterial growth due to intestinal stasis.

Acute problems/emergencies

Acute gastrointestinal bleeding

Gastrointestinal (GI) bleeding is a major cause of morbidity and mortality, with 80% of cases involving the upper GI tract and 20% the lower GI tract. GI bleeding is a common medical emergency. There are many causes, with the most common arising from peptic ulcer disease.

The incidence rate of 1.33 cases/1000 population equates to approximately 85,000 cases/year in the UK, or one gastrointestinal bleed every 6 minutes (NCEPOD 2015). Patients with any acute GI bleed should only be admitted to hospitals with 24/7 access to on-site endoscopy and interventional radiology. Gastric erosion/acute stress ulceration can be another complication associated with any critically ill patient, with lesions ranging from mild erosion to acute ulceration and perforation.

In particular, bleeding resulting from ruptured oesophageal or gastric varices has a high mortality rate (NCEPOD 2015). Acute variceal bleeding is a serious complication of portal hypertension which is, in turn, a result of chronic liver disease (as opposed to acute liver failure). Haematemesis and **melaena** are the most common presentations of acute upper GI bleeding, with fresh blood from the rectum indicative usually of lower GI bleeding. A massive GI bleed will lead to the signs and symptoms associated with *hypovolaemic shock* (e.g., tachycardia, hypotension, pallor, sweating, cyanosis, mental confusion and oliguria) (see Table 10.4).

The principles of immediate management centre on the aims:

- Resuscitate (with blood transfusion and fluids).
- Control active bleeding.
- Prevent recurrence of haemorrhage.

Remember

By the time that the patient has changes in their observations, they will have already lost at least 20% of their circulating volume.

The incidence of *non-variceal bleeding* (e.g., peptic ulceration) has been significantly reduced in the last few decades. Drugs that modify gastric sections, such as proton pump inhibitors (for example, omeprazole) have had a marked effect at reducing peptic ulcer disease along with *Helicobacter pylori* eradication and reduction in non-steroidal anti-inflammatory drug NSAIDS (Siau et al. 2017). Patients will be assessed for requirements of blood and plasma expanders via large bore cannulae, with close monitoring of cardiovascular and fluid balance status. Once the patient is stable, early endoscopic intervention is required to identify the source of bleeding with subsequent endoscopic therapy using techniques such as adrenaline injection, thermal treatments or placement of a haemoclip (Siau et al. 2017). Rebleeding occurs on 13–23% of cases. Surgery may be necessary if the bleeding continues (National Institute for Health and Care Excellence (NICE) 2016; Tripathi et al. 2015).

Patients with a *variceal bleed* are more likely to need further intervention due to a high risk of recurrent bleeding, with 15–30% rebleeding in the six weeks following initial bleed (Siau et al. 2017). In addition to fluid resuscitation and close monitoring, the patient with a variceal bleed is likely to require any of the following interventions:

- Pharmacological control with Terlipressin (NICE 2016) to reduce portal blood pressure.
- Prophylactic antibiotic therapy (NICE 2016) to prevent infection, which is common after upper gastrointestinal bleeding in patients with cirrhosis.
- Endoscopic variceal ligation (EVL), which involves rubber bands placed so that they strangulate the bleeding varices.
- Transjugular intrahepatic portosystemic shunt (TIPS), which is a procedure whereby a catheter is inserted into the portal vein (under radiological guidance) and a stent is then inserted between the portal vein and the systemic circulation, thereby reducing portal blood pressure. This latter intervention is reserved for patients with recurrent bleeding not controlled by band ligation (NICE 2016).

Lower gastrointestinal bleeding is more common in the elderly; its presentation can range from minor bleeding to a life-threatening haemorrhage, with an associated mortality of 5% (NCEPOD 2016). Most cases of lower GI bleeding are self-limiting, responsive usually to resuscitative approaches including fluid and blood administration.

Nursing care of the patient suffering from both upper and lower Gastrointestinal bleeding centres around obtaining robust intravenous access with large bore cannulae, management of the administration of blood and fluids, frequent and thorough assessment of fluid balance status, facilitation of endoscopic investigations and managing of the patient's comfort and dignity throughout the episode. Nursing assessment should focus on assessment indicators such as blood pressure, pulse rate, rhythm, perfusion, urine output and level of consciousness, using NEWS to guide assessment of deterioration risk.

Acute pancreatitis

Its close proximity to the gall bladder and common bile duct make the pancreas particularly vulnerable to inflammation when these are diseased, with one of the most common causes of acute pancreatitis being gallstones or biliary tract obstruction. The second most common cause of acute pancreatitis is alcohol abuse. The underlying pathophysiology for this is unclear, but may be due to irritation causing spasm and obstructing the flow of secretions, trapping enzymes within the pancreas. Regardless of the cause, inflammation in the pancreas causes trypsin to be improperly secreted and trapped within the pancreas itself, causing auto-digestion and compounding inflammation. Patients who presented with alcohol-related acute pancreatitis are usually younger than those with gallstones or an unknown aetiology (NCEPOD 2016).

Most patients with pancreatitis have a mild episode, but 10–20% of cases are of sufficient severity to cause a systemic inflammatory response syndrome, with complications including pancreatic cell death, sepsis, and hypovolaemic shock. Hypovolaemia in severe pancreatitis is due to body fluids being diverted to the pancreas in response to an overwhelming inflammatory response and blood loss as the pancreas is digested by its own enzymes. In view of these complications, it is recommended that patients with severe acute pancreatitis should be managed in a high dependency unit or intensive therapy unit with full monitoring and systems support (Tenner et al. 2013; Mehmood et al. 2019).

The main symptom of acute pancreatitis is sharp, twisting, deep upper abdominal pain, which may radiate through the back and is worse usually when supine. Other symptoms include nausea, vomiting, loss of appetite, diarrhoea, pyrexia and in some cases, jaundice (see patient assessment). A diagnosis of acute pancreatitis should include at least two of the following features: acute abdominal pain typical for pancreatitis, elevated lipase or amylase at least three times above normal and characteristic findings on CT scan (NICE 2018).

Unfortunately, patients with pancreatitis or liver failure can be stigmatised by a public misconception that these conditions are linked exclusively to high levels of alcohol consumption.

The goals of management include supportive care, limitation of systemic complications and prevention of infection if necrosis is present. All patients will need close monitoring, intravenous hydration and analgesia, with nasogastric suction being indicated for relief of nausea, vomiting and ileus. The nurse caring for an acute pancreatitis case must advocate for and manage nutrition. Current guidelines recommend cautious oral intake once nausea and vomiting has resolved, with alternative nutritional support (enteral and parenteral) to be coordinated within 72 hours of presentation (NICE 2018).

Liver failure

Acute hepatic dysfunction can be classified according to the time interval between the onset of jaundice and encephalopathy, with hyperacute being less than 7 days, acute being 8–28 days and subacute being 29 days–12 weeks. Additionally, patients may have stable chronic liver disease that decompensates acutely. The most common causes of acute liver failure are drug-induced (e.g., Paracetamol) and acute viral hepatitis. Other causes are included in Table 10.1.

The main manifestations and problems of liver failure are summarised in Table 10.2.

Liver blood tests include

- Bilirubin.
- Albumin.
- Prothrombin time (PT) and INR.
- Alkaline phosphate (ALP).
- Liver enzymes: AST, ALT, γ-Glutamyltransferase (GGT).

Table 10.1 Causes of acute liver failure

Viral	Hepatitis, A, B, C, D and E Herpes virus Adenovirus Epstein-Barr virus Cytomegalovirus
Drug-induced	Paracetamol (Acetaminophen)
Toxins	Amanita (death cap) mushrooms Organic solvents Phosphorus poisoning
Metabolic disorders	Acute fatty liver of pregnancy Reye syndrome
Vascular	Acute circulatory failure (shock) Budd-Chiari syndrome Veno-occlusive disease
Miscellaneous	Wilson's disease (Cu accumulation) Autoimmune hepatitis

Table 10.2 Summary of main manifestations and problems of liver failure

Hepatic encephalopathy

The cause of hepatic encephalopathy is unclear, but the patient will present with alteration in conscious level resulting from a raised ICP due to cerebral oedema. The level of reduction in conscious level is classified as below:

- Grade I: altered mood, impaired intellect, reduced ability to concentrate and impaired psychomotor function, but rousable and coherent.
- Grade II: inappropriate behaviour, increased drowsiness and confusion, but rousable (may have asterixis (liver flap) and dysarthria).
- Grade III: stuporous, somnolent, but rousable, often disorientated, agitated and aggressive.
- Grade IV: coma, unresponsive to painful stimuli.
- In extremis, the patient may have fixed, dilated pupils and exhibit manifestations of brain herniation.

Coagulopathy

Liver failure will result in a coagulopathy due to reduced levels of fibrinogen, Vitamin K and clotting factors.

Cardiovascular instability

Patients may become cardiovascularly unstable (hypotensive and tachycardic) due to endotoxaemia, which causes vasodilation and a compensatory increase in cardiac output.

Increased risk of infection

This is due to suppression of immune function and impaired neutrophil and Kupffer cell functions.

Renal failure

Deteriorating liver function can affect the circulation to the kidneys, resulting in renal failure. The mechanism behind hepatorenal syndrome is poorly understood, but it is believed that the vasoconstriction in the kidney causes this, rather than structural tissue damage.

Hypoglycaemia

The liver plays an important role in blood glucose control, and in impairment, glycogen will not be broken down into glucose, and the production of new glucose will not occur.

Acid base and electrolyte disturbance

Hypokalaemia, hypomagnesaemia, hyponatraemia, hypophosphataemia and hypocalcaemia can all occur in relation to liver failure. A metabolic alkalosis can result from vomiting, or the patient may have a metabolic acidosis if secondary to paracetamol overdose or lactic acid excess.

Abnormal liver blood tests

The patient in liver failure will also have abnormal blood results that detect deterioration in liver function. These have previously been referred to as liver function tests (LFTs), but as LFTs include elevations of hepatobiliary liver enzymes that indicate ongoing injury rather than functional changes, the term 'abnormal liver blood test' is now used (Newsome et al. 2017). These are summarised below:

- *Indicators of abnormal function*: abnormal clotting (e.g., prolonged PT or increased INR). Clotting factors are synthesised in the liver and there is a reduction in circulating clotting factors with the degree of prolongation of PT being used as a prognosticator. Serial tests need to be analysed with platelets and FFP being administered only if bleeding actively.
- *Assessment of damage*: liver enzymes are raised. These exist normally within liver cells, but will leak into the plasma when damaged (e.g., AST, Aspartate transaminase and ALT, Alanine aminotransferase [most specific for liver damage]).
- *Excretory capacity*: bilirubin is increased in obstruction (direct/conjugated) or erythrocyte breakdown (indirect/unconjugated). At a level above 50 umol/L, jaundice will be apparent.

Other: gamma GT is an inducible enzyme resulting from cell damage (often due to alcohol). ALP (alkaline phosphatase) can be increased in obstructive jaundice, reflecting cholestasis.

Abnormal liver blood test?

The extent of the abnormality does not always reflect the extent of the damage

A comprehensive analysis of abnormal blood tests and additional investigations will be required, such as:

- Abdominal ultrasound.
- Hepatitis B & Hepatitis C screening.
- Autoantibodies, immunoglobulins.
- Ferritin and transferrin saturation.
- HbA1c.

(Newsome et al. 2017)

Intestinal obstruction

A low albumin level can be a contributory cause of generalised oedema or ascites, as albumin (and other plasma proteins) provide an oncotic pressure, keeping fluid in the circulation. Low levels of circulating plasma proteins will tend towards fluid remaining in the tissues rather than being drawn back into the intravascular space.

Obstruction can occur in either the small or large bowel and if untreated, can lead to perforation and peritonitis. Mechanical obstruction can be caused by tumours, impacted foreign bodies, impacted faeces or gall stones, or by strictures. Additionally, it may be caused by volvulus, intussusceptions, adhesions or hernias. Clinical presentation depends on the level of obstruction. Proximal obstructions tend to cause colicky abdominal pain and early vomiting, whereas in distal obstructions, abdominal distension and constipation are more common. In either case, patients may present with manifestations of hypovolaemia as fluid is sequestered into the gut.

Nursing assessment

A systematic approach to assessment is essential in order to quickly identify any problems in the deteriorating patient. Using ABCDE provides a sound basis for prioritising issues, and these should be managed as they arise.

The *airway* should be assessed for patency, patients with acute liver failure, pancreatitis or severe bleeding may have a deteriorating level of consciousness, and airway protection may be required. Patients with persistent vomiting are at risk from aspiration or upper airway obstruction. Assessment of *breathing* is important to identify signs of compromise, for example, the patient with a gastrointestinal emergency may present with hypoxaemia and tachypnoea requiring supplemental oxygen administration. The *circulation* may be compromised by gastrointestinal emergencies associated with hypovolaemia, as evidenced by a combination of cold peripheries, reduced capillary refill time, tachycardia, weak pulse, hypotension, oliguria, etc. Gaining intravenous access is a priority to enable rapid fluid administration as necessary. These interventions should be initiated prior to proceeding to the next assessment in the sequence. *Disability* assessment includes level of consciousness as well as determining blood glucose level. *Exposure* review involves assessment of the abdomen and interpreting blood results to help ascertain the cause of an acute deterioration. NEWS 2 guides the nurse as to the appropriate care escalation required (see Table 10.3 for a summary of patient-assessment findings related to specific gastrointestinal emergencies).

The most common GI symptoms are abdominal pain, heartburn, nausea and vomiting, altered bowel habits, GI bleeding and jaundice. Additional symptoms may include: dysphagia, anorexia, weight loss and fatigue.

Abdominal pain

Abdominal pain can be due to a wide range of causes (see Table 10.4). Regardless of the cause, it must be assessed consistently and thoroughly by the nurse to determine important characteristics, improvement or deterioration, and this must be communicated promptly to the medical team. Utilising established pain assessment tools, such as the 1–10 scale and OLD CART pneumonic, can assist the nurse in measuring change in the pain status. Pain may originate from inflammation of the peritoneum (peritonitis), inflammation of the bowel (e.g., gastro enteritis), dilatation of the bowel (e.g., gastro enteritis) or inflammation of any organ within the abdomen (e.g., pancreatitis, cholecystitis, etc.). Additionally, pain may be initiated by other body areas in the form of referred pain (thorax, spine, genitalia), metabolic conditions (diabetes, uraemia, hypercalcaemia) or neurogenic disorders (herpes zoster). Finally, abdominal pain may be psychogenic in origin.

Table 10.3 Patient assessment utilising an ABCDE approach

	Variable	*GI bleed*	*Pancreatitis*	*Acute liver failure*	*Bowel emergency(inflammation, perforation, obstruction)*
A/B	• Airway patency • Respiratory rate and pattern • $Sp0_2$	• Risk of airway obstruction with haematemesis. • Tachypnoea due to hypoxia.	• Tachypnoea and dyspnoea due to pain and proximity of pancreas to diaphragm.	• Tachypnoea, shallow breathing due to respiratory compromise secondary to discomfort affecting diaphragm. Possibly secondary to a metabolic acidosis.	• Tachypnoea, shallow breathing due to respiratory compromise secondary to pain affecting diaphragm and ability to breathe properly.
C	• BP • Pulse • Capillary refill time (CRT) • Skin • CVP • Urine output	• Hypovolaemia due to haemorrhage causing hypotension, tachycardia, cool and clammy, oliguria.	• Hypovolaemia due to sequestration of fluid around inflamed pancreas (hypotension, tachycardia, cool and clammy, oliguria). • ST segment changes on ECG. • Pyrexia due to inflammatory processes or infection.	• 'Vasodilatory' shock due to endotoxins and/or sepsis hypotension, tachycardia, warm to touch, oliguria. • Oliguria may also be due to acute kidney injury (AKI) secondary to liver failure.	• Evidence of hypovolaemia (hypotension, tachycardia, cool and clammy, oliguria), if ongoing diarrhoea and vomiting.
D	• GCS • Pain assessment	• Reduced level of consciousness, if severe haemorrhage.	• Severe abdominal pain. • Worse on lying down.	• Reduced level of consciousness (LOC) due to encephalopathy.	• Pain may be constant in inflammation or perforation leading to peritonitis, or colicky in nature with intestinal obstruction.
E1	• GI assessment	• Haematemesis with upper GI bleed. • Melaena with lower GI bleed.	• Distended abdomen. • Possible bruising on flanks (Turners sign), umbilicus (Cullen's sign or groin [Fox sign]).	• Distended abdomen with tender, palpable liver due to enlargement.	• Distended (and taut) abdomen. Bowel sounds may at first be high-pitched, 'tinkling' and later be absent. • Vomiting and/or diarrhoea/ constipation. Fresh blood in stool from lower GI bleed, melaena.
E2	• Temperature • Blood results	• Drop in Hb	• May rise with inflammatory response. • Elevated serum amylase and lipase. • Hyperglycaemia. • Hypomagnesaemia in alcoholic pancreatitis. • Hyperkalaemia due to metabolic acidosis and renal failure (AKI). • ↑ Bilirubin and jaundice due to effects on common bile duct.	• Deranged LFTs. • Elevated enzymes (AST and ALT). • Low albumin. • Deranged clotting. • Elevated lactate (and metabolic acidosis). • Hypoglycaemia. • Elevated Cr and Urea if AKI developing. • Low levels of potassium, magnesium, sodium, phosphates and calcium may occur. • Jaundice due to elevated bilirubin levels.	• May rise with inflammatory response/ infection. • Elevated lactate and metabolic acidosis on ABGs, if ischaemic bowel present.

(*Continued*)

Table 10.3 Continued

	Variable	*GI bleed*	*Pancreatitis*	*Acute liver failure*	*Bowel emergency(inflammation, perforation, obstruction)*
E3	• Other: • Medical Scoring Systems	• Use Rockall Numerical Risk Scoring System (a prognostic score utilising age, degree of shock, and comorbidities).	• Use Atlanta classification Pancreatitis Outcome Prediction score (POP) (or Ranson's criteria, if alcohol-induced pancreatitis) for scoring severity of pancreatitis.	• Use Child-Pugh scoring or MELD for severity of liver failure. • Use Kings Criteria for indications for liver transplant.	

Table 10.4 Abdominal pain by location

Right upper quadrant	**Epigastric**	**Left upper quadrant**
Cholecystitis	Peptic ulcer	Splenic rupture
Cholangitis	Gastritis	Splenic abscess
Pneumonia	Pancreatitis	Gastritis
Hepatitis	Myocardial infarction	Gastric ulcer
Subphrenic abscess	Pericarditis	Pancreatitis
	Oesophagitis	Subphrenic abscess
	Ruptured aortic aneurysm	
Right lower quadrant	**Periumbilical**	**Left lower quadrant**
Appendicitis	Appendicitis (early)	Diverticulitis
Salpingitis	Gastroenteritis	Salpingitis
Inguinal hernia	Bowel obstruction	Inguinal hernia
Ectopic pregnancy	Ruptured aortic aneurysm	Ectopic pregnancy
Inflammatory bowel disease		Inflammatory bowel disease
Non-localised pain		
Gastroenteritis	Mesenteric ischaemia	Bowel obstruction
Irritable bowel syndrome	Peritonitis	Metabolic disease
Diabetes	Malaria	Psychiatric disease

Using OLD CART to assess abdominal pain caused by acute appendicitis, the nurse may anticipate the following responses from the patient:

Onset: slow onset of dull pain progressing to severe pain.
Location: near the navel to begin with and moving towards the right lower abdomen as the condition progresses.
Duration: constant from onset of first feelings of pain.
Characteristic: starting with a dull visceral pain progressing to peritoneal pain in the right lower quadrant.
Aggravating/relieving factors: worsens prior to vomiting.
Radiation: pain can radiate to the navel or the back; in males, pain can radiate to the right testicle.
Timing: pain is constant, as the source is related to inflammation of the peritoneal cavity.

(Alvarado 2018)

The acute abdomen

The term "acute abdomen" describes a syndrome of acute abdominal pain with accompanying signs and symptoms that focus attention on the abdomen. There are many causes of an acute abdomen, both abdominal and extra abdominal. These can be classified into:

- *Infective/inflammatory*: specific organs may be inflamed, for example, as in acute cholecystitis, acute pancreatitis, acute appendicitis or pelvic inflammatory disease. Peritonitis is defined as inflammation of the peritoneal membrane. Causes include physical damage, chemical irritation and bacterial invasion, for example, following perforation of the bowel. Peritonitis can be a complication of any surgery in which the peritoneal cavity is breached, or any disease that perforates the walls of the stomach or intestines. Continued inflammation will be associated with guarding and rebound tenderness. The spread of infection throughout the abdominal cavity will lead to generalized abdominal wall rigidity and manifestations of sepsis.

- *Obstructive*: this occurs when a hollow lumen has a blockage which interferes with its normal motility pattern. For example, biliary colic, when the cystic duct is blocked by a gall stone, or renal colic due to an obstructing ureteric calculus. Intestinal obstruction will result in abdominal colic, vomiting and progressive constipation. If neglected, it will lead to perforation, peritonitis and signs of an acute abdomen.
- *Haemorrhagic*: this is not the commonest cause of acute abdominal pain, but is frequently serious. The pain will be due to the presence of blood in the peritoneal cavity.
- *Other Causes*: abdominal pain may be present in a variety of other conditions e.g., pneumonia (arising from parietal pleura), subphrenic abscess, myocardial ischaemia, diabetic ketoacidosis, hypercalcaemia, porphyria or psychogenic factors.

Look, listen and feel (inspection, auscultation, palpation) of the acute abdomen

Look (inspection)

A patient with an acute abdomen often exhibits pallor and anxiety, is sweating, and tachypnoeic. The patient should be assessed for pyrexia and signs of shock (hypovolaemic or septic). With colic, the patient will be restless. In acute pancreatitis, bruising may be present in the flanks (Grey-Turner's sign) and/or around the umbilicus (Cullen's sign). Inspection would also include the noting of striae (stretch marks) and surgical scars.

Apart from obesity, a distended abdomen might suggest ascites or intestinal obstruction. In obesity, the abdomen will be enlarged but not tense, whereas ascites or intestinal obstruction will result in the skin over the abdomen being taut. In extremis, this can result in Abdominal Compartment Syndrome (ACS), whereby the intra-abdominal pressure is so high that it compresses the kidneys and other abdominal structures and may impact on the diaphragm, compromising breathing. If the high pressure progresses, renal function may be compromised.

Listen (auscultation)

Bowel sounds may be high-pitched in intestinal obstruction or absent in the presence of an ileus or peritonitis. Ileus is a failure of peristalsis. The presence or absence of bowel sounds should be interpreted with caution, as it is possible to have sounds present with poor gut functioning and vice versa. Bowel sounds should therefore be interpreted in context with other indicators of bowel function such as distension, pain, gastric aspirate, vomiting and diarrhoea.

Feel (palpation)

Palpation of the acute abdomen may cause brief but intense pain for the individual being examined. It is important, therefore, that this is not repeated unnecessarily. Only health care professionals competent in abdominal palpation and with relevant diagnostic skills perform this assessment, unless under direct supervision. Local areas of tenderness may be identified on palpation, with rebound tenderness or guarding present as underlying pathology worsens. A palpable mass may indicate a neoplasm or hernia and, if in the right iliac fossa, may indicate Crohn's disease or an appendix abscess. A pulsatile mass may be identified in the presence of an abdominal aortic aneurysm.

CASE STUDY 10.1 MR HARVEY: PART 1

Initial Assessment

It is 09:00 and you are caring for Mr Harvey, aged 60, who has been admitted to the Admissions Ward via A&E, where he presented following an episode of haematemesis at home. He has a history of chronic liver failure due to cirrhosis of the liver (caused by Hepatitis C). He has not vomited any more blood since admission and is awaiting a diagnostic endoscopy.

On approaching Mr Harvey you notice that he is sitting comfortably in bed. You introduce yourself, wash your hands, pull the screen around you and ask him if he is happy to perform an assessment. Mr Harvey agrees. He is anxious about having vomited blood, so you check that an empty bowl and tissues are within reach and that the suction equipment is working, in case Mr Harvey has another episode of haematemesis.

Airway/breathing

Mr Harvey is able to talk in whole sentences and is cooperative in answering questions. You assess his airway as patent. You document that Mr Harvey has a respiratory rate of 28 breaths per minute and observe his breathing to be shallow; he is not using any accessory muscles of respiration. He has a nasal cannula in place with 2L/min oxygen and his saturations are 96%. On auscultation, he has clear, bilateral air entry to both bases with no wheeze or additional sounds.

As Mr Harvey is currently within his prescribed oxygen targets (94–98% Scale 1 on NEWS), and as you have verified presence and functionality of his suction equipment, you decide to move on further with your assessment. You document Mr Harvey's respiratory rate, saturations and use of supplemental oxygen on the NEWS 2 chart.

Breathing NEWS 3 + 0 + 2 = 5

Circulation

He has warm peripheries, you note two large bore peripheral cannulae in situ, and he is receiving 100mL/hour of Hartmann's Solution (as he is nil by mouth). Two cannulae have been placed as a precaution, in case Mr Harvey needs urgent fluid administration. You measure Mr Harvey's pulse of 110 beats per minute, which is regular and strong, BP 112/60 mmhg and a capillary refill time of 3 seconds. He has passed 150mL of urine (using a bottle) over the past 3 hours.

Circulation NEWS 0 + 1 = 1

It is good practice to site a second cannula in a patient who may need intravenous (IV) fluids in an emergency: "One to use and one to lose".

Disability

You conduct an ACVPU assessment and find Mr Harvey to be alert, orientated, fully cooperative and in no pain. His blood sugar on admission is 5mmol/L.

Disability NEWS = 0

Exposure

His temperature is 37.1°C. Mr Harvey appears underweight, but he has a distended abdomen. In view of Mr Harvey's history of chronic liver failure, it is likely that this is due to ascites (collection of fluid in the abdominal cavity), which may be contributing to his tachypnoea, as the fluid collection may compromise diaphragmatic function. A large bore nasogastric tube is in situ. This has been placed to a) determine whether active bleeding is still evident; and b) to empty blood from the stomach prior to endoscopy. You note that although Mr Harvey's skin is intact, it has a slight yellow tinge. This may be due to jaundice, and the bilirubin level should therefore be checked when blood results are available.

Exposure NEWS = 0

Total NEWS = 6

Whilst Mr Harvey appears to be quite comfortable and stable, you recognise that his NEWS 2 is high (total of 6) and his condition can change from stable to unstable quickly. This requires an **urgent response**. You report Mr Harvey's NEWS score to the nurse in charge, who will contact the SpR. You stay with Mr Harvey to check his observations.

Mr Harvey is weighed, and this is documented carefully, as daily weights in a patient with ascites can provide a guide to increased fluid formation or retention. In respect to Mr Harvey being underweight, you calculate his BMI to be 18 and note that a referral to a dietician should be made. The nurse is also aware that chronic poor nutritional status may impact adversely on prognosis.

Care escalation

The SpR, given Mr Harvey's history and presentation, makes a provisional diagnosis of ruptured oesophageal varices. This is a complication of chronic liver disease, as is ascites. There is a high risk of Mr Harvey re-bleeding, and therefore, he is now booked for an emergency endoscopy and intervention as relevant. It is possible also that his chronic liver disease has become 'decompensated', i.e. 'acute on chronic'. If this is substantiated, he is at even greater risk of re-bleeding from his varices, due to a coagulopathy. The nurse will therefore check Mr Harvey's blood liver tests to look for abnormalities in clotting profile and full blood count when they are available. The team are happy to support Mr Harvey on the ward, pending endoscopy.

You commence 15-min observations and instigate a fluid balance chart. You reassure him that you will be monitoring his condition closely.

Maximising GI status

Monitoring of fluid balance

The most important nursing intervention in relation to gastrointestinal emergencies is monitoring fluid balance, as most of these situations will result in hypovolaemia. The

Table 10.5 Blood losses

	Minimal	*Mild*	*Moderate*	*Severe*
%	10%	20%	30%	40%+
Volume lost	500mL	1000mL	1500mL	2000mL+
HR	Normal	100–120	120–140	140+
BP systolic	Normal	Postural drop	<100	<80
Urine Output	Normal	20–30mL/hr	10–20mL/hr	Anuric
Mental Status	Normal	Normal	Restless	Impaired LOC
Peripheral	Normal	Cool/pale	Cool/pale	Cold/clammy

early identification of fluid losses and timely administration of appropriate fluid replacement will prevent the deteriorating patient from developing hypovolaemic shock. Nurses are directly responsible for monitoring patients of all ages for actual or potential fluid and/or electrolyte disturbance, and the NMC (2018) requires these assessments to be performed accurately by using appropriate diagnostic and decision-making skills.

Table 10.5 gives an overview of how clinical parameters may change as blood/fluid is lost. In the case of haemorrhage (e.g., from a variceal bleed), routine observations may remain stable until they have suffered a blood loss of at least 20% of their circulating volume, equating to a litre of blood.

Although we should drink approximately 2 litres of fluid daily, most hospitalised patients will not achieve this, due to change in normal habits, lack of available fluids, general malaise, nausea, vomiting and diarrhoea. Additionally, many GI patients will also be nil by mouth. The importance of keeping accurate fluid balance charts **cannot** be overemphasised.

Impaired, or lack of, reabsorption (e.g., vomiting and diarrhoea) will result in fluids being lost from the body, leading to hypovolaemia. Fluids may also be lost via drains (e.g., biliary drains and nasogastric tubes on free drainage) or due to the disease process (e.g., sequestration of fluid in pancreatitis).

The pyrexial patient will have increased insensible fluid losses, which will further exacerbate hypovolaemia. These additional fluid losses need to be taken into consideration when calculating fluid replacement.

CASE STUDY 10.2 MR HARVEY: PART 2

You receive Mr Harvey's blood results back from the lab:

	Result	*Normal range*
INR	2	*1*
Prothrombin time	30 seconds	*12–14 seconds*
Platelets	62 x 10^9/L	*130–450 x 10^9/L*

Hb	8.1g/dL	*13–16 g/dL in men*
WBC	13.9 x 10^9/L	*4.4–10 x 10^9/L*
Sodium (Na^+)	130mmol/L	*135–145mmol/L*
Potassium (K^+)	3.8mmol/L	*3.5–5.0mmol/L*
Bilirubin	60umol/L	*5–17umol/L*
AST	133U/L	*5–40U/L*
ALP	89U/L	*5–40U/L*
Albumin	22g/L	*35–50g/L*
Urea	17mmol/L	*3–6mmol/L*
Creatinine	170umol/L	*60–120umol/L*

Nursing interpretation of blood results:

Clotting Profile: bleeding time is high and platelets are low, indicating abnormal liver function and adding a critical aspect to the variceal bleed, should it reoccur.

Haemoglobin: this is low, confirming anaemia in the context of blood loss. The nurse will anticipate the administration of a blood transfusion. Clotting products will be administered (in addition to the blood), if bleeding actively.

Abnormal: all indicators are elevated, indicating damage to liver cells and progression of cirrhosis. Bilirubin levels are elevated due to the liver being unable to process bilirubin, resulting in it remaining in the circulation and manifesting as jaundice. Liver enzymes (AST and ALP) are moderately elevated as a result of liver cell damage. Albumin levels are low, confirming liver damage and providing a cause for ascites.

The elevated urea and creatinine suggest renal dysfunction, which may be pre-existing or due to hepatorenal syndrome.

In response to the above blood results, you ensure the presence of intravenous access, discuss the possibility of a blood transfusion with Mr Harvey, and answer his questions, collect the equipment you will need to administer a blood transfusion and manage your time with your other patients appropriately to ensure you will be available to undertake this task.

Two hours later

Mr Harvey's observations are as follows:

Airway and breathing: respiratory rate is 32 breaths per minute, oxygen saturations are 91%, on 2L of oxygen therapy. As you are aware of BTS Guidelines (2017) of target saturations of 94–98%, you increase Mr Harvey's oxygen flow to 4L/min and make a mental note to reassess his saturation in a few minutes.

Breathing NEWS 3 + 3 + 2 = 8

Circulation: BP is 88/55. Pulse is 130 beats per minute (regular but thready) and cold peripheries

Circulation NEWS: 3 + 2 = 5

Disability: Mr Harvey says that he feels very nauseous and has a metallic taste in his mouth. The nausea could be due to accumulating blood in the stomach and hypotension. He is, however, fully alert; his blood glucose was not rechecked.

Disability NEWS = 0

Exposure: temperature 36.1°C.

Total NEWS = 13

You inform the doctor for an **emergency response** of the changes, as per NEWS protocol, and are aware that the trend in his observations (in conjunction with the nausea) indicates that he is bleeding. The critical care team are informed, as an ITU admission may be required.

Mr Harvey is reviewed immediately by a senior doctor who confirms your concerns. An ABG is taken, a urinary catheter inserted and intravenous lines are checked for patency. Immediate transfer to the Endoscopy Suite is arranged. Fifteen minutes later, Mr Harvey has a haematemesis of approximately 600mL of blood. His airway remains patent (there is a possible risk of airway obstruction) and the nurse assesses his level of consciousness and finds that he is still able to speak clearly.

He is prescribed two units of blood, which you commence after following the trust policy on checking procedures, and he is placed on 15-minute observations, in view of his haematemesis and the blood transfusion. Fresh, frozen plasma FFP and platelets are prescribed to treat his condition, as clotting products are absent from transfused blood.

You accompany him to his endoscopy, continuing the blood products administration and 15-minute observations. He also has pulse rate and oxygen saturations displayed via a pulse oximeter.

Mr Harvey has an endoscopy which confirms variceal bleeding. Four varices are banded (Endoscopic Variceal Ligation) to stop the bleeding, and he becomes more stable, returning to the admissions ward for reassessment.

Nausea and vomiting

Acute nausea, with or without vomiting, is a common symptom. Nausea is described as a sensation of imminent vomiting and vomiting (emesis) is the forcible expulsion of the stomach contents through the mouth. The strongest triggers are irritation (gastritis, infection or presence of blood) and also distension of the stomach, with many causes (see Table 10.6). The trigger to initiate vomiting is located in the brain, explaining why many neurological conditions can also induce symptoms of nausea and vomiting.

Nasogastric aspirate

Mendelson's syndrome

This is a chemical pneumonitis caused by aspiration of gastric contents. It was first described by Mendelson in 1946, in relation to obstetric anaesthesia. It is considered that as little as 25 mL of gastric contents can cause significant damage.

Monitoring colour, consistency, and amount of content aspirated from a nasogastric tube is an important aspect of nursing care. Contents of the GI system are aspirated either via a suction system or manually by the nurse, with a large syringe. There is no definitive

Table 10.6 Causes of acute vomiting

GI tract	Peritonitis
	Bowel obstruction
	Acute pancreatitis
	Acute cholecystitis
	Acute appendicitis
	Mesenteric ischaemia
CNS	Raised intracranial pressure
	CNS tumours
	Meningitis
	Vestibular disorders/travel (motion sickness)
	Cerebral abscess
	Subarachnoid haemorrhage
	Head injury
	Migraine
Drugs	Chemotherapy
	Antibiotics/antivirals
	Narcotics
	Analgesics
Infections	Gastroenteritis (food poisoning, e.g., salmonella)
	Epidemic, e.g., Norwalk virus
	Hepatitis viruses
	Non-GI tract infections
Endocrine	Diabetic ketoacidosis
	Adrenal insufficiency
	Hypercalcaemia
	Uraemia
Miscellaneous	Ethanol abuse
	Recreational drug abuse
	Radiotherapy
	Pregnancy (hyperemesis gravidarum)
	Post myocardial infarction/CCF
	Carcinoma
	Postoperative

level at which the amount of aspirate indicates a problem with gut function, however, any amount over 200 mL at 4 hours, is generally taken as a cue to consider slowing or discontinuing feeding.

Diarrhoea

This is defined as a reduced consistency (or increased liquidity) of the faeces. Physiologically this will be due to inadequate reabsorption of water by the bowel (and/or increased mucus secretion) as the contents transit. There is an extensive differential diagnosis, however, including: infective (bacterial, viral, parasitic and toxins), inflammatory bowel disease (e.g., Crohn's, ulcerative colitis), drugs (antibiotics, ACE inhibitors, chemotherapy, laxatives), faecal impaction with overflow and, in the critically ill: altered gut motility and paralytic ileus.

Nursing management should focus upon close monitoring of cardiovascular and fluid balance status (early recognition of hypovolaemia) and a fresh stool sample sent for culture and sensitivity (in particular to exclude *Clostridium Difficile* enterotoxin, which is one of the most common nosocomial infections). Nursing care for this condition focuses on providing the patient with safe and easy access to toileting facilities, infection control measures, maintaining patient comfort and dignity and preserving perianal skin integrity throughout. The nurse must consider that a patient will have urgency with bowel movements, and this may compromise their safety in getting in and out of bed to the toilet; care must be taken to ensure the patient does not fall.

Pharmacology for GI problems

Stress ulceration medication

- H2 receptor antagonists: e.g., Ranitidine. These drugs suppress acid secretion by competing for the histamine receptor on the parietal cell.
- Proton pump inhibitors: e.g., Omeprazole or Lansoprazole. These are acid-suppressing agents, as they block the final pathway of acid secretion by the parietal cell, i.e. the proton pump. These are indicated for patients with major peptic ulcer bleeding following endoscopic intervention.
- Sucralfate: this increases mucus secretion, mucosal blood flow and local prostaglandin production. These effects protect the mucosa against damage by acid or pepsin. It forms a protective barrier over the gastric mucosa (but does not alter gastric ph. It is given via nasogastric (NG) tube (1 g every 4–6 hours).
- Antacids: antacids given hourly via NG tube can maintain gastric alkalinisation. These can contain magnesium, aluminium, calcium or sodium with problems resulting from excessive intake. They are used rarely now.

Anti-emetics

- Ondansetron: a serotonin 5-HT3 receptor antagonist (IV, IM or orally administered).
- Prochlorperazine (Stemetil): this is antidopaminergic and is particularly useful for vestibular vomiting. Administered IM.
- Cyclizine: this is a histamine H1 receptor antagonist and is effective for motion sickness and vestibular causes and where there is a contraindication to Prochlorperazine, e.g., Parkinson's Disease. Side effects include tachycardia.
- Domperidone: this is a dopamine receptor antagonist, useful for a wide range of causes of nausea and vomiting.

Nutritional support

According to NICE (2017), nutritional support should be considered in people who are malnourished or are at risk of malnutrition. All acutely ill patients, and particularly those with gastrointestinal disorders in whom feeding by normal methods is challenging (e.g., during gastrointestinal emergencies), are at risk of malnutrition. A degree of malnutrition is extremely common in most hospitalised patients. It is estimated that around 30% of hospitalised patients aged 65 or over are malnourished, and that this is frequently undiagnosed (British Association of Parenteral Nutrition (BAPEN) 2014). Poor nutritional status will also adversely affect mortality, morbidity and overall prognosis, for example, the patient with chronic liver failure and cachexia is likely to fare less well when undergoing liver transplantation than a patient with liver failure who is well-nourished.

Nutrition may be administered artificially, either enterally or parenterally, with both routes being compared and contrasted in Table 10.7.

Enteral nutrition (EN)

A 'never event'

It should **never happen** that a patient is fed via a misplaced nasogastric tube, as correct tube position should always be checked prior to commencing feeding. The Gold Standard for confirming tube position is CXR and the use of pH testing strips.

NICE (2017) NHS Improvement (2016)

Enteral feeding tubes can be placed into the stomach, duodenum or jejunum. Enteral feeding guidelines have shown evidence in favour of early institution of feeding and the of continuing delivery of food via the GI tract to be efficacious in the majority of the hospital population. The nurse, though, needs to be cognisant of the potential risks involved. NHS Improvement (2016) found, on reviewing incidence reports, that 32 patient deaths occurred where errors in nasogastric tube placement checking had been reported. Competency-based training for nursing staff on tube placement, with good recording processes to include all safety checks, is necessary to ensure safe and effective care. Those health care professionals, including medical staff that check CXR for tube placement, also require competency-based training, as misinterpretation of CXRs is a common error. NICE (2017) suggest all nasogastric tube positions should be confirmed after placement and *before each use* with pH-graded paper (and CXR, as necessary).

Aspiration of stomach contents

Aspiration pneumonia occurs if stomach contents are aspirated into the lungs. This can result in an acute lung injury which may be fatal. There is an increased risk of aspiration associated with a reduced level of consciousness, absent cough/gag reflexes, delayed gastric emptying, paralytic ileus or by simply having an enteral feeding tube in situ. Strategies to minimise the risk of aspiration include monitoring nasogastric aspirates, nursing patients upright (45%) and confirming and monitoring tube positioning.

Parenteral nutrition (PN)

Although enteral nutrition is favoured, PN is an alternative when it is not possible to use other routes or enteral nutrition has failed. ESPEN (2019) recommend, in their guidelines on parenteral nutrition, that all patients receiving less than their targeted enteral feeding after two days should be considered for PN, which should be administered in the form of a complete 'all in one bag'. For a comparison of enteral and parenteral routes see Table 10.7

Conclusion

An insight into the common gastrointestinal emergencies will assist the nurse in recognising and responding to the deteriorating patient with these problems. In particular, an

Table 10.7 Comparison of enteral and parenteral routes

	Enteral nutrition (EN)	*Parenteral nutrition (PN)*
Advantages	• As it uses the natural route, it is considered more physiologically normal. • It is relatively cheap (and simple). • Does not require vascular access. • Preserves gut mucosal integrity. • Stimulates immune barrier function. • May prevent bacterial translocation.	Greater potential for successful absorption of nutrients.
Disadvantages	• Associated with diarrhoea. • Inadequate feeding if interrupted for procedures or if patient not absorbing. • Increased risk of nosocomial pneumonia. • Not all patients will be capable of absorbing feed.	• Relatively expensive. • Requires vascular access. • Needs individualised calculations for constitution of feed.
Complications	• The tube may become knotted or blocked. • Aspiration. • Incorrect placement. • Nasopharyngeal erosions and discomfort. • Sinusitis. • Oesophagitis. • Tracheoesophageal fistula. • Abdominal distention. • Ruptured oesophageal varices. • May cause nausea and vomiting. • Risk of aspiration. • Diarrhoea. • Abdominal distension and cramping. • Constipation. • Hyperglycaemia. • Hypercapnia (due to high level of carbohydrate). • Electrolyte and trace element abnormalities.	Risks associated with central line placement (pneumothorax, catheter misplacement, etc.) • Infection. • Metabolic complications, such as hyperglycaemia, hypoglycaemia and hyperlipidaemia. • Hepatic dysfunction. • Acid base disturbance. • Electrolyte disturbance. • Risk of 'refeeding syndrome'.

understanding of the disordered pathophysiology will support the nurse in a systematic assessment of the patient and an appreciation of the rationale for the patient's presentation, signs and symptoms. Gastrointestinal emergencies often result in increased fluid losses and disruption to the normal secretion and reabsorption of bodily fluids culminating in hypovolaemia and hypovolaemic shock. Therefore, fluid balance assessment is of paramount importance and is a vital role for the nurse in caring for these patients.

Glossary 

Ascites Excess fluid that has accumulated in the peritoneal cavity. Comes from the Greek 'askites', 'bag like'. It can also be called hydroperitoneum.

Asterixis This is the term for hepatic flap (of the hands). The word comes from 'without fixed position'. When the patient with hepatic encephalopathy stretches out their hands, they have jerky irregular flexion/extension of the wrist. It is thought to be due to the interference with the inflow of joint position sense to the brain stem. Although characteristic of liver failure, it can also occur in cardiac, respiratory and renal failure.

Bacterial translocation of the gut Passage of indigenous bacteria from the GI tract to the systemic circulation. This can be due to a breach of mucosal barrier, impaired immune defence mechanisms and/or bacterial overgglossentryth.

Bile Bile (or gall) is fluid produced by the liver (and stored in the gall bladder) that is used to digest fats in the duodenum.

Chyme From Greek 'khymos', meaning 'juice'. This is semifluid, partly digested food expelled by the stomach into the duodenum.

Cirrhosis From Greek 'kirrhos', meaning 'yellowish or tawny', which is the colour of the diseased liver. Cirrhosis is the consequence of chronic liver disease, whereby the liver tissue is replaced by fibrosis and scar tissue.

Endocrine From Greek 'endo', meaning 'inside' and 'crinis', 'to secrete'. The endocrine system secretes hormones into the circulation to elicit a response in target organs.

Exocrine Exocrine glands secrete their products into ducts, e.g., stomach, pancreas or liver.

Haematemesis Vomiting of blood ('haem', blood and 'emesis', vomiting).

Melaena This is the black, tarry faeces associated with gastrointestinal haemorrhage. The black ('melan') colour is caused by the oxidation of iron in the haemoglobin during the passage through the ileum and colon.

Pancreatitis Inflammation of the pancreas that may either be acute or chronic.

Paralytic ileus Disruption in the normal propulsive ability of the gastrointestinal tract.

Peristalsis Contraction and relaxation of muscles, which propagates in a wave down a muscular tube. From Greek 'peristallein' (to wrap around), from 'peri' (around) and 'stallein' (to place).

Peritonitis Inflammation of the peritoneum – the membrane which lines part of the abdominal cavity and viscera.

Sengstaken-Blakemore Tube This is used in upper GI tract bleeding. It consists of a tube with two balloons, one of which is inflated against the walls of the oesophagus and the other in the stomach, the purpose of which is to apply pressure to bleeding points.

Translocation of bacteria The movement or translocation of bacteria from the gut, to the tissue outside the gut wall, such as lymph nodes, liver or bloodstream

Varices Varices are distended veins. From the Latin 'varix', meaning twisted veins.

Venturi masks These oxygen masks are so named because they utilise a 'venturi effect', which is to entrain air to mix with piped oxygen to achieve a specified oxygen percentage being delivered to the patient (fixed performance oxygen).

TEST YOURSELF

1 Reflux of gastric contents into the oesophagus can cause ulceration because gastric contents are:
   a. Acidic
   b. Alkaline

2 In liver failure, low levels of plasma proteins can predispose to:
   a. Oedema
   b. Ascites
   c. Jaundice
   d. Infection

3 The most common causes of pancreatitis are ____________________ and ____________________.

4 Liver tests include:
   a. Clotting profile
   b. AST
   c. Electrolytes
   d. Bilirubin

5 All of the following are signs of hypovolemia except:
   a. Tachycardia
   b. Hypotension
   c. Tachypnea
   d. Increased urine output

6 The vomiting centre is in the:
   a. Medulla
   b. Frontal lobe

7 A necrotic pancreas may be evidenced by:
   a. A high white blood cell count
   b. A low haemoglobin
   c. A metabolic acidosis
   d. Pyrexia

8 Epigastric pain may typically be due to:
   a. Gastritis
   b. Ectopic pregnancy
   c. Myocardial infarction
   d. Inguinal hernia

9 Nursing care of the patient with diarrhoea includes all of the following except:
   a. Maintaining skin integrity
   b. Ensuring safe access to toilet facilities
   c. Administration of enema to cleanse the bowel
   d. Maintaining strict infection control and handwashing

10 Patients with diarrhoea always have a sample sent for C&S to test for which common nosocomial infection? ______________________

11 The correct term for vomiting blood is __________________ and coughing blood is __________________.

Answers

1 a
2 a, b, d
3 gall stones, alcohol
4 a, b, d
5 d
6 a
7 a, c, d
8 a, c
9 c
10 *Clostridium Difficile*
11 haematemesis, haemoptysis

References

Alvarado A. (2018). *Clinical Approach in the Diagnosis of Acute Appendicitis, Current Issues in the Diagnostics and Treatment of Acute Appendicitis*. doi:10.5772/intechopen.75530. Available from https://www.intechopen.com/books/current-issues-in-the-diagnostics-and-treatment-of-acute-appendicitis/clinical-approach-in-the-diagnosis-of-acute-appendicitis.

British Association of Parenteral Nutrition (BAPEN). (2014). *Nutrition Screening Surveys in Hospitals in the UK 2007–2011: A Report Based on the Amalgamated Data from the Four Nutrition Screening Week Surveys Undertaken by BAPEN in 2007, 2008, 2010 and 2011*. Available from https://www.bapen.org.uk/pdfs/nsw/bapen-nsw-uk.pdf. Accessed August 2019.

British Thoracic Society. (2017). BTS guideline for oxygen use in adults in healthcare and emergency settings. *Thorax: An International Journal of Respiratory Medicine*, 72(Supplement 1), ii1–ii90.

ESPEN (European Society for Clinical Nutrition and Metabolism). (2019). ESPEN guidelines on parenteral nutrition: intensive care. *Clinical Nutrition*, 38(4), 48–79. Available from https://www.espen.org/files/ESPEN-Guidelines/ESPEN_guideline-on-clinical-nutrition-in-the-intensive-care-unit.pdf. Accessed August 2019.

Mehmood A, Ullah W, Chan V and Rongold D. (2019). The assessment of knowledge and early management of acute pancreatitis among residents. *Cureus*, 11(4). doi:10.7759/cureus.4389. Available from https://www.ncbi.nlm.nih.gov/pmc/articles/PMC6561519/.

National Confidential Enquiry into Patient Outcome and Death. (2015). *Time to Get Control? A Review of the Care Received by Patients Who Had a Severe Gastrointestinal Haemorrhage*. Available from https://www.ncepod.org.uk/2015report1/downloads/TimeToGetControlSummary.pdf.

National Confidential Enquiry into Patient Outcome and Death. (2016). *Treat the Cause A Review of the Quality of Care Provided to Patients Treated for Acute Pancreatitis*. Available from https://www.ncepod.org.uk/2016report1/downloads/TreatTheCause_summaryReport.pdf.

National Institute of Health and Care Excellence (NICE). (2012 updated 2016). *Acute Upper Gastrointestinal Bleeding in Over 16s: Management*, Cg 141. National Institute for Clinical Excellence. Available from https://www.nice.org.uk/guidance/cg141.

National Institute for Health and Care Excellence (NICE). (2017). *Nutritional Support in Adults: Oral Nutrition Support, Enteral Tube Feeding ad Parenteral Nutrition*, Cg 32. National Institute for Health and Clinical Excellence. Available from https://www.nice.org.uk/Guidance/CG32. Accessed August 2019.

National Institute for Health and Care Excellence (NICE). (2018). *Pancreatitis*, ng 104. National Institute for Clinical Excellence. Available from https://www.nice.org.uk/guidance/ng104/.

Newsome B, Cramb R, Davison S, Dillon J, Foulerton M, Godfrey E, Hall R, Harrower U, Hudson M, Langford A, Mackie A, Mitchell-Thain R, Sennett K, Sheron N, Verne J, Walmsley M and Yeoman A. (2017). Guidelines on the management of abnormal liver blood tests. *Gut*, 67, 1–14. doi:10.1136/gutjnl-2017-314924. Available from https://gut.bmj.com/content/gutjnl/early/2017/11/09/gutjnl-2017-314924.full.pdf.

NHS Improvement. (2016). *Patient Safety Alert Nasogastric Tube Misplacement: Continuing Risk of Death and Severe Harm NHS/PSA/RE/2016/006*. Available from https://improvement.nhs.uk/documents/194/Patient_Safety_Alert_Stage_2_-_NG_tube_resource_set.pdf. Accessed August 2019.

Nursing and Midwifery Council. (2018). *Standards for Pre-Registration Nursing Education*. NMC. Available from https://www.nmc.org.uk/standards/standards-for-nurses/standards-of-proficiency-for-registered-nurses/.

Siau K, Chapman W, Sharma N, Tripathi D, Iqbal T and Bhala N. (2017). Management of acute upper gastrointestinal bleeding: an update for the general physician. *Journal of the Royal College of Physicians Edinburgh*, 47, 218–230. doi:10.4997/JRCPE.2017.303. Accessed August 2019.

Tenner S, Baillie J, De Witt J and Vege SS. (2013). Management of acute pancreatitis. *American Journal of Gastroenterology*, 108, 1400–1415.

Tripathi D, Stanley AJ, Hayes PC, et al. (2015). UK guidelines on the management of variceal haemorrhage in cirrhotic patients. *Gut*, 64, 1680–1704.

11 The patient with acute endocrine problems

Muili Lawal

AIM

The aim of this chapter is to identify key roles and functions of the endocrine system to appreciate how altered physiology can disrupt homeostasis and cause a medical emergency. The chapter will discuss the more commonly experienced endocrine disorders and use case studies to explore the nurse's role in recognising and responding appropriately to patients with acute endocrine problems.

OBJECTIVES

After reading this chapter you will be able to:

- Recognise the major organs involved in endocrine function.
- Identify the roles of endocrine organs in maintaining homeostasis.
- Identify the common endocrine disorders and differentiate between patient presentations.
- Understand the use of assessment and therapeutic interventions to maximise the health status of patients with endocrine disorders.
- Describe the responsibilities of the nurse in assessing, monitoring and managing patients with acute endocrine disorders.

Introduction

Although most endocrine emergencies occur rarely, diabetic emergencies are witnessed by most nurses caring for patients within the hospital setting. People with diabetes are at greater risk of comorbidity and anecdotal evidence suggests that it can increase the burden of ongoing Covid-19 pandemic infection. Therefore, it is important for nurses to have insight into glucose metabolism and control coupled with their responsibilities in monitoring and managing this aspect of patient care. These principles are paramount not only during emergency situations, but routinely, as the monitoring and control of blood glucose is frequently part of patient management. Uncommon presentations of acute endocrine malfunction include thyrotoxicosis and adrenal insufficiency. All these can present with severe patient deterioration, so a basic understanding of the endocrine system and associated hormones is required.

Applied physiology

Overview of the endocrine system

The endocrine, nervous and immune system work in harmony to regulate the internal and external environment of human beings. The endocrine system is composed of various glands that are widely dispersed throughout the body, and they secrete chemical messengers called hormones (Brashers and Huether 2017). The major endocrine glands are the pituitary, thyroid, parathyroid, thymus, pancreas, adrenal, ovaries and testes. The endocrine structure and function witness some changes due to the ageing process (Brashers and Huether 2017). In contrast to the exocrine glands, which discharge their products via ducts into the external environment, e.g., pancreatic juice, the endocrine glands, which are ductless, synthesise and release hormones directly into the circulation. Figure 11.1 identifies the position of the major endocrine glands and the hormones they produce.

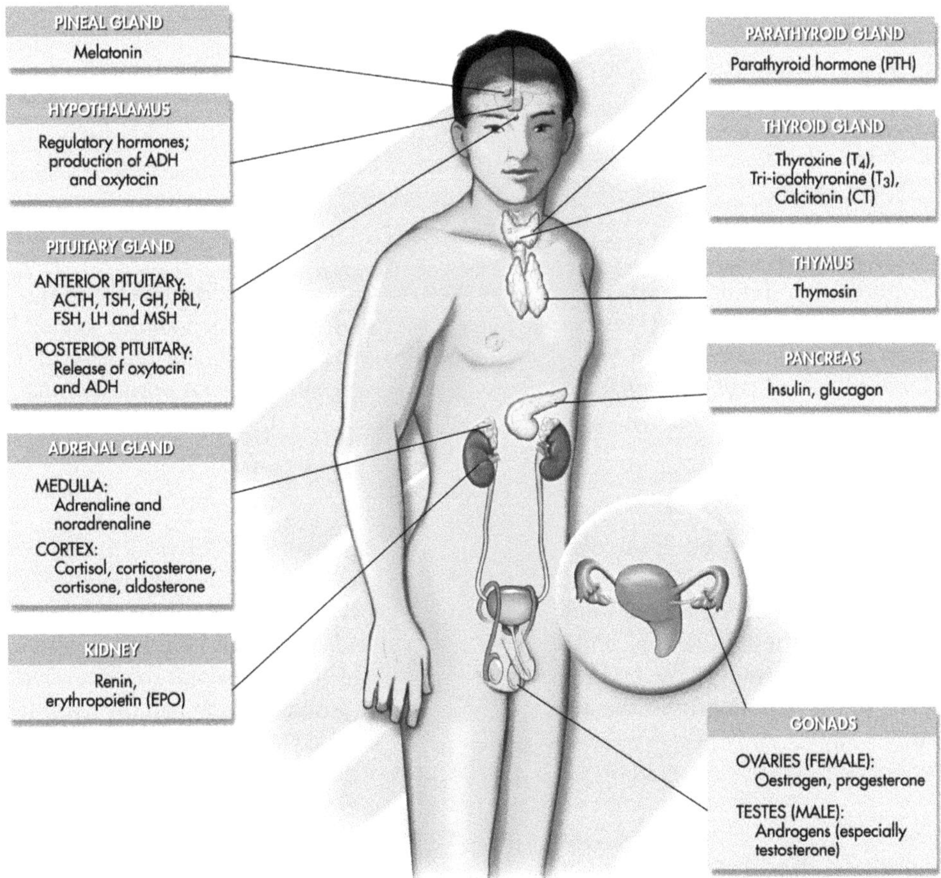

Figure 11.1 The position of the major endocrine glands and the hormones they produce.

Hormones have a wide variety of functions, and their effects can last for minutes, hours or even days. Hormones are composed predominantly from amino acids or sometimes cholesterol, as with the steroid hormones. They affect organs that have hormone-specific receptors, and these are known as target cells for that hormone. Circulating hormones activate the target cells directly, and the degree of response is related to total blood concentration. The more hormone circulating, the greater the target cell activity, though some hormones can have powerful effects at a very low concentration. Hormones are broken down rapidly either within their target cells or by the liver and kidney. The functions of the endocrine organs that may be involved in a medical emergency are summarised in Table 11.1.

The hormones have a wide influence on body processes, such as reproduction, maintenance of fluid and electrolyte balance, cellular growth and metabolism (Dixon and Salamanson 2006). The hormonal regulation helps to initiate adaptive responses to emergency demands and therefore assist to maintain an optimum internal environment. The endocrine glands respond to specific signals, and hormone production by each endocrine gland is finely balanced. The regulation of hormone release is controlled by negative and positive feedback. Both feedback systems help to maintain balance between physiological production and bodily demand (Lawal 2008). The negative feedback control loops are inhibitory (oppose the change) while positive feedbacks are stimulatory (potentiate the change). Most homeostatic feedback systems are negative feedback, e.g., blood glucose control, and an example of a positive feedback mechanism is uterine contraction during childbirth. Endocrine disorder is characterised by either underproduction or overproduction, and common endocrine imbalance are discussed below.

Structure and function of the endocrine glands

The hypothalamic-pituitary axis (HPA) forms the structural and functional basis to integrate endocrine and neurologic systems, which is referred to the neuroendocrine system. The hypothalamus is connected to the pituitary via the pituitary stalk and regulates the two lobes by neural and hormonal pathways. The HPA produces several hormones that affect other body functions, such as the thyroid and adrenal gland.

The hypothalamus

The hypothalamus, located in the diencephalon, is an important link between the nervous system and the endocrine system. It is involved in many of the normal physiological mechanisms that contribute to homeostasis, such as temperature control, thirst and hunger reflexes. The hypothalamus controls the pituitary gland, which, in its turn, regulates most of the other glands in the endocrine system. Figure 11.2 demonstrates the extensive influence of the hypothalamus, the anterior and posterior pituitary gland and their target organs.

The pituitary

The pituitary gland has an important role in the control of other glands. It has two lobes, anterior and posterior, producing several hormones that are summarised in Table 11.1.

Table 11.1 Summary of the hormones of the endocrine system and their effects

Tissue	*Hormones*	*Target/effect/function*
Hypothalamus	TRH (thyrotropin-releasing hormone) DA (dopamine) (or prolactin-inhibiting hormone) GHRH (growth hormone-releasing hormone) SS (somatostatin) (or GHIH growth-hormone inhibiting hormone) GnRH (gonadotropin-releasing hormone) CRH (corticotrophin-releasing hormone)	• Stimulates TSH (thyroid-stimulating hormone) release from the anterior pituitary. • Stimulates prolactin release from the anterior pituitary. • Inhibits prolactin release from anterior pituitary. • Stimulates GH (growth hormone) release from the anterior pituitary. • Inhibits GH release from the anterior pituitary. • Inhibits TSH being released by the anterior pituitary. • Stimulates FSH (follicle-stimulating hormone) release from the anterior pituitary. • Stimulates LH (luteinising hormone) release from the anterior pituitary. • Stimulates ACTH (adrenocorticotrophic hormone) release from the anterior pituitary.
Pituitary gland: anterior lobe	ACTH (adrenocorticotrophic hormone) TSH (thyroid-stimulating hormone) GH (growth hormone) FSH (follicle-stimulating hormone) LH (luteinising hormone) Prolactin	• Stimulates the adrenal cortex – specifically targets cells that produce glucocorticoids, which influence glucose metabolism. • Targets the thyroid gland with subsequent release of thyroid hormones T4 (thyroxine) and T3 (triiodothyronine). • Stimulates cell growth and replication. • Affects follicle development in females – stimulates oestrogens by ovarian cells. • Stimulates cells in tubules where sperm differentiate. • Induces ovulation in females and androgens including testosterone in males. • Stimulates milk production by the mammary glands.
Pituitary gland: posterior lobe	ADH (antidiuretic hormone) Oxytocin	• Increases the absorption of water in the distal tubule and collecting duct in the kidney. • Stimulates smooth muscle in the wall of the uterus promoting labour and delivery.
Pineal gland	Melatonin	• Control of 'biological clock'.
Thyroid gland	T4 (thyroxine) T3 (triiodothyronine) Calcitonin	• Directly affect the mitochondria in cells and therefore metabolic rate. • Regulation of calcium concentration in body fluids.
Parathyroid	PTH (parathyroid hormone)	• Regulation of calcium concentration in body fluids.
Thymus	Thymosins	• Role in immunity.
Adrenal glands	Adrenal medulla: Produce 2 hormones: adrenaline (epinephrine) and noradrenalin.	• They both potentiate the fight or flight response.
	Adrenaline Noradrenaline	• Accelerates the utilisation of cellular energy and mobilisation of energy reserves, e.g., increase metabolic rate.

(*Continued*)

Table 11.1 Continued

Tissue	*Hormones*	*Target/effect/function*
	Adrenal cortex: Produce 3 groups of steroids: Mineralocorticoids Glucocorticoids and Sex hormones	• Mineralocorticoids, e.g., aldosterone secretion targets cells that regulate the sodium and potassium ions in excreted fluids.
	Glucocorticoids	• Glucocorticoids, e.g., cortisol regulates metabolism of fat, protein and carbohydrates.
	Sex hormones	• Sex hormones: androgens, oestrogens and progesterone influence reproductive functioning.
Pancreatic (Islets of Langerhans)	Insulin	• Lowers blood glucose levels by increasing the rate of glucose uptake and utilisation by cells.
	Glucagon	• Raises blood glucose levels by increasing rates of glycogen breakdown and glucose release by the liver.
	Somatostatin	• Inhibits insulin and glucagon release by the pancreas, also suppresses exocrine secretion by the pancreas.
	Pancreatic polypeptides (PP)	• Self-regulates endocrine and exocrine pancreatic activity.
Gonads	Male testes: androgens Female ovaries: oestrogens	• Affects reproductive functioning. • Secondary sexual characteristics.

The **anterior pituitary** is under the control of the hypothalamus, but also acts independently. The hormones most likely to be related to a medical emergency are:

- Adrenocorticotrophic hormone (ACTH).
- Thyroid stimulating hormone (TSH).

The anterior pituitary gland produces adrenocorticotrophic hormone (ACTH) in response to corticotrophin-releasing hormone (CRH) released by the hypothalamus under the neural influence of the sympathetic nervous system. ACTH causes the adrenal cortex to secrete glucocorticoid hormones such as cortisol (hydrocortisone). Glucocorticoid receptors are widely present in most body tissues. The major functions of cortisol are:

- Increased gluconeogenesis.
- Inhibition of glucose utilisation.
- Fatty acid mobilisation and catabolism by muscle cells.
- Modification of the body's response to injury.

These represent a metabolic response to stress and oppose the action of insulin.

The anterior pituitary produces thyroid-stimulating hormone (TSH) in response to thyrotropin-releasing hormone (TRH) from the hypothalamus. TSH targets the thyroid gland, resulting in rising levels of thyroid hormones (T4 thyroxine, T3 triiodothyronine). Thyroid hormones control cell metabolism and growth. The posterior lobe of the pituitary is an extension of the hypothalamus and contains hypothalamic neurones that are specialised to secrete hormones rather than neuro-transmitters. The hormone most likely to be related to a medical emergency is antidiuretic hormone (ADH). Antidiuretic hormone (ADH), also known as vasopressin is sythesised in the hypothalamus, but is actually released from the posterior pituitary. It is released in response to several different stimuli, but most importantly to a change in the solute concentration of the blood or a change in blood pressure. Osmoreceptors are situated in the hypothalamus and respond to the changes in tonicity (effective osmolality) of extracellular fluid. If the tonicity rises, then ADH release is stimulated, and the kidneys will increase reabsorption of water, resulting in concentrated urine. If the extracellular fluid tonicity falls, then ADH release is inhibited, leading to reduced water reabsorption resulting in dilute urine. Osmoreceptors will respond to a change in tonicity of around 2%. Baroreceptors are situated in the right atrium and carotid sinus. They respond to changes in intravascular volume. A reduced

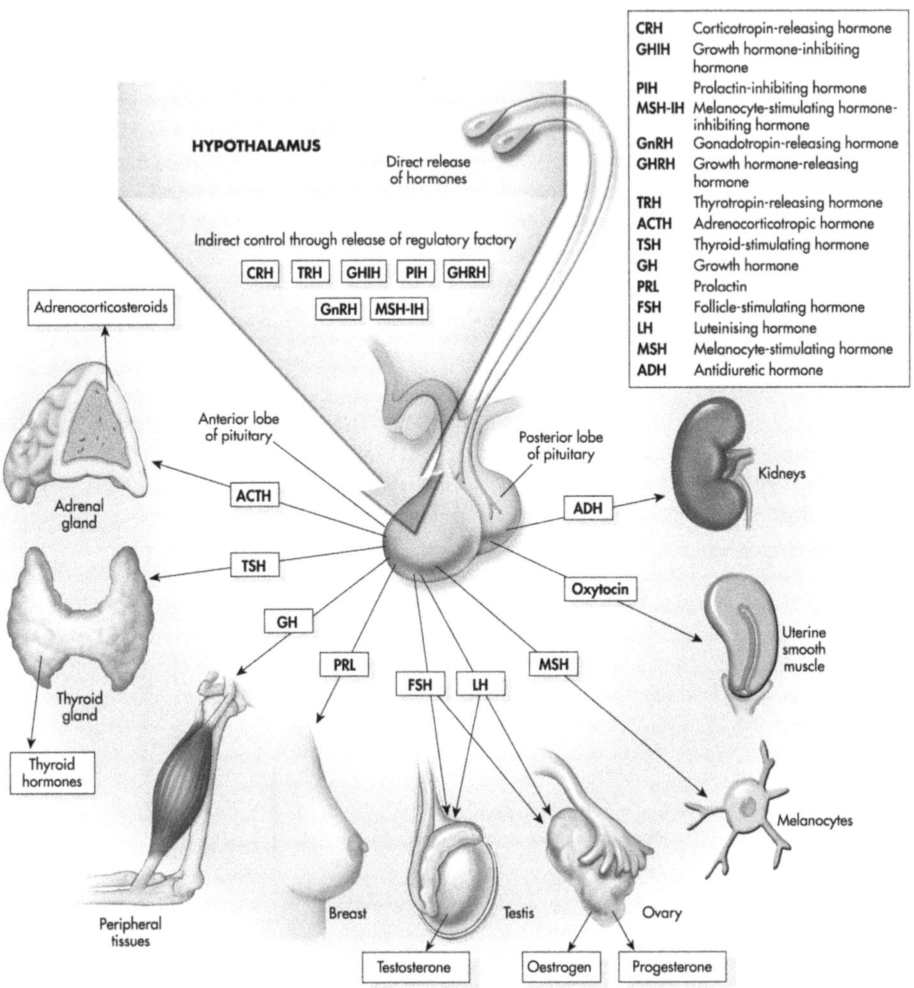

Figure 11.2 The hypothalamus, anterior and posterior pituitary glands, their targets and associated hormones.

circulating volume will result in increased ADH release, and an increased circulating volume will inhibit ADH release. Baroreceptors require a 10% change in circulating volume before they respond. In some circumstances, baroreceptors can override osmoreceptors because the control mechanism will attempt to maintain intravascular volume at the expense of normal extracellular fluid osmolality.

The thyroid gland

The thyroid gland is composed of two lobes joined by an isthmus. It is located in the lower part of the neck anterior to the trachea, inferior to the thyroid cartilage (see Figure 11.3) and has an extensive arterial blood supply. When viewed under the microscope, the thyroid gland is composed of closely packed follicles which comprise epithelial cells enclosing a colloid-filled space. These functional units synthesise, store and secrete thyroid hormones. Thyroid cells form the wall of each follicle, and these cells enlarge as their metabolic activity increases. This accounts for the gland becoming visible (goitre) in certain thyroid disorders. In addition to supporting cells, the thyroid also contains C cells which synthesise calcitonin.

Two pairs of parathyroid glands are embedded in the posterior surface of the thyroid gland (see Figure 11.3). The thyroid makes and stores thyroid hormones (T3 and T4), and it is able to hold up to a 100 days' supply. Iodine is necessary for the production of thyroid hormones. Thyroid hormones affect virtually every organ in the body and increase metabolic rate. The parathyroid glands produce parathyroid hormone (PTH), which regulates serum calcium levels. PTH secretion is stimulated when ionised serum calcium falls. This hormone influences the bones and the kidneys, leading to restoration of normal calcium levels (bone resorption and increased renal tubular calcium reabsorption, respectively).

Effects of thyroxine include:

- Stimulates basal metabolic rate, resulting in increased oxygen consumption and heat production (thermogenesis).
- CNS and cardiovascular sensitivity to catecholamines, e.g., increased heart rate and contractility.

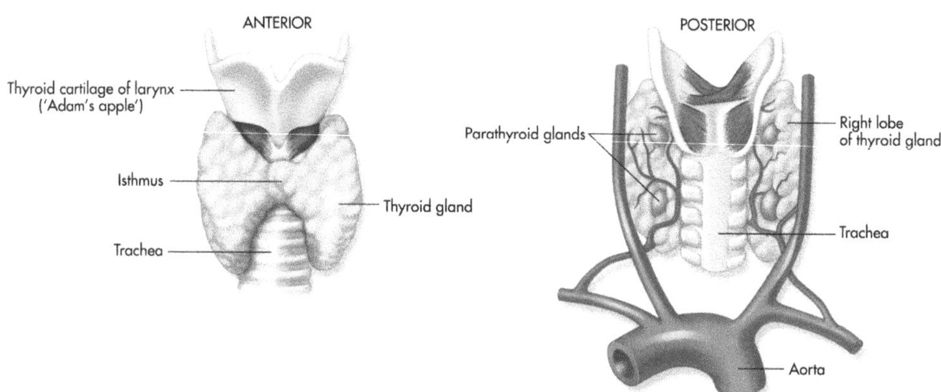

Figure 11.3 The thyroid and parathyroid glands.

- Enzyme synthesis, which promotes protein, fat and carbohydrate metabolism.
- Growth and development, e.g., of the nervous system.

PTH is one of the principal hormones that control mineral metabolism, the others being vitamin D and calcitonin. It is important that a constant ionised calcium concentration is maintained in the extracellular fluid, as key physiological functions, e.g., bone mineralisation, neuromuscular excitability, blood coagulation and cell membrane integrity, are reliant upon this state.

Most hormone production is affected by negative feedback loops, whereby the initial hormone producer reacts to subsequent levels of hormones produced by the target organ. The regulation of the production of thyroid hormone is a good example of a negative feedback loop (see Figure 11.4).

Adrenal glands

The adrenal glands are a pair of small glands situated on top of the kidneys. They are split into two regions:

- Adrenal cortex.
- Adrenal medulla.

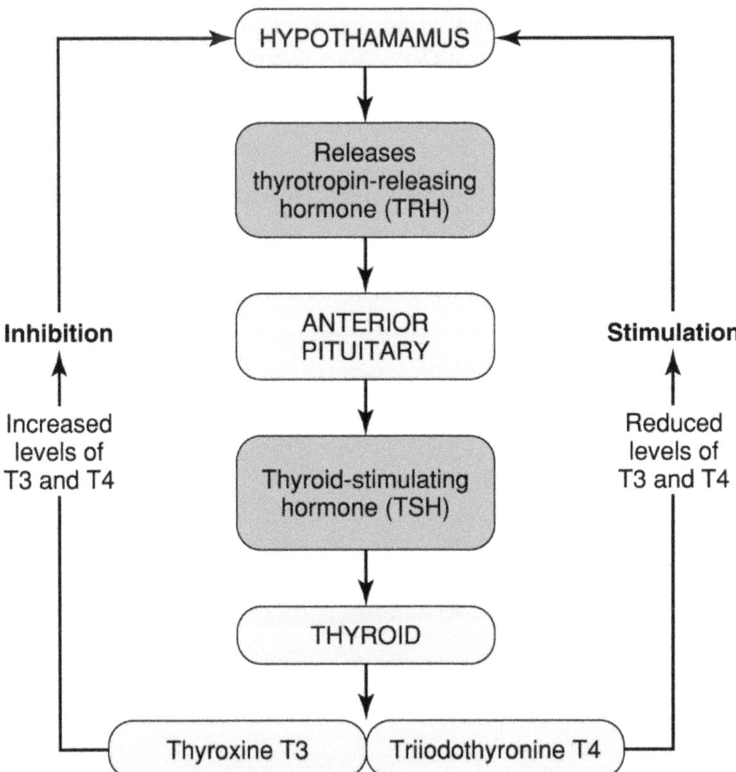

Figure 11.4 Example of a negative feedback loop.

The adrenal cortex secretes many steroid hormones, collectively known as corticosteroids. In addition to the glucocorticoids (e.g., cortisol), the other major groups of adrenocortical hormones include mineralocorticoids (e.g., aldosterone) and androgenic hormones (e.g., dehydroepiandrosterone – DHEA). Production of cortisol and androgen precursors is controlled by ACTH. The androgen precursors are converted in peripheral tissues to oestrogen and testosterone. Aldosterone production is regulated by angiotensin and potassium. This hormone is the principal sodium-retaining steroid hormone and maintains normal fluid balance and circulating volume.

The adrenal medulla is both a part of the autonomic nervous system and endocrine system. On response to sympathetic stimulation, two hormones, adrenaline and noradrenaline, are released. Adrenal medulla cells can be considered as neuronal cells that function as an endocrine gland.

Noradrenaline is both a neurotransmitter of the sympathetic nervous system and a hormone when released from the adrenal medulla. As noradrenaline and adrenaline enter the bloodstream, heart rate, blood pressure and respiratory rate increase, sweat glands become more active, the mouth becomes dry, glycogen breakdown increases, and blood glucose levels increase.

If the adrenal glands are destroyed or removed, appropriate steroid replacement will be required, including glucocorticoids and mineralocorticoids, as these are essential for life. Examples of common steroids that are commonly administered are prednisolone, hydrocortisone and dexamethasone. Steroids are used to treat inflammation, immune system disorders and prevent rejection of transplanted organs, and the side effects are listed in box 1. Steroids must not be withdrawn suddenly, as the adrenal glands need time to increase their own production of corticosteroids. Interestingly, medullary catecholamine replacement is not required, because the sympathetic nervous system can independently produce noradrenaline, which acts on adrenergic receptors, producing the characteristic sympathetic effects.

Side effects of steroids

- Weight gain (truncal obesity).
- Hair growth (hirsutism).
- Delayed wound healing.
- Diabetes.
- Muscle weakness and wasting.
- Bone thinning and osteoporosis.
- Fluid retention (oedema).
- Gastric ulceration.
- Skin thinning, acne and stretch marks.
- Suppression of all inflammatory processes and generalised reactions of inflammation (can mask signs of underlying pathology, e.g., acute abdomen).
- Increased susceptibility to infections.

The pancreas and glucose homeostasis

The pancreas is an elongated, flattened organ situated in the epigastric and left hypochondriac regions of the abdominal cavity. It is both an exocrine and endocrine gland;

the exocrine portion secretes pancreatic juice that aids the digestion of carbohydrates, proteins and fats through a duct (Waugh and Grant 2018). The endocrine component of the pancreas is a ductless gland that consists of the islets of Langerhans, which contain hormone-secreting cells. The islets of Langerhans produce three types of cells, termed alpha, beta and delta cells. The alpha cells secrete glucagon, the beta cells secrete insulin, and the delta cells secrete somatostatin. The plasma glucose level is the most important determinant of the rate of insulin release from the beta cells or glucagon from the alpha cells. High levels of glucose trigger insulin secretion and low plasma glucose leads to glucagon secretion, which in turn promotes glycogenolysis by the liver. Thus, insulin may be considered an anabolic hormone, whereas glucagon is catabolic in nature; insulin will lower blood glucose and glucagon will raise blood glucose. Insulin and glucagon have an inhibitory effect on each other, and both can be inhibited by somatostatin; thus, there is complex interplay between the three hormones. Figure 11.5 gives a summary of the control of blood glucose by pancreatic hormones and the liver. Insulin secretion can also be triggered by an increase in amino acids (e.g., a high protein meal) and ingestion of food as a result of hormones released by the gastrointestinal mucosa. There are, however, many mechanisms in place that operate both to increase and decrease circulating glucose as necessary to maintain homeostasis (Figure 11.5).

The role of the pancreas in glucose homeostasis

The specialised cells in the islet of Langerhans secret hormones which are finely balanced through sympathetic and parasympathetic stimulation to prevent the development of endocrine disorders (Waugh and Grant 2018; VanMeter and Hubert 2014). The opposing actions of glucagon and insulin regulate the blood glucose level, with glucagon raising the blood glucose level while insulin lowers the blood glucose level (Table 11.2). Insulin performs many important functions, including facilitating the transport of glucose into cells and promoting glycogen storage in the liver and muscles by activating enzymes to enable the storage of glucose. The cells preferentially use glucose for energy, facilitated by insulin. The presence of the insulin inhibits fat metabolism while glucose is utilised. In the absence of insulin (either due to low glucose levels or inadequate circulating levels of insulin), fat metabolism is increased, and free fatty acids are released into the circulation. These are used as an alternative energy source, as the cells are unable to take up glucose due to the lack of insulin. It is this mechanism that accounts for the weight loss exhibited by newly diagnosed patients with type 1 diabetes. Insulin also promotes *protein deposition in cells and tissue growth* – a lack of insulin will also lead to protein being used as alternative energy by cells. It is the utilisation by the cells of amino acids (protein) and free fatty acids that results in ketoacidosis.

The role of the liver in glucose homeostasis

The greatest amount of glucose input during the periods between meals and during the overnight fast comes from the contribution of the liver (Figure 11.6). The liver plays such an important role in glucose production, that a total hepatectomy will result in death within 24 hours due to hypoglycaemia. The liver helps to maintain blood glucose homeostasis through two general mechanisms:

- The breakdown of stored glycogen (glycogenolysis).
- The formation of glucose from non-glucose precursors (gluconeogenesis).

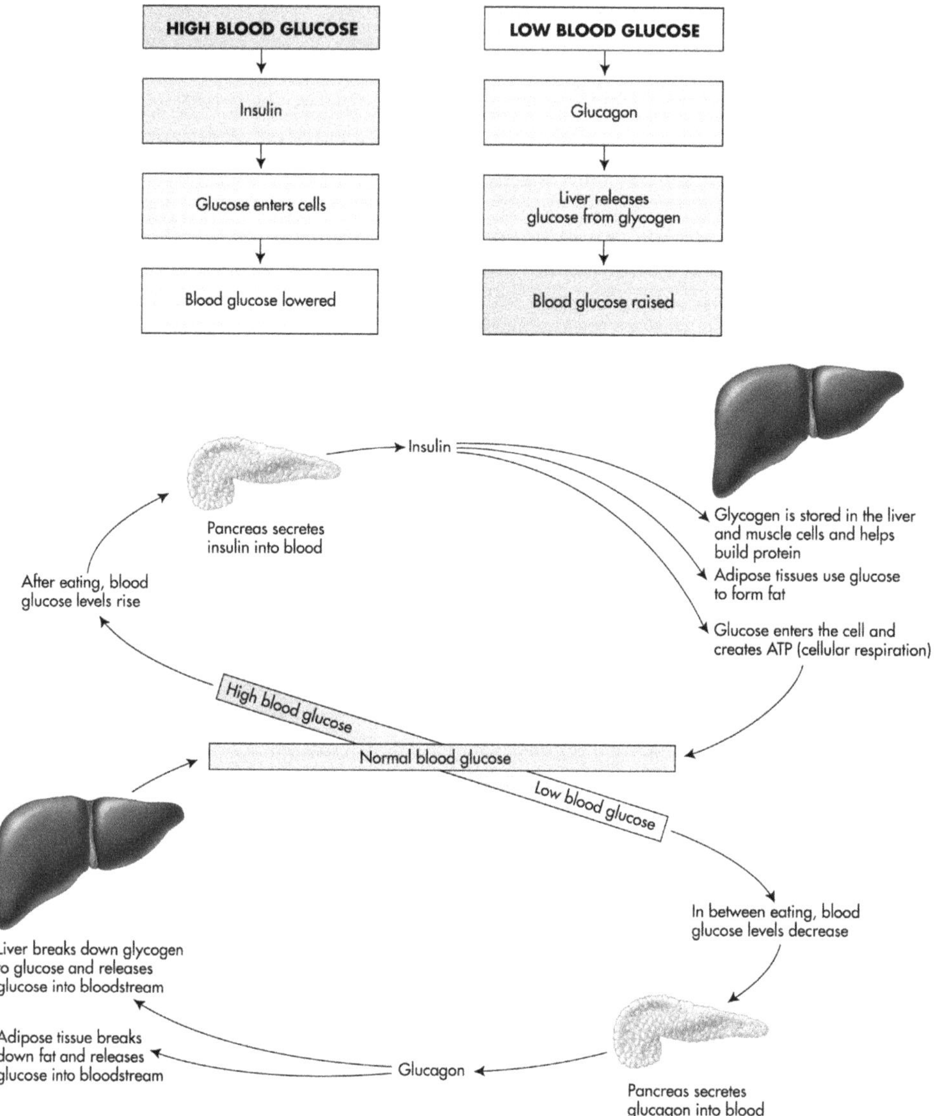

Figure 11.5 Control of blood glucose by pancreatic hormones.

If dietary glucose is available, the liver increases its store of glycogen, but this is limited to 75–100g. The minimum required by the body daily is 125–150g in order to supply the brain, for which glucose is a mandatory requirement. During fasting, the initial source of glucose is from stored glycogen, but as this is restricted, amino acids (released from tissue protein) contribute about 75g of glucose daily via gluconeogenesis. This is mostly muscle protein, but there is a degree of protein breakdown from most organs. Glycerol (released from adipose tissue) can be converted to glucose by the liver, providing a further source of glucose, but can only contribute about 20g. Finally, lactate (produced from muscle) can also be metabolised by the liver for gluconeogenesis and thus provide additional glucose.

Table 11.2 Hormonal secretions of the islets of Langerhans and their roles

Hormones	*Role*
Insulin	Decreases high levels of blood nutrients, especially glucose, but also amino acids and fatty acids, by: • Stimulating the uptake and utilisation of glucose by muscle and connective tissue. • Increasing the rate of conversion of glucose to glycogen (glycogenesis), mostly in the liver and skeletal muscles. • Increasing the uptake of amino acids by cells. • Increasing the synthesis of fatty acids and fat storage in adipose tissue (lipogenesis). • Reducing the breakdown of glycogen into glucose (glycogenolysis). • Preventing the breakdown of protein and fat.
Glucagon	Glucagon increases the blood glucose level by: • Converting glycogen to glucose in the liver and skeletal muscles (glycogenolysis). • Converting non-carbohydrates, such as amino acids, to glucose (gluconeogenesis). Glucagon secretion is stimulated by a low blood glucose level and exercise and decreased by somatostatin and insulin.
Somatostatin	Somatostatin: • Inhibits the secretion of insulin and glucagon from the pancreas and the secretion of growth hormone from the anterior pituitary gland.

Source: Waugh and Grant (2018)

The role of the kidney in glucose homeostasis

No glucose is excreted by the kidney under normal conditions. Glucose is filtered into the glomerular fluid and is reabsorbed, but in hyperglycaemia, some of the glucose will be present in the urine (glycosuria). The presence of glucose in the distal tubules raises the osmotic pressure of the urine and reduces the amount of water reabsorbed by the proximal tubule, thus resulting in an increase in urine output (polyuria) and subsequent hypovolaemia (triggering thirst – polydipsia). This accounts for these symptoms being predominant in the presentation of diabetes mellitus. Sustained hyperglycaemia will result in dehydration, with fluids and electrolytes lost from the body as a result of an osmotic diuresis.

Catecholamines in the acutely ill

Extreme physiological stressors such as infection represent a stimulus for stress response. An increase in adrenaline or noradrenaline levels due to stress of critical illness (sympathetic nervous system stimulation) or via medication infusion to manage hypotension, can result in hyperglycaemia. Catecholamines stimulate glycogen breakdown into glucose by the liver (glycogenolysis) and inhibit insulin secretion by the pancreas. A patient may therefore require an insulin infusion *temporarily* to control the high blood glucose level. The liver is also responsive to plasma glucose levels, with low levels resulting in a release of glucose (by glycogenolysis) and high levels leading to glucose uptake. However, the liver is also very

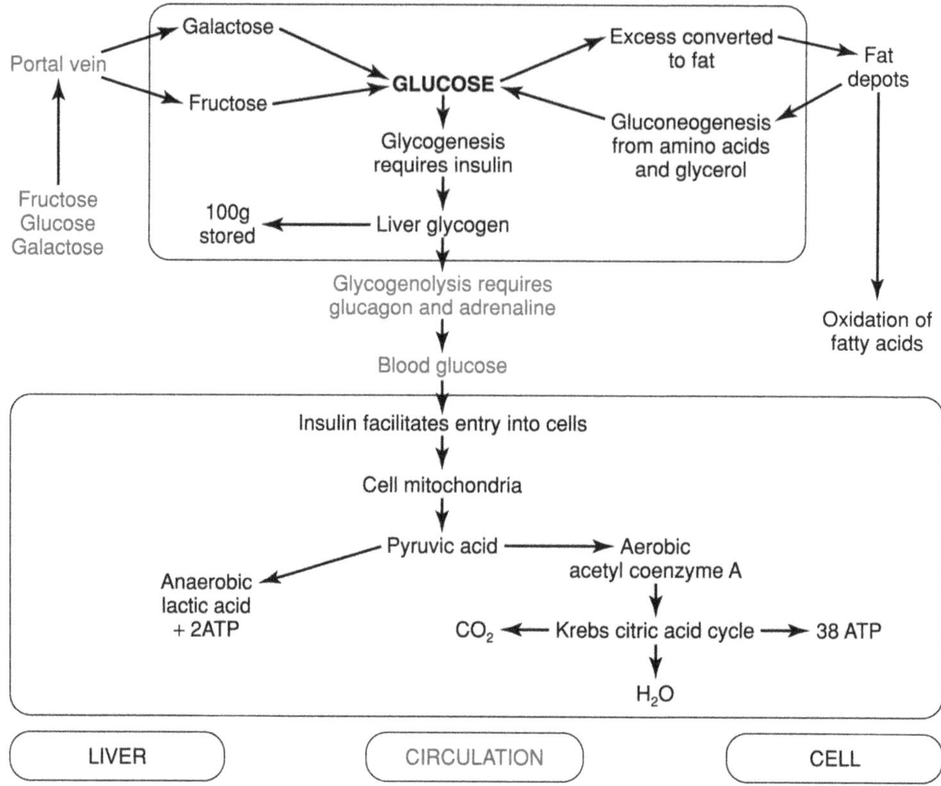

Figure 11.6 The role of the liver in glucose metabolism.

sensitive to levels of insulin (and glucagon), as glycogenolysis will continue to occur even in the face of a high plasma glucose level (as in the diabetic without insulin), identifying the importance of the hormonal influence. In the presence of insulin, however, glycogenolysis is inhibited, whereas glucagon will have the opposite effect. The physiological effects of catecholamines on glucose metabolism is summarised in Table 11.3.

Table 11.3 Physiologic effects of catecholamines

Organ/tissue	*Process or result*
Brain	• Increase glucose metabolism.
Skeletal muscle	• Increase glycogenolysis.
	• Decrease glucose uptake and utilisation (decreases insulin release).
Liver	• Increase glucose production.
	• Increase glycogenolysis.
Adipose tissue	• Increase lipolysis.
	• Decrease glucose uptake.

Source: Clayton, McCance and Takahashi (2017)

Sources of glucose

The two main sources of glucose are:

- Intestinal absorption of dietary glucose and its precursors.
- Release of glucose from the liver.

Plasma glucose levels increase with meals, rising slightly and then returning to basal levels after around two hours; therefore, both of these mechanisms are necessary for normal daily functioning. The most direct pathway for the formation of glucose is as a result of carbohydrate metabolism. As there is very little pure glucose in the diet, this results predominantly from the breakdown of the larger molecules, disaccharides and polysaccharides. The former are hydrolysed (broken down, using water to split the molecule) and absorbed rapidly, causing a prompt increase in plasma glucose concentration.

The rate of rise in blood glucose after the ingestion of foods are ranked in a glycaemic index. Carbohydrate foods that have an immediate effect on blood glucose levels are regarded as high glycaemic index, while those that have a slow effect on the blood glucose level are called low glycaemic index food. Foods containing disaccharides have a high glycaemic index. Polysaccharides enter the bloodstream more slowly, therefore having a low glycaemic index. Foods with a low glycaemic index release their energy slowly and may help those with type 2 diabetes with blood glucose control. However, a low glycaemic index diet is not recommended for children and young people with type 1 diabetes, due to limited evidence to support its effectiveness (National Institute for Health and Care Excellence [NICE] 2015).

Food with a low glycaemic index include:

- Oats.
- Lentils.
- Chickpeas.
- Carrots.
- Chocolate.

Food with a high glycaemic index include:

- Ripe fruit.
- French fries.
- White rice.
- Sugary drinks.

Proteins are metabolised to amino acids, but some are able to donate their carbon atoms for glucose formation. Glucose generation from protein or from any other non-glucose source is called gluconeogenesis. With regard to fat metabolism, triglycerides release glycerol, which can be converted readily to glucose by the liver, but this accounts only for approximately 10% of the carbon atoms available from triglycerides, and thus has only a minor role in gluconeogenesis.

Utilisation of glucose

All tissues utilise plasma glucose, with some being obligatory users that cannot mobilise alternative substances when glucose is unavailable. Nervous tissue is unable to utilise free fatty acids (FFA), which are a major circulating fuel, hence the serious neurological sequelae of hypo-glycaemia. Other tissues that require exclusively glucose include red blood cells, the intestinal mucosa and the renal medulla. When FFA levels are high, and glucose and insulin levels are low, they will switch to use FFA as their primary metabolic fuel.

Neurological consequences of hypoglycaemia:

Irritability, shakiness, confusion.
Abnormal behaviour.
Seizures.
Loss of consciousness.

Alterations in glucose homeostasis

Maintenance of plasma glucose levels within certain limits is of vital importance, because the central nervous system, including the retina, depends upon an uninterrupted supply for normal functioning, the brain being an obligate glucose user (exclusively utilises glucose, as opposed to free fatty acids or amino acids). Insulin facilitates the entry of glucose into cells; therefore, any variation of blood glucose from the normal range (both excess and deficit) that is caused by a deficiency of insulin leads to a type of diabetes, depending on the aetiology of the condition:

- Type 1.
- Type 2.
- Gestational.
- Impaired glucose tolerance and impaired fasting glycaemia.

Type 1 diabetes – insulin-dependents diabetes mellitus (IDDM) – is the result of a primary defect in the ability of the pancreatic islet tissue to respond to glucose with a release of insulin.

Type 2 diabetes, which was previously referred to as non-insulin-dependent diabetes mellitus (NIDDM), manifests as a relative insensitivity of the tissues to plasma insulin. Gestational diabetes is a pregnancy-induced diabetes, while impaired glucose tolerance and impaired fasting glycaemia is referred to as a pre-diabetes state, characterised by an elevated body glucose level, but not one high enough to prompt a diagnosis of diabetes. A summary of the characteristics of diabetes based on WHO (World Health Organisation) (2018) classification is shown in Table 11.4.

Table 11.4 Summary of diabetes

Insulin-dependent diabetes mellitus (IDDM)	*Non-insulin-dependent diabetes mellitus (NIDDM)*
Type 1 diabetes	Type 2 diabetes
• This is less common (10% of diabetics).	• This is becoming increasingly common (90% of diabetics).
• There is a sudden onset that can at any age, but mostly affecting young persons. At diagnosis the person is underweight or normal weight.	• There is a gradual onset, predominantly in adults. The person is usually overweight at diagnosis.
• Characterised by an insulin resistance (the cause of which is unknown) this may be combined with a relative reduction in insulin production.	• Characterised by a lack of insulin produced by the beta cells in the islets of Langerhans in the pancreas. This is thought to be immune-induced in the majority of cases.
• Managed by diet and oral hypoglycaemic medications.	• Managed by the administration of insulin administration.
Gestational diabetes	
This type of diabetes occurs during pregnancy (2–5% of pregnancies) and most closely resembles type 2 diabetes. This type of diabetes will often self-correct after delivery, however, affected mothers have a tendency to develop type 2 diabetes later on in life.	

IMPAIRED GLUCOSE TOLERANCE AND IMPAIRED FASTING GLYCAEMIA

Impaired glucose tolerance (IGT) and impaired fasting glycaemia (IFG) are intermediate conditions, and people with IGT or IFG are at high risk of progressing to type 2 diabetes, although this is not inevitable.

Acute endocrine problems and emergencies

Thyrotoxicosis, thyroid storm/crisis

Hyperthyroidism results from an excess of thyroid hormones (T3 and T4), with an exaggerated form being a thyroid crisis. A thyroid crisis (or storm) can be triggered by infection, surgery, trauma or any other acute episode (e.g., myocardial infarction, stroke and eclampsia), but fortunately, is very rare. An over-secretion of thyroid hormones will lead to a hypermetabolic state, resulting in hyperpyrexia, tachycardia, hypertension, agitation and tremors. The management is aimed essentially at reducing the effects of these hormones until the patient is stable. Drug therapy will include the use of:

- Beta-blockers such as metoprolol, to reduce sympathetic activity.
- Sedatives, such as chlorpromazine or haloperidol.
- Corticosteroids such as hydrocortisone, to inhibit the conversion of T3 to T4.
- Carbimazole, a specific anti-thyroid drug, inhibits enzymes that play a role in T3 and T4 production.
- Iodine is a specific antithyroid therapy used to inhibit thyroxine release and treat some forms of hyperthyroidism.

Hyperthyroidism symptoms:

- Tachycardia and tachyarrhythmia.
- BP ↑.
- Nausea.
- Hyperactivity.
- Diarrhoea.
- Agitation.
- Heat intolerance.
- Goitre.
- Exophthalmos (prominent bulging eyes).

Myxoedema and myxoedema coma

Myxoedema results from decreased thyroid hormone secretion (hypothyroidism), with signs such as bradycardia and slow mental functioning being representative of the hypometabolic state. The management strategies are focused on restoring thyroid levels, such as levothyroxine, which can take some time to stabilise and will usually be taken for life, as this is a long-term condition.

A myxoedema coma (rare, but with a high mortality) can occur in a patient with a chronic condition who is challenged by additional stress such as trauma. They may have had previous thyroid surgery or inappropriate doses of anti-thyroid medication such as carbimazole. The extreme hypometabolic condition will result in bradycardia, leading to hypotension and poor tissue perfusion, which, in turn, can result in a metabolic acidosis. Hypoventilation may result from the decreased conscious level, leading to hypercarbia and hypoxia and risking airway integrity. Other manifestations that may occur include fatigue, reduced cardiac output, an increased sensitivity to drugs, e.g., opiates, and paralytic ileus. The coma itself is likely to have been caused by multiple contributory factors, including the primary hypometabolism and secondary hypothermia, hypoxia, hypercarbia and hypoglycaemia. Management strategies are focused upon IV thyroxine replacement, support of airway, breathing and circulation requiring invasive monitoring and intensive care support.

Hypothyroidism symptoms:

- Hypothermia.
- Slow movements and thoughts.
- Fatigue.
- Excessive sleep.
- Constipation.
- Weight increase.
- Dry skin.
- Coarse hair, brittle nails.
- Goitre.
- Hoarse voice.
- Bradycardia.
- Puffy face.

Adrenal insufficiency

Addison's disease is a chronic deficiency of cortical hormones, with symptoms reflecting the lack of cortisol (muscle weakness, fatigue, hypoglycaemia, ileus, reduced immunity to infection, low cardiac output), aldosterone (polyuria, dehydration, thirst, hypovolaemia, hyponatraemia, hyperkalaemia, postural hypotension, arrhythmias) and androgens (loss of libido and body hair). The condition is controlled by lifelong hormone replacement therapy. In times of stress (e.g., surgery, trauma, infection) where the increased demand for cortisol cannot be met, a patient may develop an Addisonian crisis or acute adrenal insufficiency. The immediate management of this life-threatening emergency will include urgent rehydration and correction of the hypoglycaemia. Cortisol will need to be administered, e.g., in the form of intravenous hydro-cortisone, and the trigger for the crisis (e.g., infection) addressed.

Causes of acute adrenal insufficiency:

- Abrupt withdrawal of steroid therapy.
- Stress, trauma, infection, surgery.
- Addison's disease.
- Pituitary or hypothalamic damage.

Pheochromocytoma or catecholamine crisis

A pheochromocytoma is a (very rare) tumour of the adrenal medulla, whereby abnormally high levels of adrenaline and noradrenaline are secreted into the systemic circulation. The release of these catecholamines is intermittent, but results in headaches, tachycardia, hyperglycaemia, blurred vision, bowel disturbances and very severe hypertension. Following blood pressure stabilisation (usually with alpha- and beta-blockers), a pheochromocytoma will require surgical removal.

Diabetes insipidus (DI)

This is due to an insufficiency of ADH (antidiuretic hormone) being produced by the posterior pituitary. This can be precipitated by neuropathology affecting the hypothalamus or pituitary, or, rarely, by an insensitivity of the kidney to ADH (nephrogenic diabetes insipidus). It results in excessive water loss (polyuria), and if untreated, the patient will become profoundly hypovolaemic and hypernatraemic (as water is lost in excess of sodium). This situation is managed by the administration of desmopressin (DDAVP).

Syndrome of inappropriate antidiuretic hormone hypersecretion (SIADH)

This is characterised by excessive antidiuretic hormone (ADH) being secreted by the posterior pituitary gland. Its aetiology includes neuropathology (e.g., head injury, subarachnoid haemorrhage) or some carcinomas or infections. SIADH causes water retention (potential fluid overload) and haemodilution of solutes resulting in hyponatraemia. Initial management necessitates fluid restriction, with some situations including the administration of normal saline, but extreme care must be taken not to increase the plasma sodium by more than 12mmol/L per 24 hours (i.e., 0.5mmol per hour). It is important that SIADH is differentiated from other conditions causing hyponatraemia (e.g., cerebral salt-wasting syndrome) in which there is an accompanying hypovolaemia, as opposed to hypervolaemia, with its corresponding implications for fluid management strategies. Electrolyte imbalance is discussed in more detail in Chapter 4.

Diabetic emergencies

Endocrine emergencies account for about 1.3% of medical emergency admissions to critical care (Kerr, Wen ham and Newell-Price 2017), and the majority are related to diabetes. Early recognition and treatment of possible problems, with an understanding of glucose management, is essential for the nurse caring for patients with diabetes. However, a small-scale study by Lange and Pearce (2017) that evaluates diabetes knowledge of registered nurses found a significant gap in diabetes knowledge among some staff in the hospital trust. Similarly, National Diabetes Inpatient Audit (2018) found that 20% of hospitals in England and Wales have no specialist inpatient diabetes nurses (DISNs).

Diabetes emergencies are either due to hypoglycaemic or hyperglycaemic episodes, and the most common problems are:

- Hypoglycaemia.
- Hyperglycaemia:
  - Diabetic ketoacidosis (DKA).
  - Hyperglycaemic hyperosmolar syndrome (HHS).
  - Euglycemic diabetic ketoacidosis.

Diabetic emergencies: hypoglycaemia

Hypoglycaemia is a biochemical diagnosis based on a blood glucose of less than 4mmol/L (JBDS 2018). It may be caused by insulin overdosage, a delayed meal following administration of insulin or increased metabolic rate due to exercise or acute febrile illness. The patient who is hypo-glycaemic will exhibit autonomic symptoms such as sweating, warmth sensation, anxiety, nausea and palpitations as a result of sympathetic nervous system stimulation. Other symptoms (e.g., tiredness, poor coordination, visual disturbances, drowsiness, confusion, seizures) are due to the effects of low glucose levels upon the nervous system (neuroglycopenia). Prolonged low blood glucose levels may starve the brain of glucose, resulting in coma and possibly death. The autonomic symptoms usually occur first, with neuroglycopenia more evident with a blood glucose of less than 2.5mmol/L.

Hypoglycaemia is a serious medical condition which can either be mild (self-treated), or severe hypoglycaemia, if assistance with care is required from another person (JBDS 2018). Once a patient has had a severe episode of hypoglycaemia, they may have impaired recognition of hypoglycaemia symptoms over the subsequent 24 hours. Other factors that can contribute to hypo unawareness include having type 1 diabetes for a number of years, use of certain drugs such as beta blockers, stress, depression and alcohol consumption (Diabetes UK 2018). The risk factors for hypoglycaemia include patients on insulin or sulfonylurea treatment, strict glycaemic control, impaired awareness of hypoglycaemia, severe hepatic and renal dysfunction, sepsis, increasing age and cognitive dysfunction (JBDS 2018). It is a requirement for a patient who is unable to notice hypoglycaemia to inform DVLA if they are driving. Some studies have indicated that the annual prevalence of hypoglycaemia is between 30–40% of people with diabetes (Strachan 2014). Zaccardi et al. (2016) found an increase of 39% in hospital admissions for hypoglycaemia over a 10-year period in England.

The potential causes of inpatient hypoglycaemia include medical issues such as inappropriate administration of insulin, mobilisation after illness, major amputation of limb and nutritional issues such as missed or delayed meal, vomiting or prolonged starvation due to being nil by mouth (JBDS 2018). However, there are also occasional healthcare professional-associated hypoglycaemic induced by error.

Iatrogenic hypoglycaemia

Iatrogenic hypoglycaemia (i.e. caused by health care professionals) is preventable. Examples of iatrogenic hypoglycaemia include stopping artificial feeding (enteral or total parenteral nutrition) for procedures such as CT scan, but leaving an insulin infusion running, or giving an incorrect higher dose of insulin.

Management of hypoglycaemia

Mild episodes can be treated by consuming refined carbohydrates, such as dextrose tablets, followed by long-acting carbohydrates, e.g., biscuits. Otherwise, patients may be treated with 'GlucoGel' (30% glucose) which is a gel that is applied to the buccal mucosa. *It is contra-indicated to give anything by mouth to an unconscious patient.* In the unconscious patients, 1mg of glucagon can be given intramuscularly (IM) or intravenously (IV). Hospitalised patients may be treated with 250mL of 10% dextrose (IV) administered over a few minutes, followed by a continuous infusion depending upon local hospital guidelines. If no IV access is available, glucagon may be given intramuscularly. The administration of high concentrations of dextrose intravenously carries the risk of thrombophlebitis, therefore cannula insertion sites should be monitored closely. Whilst it is important to consult local guidance, JBDS (2018) have summarised the management of hypoglycaemia in different categories of patients, as seen below:

MANAGEMENT FOR CONSCIOUS ORIENTATED, CONSCIOUS BUT CONFUSED, UNABLE TO COOPERATE BUT ABLE TO SWALLOW:

1. Give 15–20g quick acting carbohydrate such as:
   - 5–7 dextrosol tablets. Or
   - 150–200mL pure fruit juice e.g., orange. Or
   - 3–4 teaspoons of sugar in water.
2. Repeat capillary BG 10–15 minutes. If <4mmol/L, then repeat (up to 3 times in total, if required).
3. If remains <4mmol/L after 30–45 minutes or 3 cycles, then contact medical staff and consider glucagon IM or IV, 150–200mL of 10% glucose over 15 minutes.
4. Once >4mmol/L and the person has recovered, consider long-acting carbohydrates, e.g., 2 biscuits, slice of toast or 200–300mL of milk.
5. Treat hypoglycaemia, but do not omit insulin injection if due – however, regimen may need to be reviewed.
6. Ensure appropriate documentation, continue regular BG monitoring for 24–48 hours, consider cause of hypoglycaemia, provide hypoglycaemia education or refer to Diabetes team.

MANAGEMENT OF UNCONSCIOUS AND/OR HAVING SEIZURES AND/OR VERY AGGRESSIVE:

1. Check ABCDE assessment, institute appropriate interventions and request immediate medical help.

2. If on insulin infusion, stop immediately.
3. Consider one of the following 3 appropriate options:
   a) If there is IV access, give 75–100 mL 20% glucose over 15 minutes, check BG after 10 minutes and if less than 4.0 mmol/L, repeat or give 150–200 mL of 10% glucose IV over 15 minutes, use an infusion pump if available and check BG after 10 minutes, if less than 4.0mmol/L, repeat
   b) In case of no intravenous access, give glucagon, 1mg intramuscularly, but this may take up to 15 minutes to take effect.
4. Once >4mmol/L and the person has recovered, consider long-acting carbohydrate, such as 2 biscuits, a slice of toast or 200–300mL of milk (not soya).
5. Treat hypoglycaemia, but do not omit insulin injection if due – however, regimen may need to be reviewed.
6. Consider possible cause of hypoglycaemia, document in notes and continue BG monitoring or refer to Diabetes team.

MANAGEMENT OF ADULTS WHO ARE NIL BY MOUTH:

1. For patients on a variable rate intravenous insulin infusion, adjust according to the prescribed regimen and seek medical attention. Most variable rate insulin infusions should re-commence once blood glucose level is over 4mmol/L, though adjustment of the rate may be indicated.
2. Consider one of the following options
   a) 75–100mL 20% glucose over 15 minutes, check BG after 10 minutes, and if less than 4mmol/L, give 150–200mL of 10% glucose over 15 minutes and repeat BG after 10 minutes until the patient is reviewed by the clinical nurse specialist or doctor.
   b) Hypoglycaemia may persist for up to 24–36 hours after the last dose, if the hypoglycaemia was due to long-acting insulin treatment or sulfonylurea, especially if there is a renal impairment.
3. Once >4mmol/L and the patient has recovered, consider intravenous infusion of 10% glucose at a rate of 100mL/hour.
4. Ensure appropriate documentation, continue regular BG monitoring for 24–48 hours, provide hypoglycaemia education or refer to diabetes team.

Diabetic emergencies: hyperglycaemia

Hyperglycaemia: diabetic ketoacidosis (DKA)

Diabetes ketoacidosis is a life-threatening complication of diabetes and accounts for a significant amount of all diabetes emergency-related hospital admissions. Most cases of DKA occur in patients with type 1 diabetes, but occasionally occur in type 2 diabetes. It is due to an increased demand for insulin, inadequate adjustment of insulin injection to meet the required needs of the body, severe physical or psychological stress or physical trauma without compensatory insulin and increased resistance to insulin due to various factors such as pregnancy or infection (Brashers, Jones and Huether 2017). The resultant lack of adequate insulin required to drag glucose into the cells leads to the body burning fatty acids to provide energy and thereby producing ketone bodies.

DKA is a triad of hyperglycaemia, hyperketonaemia and metabolic acidosis, thus, the diagnostic criteria are:

- Ketonaemia ≥3 mmol/L or significant ketonuria.
- Blood glucose >11 mmol/L or known diabetes mellitus.
- Bicarbonate (HCO_3) <15 mmol/L **and/or** venous pH <7.3.

In addition to elevated blood glucose, acidosis, ketonaemia and ketonuria, the signs and symptoms of DKA include vomiting, dehydration, abdominal discomfort, unusual smell on the breath, tachycardia, alteration in potassium level, confusion and coma. Both DKA and HHS (Hyperglycaemic hyperosmolar syndrome) are triggered commonly by infection, but may be secondary to trauma, myocardial infarction and non-compliance with diabetes management. These emergencies may occur also in previously undiagnosed diabetics, thus being a first presentation of diabetes mellitus. Other precipitating factors include inappropriate insulin dosage or omission, acute illness, hyperthyroidism, alcohol abuse, other co-morbidities such as pancreatitis and drugs such as corticosteroids.

Management of DKA

For management of a deteriorating patient with DKA, use the ABCDE assessment approach and respond appropriately. Early recognition is essential to promote positive patient outcome. The management of DKA in adults include rehydration, insulin therapy and potassium replacement if needed, because insulin is a potent stimulus for potassium cellular uptake (Joint British Diabetes Societies Inpatient Care Group 2013). Therefore, fluid status, blood glucose, blood ketones and vital signs need to be closely monitored.

FLUID ADMINISTRATION (MOST IMPORTANT INITIAL THERAPY)

Assess fluid status, establish intravenous access, send blood for Urea and Electrolyte, bicarbonate, plasma glucose, blood culture and venous PH. Administer 0.9% sodium, 1 litre with no potassium over 1 hour, repeat over 2 hours and check potassium level, give another 1 litre over the next 2 hours and re-check potassium level and continue close monitoring of blood glucose level and cardiovascular status. Dextrose 10% is commenced to run at 125mL/hour when capillary blood glucose is less than 14mmol/L (NICE 2015).

INSULIN THERAPY

The aim of insulin therapy is to suppress ketogenesis, reduce blood glucose level and correct electrolyte imbalance. Commence a fixed rate intravenous insulin infusion (FRII) based on 0.1 units/kg body weight and monitor blood ketones and capillary blood glucose level to determine whether adjustment is required. Avoid hypoglycaemia, and introduce dextrose regimen if blood glucose <14mmol (JBDS 2018).

POTASSIUM REPLACEMENT

Potassium is an essential mineral which helps with fluid balance regulation and electrical impulse transmission. The normal potassium level is 3.5–5mEq/L, and hypokalaemia is a life-threatening condition, but is not common in DKA. 40mmol of potassium is added per litre of normal saline if the value is between 3.5–5.5mmol/L, and a medical review is required if below 3.5mmol/L.

RESOLUTION OF DKA

Resolution of DKA is achieved when there is a rapid improvement marked with pH >7.3, bicarbonate >15mmol/L and blood ketone level <0.6mmol/L.

Hyperglycaemic hyperosmolar syndrome (HHS)

HHS is also referred to as hyperosmolar hyperglycaemic nonketotic syndrome (HHNS), and it is a rare metabolic emergency requiring prompt management. Although it can affect both patients with type 1 and type 2 diabetes, it is common among people with type 2 diabetes. Like DKA, the precipitating factors include illness or infection. Other contributory factors are undiagnosed diabetes, poorly controlled type 2 diabetes, drugs such as long-term diuretics, beta-blockers (block the release of insulin) and corticosteroids. In HHS, there is some endogenous insulin secretion that is enough to extinguish excessive lipolysis and ketogenesis, but insufficient to facilitate adequate glucose utilization. It is characterised by:

- Hypovolaemia.
- Marked hyperglycaemia (>30mmol/L) without significant hyperketonaemia (<3.0mmol/L) or acidosis (pH >7.3, bicarbonate >15 mmol/L); and
- Osmolality >320mOsmol/Kg.

The signs and symptoms include marked dehydration, elevated blood glucose level, dry mouth, skin and mucous membranes, polydipsia, polyuria and impaired consciousness levels. The goals of management are to treat the underlying cause, replace fluid and electrolyte losses and normalise the osmolality and blood glucose level. Similar to DKA, intravenous fluid management and potassium replacement are commenced, but insulin therapy is only initiated if there is a significant ketonaemia >1mmol/L or ketonuria +++ Some of the similarities and differences between DKA and HHS are presented in Table 11.5.

Euglycemic diabetic ketoacidosis (EDKA)

This is a serious medical condition characterised by increased blood ketone, metabolic acidosis, but with blood glucose level less than 11.1mmol (200mg/dL). EDKA can present a diagnostic challenge because of normoglycaemia (blood glucose level is within the normal range). The causes include infection, decrease calorie intake/fasting, pancreatitis, prolonged vomiting, diarrhoea and patient on insulin pump (Rawla et al. 2017). It is important to monitor metabolic profile, check blood glucose level, arterial blood gas, ketone level, anion gap, bicarbonate and pH value. The management is to correct dehydration with intravenous normal saline of 4–5 litres and insulin drip with dextrose containing solution to correct anion gap and bicarbonate level.

Table 11.5 Comparisons and contrasts between DKA and HHS

	Diabetic ketoacidosis (DKA)	*Hyperglycaemic hyperosmolar syndrome (HHS)*
Definitions (American Diabetic Association)	• Blood glucose >13.8mmol/L. • PH <7.30. • Bicarbonate <18mmol/L. • Anion gap >10. • Ketonaemia.	• Blood glucose >33.3mmol/L. • Ph <7.30. • Bicarbonate >15mmol/L. • Serum osmolality >320osmol/kg.
Demographics	• Most commonly younger, slimmer patients with type 1 diabetes. • Mortality less than 5% – most common cause of death in young people with diabetes.	• More commonly older, obese patients with type 2 diabetes. • Mortality 15%.
Presentation	• Rapid onset (<24 hours). • Vomiting, polyuria, polydipsia, weight loss plus abdominal pain.	• Insidious onset (several days–weeks). • Vomiting, polyuria, polydipsia, weight loss.
Physical signs	• As per hypovolaemia: tachycardia, hypotension, low CVP. • Confusion is rare.	• As per hypovolaemia: tachycardia, hypotension, low CVP. • Confusion more common.
Biochemistry	• Blood glucose rarely greater than 40mmol/L. • Ketones in urine.	• Blood glucose often greater than 50mmol/L. • No ketones in the urine.

DKA and HHS are caused by an absolute or relative deficiency of effective circulating insulin with associated increased levels of glucagon, catecholamines, cortisol and growth hormone. These result in increased glycogenolysis by the liver, generating hyperglycaemia. In DKA, the deficiency of insulin and increased counter-regulatory hormones lead to increased lipolysis and production of ketone bodies, with a resulting metabolic acidosis. The disturbed acid-base balance due to the metabolic acidosis is due to the dissociation of the H^+ ion from the ketone body acetoacetic acid. Patients with HSS do not develop ketoacidosis, but the mechanism for this is unclear.

Ketoacidosis

A metabolic condition associated with an accumulation of ketone bodies. Ketones (acetoacetic acid and beta hydroxybutyrate) result from the breakdown of free fatty acids and deamination of amino acids. Ketones can be smelt on the breath (like fruit or nail polish remover) due to acetone (from acetoacetic acid).

Differential diagnosis:

- *Diabetic ketoacidosis*: known history of diabetes.
- *Alcoholic ketoacidosis*: usually known history of alcohol abuse (no hyperglycaemia).

Starvation: ketosis (rather than ketoacidosis) (no hyperglycaemia).

Both DKA and HHS present with vomiting and a history of polyuria, polydipsia and weight loss. Patients with DKA can additionally have abdominal pain, although the underlying pathophysiology for this is unclear. Confusion is more common in HHS and believed to be related to the increase in serum osmolality rather than the hyperglycaemia. Physical signs include those associated with hypovolaemia (see patient assessment) resulting from the polyuria. This has been estimated to reach 5–8 litres in DKA and 8–10 litres in HHS (Kearney and Dang 2007). The excessive urine output leads to depletion in sodium, potassium, magnesium and phosphates. The main aims for treating both DKA and HHS are to correct dehydration, decrease the blood glucose level, correct electrolyte abnormalities and treat any precipitating causes, such as infection. Some patients with DKA or HHS will require initial management in the intensive care unit.

Hypovolaemia and urine output

Although patients with DKA or HHS will develop hypovolaemia (as a result of polyuria) they will still be passing urine. This is in contrast to patients who are hypovolaemic from other (non-diabetic) causes (e.g., haemorrhage) who will be oliguric or even anuric.

Assessment and physical examination

A systematic ABCDE approach to patient assessment is essential in order to identify problems and initiate appropriate and timely interventions (Resuscitation Council 2015). Patients with DKA may have airway problems due to deteriorating levels of consciousness. Respiratory assessment may reveal signs of hypoxaemia and respiratory distress if a chest infection is the cause of the disruption in glucose homeostasis. Tachypnoea, with deep sighing respirations, can occur as a result of respiratory compensation for the metabolic acidosis arising from their ketoacidosis. Those with DKA or HHS may be cardiovascularly unstable as a result of hyperglycaemia, because their urine output may be inappropriately high (due to excreting excess glucose accompanied by water), resulting in severe hypovolaemia and dehydration with associated tachycardia, hypotension and hypothermia. The hypoglycaemic patient is often clammy or sweaty, whereas the patient with hyperglycaemia typically appears warm and dry, hence touching the patient may be informative. Disability assessment (including blood glucose measurement) will reveal hypo- or hyperglycaemia and may demonstrate altered neurological function (confusion, weakness and reduced level of consciousness) caused by altered glucose levels. Abnormal observations should always be reported immediately, particularly adverse changes in neurological status. Finally, measurement of the blood glucose, biochemistry and electrolytes will assist in identifying the underlying cause of the endocrine dysfunction (Resuscitation Council 2015). Table 11.6 gives an account of assessment findings of people with abnormal blood glucose levels.

Table 11.6 Summary of examination and assessment

	Variable	*Hypoglycaemia*	*DKA*	*HHS*
A/B	• Airway patency. • Respiratory rate pattern. • O_2 saturations.	• Most commonly: normal respiratory rate and pattern.	• Tachypnoea. • **Kussmaul breathing** (rapid, deep laboured) due to respiratory compensation for a metabolic acidosis.	• Most commonly: normal respiratory rate and pattern.
C	• BP. • Pulse. • Capillary refill time (CRT). • Skin. • CVP. • Temperature. • Urine output.	• Sweating. • Palpitations due to sympathetic nervous system (SNS) stimulation.	• Tachycardia, hypotension, low CVP due to hypovolaemia. • Increased CRT. • Dysrhythmias due to electrolyte imbalance. • Often hypothermic. • Urine output may be inappropriately high due to hyperglycaemia.	• Tachycardia, hypotension, low CVP due to hypovolaemia. • Increased CRT. • Dysrhythmias due to electrolyte imbalance. • Often hypothermic. • Urine output may be inappropriately high due to hyperglycaemia.
D	• GCS pain assessment.	• Anxiety (due to SNS stimulation). • Tiredness, poor coordination, visual disturbances, drowsiness, confusion, coma, seizures are due to the effects of low glucose levels upon the nervous system (neuroglycopenia). • Reduced level of consciousness due to neuroglycopenia. • Low GCS.	• Confusion, lethargy, reduced level of consciousness.	• Confusion (thought to be due to increased serum osmolality).

(*Continued*)

Table 11.6 Continued

	Variable	*Hypoglycaemia*	*DKA*	*HHS*
E1	• Blood results.	• Blood glucose <3mmol/L.	• Blood glucose >13.8mmol/L. • PH <7.30 • Bicarbonate <18mmol/L. • Anion gap >10. • Ketonaemia. • Hyponatraemia. • Hypo/hyperkalaemia. • Hypomagnesaemia. • Hypo- or hypophosphatemia.	• Blood glucose >33.3mmol/L. • Ph <7.30. • Bicarbonate >15mmol/L. • Serum osmolality >320osmols/kg. • Small amount (or no) ketones. • Hyponatraemia. • Hypo/hyperkalaemia. • Hypomagnesaemia. • Hypo- or hypophosphatemia.
E2	Other.	• Nausea (due to SNS stimulation).	• Nausea, vomiting. • Abdominal pain. • Acetone smell on breath due to ketones.	

CASE STUDY 11.1 MR SHAH: PART 1

Initial assessment

Mr Shah, a 65-year-old man was brought to the Emergency department this morning with a worsening abdominal pain. He has a past medical history of type I diabetes (aged 15), which is normally well-controlled. Mr Shah is on steroid, glargine insulin 20 units daily (long-acting insulin) and Humalog (fast-acting insulin) 4–6 units three times daily. He was a lorry driver before retiring. He has been feeling very tired, lethargic and complaining of abdominal upset and loss of appetite. He recently had a flu-like illness and had been making a good recovery, but now he feels worse. He had been reducing his insulin, as he was not eating properly, and monitoring his blood glucose accordingly. The previous evening he had felt hot and unwell; early in the morning, the abdominal pain started, and by 10:00 he then came to the emergency department. He last assessed his blood glucose at midnight, and as it was raised at 13.2mmol/L (normal range normal range 4–10mmol/L). He did not want to administer his insulin as he had not eaten supper. He weighs 80Kg.

Assessment at 10:30

Airway: on assessment, you note his airway is patent, with no stridor or gurgling sound. He is able to speak, though he feels unwell. Therefore, there is no immediate airway risk, so the assessment is continued.

Breathing: his lips and oral mucosa appear dry, as he is mouth breathing, but show no evidence of central cyanosis. He is able to speak in full sentences. His breathing pattern appears a little laboured. His respiratory rate is 18/minute, with oxygen saturations of 95% and deep, equal, bilateral chest movements. He is using his accessory muscles to breath. On lung auscultation, no adventitious breath sounds are heard. His SpO_2 is within the target saturation of 94–98% set by medical staff, recommended by the British Thoracic Society guidance. There is no need to institute oxygen administration, though it is prescribed, if required. You notice a strange smell on his breath and, in light of his past medical history, are concerned this might be a sign of raised ketones.

Breathing NEWS (0 + 1 + 0) = 1

Circulation: on admission to the emergency department, his skin feels warm and dry. His capillary refill time is 2 seconds. His BP is 99/74mmHg, with a heart rate of 105, and his pulse feels regular. He reports passing urine frequently overnight and is happy to use the bottle so an accurate assessment of fluid balance can be maintained using a fluid balance chart. He feels thirsty and is drinking freely, but he also feels nauseated. You explain that you would like a sample of urine to test for glucose, ketones and infection as soon as he feels the need to pass urine. You establish IV access and take blood for venous gasses, electrolytes, glucose, ketones, renal function and infection markers.

Circulation NEWS (2 + 1) = 3

Disability: He is assessed as alert, using ACVPU (RCP 2017). He understands where he is and who you are, so no new confusion is evident. Hyperglycaemia (and hypoglycaemia) is a common cause of a reduced level of consciousness and can present with drowsiness, confusion or coma due to its effect on the nervous system (neuroglycopenia). Always check a blood glucose if a patient presents with new confusion or their level of consciousness drops.

His blood glucose is 23.5mmol/L (**normal range 4–10mmol/L**). You are concerned, as he is hyperglycaemic and reporting abdominal pain. Those with DKA can present with abdominal pain, which may be due to a primary problem causing the DKA (that requires treatment), or a symptom of the acidosis associated with DKA (Umpierrez and Freire 2002).

Disability NEWS = 0

However, the high blood glucose is a cause for concern. Bedside blood ketone testing was deemed necessary.

Exposure: Mr Shah looks flushed and uncomfortable. His temperature is recorded at 38.5°C. You are unsure of the reason for this and decide to collect sputum and urine samples when possible. The notes identify his BMI is 40, confirming obesity. His abdomen appears distended, he has regular bowel sounds on auscultation and is not constipated. However, when gently palpating the abdomen you notice guarding, and Mr Shah says 'ooh that hurts'. You do not want to continue with any further abdominal assessment, but will ask your medical colleagues to examine him, to minimise discomfort for Mr Shah.

Exposure NEWS = 1

Total NEWS = 5

Mr Shah has a high blood glucose level and ketones are present. Your concern increases when urinalysis reveals:

- +++ glucose.
- ++ ketones.
- Positive to protein and leucocytes.

You are aware that he has the potential to deteriorate rapidly. His NEWS of 5 requires urgent escalation.

Action: escalate to doctor and outreach team

SBAR used to articulate concerns regarding NEWS score of 5.

As a result of the SBAR handover, it is recommended that a second IV cannula is sited and blood cultures are taken, as per the Sepsis Trust's protocol.

Medical Review: 11:00

Given his history and presentation, a provisional diagnosis is made of diabetes ketoacidosis. A urinary tract infection is likely, and abdominal problems cannot be discounted. An arterial blood gas sample is taken for analysis also.

Initial blood results confirm suspicions.

Initial blood results

Arterial blood gas results		*normal range*	*Venous blood results*		*normal range*
pH	7.22	7.35–7.45	Na+	138mmol/L	135–145mmol/L
$PaCO_2$	3.3kPa	4.6–6kPa	K+	5.5mmol/L	3.5–5.5mmol/L
PaO_2	10.8kPa	10.5–13.5kPa	Glucose	22mmol/L	4–10mmol/L
HCO_3^-	16mmol/L	22–26mmol/L	Ketones	5.0mmol/L	<0.6mmol/L
BE	-6.1mmol/L	-2 to + 2	WCC	15.8mmol/L	4–11mmol/L
Lactate	1.8mmol/L	<2mmol	CRP	45mg/L	<10mg/L
			Urea	11mmol/L	3–7mmol/L
			Creatinine	70 mcmol/l	60–110 mcmol/L

The team discuss the blood results and patient presentation/potential problems.

No **airway** problems are noted, but if the blood glucose continues to rise, an altered level of consciousness may threaten airway integrity.

No specific **breathing** problems are identified; the low $PaCO_2$ combined with the low pH suggests a partial respiratory compensation for a metabolic acidosis. The pH of 7.22 (normal range 7.35–7.45) confirms acidosis. The lowered bicarbonate of 16mmol/L (normal range 22–26mmol/L), along with the negative BE of 6 (BE -6, normal range +/- 2), is consistent with a metabolic acidosis. The high blood glucose, the presence of ketones in the blood and urine suggests DKA. The criteria to diagnose DKA is a triad of hyperglycaemia, metabolic acidosis and hyperketonuria, which are all clinical manifestations presented by Mr Shah. The team discuss how this is caused by a deficiency of insulin, reducing the ability of the glucose to enter the cell to be broken down into energy. The liver responds by breaking down fat (lipolysis) into ketones for energy. The presence of ketones lowers the blood pH causing acidosis. This will be treated under circulation.

As SpO_2 remains within the normal range, and the extra work of breathing will reduce as the acidosis resolves, no further action is taken for breathing. The Hb is within normal range, suggesting oxygen transport is good.

Action to be taken to support **circulation and disability** include:

- Insertion of a second IV canula.
- 500mL NaCl 0.9% to be given over 15 minutes. It is decided not to include K^+ supplements in this first bag, as his serum K^+ is in the high normal range. This will be checked again in 1 hour.
- An infusion of soluble insulin, diluted with 0.9% normal saline for a concentration of 1 unit/mL, is prepared. This needs to be given at 0.1units/kg/hr. Mr Shah weighs 80kg, so the infusion is prescribed to run at $(0.1 \times 80 = 8)$ 8mL/hr. This is given via the second IV line.
- Serum glucose, ketones and K^+ to be checked in 1 hour.
- Urinary catheter inserted to monitor urine output accurately, residual of 300mL obtained, sample sent for microscopy.
- A stat dose of cefuroxime 250mg IV is given, prescribed 12 hourly.
- The usual dose of long acting insulin is administered when due.

Continuous cardiac monitoring is commenced and reveals sinus rhythm. Serum K^+ is on the high end of normal, so this needs to be closely monitored. The insulin infusion will reduce serum K^+. Urea is higher than the normal range, suggesting (as the creatinine is normal) that Mr Shah does not have renal dysfunction, but may be dehydrated. The raised WCC and CRP is consistent with infection; the source needs to be found.

Under **exposure**, Mr Shah's abdomen is assessed by the medical team. General tenderness is discovered on palpation, but with no evidence of rebound tenderness that may indicate peritonitis. The team decide to re-examine his abdomen as the treatment for DKA progresses and acidosis resolves. Paracetamol 1gm IV is prescribed and given, to reduce pyrexia and abdominal pain.

Ongoing care

The nurse feels confident to explain to Mr Shah exactly what is going on and asks if there is anybody that should be called. Mr Shah requests his daughter be informed so she can bring him in some pyjamas and toiletries. He is surprised at how quickly his blood glucose has risen. You suggest that both him and his daughter chat to the team when he is feeling better, so he can be confident in managing his diabetes, asking for help should he feel unwell in the future

Mr Shah is in the resuscitation area in the emergency department to facilitate close monitoring of his condition whilst initial interventions are in progress and a bed on the acute medical unit can be found. The initial 500mL of normal saline is complete, and the fixed rate insulin infusion is in progress. He has been given his normal dose of long-acting insulin. His urine output is looking to be good for the following hour. In light of this output, the medical team prescribe normal saline 1L with 40mmol KCL to be infused over 2 hours via a volumetric pump.

12:00

His observations are checked prior to transfer to AMU.

A and B: breathing less laboured, RR 16, SpO_2 95%.
C: BP 109/80, HR 93, urine output 200mL for last hour. K^+ now 4.7mmol/L.
D: alert, blood glucose 18mmol/L, ketones 4.5mmol/L.
E: temp 37.8°C.
NEWS = 2 (blood glucose and ketones remain raised)

The nurse is reassured but realises that Mr Shah is far from completely well, even though his NEWS is reduced. His BP has risen, and his HR is falling as a result of the IV fluid, helping to restore fluid balance. Hourly monitoring continues.

Maximising endocrine status

Insulin administration

Insulin treatment will increase glucose utilisation in peripheral tissues and also decrease glucose production by the liver. It also decreases the formation of ketones and inhibits the release of free fatty acids (FFAs), thereby correcting the metabolic acidosis. The ultimate aim is to achieve a blood glucose between 10–15mmol/L over 24–48 hours. The use of insulin may lead to hypokalaemia, as it facilitates movement of potassium into cells. Close electrolyte monitoring is therefore essential, and replacement is administered to maintain serum potassium between 4–5mmol/L.

National Patient Safety Agency (NPSA) insulin safety guidance (2010)

Recommendations to reduce the number of wrong dose incidents involving insulin:

- All insulin bolus doses should be measured and administered using an insulin syringe (not intravenous syringe).
- The term 'units' should be used at all times (not U or IU).
- Training programmes should be in place for all health care professionals involved in the administration of insulin.

The transition from insulin infusion to the subcutaneous route is challenging, but should be attempted once the patient is stable and is able to eat and drink.

Glycaemic control

Normal fasting blood glucose levels are 3.5–5.5mmol/L, fluctuating to 7–9mmol/L following a meal. Insulin infusions are titrated against a sliding scale of blood glucose, aiming usually for a blood glucose within the 'normal range'. It is well recognised that hyperglycaemia is toxic: Falciglia et al. (2009) demonstrated an increase in mortality of ICU patients with a blood glucose of greater than 6.1mmol/L which was unrelated to illness severity. However, such tight control over blood glucose brings logistical challenges with the frequency of monitoring of blood glucose, and more importantly, a risk of iatrogenic hypoglycaemia, which can be harmful. A blood glucose of 2.2mmol/L is associated with a six-fold increase in mortality, and lower levels could be fatal. Hence, local recommendations are to maintain a blood glucose between 4 and 10mmol/L, rather than strictly between 4 and 6mmol/L in the critical care setting (see NICE-SUGAR Study 2009).

NICE-SUGAR Study (2009): a large randomised controlled trial

On admission to intensive care, patients were randomised to:

- Either maintain intensive glucose control of between 4.5–6.0mmol/L;
- Or conventional glucose control of less than 10mmol/L.

Although there was no difference between the two groups regarding length of stay on intensive care, the conclusion of this large multi-centre international trial was that intensive glucose control increased mortality among adults in intensive care. There were also significantly more episodes of severe hypoglycaemia (less than 2.2mmol/L) in the group with intensive glycaemic control (6.8% versus 0.5%) and increased morbidity.

Fluid and electrolyte management

Fluid administration for hypovolaemic patients (DKA and HHS) commonly includes using isotonic/normal saline (0.9% NaCl), but hypernatraemic patients may need half normal saline (0.45% NaCl). Correcting the fluid deficit will increase the intravascular volume and lower the plasma osmolality and blood glucose levels by dilution. The infusion rate will depend upon the circumstances, but the initial aim would be to correct the hypovolaemia within 24 hours.

Hyperglycaemia and serum sodium

Measured serum sodium needs to be recalculated in hyperglycaemia to obtain a 'true sodium level'. This is because extracellular osmolality rises in the presence of excess glucose (as it is slower to enter cells if there is a relative lack of insulin), with water accompanying the glucose into the extracellular fluid. As the extracellular fluid is diluted, the sodium concentration falls. This is described as a translational hyponatraemia because there is no change in total body water. The sodium level will not need to be treated, as this will correct itself as the glucose level normalises.

The chronicity of the situation should be considered with acute hyponatraemia (<48 hours) being more amenable to a faster correction than a longstanding condition, however, plasma sodium levels should not be increased faster than 12mmol per 24 hours.

Hypokalaemia will need correction, particularly with respect to patients receiving insulin, to attain levels between 4–5mmol/L. Patients who are hypokalaemic due to polyuria are at risk of having their hypokalaemia exacerbated iatrogenically when large fluid volumes are administered, as they will be haemodiluted. Fluid administration, in these circumstances, should therefore include a potassium supplement. Phosphate depletion is common in DKA, but replacement is seldom required.

Pharmacological interventions

The pharmacological management (hypoglycaemic agents) options include:

- *Sulphonylureas*: e.g., glibencamide, gliclazide, chlorpropamide, tolbutamide. These drugs lower blood glucose levels by increasing insulin production by the pancreas. They may also increase the sensitivity of the tissues to insulin. Drug interactions may include NSAIDs (including aspirin) enhancing the effect and thiazide diuretics reducing efficacy.
- *Metformin*: this belongs to a group of chemicals called biguanides. The mechanism of action is not understood fully, but it may stimulate uptake of glucose into muscle and reduce glucose release from the liver. It is most commonly prescribed in conjunction with a sulphonylurea if a patient is not responding to the latter alone.
- *Thiazolidinediones*: e.g., pioglitazone, rosiglitazone, which belong to chemicals called glitazones. They appear to reduce tissue resistance to insulin and are usually administered alongside a sulphonylurea or metformin.
- *Prandial (relating to a meal) glucose regulators*: nateglinide and repaglinide have differing mechanisms of action, but both are unique in that they act postprandially (after eating) to stimulate insulin release by the pancreas.

- *GLP-1 agonist (Glucagon like peptide 1 receptor agonist)*: e.g., exenatide, liraglutide, lixisenatide, which stimulate insulin release, suppress glucagon, slow gastric emptying, offer sense of satiety and fullness and lead to reduced food intake.
- *DPP-4 inhibitors or gliptins*: a class of oral hypoglycaemics that block the enzyme dipeptidyl peptidase-4 (DPP-4). Examples of DPP-4 agents are sitagliptin, vildagliptin, saxagliptin, linagliptin and alogliptin.
- *Sodium-glucose co-transporter-2 (SGLT2) inhibitors*: also called gliflozins, e.g., dapagliflozin, canagliflozin and empagliflozin; they block glucose re-absorption in the kidney and thereby increase urinary glucose excretion (glycosuria) to reduce blood glucose level.

CASE STUDY 11.2 MR SHAH, TYPE I DIABETIC: PART 2

Mr Shah, with type 1 diabetes, was admitted to the emergency department this morning with abdominal pain and was feeling generally unwell. He was found to have diabetic ketoacidosis and initial treatment with fluids and a fixed insulin infusion were started at 11:00.

Diabetic ketoacidosis is a life-threatening medical condition characterised by hyperglycaemia, osmotic diuresis, metabolic acidosis, glycosuria, ketonuria and dehydration. It is due to an increased demand for insulin, inadequate adjustment of insulin injection to meet the required needs of the body, severe physical or psychological stress or physical trauma without compensatory insulin and increased resistance to insulin due to various factors such as pregnancy or infection (Waugh and Grant 2018). Other precipitating factors include inappropriate insulin dosage or omission, acute illness, hyperthyroidism, alcohol abuse, other co-morbidities such as pancreatitis and drug such as corticosteroids.

Mr Shah had recently been unwell, possibly has a new urinary tract infection and has not stuck to his normal insulin regimen, which could have contributed to his DKA development. Ketoacidosis has resulted in increasing hyperglycaemia, polyuria, dehydration, hypovolaemia and electrolyte imbalance. If not treated in a timely manner, confusion, coma and death may ensue (Waugh and Grant 2018). Diabetic ketoacidosis accounts for a substantial amount of all diabetes-related hospital admissions.

A key indication for managing type 1 diabetes is the need for exogenous insulin due to progressive destruction of beta cells leading to insulin insufficiency. With lack of circulating insulin in the system, Mr Shah underwent a series of compensatory mechanisms which led to lipolysis and, consequently, ketones in the blood. Hyperglycaemia-induced osmotic diuresis can also lead to dehydration and electrolyte imbalance. Other manifestations of DKA are Kussmaul respiration (deep sighing breaths), acetone breath, nausea, vomiting and coma. Depending on individual compensatory reserve, DKA can develop as early as 24 hours. Noncompliance to insulin therapy accounts for a significant number of DKA cases, and this could be a contributory cause in this case.

The foci of management of DKA in adults are: rehydration, insulin therapy and potassium replacement, as insulin is a potent stimulus for potassium cellular uptake (Joint British Diabetes Societies Inpatient Care Group 2013; NICE 2015). Therefore, Mr Shah's fluid status, blood glucose, blood ketones and vital signs were being closely monitored. The aim of treatment is to reduce blood ketones by 0.5mmol/L/hr and blood glucose by at least 3mmol/L/hr.

He was transferred to the higher monitoring bay of the AMU, under the care of diabetologist and the diabetes specialist team. The National Service Framework emphasises the importance of skilful management of diabetes emergencies, DKA inclusive (DH 2001).

13:00: higher monitoring bay, AMU

A and B: breathing, RR 16, SpO_2 95%.
C: BP 110/80, HR 91, urine output 150mL for last hour. K^+ now 4.1mmol/L.
D: alert, blood glucose 13mmol/L, ketones 3.9mmol/L.
E: temp 37.8°C.

NEWS 2 = 2

Mr Shah seems to be progressing well, with a stable NEWS of 2. He is beginning to feel better, and he thinks the paracetamol has helped his abdominal pain. Further blood test results at 13:00 are below.

Blood test results at 13:00

Arterial blood gas results		*normal range*	*Venous blood results*		*normal range*
pH	7.29	7.35–7.45	Na^+	142mmol/L	135–145mmol/L
$PaCO_2$	4.3kPa	4.6–6kPa	K^+	4.1 mmol/L	3.5–5.5mmol/L
PaO_2	10.8kPa	10.5–13.5kPa	Glucose	13 mmol/L	4–10mmol/L
HCO_3^-	18mmol/L	22–26mmol/L	Ketones	3.9 mmol/L	<0.6mmol/L
BE	-4.1mmol/L	-2 to + 2	WCC	15.8mmol/L	4–11mmol/L
Lactate	1.6mmol/L	<2mmol	CRP	40mg/L	<10mg/L
			Hb	132g/L	130–160mg/L
			Urea	13mmol/L	3–7mmol/L
			Creatinine	75mcmol/l	60–110mcmol/L

Ensuring fluid balance

Fluid replacement is the priority in DKA, as an osmotic diuresis causes fluid depletion with negative cardiovascular effects. Mr Shah was initially tachycardic and hypotensive. 1500mL of IV saline helped replace the volume lost, and his NEWS fell from 5 to 2. NICE (2015) suggest IV fluid therapy should be continued until the deficit is replaced and to maintain fluid balance thereafter. An accurate fluid balance chart is essential, as, if too much fluid is given, the rare, but often fatal, condition of cerebral oedema may develop. This is not common in Mr Shah's age group, being a higher risk for children and young adults.

Ensuring serum potassium balance

The falling serum K^+, despite giving supplemental potassium with the IV fluids, is noted. The litre of normal saline with 40mmol KCL given over 2 hours is nearly complete, and the blood results suggest the potassium supplement should continue with the next bag. Therefore, medical review was sought. There are several factors at play here:

- Initially, when acidosis is present (pH<7.35) the serum K^+ will be raised. The competing H^+ and K^+ ions mean more K^+ leaves the cell (as H^+ enters) into the blood, raising serum K^+. This can be seen in the first blood result with the K^+ of 5.5mmol/L.
- As serum pH moves towards normal, H^+ reduces and potassium enters back into the cell, reducing serum K^+.
- The fixed-rate insulin infusion facilitates entry of glucose into the cell along with K^+, thereby reducing not only blood glucose, but serum K^+ also.

It can be seen in this case study that the serum potassium is gently falling in spite of IV potassium supplements, but currently remains within a safe range. In short, close monitoring of serum potassium is essential in DKA, as large variations in a short time span can cause fatal cardiac arrhythmias. Cardiac monitoring in the initial management can help early detection of arrhythmia.

Ensuring blood ketone and glucose balance

Mr Shah's blood glucose has now fallen below 14mmol/L. His blood ketones are reducing, but remain raised. Note that the serum pH is also rising to near normal range as the ketones are being excreted. As per NICE (2015) guidance, 10% glucose at 125mL/hr is given in addition to the normal saline infusion. This is to enable insulin infusion to continue, until the blood ketone concentration is <0.6mmol/L and serum pH is >7.3. As this stage is reached, Mr Shah should be able to eat and drink normally, be given a subcutaneous fast-acting insulin and a meal, with the insulin infusion stopping soon after. Blood glucose and ketone monitoring should be performed hourly for the first 6 hours (NICE 2015).

The abdominal pain that prompted his hospital attendance improved as his DKA resolved. Whilst abdominal pain can be a symptom of the acidosis associated with DKA, further investigation is required, as problems such as pancreatitis, hepatitis and pyelonephritis may be an underlying cause (Bello et al. 2018).

Resolution of DKA has been achieved when:

- pH >7.3.
- Bicarbonate >15mmol/L.
- Blood ketone level <0.6mmol/L.

Mr Shah and his family will need support in continuing management of his diabetes, both during his hospital stay and on discharge.

This is an example of a patient with DKA who was well-managed on admission. The probable trigger of the event, a UTI, was treated promptly. It is interesting to note that the NEWS score of 2 during his recovery indicated improvement, but close monitoring was still required as he remained at risk of deterioration. NEWS is a guide for assessment of deterioration risk, but should not replace the health care professional's clinical judgement.

Conclusion

The aim of this chapter is to provide an insight to common endocrine disorders, because nurses are often confronted with the challenges of managing this group of patients. A prompt diagnosis is important in the hospital setting; it is claimed by Kearney and Dang (2007) that, with improved care and early detection, DKA and HHS can be prevented entirely. Certainly, awareness and prompt recognition of these conditions will promote better outcomes in such patients (Kisiel and Marsons 2009). Fortunately, DKA and HHS are relatively uncommon, however, the diabetic emergency of hypoglycaemia is more frequently encountered, so this situation requires particular insight and awareness by nurses into the importance of their role, as many hypoglycaemic episodes are iatrogenic in causation and are associated with increased morbidity and mortality. Nurses have a key role to play in the care of patients with acute endocrine problems, and it is important for nurses to respond appropriately, recognise their limitations, call for assistance and make appropriate referral when necessary.

Glossary

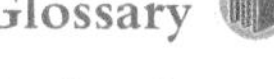

Endocrine From Greek *endo* inside and *crine* to secrete. The secretion of hormones via ductless glands directly into the bloodstream.

Exocrine *Exo* = outside. Secretion of chemicals via glands with ducts.

Gluconeogenesis Metabolic pathway resulting in the generation of glucose from non-carbohydrate sources such as lactate, glycerol and glucogenic amino acids.

Glycogenolysis Conversion of stored glycogen to glucose by the liver.

Glycosuria Presence of glucose in the urine.

Ketoacidosis A metabolic condition associated with an accumulation of ketone bodies. Ketone bodies are the breakdown product of free fatty acids and the result of deamination of amino acids.

Kussmaul breathing Rapid, deep, laboured breathing due to respiratory compensation for a severe metabolic acidosis. This can arise from either ketoacidosis or renal failure. Named after Adolf Kussmaul, a nineteenth-century German doctor.

Neuroglycopenia A deficiency of glucose in the brain as a result of hypoglycaemia. This adversely affects the functioning of neurones.

TEST YOURSELF

1 Which of the following is not produced by the anterior pituitary gland?:
   a. Growth hormone
   b. Adrenocorticotrphic hormone
   c. Antidiuretic hormone
   d) Follicle stimulating hormone

2 Unused glucose is stored in the liver as:
   a. Glycerol
   b. Glucagon
   c. Glycogen
   d. Glucose

3 Which of the statements is false
   a. All individuals with diabetes are at risk of hypoglycaemia
   b. Individuals with diabetes treated with biguanide only are not at risk of hypoglycaemia
   c. Individuals with diabetes treated with exogenous insulin administration are at risk of hypoglycaemia
   d. Individuals with diabetes treated with GLP-1 Agonist are at risk of hypoglycaemia
4 A body fluid is acidic when the hydrogen ion concentration (PH) is:
   a. Above 10.5
   b. 2
   c. Below 10
   d. None of the above
5 One of the following four options is not a symptom of Euglycemic diabetic ketoacidosis (EDKA)?
   a. Blood glucose level of less than 11.1 mmol
   b. High blood glucose level of above 12 mmol
   c. Metabolic acidosis
   d. Increased level of blood ketone
6 An increase in plasma blood glucose results in:
   a. Increased insulin and increased glucagon secretion by the pancreas
   b. Decreased insulin and increased glucagon secretion by the pancreas
   c. Increased insulin and decreased glucagon secretion by the pancreas
   d. Decreased insulin and decreased glucagon secretion by the pancreas
7 Diabetes insipidus is due to:
   a. Insufficiency of antidiuretic hormone
   b. Excessive production of antidiuretic hormone
   c. Underproduction of insulin
   d. Thyroid insufficiency
8 Which of the following symptoms is not a manifestation of autonomic neuropathy?
   a. Erectile dysfunction
   b. Inability to recognise hypoglycaemia
   c. Sweating abnormalities
   d. Sudden increase in blood pressure
9 Which of the following is a life-threatening complication of hyperthyroidism?
   a. Thyroid storm
   b. Myxoedema coma
   c. Diabetic ketoacidosis
   d. Grave's disease
10 Insulin is produced by:
   a. Beta cells in the pancreas when the blood glucose level is low
   b. Alpha cells in the pancreas when the blood glucose level is low
   c. Beta cells in the pancreas when blood glucose level is high
   d. Alpha cells in the pancreas when the blood glucose level is high

11 The acute complications of diabetes are:
   a. Hypertension and hyperglycaemia
   b. Retinopathy and diabetic foot ulcer
   c. Hyperosmolar hyperglycaemia syndrome and hypoglycaemia
   d. Erectile dysfunction and nephropathy

12 Hameedat, a 25-year old lady, is 24 weeks pregnant with her first pregnancy. Her body mass index is 35 and she has a family history of diabetes. Her glucose tolerance test indicates a higher value above the normal range and her sister recently had a baby with a high birth weight. Based on her history and test result, what would you suggest as her diagnosis?
   a. Type 1 diabetes
   b. Pre-diabetes
   c. Gestational diabetes
   d. Type 2 diabetes

Answers

1 c
2 c
3 b
4 b
5 b
6 c
7 a
8 d
9 a
10 c
11 c
12 c

References

Bello, A., Gago, M., Fernandes, F., Oliveira, M. (2018). Abdominal pain in diabetic ketoacidosis: beyond the obvious. *Journal of Endocrinology and Metabolism*, 8(2–3), 43–46.Accessed from https://www.jofem.org/index.php/jofem/article/view/494/284284305.

Brashers, V. L., Huether, S. E. (2017). Mechanisms of hormonal regulation. In Huether, S. E., McCance, K. L., (Eds.), *Understanding Pathophysiology*, 6th Edition. St Louis, MO, USA: Elsevier, pp. 439–459.

Brashers, V. L., Jones, R. E., Huether, S. E. (2017). Alterations of hormonal regulation. In Huether, S. E., McCance, K. L., (Eds.), *Understanding Pathophysiology*, 6th Edition. St Louis, MO, USA: Elsevier, pp. 460–489.

Clayton, M. F., McCance, K. L., Takashashi, L. K. (2017). Stress and disease. In Huether, S. E., McCance, K. L., (Eds.), *Understanding Pathophysiology*, 6th Edition. St Louis, MO, USA: Elsevier, pp. 214–232.

Department of Health. (2001). *National Service Framework for diabetes*. London: DH

Diabetes UK. (2018). *Diabetes Ketoacidosis (DKA)*. Available from https://www.diabetes.org.uk/guide-to-diabetes/complications/diabetic_ketoacidosis. Accessed 20 October 2019.

Dixon, K., Salamonson, Y. (2006). Disorders of the endocrine system. In Chang, E., Daly, J., Elliott, D., (Eds.), *Pathophysiology Applied to Nursing*. Australia: Elsevier Mosby, pp. 79–104.

Falciglia, M., Freyberg, R., Almenoff, P. (2009). Hyperglycaemia-related mortality in critically patients varies with admission diagnosis. *Critical Care Medicine*, 37, 3001–3009.

Joint British Diabetes Society for Inpatient Care (JBDS-IP). (2013). *The Management of Diabetic Ketoacidosis in Adults*, 2nd Edition. Available from https://www.diabetes.org.uk/resources-s3/2017-09/Management-of-DKA-241013.pdf.

Joint British Diabetes Society for Inpatient Care (JBDS-IP). (2018). *The Hospital Management of Hypoglycaemia in Adults with Diabetes Mellitus*, 3rd Edition. Available from http://www.diabetologists-abcd.org.uk/JBDS/JBDS_HypoGuideline_FINAL_280218.pdf. Accessed 20 October 2019.

Kearney, T., Dang, C. (2007). Diabetic and endocrine emergencies. *Postgraduate Medical Journal*, 83, 79–86.

Kerr, D. E., Wenham, T., Newell-Price, J. (2017). Endocrine problems in the critically ill 2: endocrine emergencies. *British Journal of Anaesthesia*, 17(11), 377–382.

Kisiel, M., Marsons, L. (2009). Recognising and responding to hyperglycaemic emergencies. *British Journal of Nursing*, 18(18), 1094–1098.

Lange, C., Pearce, R. (2017). Exploration of diabetes knowledge among registered nurses working in an NHS trust. *Journal of Diabetes Nursing*, 21(6), 203–207.

Lawal, M. (2008). Management of diabetes mellitus in clinical practice. *British Journal of Nursing*, 17(17), 1106–1113.

National Diabetes Inpatient Audit . (2018). *Key Facts: Hospital Characteristics Report in England and Wales*. Available from https://files.digital.nhs.uk/D9/2BEDFE/NaDIA%202018%20-%20Full%20Report%20V1.0.pdf. Accessed 20 October 2019.

NICE-SUGAR Study. (2009). Intensive versus conventional glucose control in critically ill patients. *New England Journal of Medicine*, 360, 1283–1297.

NICE. (2015). *Type 1 Diabetes in Adults: Diagnosis and Management* (NG17). Available from https://www.nice.org.uk/guidance/ng17. Accessed 27 October 2019.

NPSA (National Patient safety Agency). (2010). *New Insulin Safety Guidance Issued to Reduce Wrong Dosages*. Available from www.npsa.nhs.uk. Accessed 17 June 2010.

Rawla, P., Vellipuram, A. R., Bandaru, S. S., Raj, J. P. (2017). Euglycemic diabetic ketoacidosis: a diagnostic and therapeutic dilemma. *Endocrinology, Diabetes & Metabolism*. doi:10.1530/EDM17-0081. Available from http.www.edmassereports.com. Accessed 16 June 2019.

Resuscitation Council UK. (2015). *Resuscitation Guidelines*. Available from www.resus.org.uk.

Royal College of Physicians (RCP). (2017). *National Early Warning score (News) 2 – standardising the assessment of acute illness severity in the NHS*. London: RCP.

Strachan, M. W. J. (2014). Frequency, causes and risk factors for hypoglycaemia in type 1 diabetes. In Frier, B. M., Heller, S. R., Mccrimmon, R. J., (Eds.), *Hypoglycaemia in Clinical Diabetes*, 3rd Edition. Chichester: John Wiley & Sons Ltd.

Umpierrez, G., Freire, A. (2002). Abdominal pain in patients with hyperglycemic crises. *Journal of Critical Care*, 17(1), 63–67.

VanMeter, K. C., Hubert, R. J. (2014). *Gould's Pathophysiology for the Health Professions*, 5th Edition. St Louis, MO, USA: Elsevier.

Waugh, A., Grant, A. (2018). *Ross and Wilson Anatomy and Physiology in Health and Illness*, 13th Edition. Edinburgh: Elsevier.

WHO. (2018). *Diabetes: Key Facts*. Available from https://www.who.int/news-room/fact-sheets/detail/diabetes. Accessed 20 October 2019.

Zaccardi, F., Davies, M. J., Dhalwani, N. N., Webb, D. R., Housley, G., Shaw, D., Hatton, J. W., Khunti, K. (2016). Trends in hospital admissions for hypoglycaemia in England: a retrospective, observational study. *The Lancet*, 4(8), 677–685.

Further reading

Diabetes UK. www.diabetes.org.uk.

International Diabetes Federation. www.idf.org.

12 The immune and lymphatic systems, infection and sepsis

Michelle Treacy, Caroline Smales and Helen Dutton

AIM

The aim of this chapter is to provide you with insight and understanding of the immune and lymphatic systems, as well as understanding the nurse's role in the recognition and management of patients who are at risk of acute deterioration due to altered immunity and sepsis.

OBJECTIVES

After reading this chapter you will be able to:

- Review the components and function of the lymphatic and immune systems and outline their purpose.
- Review the types of infective microorganisms, methods of infection transmission and infection control strategies, considering the nurse's role in reducing infection.
- Describe the pathophysiology and immediate management of allergy and anaphylaxis.
- Review the pathophysiology of sepsis and understand the contribution of the Surviving Sepsis Campaign to the current evidenced guidelines and care-bundle approach for sepsis and sepsis management.
- Understand the nurse's role in the systematic assessment of the patient who has problems with immunity and/or sepsis.
- Consider management and supportive interventions in order to maximise recovery from immunity and sepsis-related illnesses.

Introduction

This chapter will review the important cellular and chemical components that seek and destroy invading microorganisms in order to protect the body from infection. This coordinated response is the role of the immune and **complement** systems and, in combination with the body's natural, defences, protects from a multitude of microbes. The body's response to infection will be explored, reviewing the pathophysiology of fever, the activation of the inflammatory response and problems of allergy and anaphylaxis. The spread of microbes and the role of health care professionals in actively preventing the spread of health care-associated infections (HCAIs) will also be discussed. The role of the nurse is crucial in recognising the early signs of infection and in the delivery of evidence-based care to those who experience acute deterioration from problems related to immunity and infection.

Applied anatomy and physiology

The body contains a remarkable array of cells, proteins and complex networks of interrelated hormones and chemicals which provide constant surveillance of our body for any signs of invasion from microbial or other organic substances, e.g., pollen, that might cause harm. This array is collectively known as the immune system. It alerts our defence systems when microorganisms are breaching our natural defences and provides the first line of defence. For the immune system to function rapidly and effectively, it must have a transport network that delivers the immune response to its target location: that system is called the lymphatic system.

The lymphatic system

The lymphatic system is sometimes neglected and underestimated, silently going about its functions. It is closely linked to the cardiovascular system, providing an open-ended comprehensive network of drainage, defence and the storage of white cells.

The lymphatic system consists of lymphatic (lymphoid) tissue, capillaries and vessels, lymph nodes and collecting ducts. The organs of the lymphatic system are the spleen, thymus and the tonsils, which are located in the posterior aspect of the oral cavity and nasopharynx and are the smallest lymphoid organs (see Figure 12.1). All are interconnected by lymph capillaries, which run alongside blood capillaries, reabsorbing any excess interstitial fluid and escaped plasma proteins into the lymph fluid and back into the venous system. This is important in maintaining fluid balance between the interstitial and vascular fluid compartments.

The lymphatic system recycles approximately 2–4L per day of interstitial fluid back into the bloodstream (Marieb and Hoehn 2016). Lymphatic vessels, like peripheral veins, contain valves which ensure the one-way movement of lymph back into the venous system. Lymph fluid drains into collecting vessels, then into several lymphatic trunks and finally into two main collecting ducts:

- The right lymphatic duct.
- The thoracic duct.

The right lymphatic duct drains the right upper arm, the right side of the head, thorax, subclavian and jugular regions and opens into the right subclavian vein. The larger thoracic duct drains into the left subclavian vein. Over two-thirds of lymph from the body drains into this duct via the right lymphatic duct.

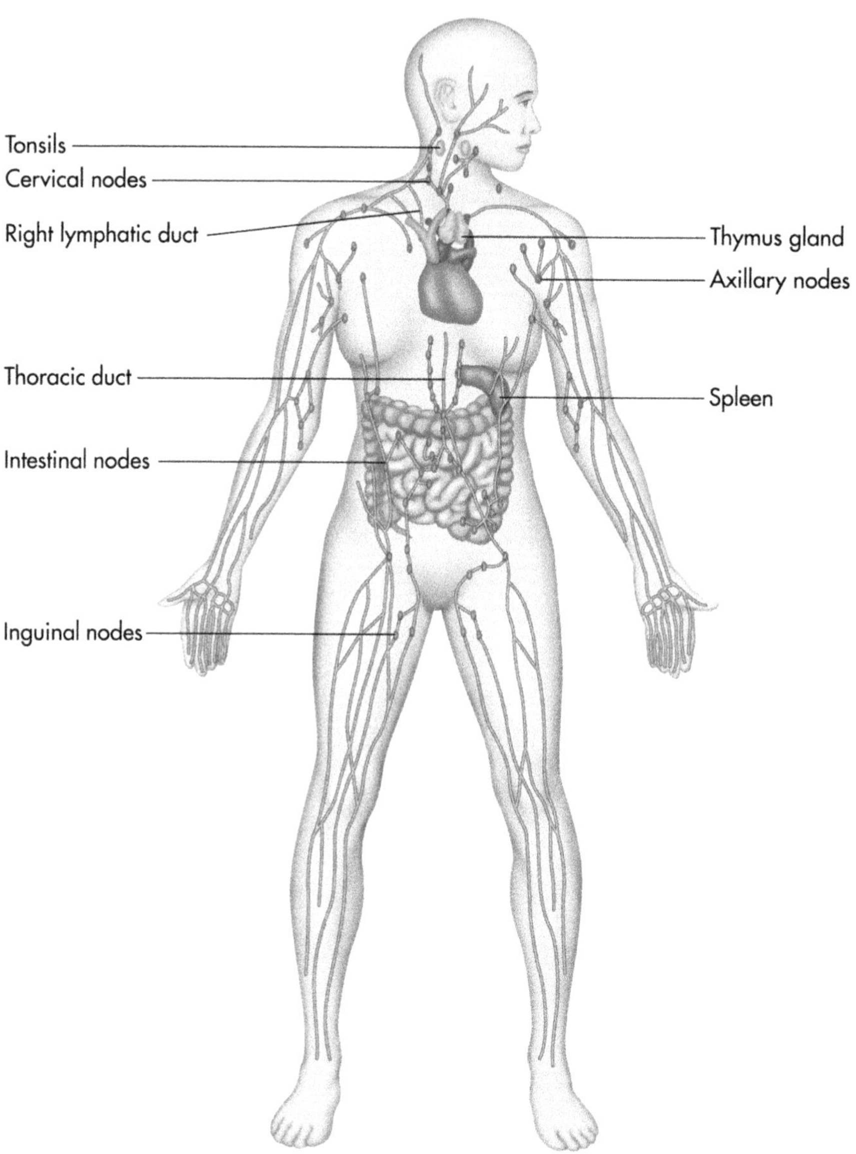

Figure 12.1 The lymphatic system.

Thus, circulation of lymph fluid follows the pattern given in Colbert et al. (2012):

Blood
↓
Tissue
↓
Lymphatic capillaries
↓

Lymphatic vessels
↓
Lymph nodes
↓
Collecting ducts
↓
Lymphatic trunk
↓
Subclavian veins
↓
Blood

Lymphocytes

Lymphocytes are the cells of the lymphatic system. Produced in the bone marrow, they form part of the cell-mediated response to antigens. As their name suggests, they spend most of their life cycle, which is about 2–4 years, within the lymphoid tissues. There are different types and sizes of lymphocytes, T cells and B cells. T cells are produced in the bone marrow, but are matured (or become immunocompetent) within the thymus. B cells are also produced in the bone marrow, but remain there to mature and become immunocompetent (see Figure 12.2). The T and B cells are exposed to antigens, normally in the lymphoid tissue, where they differentiate and mature. Within the T and B cell population, there are a range of cells with differing functions. B cells mediate the humoral or antibody response and T cells mediate the cellular immune response.

Lymphoid tissue

Lymphoid tissue is composed of reticular connective tissue, which provides support for lymphocytes and macrophages. These lymphocytes and macrophages can quickly squeeze through the capillary walls to circulate in the blood. This recirculation of lymphocytes between the blood, lymphatic tissues and organs is vitally important in exposing many lymphocytes to an invading pathogen or antigen. Depending on the route of entry the antigen, will be conveyed from the site of infection to the lymphatic tissues, where antigen-presenting cells, e.g., dendritic cells of lymphoid tissue and macrophages, are waiting to phagocytose the **microbes** and present the microbial antigen on their surface for antibodies to respond to. Antigens causing a tissue infection will be conveyed to the appropriate draining lymph nodes: the lymph node effectively closes down to retain the antigen-specific cells within the lymph node, thereby containing the infection within a small area (Stewart 2012). This causes swollen, painful lymph nodes, as experienced with an infection within the tonsils (tonsillitis). Cancerous cells can also be trapped within the lymph node: the node may become swollen but not painful, which is a useful sign in differentiating between infection and cancer.

Within the small intestine are collections of lymphoid tissues or nodules called Peyer's patches. Similar nodules are also found within the appendix. They are well-situated to detect and destroy any pathogenic bacteria found within the intestine, preventing these bacteria from trans-locating or crossing the gastrointestinal wall. These tissues or nodules are collectively called mucosa-associated lymphatic tissue (MALT), and along with the tonsils and nodules within the bronchi, they protect the respiratory and digestive systems from a continuous barrage of **pathogens**.

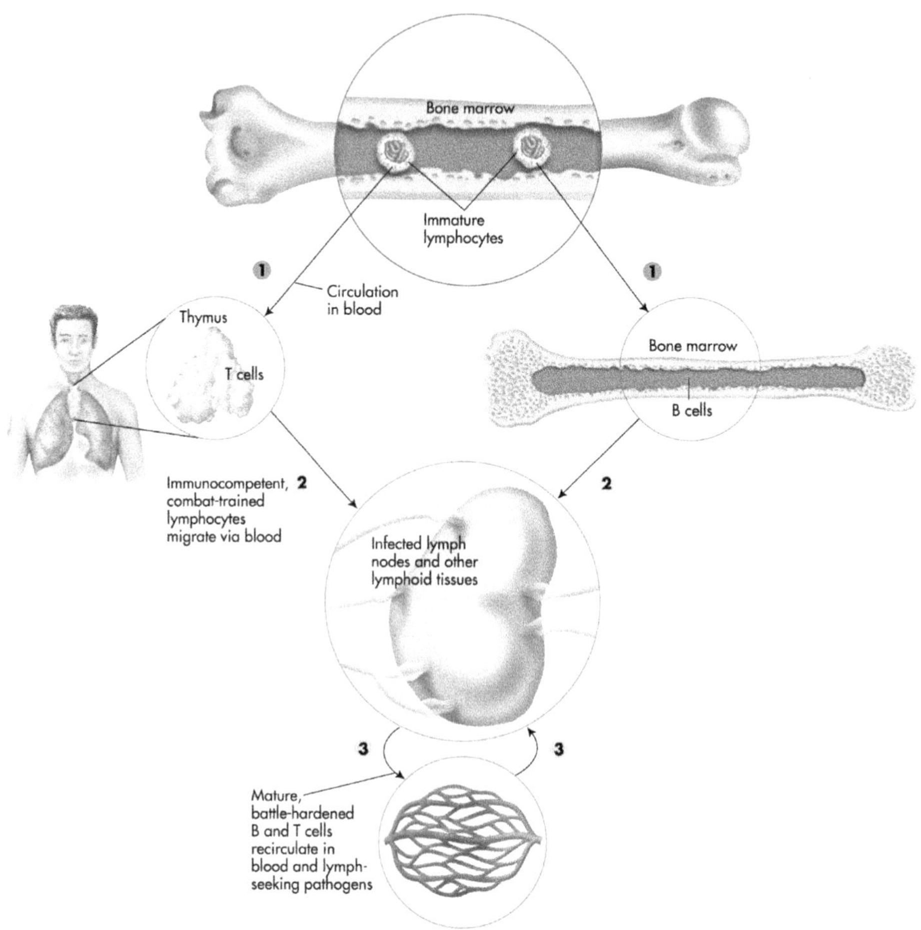

KEY:

1 Site of lymphocyte origin: some lymphocytes are sent to the thymus where they become T cells, while others remain in the bone marrow to become B cells. These cells are now much like soldiers in bootcamp that have learned their combat training but have yet to face the real enemy.

2 Sites of development of immunocompetence as B or T cells: an infection occurs and these cells are now given their marching orders to travel to the site of need. This is usually in the lymphoid tissue where the antigen challenge (the enemy has arrived) and the lymphocytes get placed into actual battle.

3 Site of antigen challenge and final differentiation to mature B and T cells: now the battle-hardened lymphocytes can competently patrol the rest of the body through the blood and lymph system, seeking out the enemy.

Figure 12.2 Lymphocyte differentiation and activation.

Lymph nodes

Lymph nodes range from the size of a pinhead to a small grape; they are strategically placed in vulnerable regions such as the digestive, respiratory and reproductive areas. Loaded with lymphocytes, they are ready to destroy harmful pathogens. Lymph nodes act like sieves, filtering the fluid and returning it cleansed of harmful microbes back into the lymphatic and circulatory systems. The lymph nodes are found mainly in the neck (cervical) under the armpits (axillary), in the groin (inguinal) and within the pelvis and abdominal and thoracic cavities (see Figure 12.1) (Colbert et al. 2012).

The spleen

The spleen is located just under the diaphragm in the upper left quadrant of the abdominal cavity, curving around the anterior aspect of the stomach; it is supplied by the splenic artery which enters at the hilus. The main functions of the largest lymphoid organ are:

- Surveillance for infection;
- Lymphocyte propagation;
- Filtering and cleaning of the blood from blood-borne pathogens and **toxins**;
- Storage of platelets and removal of ageing, faulty platelets and red blood cells and the extraction and storage of iron for the production of haemoglobin.

Ruptured or damaged spleen

If the spleen is damaged it must be removed, as haemorrhage from the splenic artery is life threatening.

Post-splenectomy (asplenism), the patient is at risk of developing serious life-threatening infections.

The main infectious organisms to cause death are:

- Pneumococcus.
- Haemophilus influenzae.
- Meningococcus.

Vaccines exist to protect against these organisms, and these, with regular boosters and health education, are essential to reduce the risk of serious infection.

The spleen is made up of areas of white and red pulp. The white pulp regions congregate around the splenic artery and blood sinuses and are primarily concerned with the immune surveillance function and the production of lymphocytes, when required. The red pulp region removes worn-out blood cells, platelets and pathogens. The spleen has a very thin outer capsule, and any blunt trauma may cause the spleen to rupture, potentially leading to life-threatening haemorrhage. If the spleen is removed (splenectomy), its function is taken over by the liver and bone marrow.

The thymus

The thymus is located in front of the aortic arch behind the sternum. In children, the thymus is very large, as it is very active fending off many new infections, but with increasing age, the immune system matures, and the thymus shrinks or may even disappear. The cells of the thymus are primarily lymphocytes. The primary function of the thymus is to secrete thymosin and thymopoietin, which bring about the maturing and immunocompetence of T cell lymphocytes.

Immunity

There are two types of immune defence systems:

- **Innate** or natural immunity.
- Adaptive or acquired immunity, which is specific to each person.

Immunity and natural defences

We are born with our own inherent immune system or innate immunity, which is made up of passive immunity and natural defences.

Passive immunity

Passive immunity is part of the innate immunity or non-specific immunity and has no memory; it can recognise our own cells (self) or antigens, but cannot recognise a pathogen that has previously invaded the body. The foetus acquires some immunity via the placenta: this is called passive immunity and lasts for about 3–6 months; the main antibody which is able to cross the placenta is **immunoglobulin** IgG. Although the time period for providing this passive immunity is limited, it is important at a time when the immune system is immature. After about six months, infants are more prone to respiratory and gastric infections, and this is in part due to the loss of foetal antibodies before the B and T lymphocytes are fully immunocompetent.

The respiratory syncytial virus (RSV) causes **croup** and bronchiolitis in the first few months of the infants' life, despite the presence of IgG from the mother.

Natural defences

One of the natural defences of the body is the skin; the largest impermeable organ in the body, it provides our first line of protection against a barrage of potentially harmful microorganisms. It contains three layers – the epidermis, dermis and hypodermis – in which there are motor and sensory nerves, hair follicles and sweat glands (see Figure 12.3). The epidermis is heavily keratinised; keratin is a protein that is resistant to bacterial toxins and **enzymes** (Stewart 2012). The dermis also produces sweat and sebum from sebaceous glands which contain lactic and fatty acids (Stewart 2012). The epidermis also contains Langerhans cells that are involved in the natural defences. The low pH of between 3 and 5 is acidic and inhibits the growth and survival of non-**commensal** bacteria. An exception to this is *Staphylococcus aureus*, a salt-resistant, gram-positive organism and opportunistic skin pathogen. *Staph. aureus* is found in the nose in about 30% of healthy people (Humphreys 2012). The cocci exist in clusters, causing many soft tissue infections by invading hair follicles and sebaceous glands. This can manifest as surgical wound infections, **abscesses** or boils. They can also produce pneumonia. *Staph. aureus*

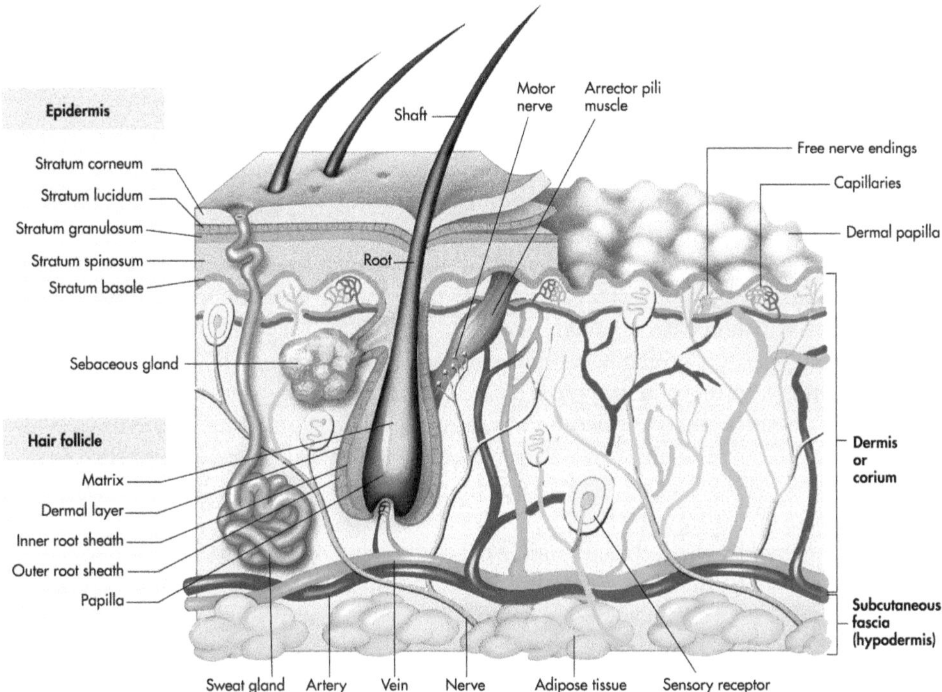

Figure 12.3 The layers of the skin.

can also release **enterotoxins** that, when ingested, cause food poisoning and other toxin-mediated diseases, such as toxic shock syndrome and scaled skin syndrome. Some strains of *Staphylococcus aureus* are resistant to many of the antibiotics used to eradicate the bacterium. MRSA infections are a particular problem in large hospitals, where stringent hygiene measures are needed to prevent it spreading between patients; although stringent measures put into place have reduced serious MRSA infections such as bacteraemia, unfortunately, methicillin-sensitive *Staphylococcus aureus* has increased and can still cause significant healthcare-associated infections.

Meticillin-resistant Staphylococcus aureus (MRSA)

Staph. aureus began to develop resistance to penicillin in the early 1950s, and since then it has developed resistance to gentamicin and vancomycin (VRSA) and is now referred to as Meticillin (renamed from Methicillin in 2005)-resistant *Staphylococcus aureus*. Globally, there have been many worldwide outbreaks of MRSA. Those most at risk are:

- The critically ill.
- Those on dialysis.
- Oncology patients.
- Immunocompromised patients.
- Patients with prosthetic heart valves.
- Patients with indwelling venous catheters.

Due to the concerns of the rising incidence of MRSA bacteraemia, mandatory enhanced surveillance was instigated in April 2001 by the Department of Health. This surveillance, together with other strategies, such as screening and decolonisation programmes, improved environmental cleaning and hand hygiene, has been very successful, and rates of MRSA bacteraemia have reduced significantly and remain low. However, in 2011, this surveillance was expanded to include MSSA (Meticillin-sensitive *Staphylococcus aureus*) bacteraemias, amid rising rates which continue to this day. In 2016–17, the rate of MSSA bacteraemia was 20.8 cases per 100,000 population. In 2017–18, this had increased to 21.6 cases per 100,000 population (Public Health England 2017).

All openings into the body are protected by mucus membranes which secrete acids, enzymes and sticky fluids to protect the tissues underneath from microorganisms. The respiratory tract is protected by several naturally occurring mechanisms; the columnar cells in the nasal passages project 200–250 cilia which beat up to 1500 times per minute, humidifying, filtering and trapping particles and dust in a gel-like substance (see Figure 12.4). The mucociliary escalator constantly expels debris forward to the nose. This mechanism is assisted by the physical acts of coughing and sneezing, expelling debris (sputum) from the deeper areas of the lungs into the upper airways, where it can be coughed out or swallowed.

Eyes are protected by the lacrimal fluids, or tears, which contain the enzyme lysozyme, also found in saliva. Both fluids neutralise bacteria, especially gram-positive organisms inhibiting bacterial growth. Saliva also contains IgA antibodies and defensins, which act as a local antibiotic and stimulate the release of neutrophils if the oral mucosa is damaged. Lysozyme is secreted by leucocytes and is also found in the genitourinary tract. Combined with the regular flushing of urine, this protects the urinary tract from pathogens.

Defensins are a group of small antimicrobial peptides occurring in neutrophils and macrophages.

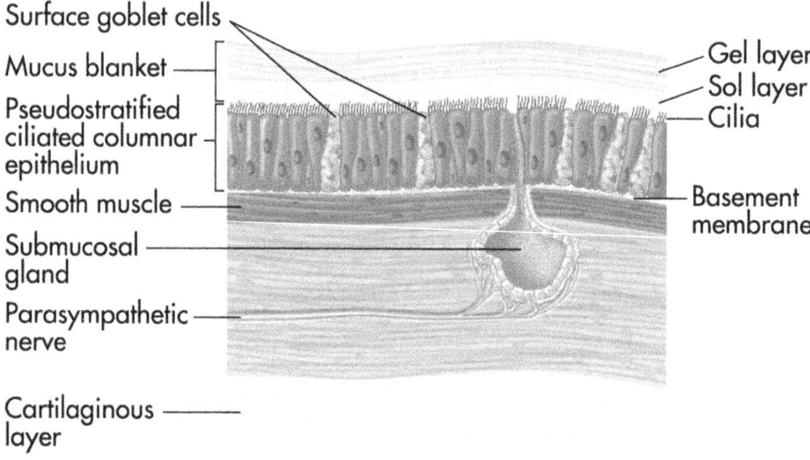

Figure 12.4 The mucociliary escalator.

The stomach is protected by the production of hydrochloric acid (HCl) from parietal cells. The acidity or pH of the gastric juices is about 1.5–3.5, which kills many ingested pathogens. The opposite occurs in the small intestine, where the pH is very high (pH 8–9). This alkaline state again destroys most pathogens, with the exception of typhoid and cholera.

Vaginal secretions produce lactobacilli, which can form lactic acid, creating an acidic environment within the vagina. The vaginal secretions have a pH of 4–5. Semen also contains chemicals that protect from invasion.

Humans are host reservoirs for a number of commensal microorganisms, for example *Escherichia coli* (*E. coli*) and natural flora that exist either in the gastrointestinal system or on the skin. There is a fine balance between host and commensal organisms and this relationship is important to maintain health. When an imbalance occurs, or the commensal enters into an area where it is not usually present, such as *E. coli* entering into the urinary tract, an infection can occur. These organisms, called opportunistic pathogens, can pose serious consequences for those who have undergone surgical treatments such as joint replacement or those who are immunocompromised.

As previously mentioned, despite MRSA bacteraemias decreasing, MSSA have been increasing, and so, too, have gram-negative microorganisms causing bacteraemia. *Escherichia coli* (*E. coli*), being one of the commonest, has increased significantly. The rate of *E. coli* cases per 100,000 population has risen from 60.4 in 2012–13 to 74.3 in 2017–18 (Public Health England 2018). In 2017, the Secretary of State for Health, Jeremy Hunt, launched an ambition to reduce gram-negative bacteraemias by 50% by 2021, with an initial focus on *Escherichia coli* (PHE/NHS Improvement 2017).

In essence, any natural opening has several mechanisms to protect the delicate membranes from invasion. The natural defence systems, combined with our complex molecular and chemical immunity, largely protect from infection. When the natural defences are breached, a complex range of components are released to counteract invasion. The blood components of immunity and how they become activated will now be considered.

Major groups of leucocytes

Once the natural barriers have been breached, the innate system is instantly activated, targeting the source of infection with a barrage of white cells or leucocytes. Leucocytes are formed in the bone marrow and make up the white cells that comprise the white cell differential. White cells are activated when they come in to contact with damaged cells and tissues, complement proteins, antibodies and chemicals released by bacterial cells.

Normal serum values for white blood cell count (WBCC) and white blood cell count differential:

- WBCC: 4–11 × 10^9/L.
- Neutrophils: 2–7.5 × 10^9/L.
- Lymphocytes: 1.5–4 × 10^9/L.
- Monocytes: 0.2–0.8 × 10^9/L.
- Eosinophils: 0.04–0.4 × 10^9/L.
- Basophils: 0–0.1 × 10^9/L.

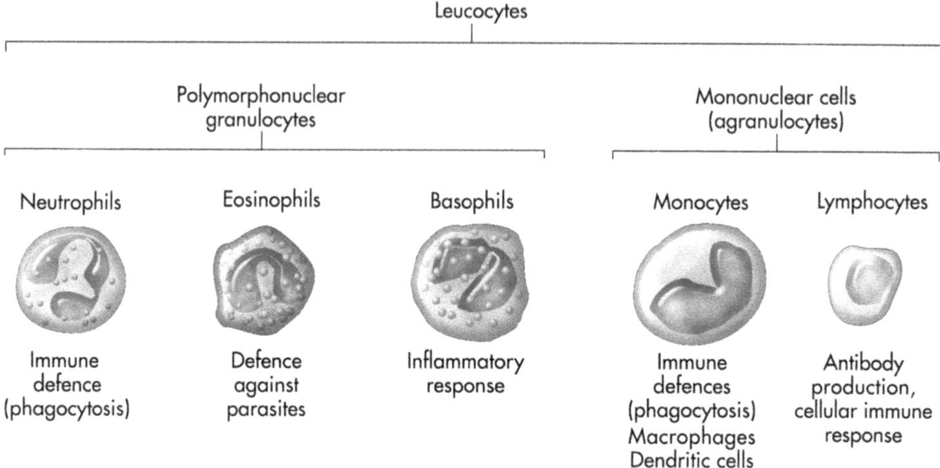

Figure 12.5 Major leucocytes.

Figure 12.5 shows the 5 major leucocytes or white blood cell groups: the 5 major leucocytes are listed below and are the normal values for white blood cell count.

1 Neutrophils.
2 Eosinophils.
3 Basophils.
4 Monocytes.
5 Lymphocytes.

Neutrophils

Neutrophils, eosinophils and basophils are polymorphonuclear granulocytes (i.e. they contain cytoplasmic granules), of which the most abundant are neutrophils. They are the first cells to arrive at the scene of infection or tissue damage. Their primary function is phagocytosis; that is, they act as scavengers, engulfing and destroying microbes. On ingestion of the microbe, the phagocyte's cytotoxic enzymes digest the organism (Marieb and Hoehn 2016). Neutrophils clump together around sites of tissue injury, releasing chemicals (**cytokine**s) which stimulate other immune cells to be activated. This stimulation causes local inflammation. A more severe inflammatory response during a bacterial infection may cause the death of the neutrophils; this cell debris forms pus or a wound infection, which occurs at the site of tissue injury. A full blood count is performed as part of the clinical assessment to diagnose the presence of infection; leucocytosis or elevated white count confirms the presence of infection. Alternatively, a low white cell count, or leucopenia, can be seen in immunocompromised patients, those with cancer or those with a very severe infection.

Leucopenia

Low WBC count $<3.7 \times 10^9$/L, caused by typhoid, viral infections.

(Blay 2011)

Leucocytosis

Elevated WBC count $>11 \times 10^9$/L, caused by a multitude of infections, e.g., meningitis, influenza, autoimmune diseases or mechanical bowel perforation.

(Blay 2011)

Basophils

The main function of basophils (see Figure 12.5) is to promote inflammation, but they are also involved in anaphylactic reactions. Basophils can leave the bloodstream to enter sites of tissue damage; when they do this, they transform into mast cells. Mast cells are found in connective tissue and in the mucosa and release **histamine** and **heparin**. Heparin is an anticoagulant and contributes to the inflammatory response, and histamine is a vasoactive amine causing vasodilation of the arteriole/capillary vascular bed and enlargement of the intracellular pores in the capillary membrane. This increases pooling of blood in the area of tissue damage. The systemic vascular resistance is lowered, which manifests as hypotension or low blood pressure if a significant area of capillary bed is affected. In response to this, the patient develops a tachycardia. In anaphylactic reactions, histamine release increases vascular capillary permeability, causing local **oedema**, which may exacerbate breathing problems and potentially cause obstruction of the airway.

Eosinophils

Eosinophils are phagocytic in nature; they counteract the chemical effects of histamine to reduce the effects of the inflammatory response. They have a role in fighting parasitic worm invasion. Both basophils and eosinophils have low cell counts unless activated by pathogens (see Figure 12.5).

Mononuclear cells

There are two main types of mononuclear cell (agranulocytes): monocytes and lymphocytes (see Figure 12.5); they have very little granular matter. The mature form of the monocyte that has left the bone marrow is a macrophage. Macrophages can survive for many months; they are phagocytic in nature and leave the bloodstream to enter tissues in later stages of infection. Macrophages release chemicals such as prostaglandins, complement, interferon and cytokines such as tumour necrosis factor (TNF), which are important in stimulating T and B lymphocytes as part of the innate immune response.

Macrophage from Greek: *macro* = big, *phage* = eat.

Dendritic cells

These are modified phagocytic monocytes or antigen-presenting cells (APCs). They, with similarly acting white cells, form the link between the innate and adaptive immune systems. They have an important function in ingesting pathogens and then placing the foreign antigens into their own cell membrane. This process triggers the adaptive immune system when they enter the lymph nodes searching for the lymphocytes that match the antigen.

Natural killer cells

These are large granular lymphocytes, belonging to the natural defences and innate immunity; their origin is unknown, and they have no memory; they constitute <1% of the total leucocyte count and are activated by interferon and cytokines. Natural killer (NK) cells are like vigilantes, killing indiscriminately by releasing chemicals and enzymes that target the invader cell membranes, damaging the membrane and causing holes to appear. They naturally kill all manner of cells from cancer cells, viruses and even body cells if the host's cell is infected with a virus. Natural killer cells also stimulate the inflammatory response by releasing chemicals.

Interferons

Interferons were first discovered in 1957. There are three types of these naturally occurring antiviral agents, α-interferon (IFN-α) (β-interferon (IFN-(β) and γ-interferon (INF-γ). They belong to the family of cytokines and are produced in response to viral infections by T cells. Interferons have myriad complex actions that ultimately inhibit viral replication and transcription phases, alter the production of proteins and cell functions and mediate other immune responses.

The complement system

The complement system is part of the innate and adaptive immune response; it is involved in the destruction (lysis) of bacteria, caused by the combination of antibody and protein activation in the blood. Like all cascade systems, it provides a rapid and augmented response. The proteins are inactive until triggered by pathogens. There are at least 20 proteins involved in the complement system. Some of them are labelled as follows; C1–C9, factors B, D and P. There are other proteins included in the system, e.g., regulatory proteins, that are not usually specifically identified (Colbert et al. 2012). There are two pathways: the classical pathway and the alternative pathway. The classical pathway is activated by forming an antigen–antibody complex as previously described. Once this has formed, one of the proteins from the complement system attaches itself to the complex; this is called complement fixation (Colbert et al. 2012). The alternative pathway is the interaction between bacterial membrane surfaces and factors B, D and P. The complement pathway is a sequential cascade system amplifying the immune response to bring about a variety of mechanisms with the aim to cause bacterial death or lysis. The following mechanisms also assist with this process:

- The process of *opsonisation* prepares the bacteria by coating the antigen with opsonin; this enables phagocytic cells to attach more quickly to begin the process of phagocytosis.
- The release of chemicals or *chemotaxis* by white blood cells and microorganisms attracts macrophages and other phagocytes to the pathogens like bees to a honeypot.

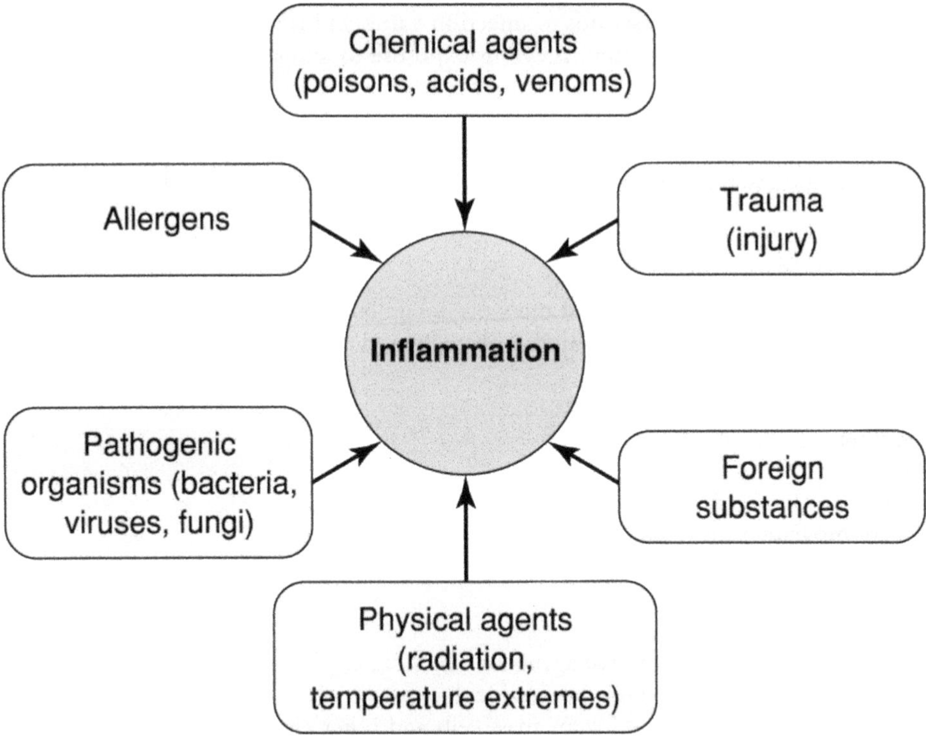

Figure 12.6 Causes of the inflammatory response.

- Inducing localised, and in severe cases systemic *inflammation* is essential to activate and convey white blood cells and platelets to the area so that the process of removing pathogens and cell debris can begin.

There are several causes that trigger the inflammatory response: see Figure 12.6 to review the aetiologies. Inflammation is part of our innate immunity response, playing an important part in our adaptive immunity.

C-reactive protein (CRP)

C-reactive protein (CRP) is a blood protein and member of the class of acute phase proteins (Goering et al. 2013). It increases dramatically during inflammation and is therefore one of the inflammatory markers used to identify **sepsis** and **infection**. CRP is synthesised by the liver and therefore its production is reduced in liver disease. Normal CRP levels are below 3.0mg/L, but can vary from lab to lab. The level can be raised to between 40–200mg/L in the presence of active bacterial infection and inflammation. In severe infections, the levels can be more than 200mg/L. Some types of bacterium, dying or dead cells release a substance called phosphocholine; CRP binds to this so that the complement system can be activated. It also enhances macrophage phagocytosis and opsonisation processes, as previously described.

Activation of the immune system

The way in which the body responds to infection varies and is related to several factors, such as our own genetic disposition, previous exposure to antigens and the pathogenicity or virulence of the organism. Inflammatory responses also vary: some individuals may exhibit an excessive immunological response which can cause many problems and, in some cases, may actually lead to death, such as in **anaphylaxis** or hypersensitivity to allergens. Inflammation is another innate immune response and is described below.

Inflammatory response

The inflammatory response is a natural and well-documented tissue response to a number of agents (see Figure 12.6). Inflammation is characterised by the following clinical signs:

- Redness of the skin or erythema.
- Swelling.
- Heat.
- Pain.
- Loss of movement or reduced function.

Pathophysiology of inflammation

On exposure to one of the causative agents of infection, capillaries surrounding damaged tissues and cells become increasingly permeable due to a variety of mechanisms. IgE mediates histamine release from basophils or mast cells and other chemical mediators such as 5-hdroxytryptamine, and bradykinins from neutrophils and prostaglandins released by the injured tissues increase capillary vascular permeability, ultimately causing arteriolar vasodilation. This increased blood supply to the damaged area and chemoattractants released by tissue damage encourage neutrophils and other cells to the site to begin the process of phagocytosis. The metabolic activity of the inflammatory cells increases the temperature within the tissue creating heat; as the inflammatory process evolves, redness (erythema) or hyperaemia and swelling caused by oedema from the increased leakage of vascular fluid develops. Swelling and pain caused by the interaction of bradykinin and prostaglandins

Cytokines

Cytokines are secreted by certain cells of the immune system and have an effect on other cells. They can be seen as chemical messengers that help coordinate or improve the immune response. Key cytokines are:

- **Tumour necrosing factor** (TNF): a protein produced mainly by monocytes and macrophages, especially in response to endotoxins. It mediates inflammation and induces destruction of some tumour cells and the activation of white blood cells.
- **Interferon (IFN)**: a protein released in response to the entry of a virus; it has the ability to inhibit or interfere with virus replication. There are three types of interferons: alpha, beta, and gamma.
- **Interleukins (ILS)**: influence immune response by regulating cell growth, differentiation, and motility.

result in loss of movement or function. Toxins are diluted by the increase in fluid in the area and combined with the effect of complement proteins, lymphocytes and macrophages; microbes are contained and removed from affected tissues. Chemotaxis encourages more leucocytes into the area to neutralise and engulf pathogens and remove debris: as this progresses, a **fibrin** mesh is created to contain the spread of infection. Coating the antigens with opsonins and the effects of complement proteins enables macrophages to identify intruders for phagocytosis. The stimulation of cytokines, such as tumour necrosing factor, interferon and interleukins, which are secreted by certain cells of the immune system, has an effect on other cells and helps to coordinate or improve the immune response.

The acute inflammatory process can result in either the complete resolution of the infection and the return of normal function, or the acute phase moves into a chronic phase, with resistant infections, colonisation, scarring and pus-producing abscesses that become difficult to treat, often due to their inaccessibility. In addition, leukotrienes, a family of inflammatory mediators produced in leucocytes, can also help with the immune response, however, they can also induce asthma and other inflammatory disorders; as in the case of asthma, they can be released by mast cells and bring about bronchoconstriction.

Pathophysiology of fever

Changes in the body's ability to control its own temperature can occur when infection develops. Fever or **pyrexia** is derived from the Latin word *febris*, or febrile. Fever occurs when the body temporarily fails to maintain the temperature within normal limits. Fever accelerates tissue metabolism and the activity of defences. The set-point is elevated by 1–2°C and is a symptom of many medical conditions and one of the oldest indicators of disease. In response to a stimulus, such as inflammation or the release of endotoxins from bacteria, leucocytes release endogenous pyrogens, 'fire starters', or cytokines into the bloodstream. These chemicals act directly on the thermostat or 'set-point' in the hypothalamus, causing the release of prostaglandin and elevating or resetting the hypothalamic set-point to a higher level. However, hypothermia, a lower-than-normal body temperature, can occur and is often a bad sign, especially in sepsis. 20% of septic patients present with hypothermia rather than hyperthermia, making a drop in temperature an important sign to note. Sepsis patients with hypothermia have twice the mortality of those who are normothermic or pyrexial (Kushimoto et al. 2013; Drewry et al. 2015; Wiewel et al. 2016). The mechanism of sepsis-induced hypothermia, though, is poorly understood. Scientific literature suggests it is the dis-regulated inflammatory cytokine responses, as well as physiological alterations of the temperature regulation centre in the hypothalamus, that are responsible for this response.

Normal body temperature

Temperature has a narrow range: between 35.6–37.8°C, despite changes in air temperature.

Body temperature fluctuates 1°C in 24 hours, being at the lowest in the early morning and highest in the early evening.

Fever or pyrexia can be defined as the following:

- Low grade: 38–39°C.
- Moderate: 39– 40°C.
- High grade: more than 40°C.

Hyperpyrexia is defined as a temperature greater than 42°C and is classed as a medical emergency. A temperature above 41°C can result in convulsions or seizures; the upper limit for human life is 43°C, and at this point, proteins and cells denature and are unable to function normally.

Fever has several functions. Its primary aim is to increase the **basal metabolic rate** so that bacterial growth is inhibited; most organisms cannot tolerate extremes of temperature or temperatures in excess of 37°C. A raised temperature increases the rate of elimination of toxins, and tissue repair is heightened, all of which assist the body's defence mechanisms to fight invading pathogens. Eating is inhibited and proteins are denatured at higher temperatures, which can result in irreversible brain damage. An increase in temperature increases enzymatic reactions; thereby, each rise in temperature of 1°C can result in a 10% increase in cellular chemical reactions, an increase in the heart rate by 10 beats/minute and an increase in the respiratory rate.

THE STAGES OF FEVER

There are three stages in the life cycle of a fever:

- *Stage 1*: the cold or 'chilly' heat-generating stage.
- *Stage 2*: heat maintaining.
- *Stage 3*: the defervescence stage, where the thermostat has been reset to a lower level and the body now attempts to lose heat.

During the cold phase, heat-production mechanisms such as shivering and vasoconstriction are activated and conserve body heat. This may last for 10–40 minutes causing a rapid, steady rise in temperature. The basal metabolic rate (BMR), heart and respiratory rates are also increased. The patient can feel chilly and experience goose bumps, and sweating ceases.

The second stage is heat maintaining, the length of time spent in this phase depends on how long it takes to eradicate the pyrogen. Patients with severe infections and/or resistant microorganisms may remain in this phase for several weeks. The body now attempts to balance heat loss and heat-production mechanisms. The patient is flushed, hot, tachycardic, thirsty and possibly tachypnoeic. They may complain of headache and loss of appetite. Some patients may have a seizure. The hot stage ends when the cause of the fever has been eliminated, resulting in a decrease in the hypothalamic set-point to normal.

The final stage is the defervescence, or heat-dissipating stage; this is when the hypothalamic set-point is returning to normal. The body now employs the heat-loss mechanisms of vasodilation, sweating and inhibition of heat-producing mechanisms to lower the temperature. The patient usually feels hot during this phase.

CAUSES OF FEVER

There are many causes of fever:

- Infection, e.g., bacterial, viral, fungal or protozoan.
- Autoimmune diseases such as lupus erythaematous.
- Inflammatory bowel disease.
- The breakdown of red blood cells, or **haemolysis**, from surgery can induce a temperature postoperatively.
- Myocardial infarction.

- Crush syndrome as a result of rhabdomyolysis.
- Drugs can also cause a 'drug fever', either as a direct consequence of the drug or as an adverse reaction to the drug (e.g., allergic reaction to antibiotics). Discontinuation of some drugs, for example heroin withdrawal, can induce a fever.

Adaptive immunity

Adaptive or specific immunity is the second line of defence. Once the natural defences have been breached or failed to control the invasion, the immune system attempts to instigate containment and control by limiting the spread of infection and ultimately destroying the pathogens. The cells involved in providing this defence are lymphocytes and macrophages, which contain the body's memory bank. Adaptive immunity is long-lasting, but can be affected by the ability of microorganisms to change and adapt so that they are not recognised by the immune system. It is important to appreciate that the response of the immune system depends on the nature of the infection or antigen, the route of entry into the body and the individual response, which varies between individuals and populations. The response can be systemic or localised to one region, organ or tissue. For the purposes of clarity, the humoral and cell-mediated branches of the adaptive immune system will be considered separately.

Antibodies are the substances that bind to the antigens.
Antigens are substances that stimulate the host's lymphoid cells and tissues to mount a specific direct response to the antigen and not to an unrelated substance.

Antibodies

The memory of previous pathogens or antigens is contained within antibodies, which have specific sites that recognise past exposure to an antigen. Antibodies are soluble gamma globulin proteins that are classed as immunoglobulins. Their function is to hold the 'memory' of previously experienced pathogens and to recognise them.

Antibodies are large proteins produced by B lymphocytes, of which there are five classes: IgA, IgD, IgE, IgG, IgM.

All have different functions, are slightly different in structure and are found in different parts of the body. They are stimulated in response to foreign antigens. The most abundant is IgG and the largest is IgM (see Table 12.1).

Humoral immunity

B cells or B lymphocytes are responsible for humoral or antibody-mediated immunity and form part of the adaptive immune response. There are two types of B cell:

- Plasma cells, which produce antibodies; the primary response.
- Memory B cells, stored in lymph nodes, which remember pathogens, allowing a much faster response to a second or subsequent exposure to the pathogen; the secondary response (see Figure 12.7) (Colbert et al. 2012).

When an antigen or 'foreign' substance is detected, B cells or plasma cells (found in lymphoid tissue) are stimulated to secrete large quantities of antibodies, which bind to specific antigens, forming the antigen–antibody complex. Each antibody has a specific adapter

Table 12.1 Immunoglobin classes

Class	*Generalised structure*	*Where found*	*Biological function*
IgD		Virtually always attached to B cell.	Believed to be cell surface receptor of immunocompetent B cell; important in activation of B cell.
IgM	J chain	Attached to B cell; free in plasma.	When bound to B cell membrane, serves as antigen receptor; first Ig class *released* to plasma by plasma cells during primary response; potent agglutinating agent; fixes complement.
IgG		Most abundant antibody in plasma; represents 75% to 85% of circulating antibodies.	Main antibody of both primary and secondary responses; crosses placenta and provides passive immunity to foetus; fixes complement.
IgA	J chain	Some (monomer) in plasma; dimer in secretions such as saliva, tears, intestinal juice and milk.	Bathes and protects mucosal surfaces from attachment of pathogens.
IgE		Secreted by plasma cells in skin, mucosae of gastrointestinal and respiratory tracts and tonsils.	Binds to mast cells and basophils and triggers release of histamine and other chemicals that mediate inflammation and certain allergic responses.

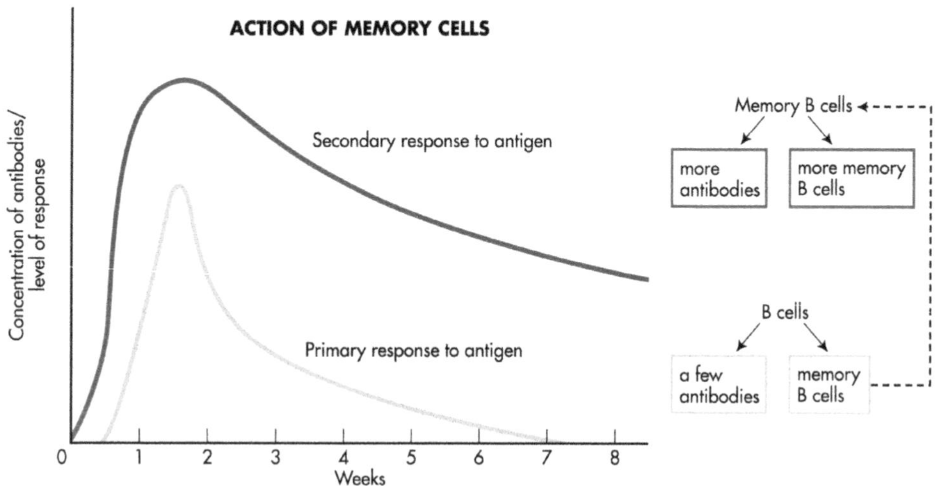

Figure 12.7 Primary and secondary responses to antigen.

site, epitope, or 'lock', that fits a particular antigen, or 'key'. Each antibody recognises the shape of the antigen to which they are programmed to bind.

Antibodies or immunoglobulins have a number of functions and effects:

- On activation, they bind to the pathogen, causing clumping or agglutination.
- Once bound, they act as opsonins, identifying or signalling that particular antigen for phagocytosis.
- Binding triggers the production of identical plasma cells or clones, which all produce the same antibody; this is called clonal expansion.
- Phagocytosis and the complement cascade system are also activated.

Antibodies are unable to enter cells; therefore, in viral infections, they can be ineffective, especially against viruses that spread directly from cell to cell. Antibodies can bind to the surface of infected host cells via epitopes, which may affect the viral replication processes. Antibodies can also block the virus attaching to the host cell; this reduces the likelihood of penetration and accumulation of the virus and limits infection spread. If the virus is conveyed via the bloodstream, then the virus can be neutralised before it reaches its target organ, e.g., poliovirus (Stewart 2012). The common cold (coryza) virus targets the respiratory mucosa. Antibodies are ineffective against the virus, as they are not present in the mucosa membranes and secretions.

Experiencing a childhood disease such as chickenpox, caused by the *Varicella zoster* virus, produces antibodies and renders the body immune to chicken pox via the humoral immunity system. Unfortunately, there is limited immunity from the common cold, as we do not possess antibodies to all the viruses that can cause the common cold.

Cell-mediated immunity

T cells are produced by the red bone marrow and matured in the thymus gland. The four main types of differentiated T cell are:

- T helper inducer T cells (T4).
- Cytotoxic T cells (T8).
- Memory T cells.

Regulatory (formerly known as suppressor cells) T cells (T8) make up about 80% of all lymphocytes and are activated when an antigen binds to the T cell surface receptor site. They then undergo rapid proliferation and

differentiation into one of the following, depending on the nature of the antigen:

- T helper cells respond by secretion of interleukins or messenger proteins, promoting the proliferation of B lymphocytes, other T lymphocytes and natural killer cells to phagocytose.
- T helper cells also promote the maturation of B cells and T lymphocytes, once interleukins have been released.
- Cytotoxic T cells recognise and destroy cells infected by viruses and cells altered by cancer.

- Memory cells continue to exist after an infection has resolved. They remember antigens and quickly expand if the infection is encountered again.
- T suppressor or regulatory cells downregulate the immune response when the objective has been achieved.

Autoimmunity

The immune system is a complex and dynamic system, in which the ability to recognise 'self ', i.e. the body's own cells and tissues, is hugely important. Failures in this mechanism, which are multifactorial, can lead to the development of autoimmune diseases such as systemic lupus erythematosus (SLE). Other abnormal responses mediated by the immune system are allergic reactions to blood products, antibiotics and other allergens. The suppression of the immune system post-tissue and -organ transplantation is essential in order to prevent rejection of 'foreign' tissue. With age, the immune system is less efficient, and therefore, older people become more prone to cancer and other diseases. This may be one of the reasons why there is an increase in malignancy as we get older. The role of the immune system in the development of malignancy is part of ongoing research into cancer (Michaud, Houseman and Marsit 2015).

Microorganisms

There are several organisms that can cause serious illness and even death. Understanding and appreciating the properties of microorganisms can only enhance knowledge and assist practitioners in understanding how healthcare-associated infections (HCAI) may occur and our role as nurses in reducing the risk to patients.

Even though humans have daily contact with millions of bacteria and viruses, the effectiveness of natural defences and immunity systems results in very few serious infections or diseases. To understand the nature of infection and sepsis, it is important to have some understanding of the important bacteria, viruses, fungi and protozoa that affect patients. It must be remembered that the influence of foreign travel will also predispose travellers to other infections that are not common to Western Europe. This section is designed to give a brief overview of common organisms seen in UK hospitals and not the vast array of other microbes seen around the world.

Commonly used terms

It is helpful to review the meaning of commonly used terms related to microbiology and infection.

- *Contamination*: soiling of inanimate objects or living material, e.g., medical equipment, with potentially harmful infectious matter. Wounds are considered contaminated if there are organisms on the surface of the wound bed but there is no replication or host response. Contamination can easily be removed with appropriate wound cleansing or environmental decontamination.
- *Colonisation*: presence of multiplying organisms in the tissue producing no or only minimal host response. Unlike the above, colonised organisms are not easily removed with standard wound cleansing, however, as long as the wound is managed appropriately, this does not adversely affect wound healing.

- *Infection*: presence of a microorganism in the tissues that causes a host response and classic signs and symptoms, including, redness, heat, swelling and temperature.
- *Bacteraemia*: the presence of bacteria in the bloodstream, which may not result in symptoms, as the immune system is able to clear the bacteria. It may result from ordinary activities such as vigorous toothbrushing, or from infections such as pneumonia or a urinary tract infection that travels and seeds itself in the blood.
- *Septicemia*: a serious bloodstream infection (also known as blood poisoning) that occurs when a bacterial infection elsewhere in the body, such as the lungs or skin, enters the bloodstream.
- *Sepsis*: is defined as life-threatening organ dysfunction caused by a **dysregulated host response to infection**. Organ dysfunction risk can be identified as an acute change in total SOFA score ≥2 points, consequent to the infection (Singer et al. 2016).
- *Pathogenicity*: the capacity of an organism to cause disease.
- *Virulence*: the ability power of an organism to cause disease. This is dependent on how large the inoculation dose is and the ability of the microorganism to invade the host's defences.
- *Hospital*, or '*nosocomial*' *infection*: an infection acquired by patients or hospital staff in a hospital setting.
- *Nosocomial infection*: an American term used to describe an infection acquired by patients or hospital staff in a hospital setting.
- *Healthcare-associated infection (HCAI)*: a more recent and broader term that acknowledges modern day healthcare occurs in a range of settings, not just a hospital, and is defined as infection that occurs as a result of contact with the healthcare system in its widest sense – from care provided in a person's own home to general practice, nursing home care and care in acute hospitals.
- *Cross-* or *exogenous infection*: infection transferred from the clinical environment, including surfaces and equipment as well as staff, other patients and visitors.
- *Self-* or *endogenous*: infection caused by microbes that the patient carries, our own normal bacterial flora.
- *Source*: a place where pathogenic organisms are growing, e.g., food poisoning from contaminated food or a collection of pus within a cavity or tissues.
- *Reservoir*: a place where pathogens can survive and then be transferred to patients directly or indirectly, e.g., blood pressure cuffs that have been inadequately cleaned prior to use on patients, but is not where they originally came from.

Classification of microorganisms

Microorganisms are classified according to their structure and shape or **morphology**, spore-forming or slime-producing properties. The main classes of microorganisms that are associated with or are medically important to humans are viruses, bacteria, protozoa, fungi and moulds and parasitic worms. Although not microscopic the last group come under the general heading of microbiology.

A group of infectious proteins called prions are also included because of their microscopic and infectious nature. The proteins remain controversial, but are implicated in a number of encephalopathies such as variant Creutzfeldt–Jakob disease (see Table 12.2).

Table 12.2 Microorganisms: structure and examples

Microorganism	*Structure/characteristics*	*Examples and diseases*
Viruses	• Smaller than bacteria and can only be seen under an electron microscope, varying in size from 10–300nm. • Contain a strand of nucleic acid, either DNA or RNA, which is enclosed in a protein coat or capsid. • Viruses replicate inside the host cell and contain few enzymes.	*Herpesviridae* family causes: • Herpes simplex. • *Varicella zoster* (chickenpox and shingles). • Cytomegalovirus. • Hepatitis B virus. • Papovaviruses associated with malignancy (cervical cancer). • Retroviruses which cause HIV (HTLV-1) causing AIDS. Some of the most serious infections known to man are caused by filovirus, which causes Ebola and Marburg viruses.
Bacteria	Bacteria are classified according to four main properties including their shape, which is divided into the following: • Cocci (spherical). • Bacilli (rod-shaped). • Coccobacilli (short rods). • Spiral-shaped (spirochetes). Other determinants include: 1 Whether they require oxygen (obligate aerobes). 2 Not requiring oxygen (obligate anaerobes). 3 Gram stain, either gram positive or gram negative. 4 Those that are acid/alcohol fast such as *Mycobacterium*, of which the most important human pathogen is *M. tuberculosis*, or TB. 5 Bacteria that form spores, such as *Clostridioides difficile*.	• *Staphylococcus aureus* (Gram-positive), causes superficial and deep tissue infections. • *Streptococci pneumoniae* causes meningitis, pneumonia, septicaemia. • *Clostridioides spp.*, Gram-positive bacilli producing spores and are anaerobic, causes gas gangrene and muscle infections, tetany. • Chlamydia, sexually transmitted infection. Important Gram-negatives: • *Pseudomonas aeruginosa* (pneumonia in CF), opportunistic infection producing blue-green distinctive pus. • *Escherichia coli*, Gram-negative bacillus causing meningitis, septicaemia and commonly urinary tract infections (UTI). • *Shigella*, causes mild dysentery. • *Klebsiella*, causes UTI wounds infections.
Protozoa	Unicellular animals.	e.g., *Plasmodium spp.*, which causes malaria.
Fungi	Classification is based on reproductive and morphology characteristics.	• Immunocompromised patients are very susceptible to *Candida albicans* (thrush) and, more recently, Candida auris. • *Aspergillus* can cause a serious lung infection. • *Cryptococcus* is associated with HIV infections.
Prions	Proteins without their own nucleic acid, resistant to heat and chemical disinfectants.	Transmissible spongiform encephalopathies (TSE) are rare neurological degenerative conditions causing dementia and destruction of brain tissue, e.g., the fatal Creutzfeldt–Jakob disease (CJD), related to bovine spongiform encephalopathy (BSE).

Gram staining to aid identification

Bacteria are classified in a number of different ways. In the laboratory, they are stained using a Gram stain; Gram-positive organisms will retain the dye and stain a deep violet colour, and Gram-negative organisms lose the violet stain but appear pink, as they take up a red counter-stain as part of the gram-staining process. The staining process is useful because the Gram-positive and Gram-negative organisms respond to different antibiotics.

Vulnerability to infection

Normally the immune system's complex mechanisms are extremely effective at maintaining health by destroying invading pathogens. However, there are a number of factors that increase vulnerability to infections, and these high-risk groups require close monitoring to detect early signs of infection. Risk relates to both the patient and to treatment-related factors (see Table 12.3). These vulnerable groups are at high risk from developing infection, both in the community and in the hospital setting. Once infection has developed, the greater the chance the patient will go on to develop sepsis, where the patient's immune system is overwhelmed and cannot mount a sufficient response to overcome the infection, and the patient goes into **septic shock**. Septic shock is associated with a high mortality rate of around 40 percent.

Healthcare-associated infection (HCAI)

It is estimated that about 1 in 7 patients develops an infection during a stay in a hospital in the UK (English surveillance programme for antimicrobial utilisation report [ESPAUR] 2017). The consequences of this for the patient are unpleasant, increasing their length of stay, causing pain, distress, loss of earnings and reducing their chances of a completely successful recovery. Whilst not all HCAI can be avoided, it has been estimated that 15–30% could be, with everyone in health care having a role to play in infection reduction.

A particular challenge for England was *Clostridioides* (name changed in 2016 from *Clostridium*) *difficile* and MRSA, with a government strategy focusing on these infections; however, more recently, Gram-negative microorganisms causing HCAIs are of greater

Table 12.3 Risk factors for infection and sepsis

Patient-related factors	*Treatment-related factors*
Extremes of age.	Recent surgical intervention.
Chronic illness, for example, diabetes, cancer, COPD.	Presence of invasive devices.
	Trauma.
Nutritional status.	Invasive diagnostic procedures.
History of infections.	Use of some drug therapies, such as steroids,
Immunosuppression.	antibiotics, cytotoxic agents.
Neutropenia.	Being a hospital inpatient.
Drug or alcohol abuse.	
Splenectomy.	

Source: Johnson and Henry (2013). In Morton, P. G. and Fontaine, D. K. (eds) *Critical Care Nursing: A Holistic Approach*, 11th ed. Philadelphia: Wolters Kluwer Health

concern, and a less targeted approach should be taken to ensure effective infection control measures aim to reduce all HCAIs (Public Health England/NHS Improvement 2017). The EPIC 3 guidelines (Loveday et al. 2014) consider standard principles for infection prevention, focusing on five areas:

1. Hospital environmental hygiene.
2. Hand hygiene.
3. Use of personal protective equipment.
4. Safe use and disposal of sharps.
5. Asepsis (new).

Evidence of contamination of the hospital environment, with pathogens of the same strain of microorganisms colonising patients, clearly indicates the importance of hospital environmental hygiene. Shared clinical equipment, such as stethoscopes and commodes, are all potential sources for contamination, so it is essential that equipment is washed thoroughly with detergent and water, or, if in an outbreak situation, hypochlorite should be considered (Loveday et al. 2014). While actual evidence of transmission of infection from the environment is not strong, it is logical to surmise that hand contamination from the environment will increase the spread of microorganisms.

Hand hygiene, with seemingly simple basic measures such as hand-washing, is widely regarded as one of the most effective ways of reducing HCAI (Gould et al. 2017), but audit demonstrates that poor hand-washing frequency and technique is often practiced by health care professionals (Gould et al. 2017). The World Health Organisation's '5 moments for hand hygiene' (WHO 2009) indicates moments where hand hygiene should occur for all health care professionals involved in direct patient contact (see Figure 12.8). Clear guidance for the procedures of hand washing and use of hand rub have been devised by the WHO (2009) and can be accessed at http://www.who.int/gpsc/tools/GPSC-HandRub-Wash.pdf.

The use of personal protective equipment such as gloves has been shown to reduce the transmission of microorganisms. It must be remembered, though, that contamination is still possible, especially during glove removal, so good hand-washing technique is still essential to prevent infection transmission (Loveday et al. 2014). Gloves are single-use items and are changed between caring for different patients. Plastic aprons are also used for a single episode of care, and disposed of as clinical waste.

Safe disposal of sharps is essential to prevent risk of blood-borne viruses such as:

- Hepatitis B virus.
- Hepatitis C virus.
- Human immunodeficiency virus (HIV).

Sharps disposal:

- Minimal handling, do not pass from hand to hand.
- Do not recap needles before disposal.
- Use sharps container, do not overfill.
- Sharps bins to be placed out of reach of children.
- Clinical and non-clinical staff need education regarding sharps disposal.

(Loveday et al. 2014)

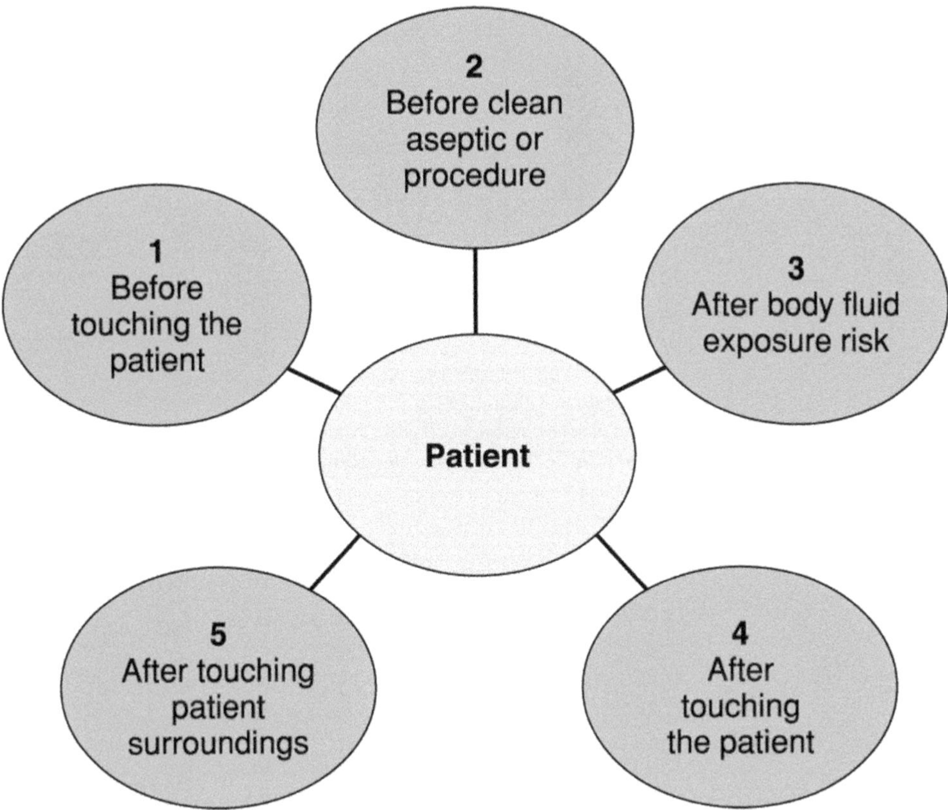

Figure 12.8 WHO 5 moments for hand hygiene. *Source*: adapted from WHO (2009).

Saving lives, high-impact interventions (HII) (DH 2017, 4th edition)

High-impact interventions (HII), first introduced in 2005, are an evidence-based approach to key clinical procedures or care processes that can reduce the risk of infection. Specific clinical activities, in the form of care bundles, have been developed to guide and audit areas of practice. A care bundle is a group of critical elements in a care process: when all elements are performed, this is associated with an improved outcome. Current HIIs related to infection control have been updated in 2017 (and are available at http://hcai.dh.gov.uk/whatdoido/high-impact-interventions/) and include:

1. Prevention of ventilator-associated pneumonia.
2. Prevention of infections associated with peripheral vascular access devices.
3. Prevention of infection associated with central venous access devices.
4. Prevention of surgical site infection.
5. Prevention of infections in chronic wounds.
6. Prevention of urinary catheter-associated infections.
7. Promotion of stewardship in antimicrobial prescribing.

Table 12.4 Central venous catheter bundle, ongoing care

1 Hand hygiene	• Decontamination immediately prior to and after every episode of patient contact, using the correct hand hygiene technique (World Health Organization's '5 moments of hand hygiene' or the NPSA 'Clean your hands campaign' is recommended).
2 Site inspection	• The site is inspected daily for any signs of infection, and this noted in the patient's record.
3 Dressing	• Use of an intact, dry, adherent transparent dressing. • Insertion site must be cleaned with 2% chlorhexidine gluconate in 70% isopropyl alcohol before the dressing is changed.
4 Catheter injection ports	• Injection ports are covered by caps or valved connectors.
5 Catheter access	• Aseptic technique is implemented for all access to the line. • Ports or hubs are cleaned with 2% chlorhexidine gluconate in 70% isopropyl alcohol before accessing catheters. • The line is to be flushed with 0.9% sodium chloride for lumens that are in frequent use.
6 Administration set replacement	• Set is replaced immediately after the administration of any blood/blood products. • The set is replaced after 24 hours following total parenteral nutrition (if this contains lipids). • Set is replaced within 72 hours of all other fluid sets.
7 Catheter replacement	• Catheter is removed when no longer required or a decision not to remove has been recorded. • Details of removal to be documented in the records (including date, location, and signature and name of operator undertaking removal).

Source: Department of Health (2017), High Impact Intervention: Central venous catheter care bundle, London: DH, pp. 2–3. Available at http://hcai.dh.gov.uk/ files/2011/03/2011-03-14-HII.

The central venous catheter care (ongoing care) bundle is shown in Figure 12.4, and is paired with a central line insertion care bundle. Each element of the bundle needs to be completed, and this can be audited to evaluate compliance. Bloodstream infections associated with central venous catheters are a major cause of morbidity (DH 2017), with 42.3% of bloodstream infections being central line-related. The care bundle is based on the EPIC guidelines (Loveday et al. 2014), and when all the elements of the bundle are performed, the risk of infection is reduced (DH 2017). Compliance with care bundles involves all health care disciplines, and a cohesive, consistent approach is required to reduce the burden of infection.

Acute problems related to the immune system

Hypersensitivity or allergic reactions

An allergen is defined as an antigen that causes an allergic reaction. The reaction may be immediate (within minutes of exposure) or delayed, depending on previous exposure, and the type of allergen, for example snake venom or insect stings. If left untreated, it can cause severe shock and circulatory collapse within 10–15 minutes. Anaphylaxis is not uncommon, incidences are rising, but death from anaphylaxis is very rare; there are approximately 20 deaths in the UK per annum from anaphylaxis (National Institute for Health and Care Excellence 2011).

Anaphylaxis is defined as an acute and rapid onset of illness with common skin manifestations, such as a urticarial rash, erythema, flushing of the skin and angioedema; there is also involvement of the respiratory, cardiovascular and gastrointestinal systems, as typically there is acute onset of bronchospasm, upper airway obstruction and hypotension; these may occur without the presence of typical skin changes (Australian Society of Clinical Immunology and Allergy 2016).

There are four types of hypersensitivity reaction: types I, II and III are mediated by antibodies and are classified as below (Weston 2013), and type IV are mediated by T cells:

- Type I (anaphylaxis, asthma and eczema).
- Type II involves IgM and IgG – caused by cytotoxic reactions which damage cells and tissues of the host, e.g., a blood transfusion reaction.
- Type III hypersensitivity reactions occur when the antibody–antigen complexes of IgM and or IgG cause inflammatory reactions within the tissues or bloodstream.
- Type IV hypersensitivity reactions are mediated by T cells and may occur over a number of hours after exposure to the allergen, e.g., eczema skin reactions occur over a number of days.

The response to an allergen is mediated by the immunoglobulin IgE. During the primary exposure, plasma cells produce large quantities of IgE which binds to mast cells. On subsequent exposure, the allergen attaches itself to the IgE antibodies on the mast cell surface; this causes the mast cells to degranulate, releasing histamine and triggering the hypersensitivity reaction, inducing a variety of effects such as allergic rhinitis or a runny nose (see Figure 12.9).

The most severe form and medical emergency is anaphylaxis – 'a severe life-threatening, generalised or systemic hypersensitivity reaction' (Resuscitation Council 2008). There are multiple triggers ranging from antibiotics and muscle relaxants to peanuts and other foods, insect stings and venom from snake bites. In children, food allergies tend to be the most common culprits. Health care practitioners who administer blood transfusions, human albumin solutions or gelatins (e.g., gelofusine), X-ray contrast media and intravenous (IV) antibiotics should be alert to the early signs of anaphylaxis, as the IV route is the fastest trigger, causing reactions within seconds.

Other culprits, especially in the elderly, are aspirin and non-steroidal anti-inflammatory drugs (NSAIDs). Many cases are not mediated by IgE and are termed idiopathic, i.e. the causative allergen is not identified (RCUK 2008).

Clinical signs and symptoms

Not all patients who have an allergic reaction will go on to develop anaphylaxis, and not all reactions are detected. Skin reactions such as urticaria (raised lumps or hives) and erythema (reddening of the skin caused by increased capillary blood flow) are common in about 80% of reactions; gastrointestinal symptoms may also be present, such as vomiting and abdominal pain (RCUK 2008).

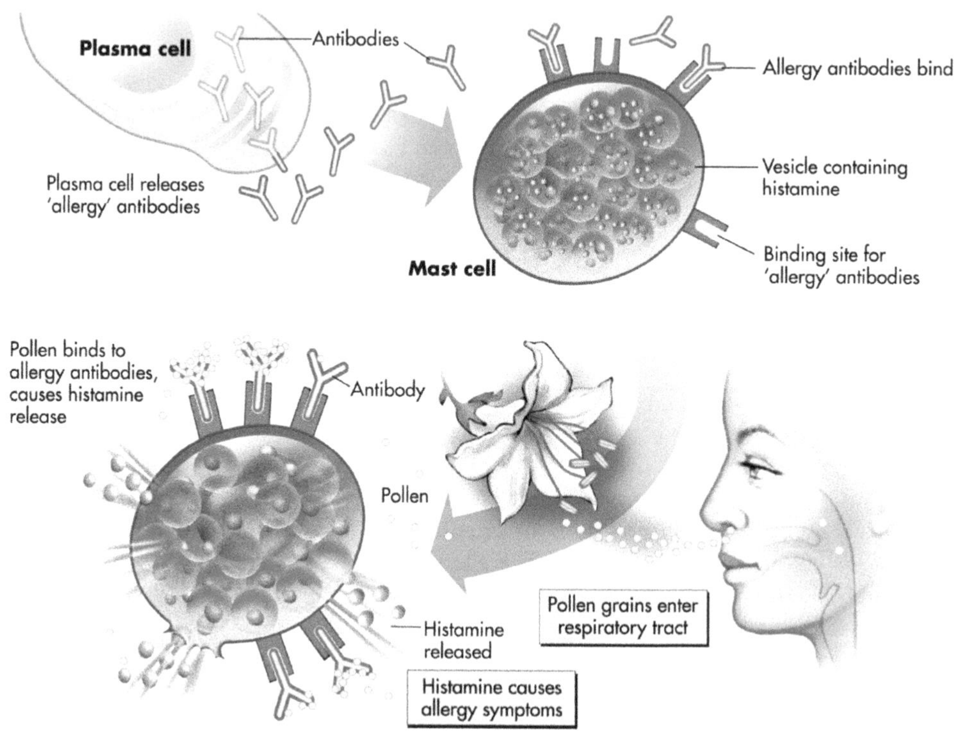

Figure 12.9 An example of local allergic reaction, allergic rhinitis.

Anaphylaxis is likely when all three of the following conditions are present together and the onset of symptoms is within a few minutes of exposure:

- Sudden onset and rapid progression of symptoms.
- Life-threatening airway and/or breathing and/or circulation problems.
- Skin and/or mucosal changes (flushing, urticaria, angioedema).

The patient will start to complain of feeling very unwell; they may become agitated and restless and may state that they have a feeling of an impending sense of doom. The symptoms, if left untreated, may rapidly progress to respiratory and cardiac arrest and death.

Rapid assessment

The patient should be rapidly assessed using the ABCDE approach. Questions should be direct and closed-ended if the patient can only answer in short sentences or singular words; the purpose is to elicit the nature of the problem, the allergen, if known, whether they have an adrenaline auto-injector or previous history of allergic reactions and how severely they may manifest. The preceding events or causative event is crucial in establishing the allergen. However, life-saving treatment such as oxygen, the administration of adrenaline and other anti-inflammatory drugs should not be delayed.

Signs and symptoms of anaphylaxis:

- Airway swelling.
- Hoarse voice.
- Stridor.
- Increased respiratory rate.
- Wheeze.
- Confusion (hypoxia).
- Central cyanosis (late sign).
- Respiratory arrest.
- Pale or flushed.
- Clammy.
- Tachycardic.
- Hypotensive.
- Dizziness/loss of consciousness.
- Cardiac arrest.
- Erythema.
- Urticaria.
- Angioedema.

Airway patency can be compromised due to rapidly swelling deep tissues of the mucus membranes and lips known as angioedema. Swelling of the tongue associated with oropharyngeal and laryngeal oedema may also threaten the airway. The patient's ability to swallow their own saliva should be assessed, and the development of a hoarse voice indicates partial airway obstruction. High-pitched inspiratory noise or **stridor** is caused by upper airway obstruction and should be immediately recognised and dealt with by summoning urgent help via the peri-arrest or cardiac arrest call systems. Under the direction of the medical team, intramuscular adrenaline and other pharmacology agents should be urgently administered. Worsening signs of airway obstruction include:

- Swelling of tongue and lips.
- Hoarseness.
- Oropharyngeal swelling.

Breathing assessment will reveal shortness of breath and respiratory difficulties. Bronchoconstriction causes wheezing, increasing the work of breathing and resulting in greater respiratory distress. Central cyanosis may be evident, although this is a late sign; the patient may become confused with the development of cerebral hypoxia. As the patient tires, respiratory arrest is possible.

Circulation

The cardiovascular system should be assessed for the following clinical signs:

- Tachycardia, with or without associated myocardial ischaemia (chest pain).
- Profound hypotension and dizziness due to peripheral vasodilation.
- Clammy, sweaty skin, flushed or pale skin depending on the reaction.

Remembering the processes for the inflammatory response, there will be increased capillary permeability leading to the sequestering of fluids in the tissues and giving rise to swelling and oedema. If left untreated, the patient may go on to develop cardiac arrest.

Disability

The neurological assessment under disability involves rapid assessment for confusion, agitation and reduced, or loss of, consciousness. An unconscious patient should already have been identified through the ABC assessment. A blood glucose should be checked, *but* should not delay or distract from more urgent, life-saving treatment, e.g., administration of adrenaline.

Exposure

Exposure of the patient is important, especially in allergic reactions, as there is a combination of both skin and mucosal changes in over 80% of reactions. The patient may complain of itchiness or urticaria from hives, or raised red lumps or weals.

The diagnosis and treatment of anaphylaxis

The priority for all health care practitioners is to recognise the early signs of allergy; know and institute the UK Resuscitation Council's anaphylaxis algorithm (2008) (see Figure 12.10), and begin aggressive treatment to prevent development of the complications of anaphylaxis.

If possible, the patient should be in a comfortable position, supine if hypotensive, or sitting up if experiencing breathing difficulties. The trigger, if known, should be removed or stopped, but this may not always be possible. Intramuscular (IM) adrenaline 1:1000 (0.5mL or 500mcgs), is the drug of choice. The best injection site is the outer aspect of the middle third of the thigh muscle, or the anterolateral aspect. Adrenaline is an alpha-receptor agonist, reversing the vasodilation, reducing oedema and dilating the bronchioles due to its beta-receptor agonist properties. Adrenaline also suppresses the release of histamine, thus reducing the vasodilatory effects. IM adrenaline can be administered, if required, every 5 minutes; the patient's response should be continuously monitored (RCUK 2008).

High-flow oxygen therapy, intravenous access and full cardiac monitoring should be established. The administration of a bolus of 500mL IV fluids and second line treatment of antihistamines such as chlorphenamine and steroids such as hydrocortisone, which shorten the reaction, should be given. Other considerations are treating for asthma-like symptoms that may involve the administration of nebulised salbutamol and ipratropium. Once the patient has stabilised, they need to be monitored closely in a critical care area for a period of time.

The nurse's role may be very varied, depending on experience. For the senior student or newly qualified nurse, it will be a supportive role, getting equipment and drugs, recording observations or, importantly, remaining with the patient and supporting and reassuring them. A more experienced nurse may cannulate the patient, prepare and administer intravenous fluids, administer the intramuscular adrenaline and carry out many other interventions.

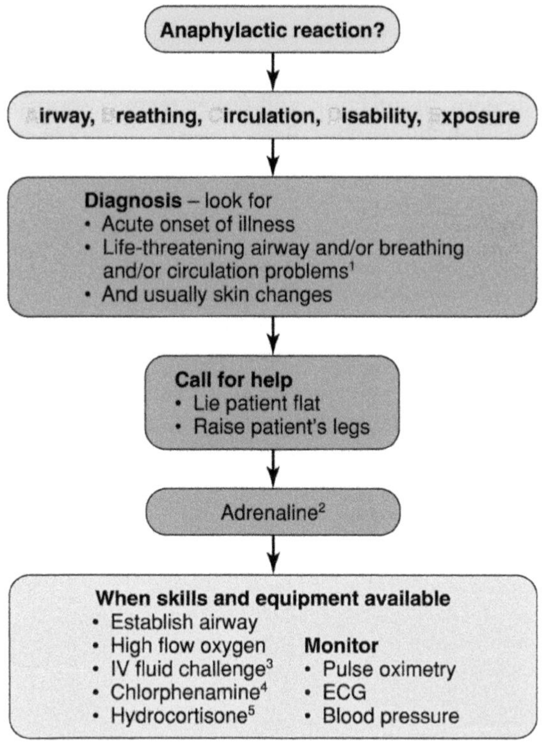

[1] **Life-threatening problems**
- **Airway:** swelling, hoarseness, stridor
- **Breathing:** rapid breathing, wheeze, fatigue, cyancsis, $SpO_2 < 92\%$, confusion
- **Circulation:** pale, clammy, low blood pressure, faintness, drowsy/coma

[2] **Adrenaline** (*give IM uniess experienced with IV adrenaline*)
IM doses of 1:1000 adrenaline (repeat after 5 min if no better)
- Adult 500 micrograms IM (0.5 mL)
- Child more than 12 years: 500 micrograms IM (0.5 mL)
- Child 6–12 years: 300 micrograms IM (0.3 mL)
- Child less than 6 years: 150 micrograms IM (0.15 mL)

Adrenaline IV to be given **only by experienced specialists**
Titrate: Adults 50 micrograms; Children 1 microgram/kg

[3] **IV fluid challenge**
Adult – 500–1000 mL
Child – crystalloid 20 mL/kg

Stop IV colloid if this might be the cause of anaphylaxis

	[4] **Chlorphenamine** (IM or slow IV)	[5] **Hydrocortisone** (IM or slow IV)
Adult or child more than 12 years	10 mg	200 mg
Child 6–12 years	5 mg	100 mg
Child 6 months to 6 years	2.5 mg	50 mg
Child less than 6 months	250 micrograms/kg	25 mg

Figure 12.10 Anaphylaxis algorithm.

Source: Resuscitation Council UK (2008) Emergency Treatment of Anaphylactic Reactions: Guidelines for Healthcare Providers. Reproduced with kind permission of the Resuscitation Council (UK).

Infection, sepsis and septic shock

Incidence

Infection can often be identified by a number of symptoms related to the infection source. The majority of individuals with an infection will either recover spontaneously or with appropriate rest, antibiotics and fluids. This demonstrates the body's well-developed immune response is appropriately regulated to respond effectively to injury/infection (Dutton and Finch 2018).

Sepsis is a global concern; it is estimated to be the leading cause of mortality and critical illness worldwide. In the United Kingdom, it is estimated that 37,000 patients die from sepsis every year, while on an international level, sepsis can cause approximately six million deaths every year, most of which are preventable (WHO 2017; NCEPOD 2015). The incidence of sepsis is increasing, most likely due to aging populations with comorbidities and greater recognition. Patients who survive sepsis often have long-term physical, psychological, and cognitive disabilities, with significant health and social care implications. Sepsis is a major cause of avoidable death in our hospitals, as early recognition and appropriate management in the initial hours after sepsis develops markedly improves outcomes. Sepsis presents a major challenge for all healthcare professionals, in terms of recognising and diagnosing infection, identifying the sepsis risk, and in the optimal and timely management of the condition with the health care resources available to them.

Definition of sepsis

Definitions of sepsis have changed over time as understanding of the condition has developed. The terms 'septicaemia' and 'blood poisoning' are often used in the public domain, but a precise universal definition is helpful for health care professionals to ensure the approach to recognition, diagnosis and treatment can be consistently applied. The European Society of Intensive Care Medicine and the Society of Critical Care Medicine's Third International Consensus (2016) agreed upon the current definition, which is applied to both clinical practice and research (Singer et al. 2016).

Infection: invasion of body tissue by a pathogen.
Sepsis: a dysregulated response to infection, causing organ dysfunction.
Septic shock: as with sepsis, but with hypotension, a serum **lactate** ≥2mmol/L, despite adequate fluid resuscitation.

Sepsis is defined as a life-threatening organ dysfunction caused by a dysregulated host response to infection. This dysregulated response means that the body's own defence mechanisms actually harm its own organs, risking organ failure and death. Previous definitions referred to this stage on the sepsis spectrum as 'severe sepsis', but this was superseded in 2016 and is now an outdated term. The definition was updated to reflect that even a small degree of organ dysfunction is associated with an increase in mortality (Singer et al. 2016). It is important to note that sepsis is the body's *dysregulated response to infection*, and not the infection per se; the organ dysfunction is evidenced by a raised serum lactate, amongst other markers. Individuals may respond to the same invading pathogen very differently; some may develop sepsis, and others may just experience an infection. Those with sepsis may go on to develop septic shock, which carries a mortality rate in excess of

40% (Singer et al. 2016). Septic shock is a subset of sepsis and is present in patients who meet the definition of sepsis, but also have persistent hypotension requiring vasopressors to maintain the MAP ≥65mmHg and a serum lactate level of ≥2mmol/L, despite adequate fluid resuscitation (Singer et al. 2016). These revised definitions help healthcare professionals to identify sepsis in a more consistent, unified and timely manner.

LACTATE AS A MARKER FOR SEPSIS

Useful lactate information

- It helps identify circulatory problems, even in the presence of a normal blood pressure (sometimes referred to as 'cryptic shock').
- Higher lactates are associated with worse outcomes.
- If lactate begins to fall with fluid therapy, then the fluid challenges are helping recovery.

Daniels and Nutbeam (2017)

Lactate is a normal product of **anaerobic metabolism** that is released into the bloodstream and metabolised by the liver. Aerobic metabolism produces energy from glucose in the form of adenosine triphosphate (ATP) in the presence of oxygen. Pyruvate (which is the end product of glycolysis), formed as part of this process, can also be metabolised without oxygen if it is not available in sufficient quantities. The end-product of anaerobic pyruvate metabolism is lactate, and this pathway is helpful in health, in terms of meeting a short-term oxygen deficit. Serum lactate, though, may be raised in a number of clinical circumstances, such as in hyperthermia, seizures, liver problems and cardiac arrest. A normal serum lactate level is less than 1mmol/L in both arterial and venous blood.

Whilst there are several reasons why lactate may be raised, usually this is due to organ dysfunction in the form of tissue hypoxia. A raised lactate alone does not diagnose sepsis, but a serum lactate greater than 2mmol/L is the evidence of organ dysfunction used to support a sepsis diagnosis and, if infection is suspected or likely, a sepsis diagnosis is confirmed. A higher lactate level, with its increasing mortality risk, has become an area of targeted treatment for sepsis/septic shock. Other tests identifying disordered renal function, and/or altered coagulation may also demonstrate the organ dysfunction of sepsis.

Identifying sepsis risk

The body is constantly at risk of infection, thus several mechanisms for preventing invasion by pathogens have evolved:

- The protective covering of the skin.
- The pH of body fluids.
- The mucociliary escalator of the respiratory tract.
- The enzyme lysosome found in tears.

These, together with the immune system, provide defence from a variety of Gram-negative and Gram-positive bacteria, viruses and fungi. If, however these homeostatic processes become overwhelmed, a complex chain of events is set in motion. This chain

Table 12.5 Risk factors for sepsis

The very young, those under 1 year of age.
Older people, who are over 75 years old.
Those people who are very frail,
Those with impaired immunity.
People who are undergoing chemotherapy.
People with diabetes.
People with sickle cell disease.
Patients who have had a splenectomy.
People taking long-term steroids.
Those receiving immunosuppressant drugs (rheumatoid arthritis).
People who have undergone surgery/and invasive procedures in the past 6 weeks.
Any breach of skin integrity (wounds, cuts, burns, blisters).
IV drug misuse.
Indwelling lines or catheters.
Women who have miscarried, post-partum haemorrhage, those who are pregnant or had a termination in the last 6 weeks.

(NICE 2016)

of events is sepsis, the body's dysregulated response to infection, which can lead to multi-organ failure and death. Those at greater risk of sepsis may have some disruption to these initial barriers to infection. For example, older people may have frail skin, are prone to injury and have delayed healing. Those with invasive surgery have their skin integrity challenged, as do those with invasive devices. See Table 12.5 for general risk factors for developing sepsis.

In clinical practice, diagnosing sepsis can be challenging even for the most experienced clinicians, as it can present with various clinical manifestations, and death can occur on timescales varying from days to just hours. The quick sequential (sepsis related) organ failure (**qSOFA**) assessment is *a rapid bedside sepsis screening tool* (Singer et al. 2016). This tool is useful as a brief screening tool, especially in areas where NEWS is not used. It is scored at the bedside without the need for blood tests, and it aims to facilitate prompt identification of infection that poses a greater threat to life. It consists of 3 warning signs that are scored to predict mortality (see Figure 12.11). A score of 2 is associated with 10% mortality and, in the presence of a suspected or known infection, a sepsis diagnosis is likely. It is important to note, though, that qSOFA is not superior to NEWS in identifying risk of sepsis (Churpek et al. 2017).

The UK National Institute for Health and Care Excellence (NICE 2016) published their first national guidance for sepsis management in order to support prompt recognition, diagnosis and management. Identifying those at risk of sepsis is a helpful first step. NICE (2016) presented a risk stratification tool with more detail than the qSOFA score, whereby patients with suspected sepsis are grouped according to risk of severe illness or death (see Table 12.6). The three groups identify those with:

- High risk criteria.
- Moderate to high risk criteria.
- Low risk criteria.

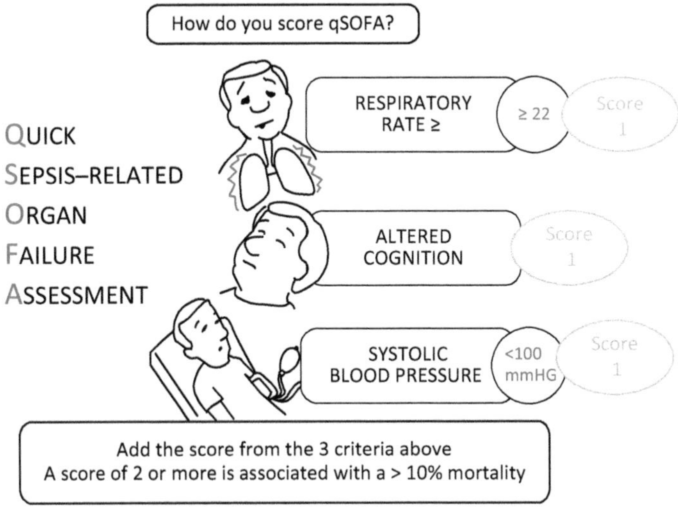

Figure 12.11 qSOFA bedside test.

Table 12.6 NICE criteria for sepsis risk management

High risk	• Objective evidence of new altered mental state. • HR >130bpm. • RR ≥ 25 or new need to ≥40% O_2 to maintain saturation >92% (>88% in known COPD). • Systolic blood pressure <90mmHg or • >40mmHg below normal. • Anuric in the last 18 hours, or, if catheterised, patient's urine output <0.5mL/kg/hr. • Mottled or ashen skin. • Cyanosis of skin, lips or tongue. • Non-blanching rash of skin.
Moderate to high risk	• History of altered behaviour or mental state. • History of acute deterioration of functional ability. • Impaired immune system. • Trauma, surgery or invasive procedures in the last 6 weeks. • RR 21–24. • HR 91–130bpm. • New on-set arrhythmia. • Systolic BP 91–100mmHg. • Anuric in the last 12–18 hours, or for catheterised patients, passed 0.5–1mL/kg/hr. • Temperature ≤36 degrees Celsius. • Signs of potential infection (redness, swelling, breakdown of wound).
Low risk	• Normal behaviour. • No high risk or moderate to high risk criteria met. • No non-blanching rash.

When assessing patients, particularly those where an infection is suspected or confirmed, the nurse needs to be aware of elements that place the patient at high risk of sepsis. It is important to note that several of the high risk criteria are associated with a higher NEWS. Notably, a new confusion, recently added to NEWS and generating a score of 3, is also viewed by NICE (2016) as high risk criteria for sepsis. Remember, NEWS advocate that with a score of 5 or more, the healthcare professional needs to 'think sepsis' (RCP 2017).

Once the risk of sepsis is established, NICE (2016) identify a flow of action/care escalation to support timely review and management.

- Patients with any 'high risk' criteria require *urgent senior clinical review* and appropriate management for sepsis such as antibiotics and fluids within 1 hour. If response to these initial interventions are poor, then Consultant medical review is recommended, with possible transfer to level 3 care.
- Those with 2 or more 'moderate to high risk' criteria require clinical review and blood results *within one hour.* If blood results reveal evidence of organ dysfunction, then they are treated as those with 'high risk' criteria.
- Those with 'low-risk' criteria only may be observed and treated according to clinical judgment.

Please note that NICE (2016) do not include neutropaenia in the high-risk criteria, which is inconsistent with established practice and other guidelines that appropriately prioritise this group for urgent treatment (NICE, 2012).

Pathophysiology of sepsis

The pathophysiology of sepsis is complex and as yet not fully understood. We have already discussed the definition of sepsis and how to identify those at risk, the following is a synopsis of some of the key elements of disordered physiology that contribute to sepsis and the clinical consequences of this. Sepsis involves changes in cell biology, biochemistry and immunology, including the activation of both pro-inflammatory and anti-inflammatory pathways in response to an invading pathogen. For sepsis to occur, there must be an *infection somewhere in the body*. The site of the infection may be anywhere, though common sites include the lungs, wound sites, the urinary tract and gastrointestinal tract.

The invading organism triggers the initial humoral response, antibodies stick to the bacterial surface, marking them for destruction by macrophages, neutrophils and monocytes. Neutrophils clump together around the destroyed pathogen, releasing chemical cytokines and stimulating elements of the immune system such as activation of the complement. This physiological response is normally *self-limiting*, but in sepsis, there is an exaggeration of this response, damaging cells tissues and organs. Sepsis develops when the pro-inflammatory response is signalled outside of the local tissue, resulting in systemic inflammation and organ dysfunction.

It is not well understood why the normal physiological response to infection becomes exaggerated in some people, with such serious consequences for mortality. It is thought that this may be due to the host response to infection, in addition to the specific invading organism. The host response is determined by the genetic make-up (genotype) of the individual and how these genes are physically expressed (phenotype). Each of us have our own phenotype, which are the observable physical or biochemical characteristics determined by both genetic make-up and environmental influences, for example, height, skin colour and weight (Bader 2016). The individual phenotype influences the nature of the immune response's impact on the septic cascade. This is determined by pathogenic load, virulence (the severity of the infection), the individual genetic characteristics and any associated patient disease (Arwyn-Jones and Brent 2019). Current studies are focusing on the improper immune response and exploring ways to support the host's immune system to reset the **hyper-inflammatory phase** into an ordered, appropriate **hypo-inflammatory** response (Zhou et al., 2019).

PRO-INFLAMMATORY AND ANTI-INFLAMMATORY RESPONSES

The hyper-inflammatory phase of sepsis is a self-reinforcing, pro-inflammatory response facilitated by sharp rises in inflammatory cytokines (such as tumour necrosis factor alpha (TNFa), interferon gamma, interleukin-1), bacterial cell wall components and activation of the complement cascade. When patients die in the first few days of sepsis, it is likely to be due to the profound hyper-inflammatory phase and resulting organ failure. Some patients are unable to initiate this acute pro-inflammatory response, and therefore their symptoms may be subtler, making the signs of sepsis difficult to detect. Changes in mentation, in the form of mild confusion may be the only manifestation.

Resolving inflammation does not occur simply as a result of stopping the pro-inflammatory response, rather, it is an active and synchronised process dependent on anti-inflammatory cytokines (those that suppress the immune system by inhibiting cytokine production). Anti-inflammatory cytokines include interleukin-1 receptor antagonist, interleukins-4, -6 and -10. Some cytokines have both pro-inflammatory and anti-inflammatory effects; it depends on the receptor they activate, see Table 12.7 for their clinical effect.

After the initial hyper-inflammatory phase, the hypo-inflammatory phase occurs, in which the anti-inflammatory response to sepsis dominates, but the problem is the patient in this phase is immunocompromised. The main focus of sepsis management is on the hyper-inflammatory phase, but the patients who survive this and go into a hypo-inflammatory phase are victim to latent, opportunistic or superimposed bacteria from which they are likely to die (Arwyn-Jones and Brent 2019). The immunocompromised patient, such as those receiving chemotherapy, are at particular risk during this stage.

CLINICAL CONSEQUENCES OF THE PRO-INFLAMMATORY RESPONSE

Pro-inflammatory mediators contribute to changes in the vascular endothelium. The permeability of the vascular endothelium normally allows movement of plasma solutes to move between the capillary, interstitial space and cells. The increase in permeability increases the movement of plasma water into the interstitial space, thus reducing the volume of the circulation. In addition, inflammatory mediators cause the blood vessels to dilate, resulting in warm, flushed peripheries, but a reduced blood pressure/perfusion pressure. Coagulation triggered initially in this process is beneficial, isolating pathogens and preventing them from entering the systemic circulation: the clots that are being formed are then broken down by normal fibrinolysis, and therefore coagulation is controlled. The loss of plasma water, though, can cause increased blood viscosity. In sepsis, a dysregulated clotting response can cause problems with tissue and organ perfusion, contributing to organ failure (Wentowski, Mewanda and Nielsen 2018).

Table 12.7 Examples of pro and anti-inflammatory cytokines released in sepsis

Mediators	*Clinical effect*
Tumour necrosis factor (TNF)	Hypotension, tachycardia, tachypnoea, hyperglycaemia, metabolic acidosis, third spacing.
Interleukin-1 (IL-1)	Fever, increased white blood cells, released amino acids from skeletal muscle, decreased systemic vascular resistance.
Interleukin-6 (IL-6)	Fever, antibody secretion.
Interleukin-8 (IL-8)	Stimulates neutrophil function and attracts inflammatory cells to site of infection/injury.
Tissue factor	Initiates blood clotting.
Interferon-y	Macrophage activation.
Interleukin-4 (IL-4)	T cell inhibition, suppression of TNF and IL-1, plus regulation of IgE and IgG secretion.
Interleukin-10 (IL-10)	Suppresses procoagulant activity.
Transforming growth factor-β (TGF β)	Promotes cell development and repair.

Sepsis

Remember, vasodilation and increased capillary permeability effectively reduces the circulating volume. Timely fluid administration is a cornerstone of sepsis management.

The very definition of sepsis requires organ dysfunction to be present. At a cellular level, tissue ischemia, cell apoptosis (cell death) and cytotoxic injury occur, and it is the cellular injury incurred in these hyper and hypo-inflammatory phases that results in organ dysfunction. Blood tests give the evidence of organ dysfunction used for the sepsis diagnosis, notably a raised serum lactate ≥2mmol/L.

Assessment of the patient with sepsis/septic shock

The ABCDE approach is used to prioritise the assessment process, treat life threatening issues and, combined with NEWS, helps detect risk of deterioration and sepsis.

During **airway** assessment the nurse will determine the degree to which the patient is able to speak and if any obstruction is apparent: secretions may lead to gurgling noises and there may be evidence of wheezing or stridor. Remember to assess the patient's cough, as it will reflect their ability to protect their airway, *provided they are alert*. Level of consciousness in sepsis may swiftly be impaired by decreased cerebral oxygenation and increased cerebral acidosis, risking airway patency.

The **breathing** status of the patient with sepsis may be compromised. Those with chest sepsis may experience increased work of breathing as lung compliance decreases, and inflammatory changes may increase airway resistance. Increased work of breathing is evident, with rapid, shallow breaths, use of accessory muscles and reluctance/inability to talk in full sentences. Assessment of RR is important, as changes in RR are significant in that an *abnormal RR alone* is widely known as an accurate indicator of clinical deterioration (Flendy, Dwyer and Applegarth 2016; Ljunggren et al. 2016). Therefore, an increased RR is often referred to as the *first sign of deterioration*; time must be given to count the RR for one full minute. Auscultation will reveal changes to airflow through the lungs caused by infection, consolidation or lower airways narrowing. Oxygen saturations may be reduced as ventilation and perfusion relationships in the lung are disrupted. It is important to maintain oxygen saturations within prescribed limits to prevent tissue hypoxia and worsening organ damage.

Arterial blood gas analysis will not only help evaluate respiratory status, but give information on the metabolic problems as a result of sepsis. Abnormalities in tissue perfusion quickly give rise to a metabolic acidosis, evidenced by a lowered arterial pH and BE/ Bicarbonate. In health, aerobic respiration meets oxygen demands, when the body has an increased demand for oxygen, such as in sepsis, the body switches to anaerobic respiration. Elevated serum lactate (the bi-product of anaerobic respiration) of more than 2mmol/L, due to ongoing tissue ischaemia, is the hallmark of sepsis. The increased acid load generated by anaerobic metabolism causes hyperventilation, with a rise in respiratory rate as the body increases carbon dioxide excretion. A chest x-ray will aid medical diagnosis and may reveal areas of patchy consolidation consistent with infection/deteriorating lung function.

Without prompt treatment, respiratory status may further deteriorate. Acute lung injury (ALI) can progress to acute respiratory distress syndrome (ARDS); the patient may start to hypoventilate and will be visibly exhausted. Widespread bronchoconstriction with poor lung compliance, a non-cardiogenic pulmonary oedema (evident on chest auscultation and through observation of frothy secretions) and a ventilation/ perfusion mismatch all contribute to a **refractory** hypoxaemia, requiring mechanical ventilation and admission to intensive care (Wentowski, Mewada and Nielson 2018).

Circulatory changes in sepsis dominate. In the early stages of sepsis, a previously healthy patient typically 'looks' well-perfused. Vasodilatation means that their peripheries are pink and warm, and their cardiac output is preserved or higher than normal as they increase their heart rate and contractility. The patient's capillary refill will be <2 seconds, and whilst the systolic pressure may not rise, a widened pulse pressure may be seen as the diastolic pressure falls. Don't be fooled, though. Their blood pressure might be already lower than ideal, and these patients will still need guided fluid resuscitation to correct their **relative hypovolaemia**. Vasodilation and relative hypovolaemia cause the heart rate to rise via sympathetic activation and an initial increase in cardiac output, but possibly failing to maintain blood pressure. The persistently leaking blood vessels reduce blood volume, further reducing BP. Heart rate rises in response to a reducing MAP. Urine output requires close monitoring, and a urinary catheter aids in the accurate assessment of hourly output. As 25% of cardiac output goes to the kidneys, renal perfusion will be affected by a reduced MAP. A urine output of less than 0.5mL/kg/hour will be secondary to a reduced glomerular filtration rate. Normal homeostatic processes like the renin angiotensin–aldosterone system and the sympathetic autonomic nervous system, will have been activated early in the septic process in an attempt to restore perfusion by fluid retention and vasoconstriction, but the numerous powerful inflammatory mediators may counter act all compensatory mechanisms by maintaining dilatation of blood vessels. The patient is at risk of developing an acute kidney injury, most likely due to pre-renal

Table 12.8 The surviving sepsis campaign bundle: 2018 update

Measure lactate level	• If lactate is more than 2mmol/L, it should be re-measured within 2–4 hours in order to guide fluid resuscitation to normalise lactate.
Obtain blood cultures prior to antibiotics	• Appropriate blood cultures are required and include at least two sets, aerobic and anaerobic. The administration of appropriate antibiotic therapy should not be delayed in order to obtain blood cultures.
Administer broad spectrum antibiotics	• Empiric broad-spectrum antibiotic therapy, with one or more IV antimicrobials should be started immediately, so as to cover all pathogens.
Administer IV fluid	• Administer 30mL/kg of intravenous crystalloid fluid; note any fluid administration beyond this requires careful assessment in order to ascertain if the patient is still fluid-responsive. This initial fluid resuscitation should be commenced immediately once sepsis is recognised, if there is hypotension and a lactate greater than 2mmol/L, it should be completed within 3 hours of commencing.
Apply vasopressors	• If blood pressure has not been restored following initial fluid resuscitation, vasopressors should then be commenced within the first hour to achieve a Mean Arterial Pressure greater than 65mmHg in order to restore adequate perfusion to the organs.

(Levy et al. 2018)

hypo-perfusion (Nagalingam 2018). Important early management strategies at this stage include antibiotics and peripheral cannulation to enable rapid fluid administration as per the sepsis care bundle (see Table 12.8).

Investigations for a patient with suspected sepsis

Lactate: initially may be venous or arterial. Serial arterial measurement may be required in septic shock to evaluate response to treatment.
Blood cultures.
Wound swabs for culture.
WCC.
CRP.
Renal function tests, urea and creatinine.
Clotting profile.
Chest X-ray.

As sepsis progresses towards *septic shock*, endothelial damage increases nitric oxide synthase production; this is a potent vasodilator released from the endothelium. Now widespread vasodilatation and persistently leaking blood vessels lead to a gross maldistribution of the circulating volume. This, together with the intravascular micro-thrombi formation, causes a further imbalance between oxygen demand and oxygen supply to the tissues. As inflammation and increased permeability persist, a marked reduction in blood flow continues. This presents as hypotension with a narrow pulse pressure and exacerbates the pro-coagulant state. The body tries to regulate this process by releasing counter-inflammatory agents such as interleukins 4 and 10 and transforming growth factor-β (TGF β), but for some patients, the inflammation and ensuing endothelial changes become overwhelming (Nagalingam 2018). It is worth noting that the capillary refill, which was initially brisk, reduces as peripheral perfusion worsens. In the early phase of sepsis, as the heart tries to compensate for the persistently low systemic vascular resistance, the cardiac output may be high. Unfortunately, as sepsis progresses to septic shock, the myocardium is exposed to the circulation of substances such as myocardial depressant factor, which is synthesised by ischaemic pancreatic tissue, directly impairing myocardial contractility (Daniels and Nutbeam 2017).

In septic shock, the patient will have not improved with initial fluid resuscitation, blood pressure may not rise, or even fall further, and serum lactate will rise or continue to be greater than 2mmol/L. Urgent senior review is required; vasopressors such as noradrenaline will be commenced to achieve a MAP >65mmHg; this requires a central line insertion and arterial monitoring of blood pressure, with transfer to a higher level of care.

Disability assessment focuses on those factors that affect neurological status. NEWS assessment requires an ACVPU assessment (alert, new confusion, verbal response, pain response or unresponsive). Confusion may be present early in the sepsis cascade, which led to the addition of 'new confusion' in NEWS (RCP 2017). A GCS assessment may be useful (see Chapter 9), as with increasing cerebral acidosis, the level of consciousness may drop to eight or below, requiring endotracheal intubation for airway protection. Blood glucose, essential for neurological function, will also rise as a result of sympathetic nervous system stimulation (fight or flight element). Gluconeogenesis and increased glycogenosis occurs in an effort to provide energy for cellular function. Hyperglycaemia can cause an immunosuppressive effect, diminishing the body's ability to mount a competent immune response; close monitoring of blood glucose is required (Wentowski, Mewada and Nielsen 2018). The Surviving Sepsis Campaign recommend initiation of a blood glucose management protocol if 2 consecutive blood glucose levels are >10mmol/L, with the target of keeping sugars at ≤10mmol/L (Rhodes et al. 2017).

Exposure The patient's temperature might rise or fall in response to infection, but it should be remembered that both hyperthermia and hypothermia will impact on the patient's metabolic rate and therefore oxygen delivery to the tissues. Traditionally, higher temperatures have been a trigger for sepsis consideration, however, patients with sepsis may be normothermic, pyrexial or hypothermic. The head-to-toe examination for those with suspected or confirmed sepsis is essential to eliminate all other possible sources of infection. A diagnosis of chest sepsis may be present, but it is possible that a urinary tract infection, pressure area or an area of infection hidden in a skin fold could cause ongoing problems. Source identification through swabs and blood cultures, with a 'best guess', appropriate antibiotic therapy initially, is an essential component of sepsis management. On further inspection, oedema due to fluid seeping into the interstitium, exacerbated by albumin also leaking through the leaky capillary endothelium, may be present. Oedema further exacerbates fluid and electrolyte imbalances. A later clinical finding may be mottled or grey-looking skin, or a petechial rash (rash that does not blanch under pressure), highlighted by NICE (2016) as high risk criteria.

Don't forget that NICE (2016) have identified a temperature **less than 36°C**, as a moderate to high risk criterion for sepsis.

NEWS allocates a score of **3** to a temperature of less than 35°C.

Ongoing problems with sepsis/septic shock require the patient to be transferred to a higher level of care, where continuous monitoring and circulatory support, with a nurse–patient ratio of 1:1, can be offered. The coagulation system is inappropriately activated, and clotting factors become depleted as a result of forming multiple clots in the capillary bed. This has several physiological effects:

- Depletion of clotting factors puts the patient at risk from spontaneous bleeding.
- Increase in clot formation increases the risk of thrombosis.

These changes herald the onset of **disseminated intravascular coagulation** syndrome (DIC), a common feature of advanced sepsis. Liver dysfunction is often a late sign in septic shock (Arwyn-Jones and Brent 2019). Further changes in respiratory, cardiac, renal, neurological and metabolic function may develop swiftly in response to the tissue hypoxia that is occurring, and the nurse needs to be diligent during the assessment process in order to detect a worsening of the patient's condition. Worsening anaerobic metabolism, decreasing ATP production and organ failure ensues. The damage is determined by the extent to which the patient's hypotension and raised lactate levels respond to the initial treatment of volume loading with crystalloid infusions (Rhodes et al. 2017). Refractory clinical states (those which are unresponsive to treatment) herald the risk of multiple organ dysfunction syndrome and ultimately death. The NMC (2018) emphasise the importance of the nurse possessing in-depth knowledge and having the ability to carry out an accurate assessment of a patient with complex problems, using appropriate diagnostic and decision-making skills. It can be seen that this is essential when caring for a patient with or at risk of sepsis. Care escalation, initial interventions and transfer to a higher level of care require the nurse to be diligent and to confidently work within the multi-disciplinary team.

THE NATIONAL EARLY WARNING SCORE AND SEPSIS

RCP (2017) recommends that sepsis is considered in any patient with a known, suspected, or high risk of infection with a NEWS score of 5 or more. These patients require an urgent clinical review with a high index of suspicion for sepsis. Patients with a NEWS2 score of 5 or more with sepsis are associated with a >3-fold-increased risk of patient transfer to ICU or death. It is stressed that patients with a NEWS score of 5 or more require the clinician to think: 'could this be sepsis?' They need to instigate an urgent escalation of clinical care, confirmatory investigations and timely treatment. NEWS is endorsed by NHS England and NHS Improvement, and its implementation has been mandated across the NHS in England, including its use to detect clinical deterioration in patients with suspected sepsis, in order to promote standardised care (NHS England 2017; RCP 2017).

CASE STUDY 12.1 PART 1

Maja is a 59-year-old lady who was admitted onto the acute medical ward with a respiratory tract infection two days ago. She is on co-amoxiclav TDS.

14:00: NEWS 4
Observations are RR 21 (2), SpO_2 94% (target 94–98%, Scale 1) (1), Pulse 95 (1), BP 113/70mmHg, (0), A (ACVPU) (0), Temperature 37.7°C (0).
The HCA reported to the RN Lucy that Maja was in bed, having a cup of tea and feeling tired. The RN asked the HCA to repeat the observations at 18:00. The HCA went to give Maja her dinner at 18:00, and prior to checking her observations, she noted that Maja was very restless and appeared sweaty. She immediately informed the RN. The RN finished with the patient they were with and went to see Maja.

18:00: the RN introduced themselves to the patient, and after gaining consent to complete an assessment, she washed her hands, donned an apron and pulled the curtains around the bed space.

Airway: Maja was alert and speaking in full, clear sentences; she was able to demonstrate a strong cough, confirming Maja could protect her airway. Maja was bringing up sputum, thick and green in colour. Maja was asked to place a sample in a sterile container to be sent for culture and sensitivity. There were no audible noises from her airway, indicating no signs of partial obstruction. The RN, now confident the airway was patent, moved on to assess breathing.

Breathing: Maja was pink in colour, signalling adequate perfusion; there was no evidence of central or peripheral cyanosis. On close examination, the RN could see that Maja was using her accessory muscles, indicating a slight increase in work of breathing. The RN counted Maja's RR for one full minute; it was 24, regular, but shallow. Auscultation of the posterior chest wall identified air entry throughout with inspiratory crackles in the right lower base. SpO_2 was now 92% on room air, the target SpO_2 was 94–98% (Scale 1 on NEWS); therefore, 4L oxygen was started via nasal specs as prescribed (O'Driscoll et al. 2017). The RN then reassessed the SpO_2, which had come up to 98%, and the RR, now 23. Once the breathing assessment was complete, the RN moved on to assess circulation.
Breathing NEWS (2 + 2 + 0) = 4
Breathing NEWS (2 + 0 + 2) = 4 after oxygen therapy.

Circulation: Maja's capillary refill was <2 seconds, indicating adequate perfusion, and she was warm to touch on all four limbs. The nurse palpated Maja's pulse for one full minute, noting a rate of 109bpm, regular yet bounding. The blood pressure was 112/65mmHg, MAP 80mmHg, pulse pressure 47mmHg, which is a wide pulse pressure, indicating vasodilation. The RN asked Maja when she had last passed urine, Maja said she wasn't sure, possibly this morning. The RN asked if Maja felt like passing urine, but she didn't. Maja reported feeling thirsty and her mouth was visibly dry; Maja was encouraged to drink water. The RN commenced a fluid balance chart and gained consent to carry out a passive leg raise. This mimics a fluid bolus of

approximately 250–300mL. Maja's HR fell to 105bpm and her BP rose slightly to 117/69mmHg, indicating a positive fluid response.
Circulation NEWS (0 + 1) = 1

Disability: Maja was alert, but in order to identify if she was confused, the RN had to determine if she was orientated to person, place and time. She asked her the following questions:
Can you tell me what my role is?
Can you tell me where you are exactly?
Can you tell me the current month and year?
Maja answered all questions correctly, confirming she was not confused. When asked if she had any pain, Maja said it was painful in her chest on coughing and she felt very tender, pointing to the lower aspect of her anterior chest wall. The RN assessed the pain using the 0–10 pain scale; Maja reported 2/10 on rest, but when coughing, the pain was 6/10. There was no analgesia prescribed.
Maja's blood glucose level was 8mmol/L, and as she had no history of diabetes, this was slightly elevated.
Disability NEWS = 0

Exposure: Maja's temperature was 38.4°C, and she reported feeling hot, therefore the top blanket was removed. Under exposure, the RN assessed Maja's skin for any rashes, sores, oedema, mottling or redness; there were no abnormalities found. Maja reported that she had last opened her bowels yesterday. The nurse completed her assessment, gave her the call bell and advised her to call if needed. The RN said she needed to review her findings and would come back to her once she had spoken with her colleagues.

Exposure NEWS = 1

The RN calculated the NEWS score, RR 24 **(2)**, SpO_2 92% on room air **(2)**, BP 112/65mmHg **(0)**, HR 109bpm **(1)**, alert **(0)**, temperature 38.4°C **(1) NEWS Score 6**.

The RN documents this score, but then must do another score to reflect the commencing of O_2 therapy; RR 23 **(2)**, SpO_2 98%, on 4L O_2 **(2)**, BP 112/65mmHg **(0)**, HR 109bpm **(1)**, alert **(0)**, temperature 38.4°C **(1)**, total **NEWS score 6** also. Both scores were recorded on the NEWS chart.

The NEWS score of 6 requires minimum hourly vital sign assessment; the medical team caring for the patient needs to be informed and to request an urgent assessment by a clinician or team with core competencies in the care of acutely ill patients. The nurse calls the medical house officer and the critical care outreach team to inform them of the patient. The RN uses the Situation, Background, Assessment and Recommendations (SBAR) tool to handover via the telephone at 18:25h.

SBAR tool used to escalate care.

Situation, background, assessment, recommendation

Situation	Hello and good evening, my name is Lucy, a registered nurse, and I am calling from medical ward 12, on floor 2. I am calling you because my patient, Maja Johnson, has a NEWS of 6.
Background	Maja was admitted onto the ward earlier this afternoon, with a respiratory tract infection, for IV antibiotics and monitoring. She has no known allergies.
Assessment	Airway is patent; she has a productive cough, and sputum is green in colour. Breathing: she is using her accessory muscles, with a slight increased work of breathing; her RR is 24, regular but shallow; SpO_2 was 92% on room air; 4L O_2 given; SpO_2 is now within target range at 98%, and RR is now 23. She has bilateral air entry with inspiratory crackles in the right lower base. Circulation: warm to touch on all four limbs; capillary refill is brisk <2 seconds; her pulse is 109bpm, regular but bounding; BP 112/65mmHg; MAP 80mmHg; pulse pressure 47mmHg, consistent with vasodilation. I did a passive leg raise, which showed a positive response to the increase in pre-load. Maja reported she last passed urine this morning; she is thirsty, and her mouth is visibly dry. Disability: Maja is alert and orientated. Blood glucose level is 8mmol/L, and she is not a known diabetic. She has pain in her lower anterior chest wall, scoring 2/10, but 6/10 on coughing. Exposure: temperature is 38.4°C. No rashes, wounds, mottling or peripheral oedema present. Bowels last opened yesterday, type 4 stool.
Recommendations	• I am concerned that Maja may have sepsis, as her NEWS score is >5, and she has a known chest infection. • I plan to take blood samples to measure her venous lactate and take peripheral blood cultures, and I will also send samples for FBC, U&Es, clotting and LFTs. • I have encouraged her to drink oral fluids and commended a fluid balance chart. • She will also require a chest C-ray. • Can you please come to review this patient, as she needs urgent assessment? Is there anything else you recommend I do in the meantime? • The house officer thanks the RN for their systematic assessment and agrees that she may have sepsis. Laura says that she will be on the ward in the next 15 minutes to review the patient.

Referring to NICE (2016) criteria for sepsis, Maja has none of the high risk criteria, but she does have 3 of the moderate to high risk criteria: raised RR, raised HR, she has not passed urine for approximately 9 hours now and she has a known respiratory tract infection. Maja's qSOFA score is 1, which indicates a mortality rate of <1 %, but is not a high risk indicator for sepsis. The lactate result will confirm/refute diagnosis and direct therapy. NICE (2016) advocates that lactate level should be measured and reviewed within 1 hour.

This is an example of good practice. The RN has identified that the patient may have sepsis and escalated care in an appropriate and timely manner. *Remember, sepsis is a medical emergency* (Brent, 2017).

Management of sepsis

In an attempt to reduce the incidence of sepsis, effective infection control policies need to be in place, with infection control teams available to support this. Previously in this chapter, we discussed how nurses have a major role in maintaining asepsis and reducing the incidence of cross-infection in health care settings. Preventing contamination of vulnerable patients, ensure invasive catheters are promptly removed when not required, and provide optimal respiratory management, including routine oral care for patients. All of these interventions help contribute towards minimising infection (WHO 2018).

To avoid progression on the continuum of infection to sepsis, comprehensive assessment skills noting key clinical indicators and timely interventions are required by the health care team, in particular the health care professionals who carry out vital signs assessment. Early recognition and treatment are essential to reduce sepsis-related mortality (RCP 2017). In hospitals, nurses are often the first to recognise deterioration in a patient. The Surviving Sepsis Campaign promotes the assessment of every patient, every shift, and every day for sepsis (Rhodes et al. 2017). It is imperative that nurses have the skills, competence and critical thinking skills to carry out systematic assessments (Treacy and Stayt 2019).

THE SEPSIS CARE BUNDLE

It is, of course, not possible to eradicate all sources of infection that the patient may be exposed to, and for this reason, a comprehensive international strategy to manage sepsis has been developed. A care bundle is a group of critical elements in a care process: when all elements are performed, this is associated with an improved outcome. Each element of the bundle needs to be completed and audited to evaluate compliance. The **sepsis 6** bundle (see below) provides a simple way of delivering the basic elements of care in a timely fashion. One study (Daniels et al. 2011) has shown that delivery of the sepsis six care bundle within 1 hour was associated with a more that 50% reduction in mortality. The sepsis bundle needs to be implemented by ward staff and clinicians in clinical practice. NCEPOD (2015) identified that management of patients with sepsis was only good in a third of cases. One broad, underlying problem was that the recognition of sepsis often requires more experience than the junior members of staff have to draw from. This emphasises the need for all staff in acute care to be able to detect signs of deterioration and escalate care accordingly (to more senior staff members), ensuring each element of the care bundle is completed in a timely manner. Failure to comply with the recommended timing of treatment will result in further patient deterioration and increased mortality. Consequently, the nurse has a key role in coordinating inter-professional interventions to ensure that this does not happen. Nursing, as a profession, needs to provide leadership and management skills in identifying the priorities for patient care, ensuring resources are used effectively (NMC 2018).

The Surviving Sepsis Campaign Bundle (2018) update, reviewed recent evidence and introduced the '1-hour Bundle'. This new bundle combines elements of previous bundles into an algorithm that emphasises the requirement for immediate treatment of sepsis to improve survival. Whilst some elements of the bundle have relatively weak evidence, others are supported with moderate quality evidence (Levy et al. 2018). The clock starts ticking from the moment *sepsis* is identified. Sepsis is a medical emergency, and all elements of the sepsis bundle are required to be completed within *1 hour* (Levy et al. 2018). The elements of the bundle are presented in Table 12.8.

THE SEPSIS 6

Sepsis 6

1. Administer oxygen: target >94% (or 88–92% for patients with COPD).
2. Take blood cultures.
3. Give IV antibiotics.
4. Give IV fluids.
5. Check serial lactates.
6. Measure urine output: may require urinary catheter.

Daniels and Nutbeam (2017)

The care bundle approach is reflected in the 'sepsis 6', with the addition of oxygen therapy and urine output assessment. This is to remind health care staff of the importance of completing the 6 essential steps within 1 hour of sepsis recognition. For each hour's delay in giving antibiotics, mortality is increased. This is a direct and simple aid memoire for 3 giving actions and 3 taking actions required on sepsis identification to support nurses in moving care forward.

Oxygen therapy supports those who are hypoxaemic, and SpO_2 should be kept within target range. There is little benefit of achieving a SpO_2 of more than 98%. Unless the lung is directly affected by chest sepsis, initially, oxygenation may not always be a problem. Later, though, acute lung injury may develop, and oxygen requirements will increase. *Blood cultures* should be taken percutaneously and from all vascular devices that have been present for more than 24 hours. Taking 2 sets percutaneously increases the capture of causative organisms. Ideally, cultures are taken before *IV antibiotics* are given, but only if that can be achieved within the 1 hour time frame. Samples from any suspect area should be taken for culture too, along with investigations such as the chest X-ray. *Fluids* are necessary to maintain the circulatory volume and cardiac output. In sepsis, fluid moves into the wrong place, from the circulation into the interstitial space and tissues, and needs replacing to maintain circulatory volume. Care must be taken, though, not to give too much fluid, as this can impair the circulation; careful monitoring is required. Choice of fluid may vary, but generally, balanced crystalloids such as Hartmann's solution or Plasma-Lyte are selected. *Lactate* must be measured, both initially and to check that fluid resuscitation is working. If the lactate remains unchanged or is increasing, this requires further care escalation to the critical care team. *Urine output* assessment can help detect early renal function decline and the adequacy of blood pressure/cardiac output. A urinary catheter may be required with hourly urine monitoring, reporting if output is less than 0.5mL/Kg/hour. An accurate fluid balance chart is essential to assess overall fluid balance.

CASE STUDY 12.2 PART 2

18:40: the house officer and outreach nurse came to review Maja. Following an ABG result, a lactate of >2mmol/L confirmed the suspected sepsis diagnosis. Management was now guided by the sepsis care bundle; all actions needed to be recorded and timed.

- Oxygen saturations remained in range on 4L oxygen via nasal specs. Maja sat in an upright position.
- A large bore cannula was inserted into the median basilica vein in left anti-cubital fossa. An initial bolus of 500mL plasma-Lyte was given over 15 minutes. Lucy ensured that Maja's saturations and respiratory rate were continuously monitored. Maja weighed 70Kg, and therefore, according to the sepsis bundle could receive up to (70 × 30mL = 2100mL) 2100mL within the next 3 hours, if required.
- Despite being on IV antibiotics already for a chest infection, a broad-spectrum antibiotic, Tazocin (piperacillin/tazobactam) 4.5g/TDS was prescribed, and first dose administered. This was until a positive culture could obtained, at which point targeted antibiotic therapy could be commenced.
- The balance of risks versus the benefit of inserting a urinary catheter were discussed, and the decision was made to catheterise. A residual of 300mL of concentrated urine was drained. Dipstick revealed specific gravity 1.010, indicating dehydration. Maja weighed 70kg, therefore the urine output was 30mL/hour, as it had been approximately 10 hours since she last voided urine. Now that we knew her urine output was <0.5mL/kg/hour, the creatinine result was needed to determine if she had an acute kidney injury.
- Paracetamol 1gm IV was given for pain management and as an antipyretic.

Initial arterial blood gas shows:

- pH: 7.34.
- $PaCO_2$: 4.2kPa.
- PaO_2: 10.9kPa.
- HCO_3^- : 20mmol/L.
- BE : -3mmol/L.
- Lactate: 2.8mmol/L.

Maja's oxygenation is adequate; she remains on 4L via nasal cannula. The lowered pH indicates mild acidosis (normal range 7.35–7.45), and paired with the negative base excess (normal range +/-2) and lowered bicarbonate (normal range 22–24mmol/L), is consistent with metabolic acidosis. The increased RR has reduced the carbon dioxide levels below their normal range (of 4.6–6kPa) and has partially compensated for the metabolic acidosis. Maja meets the criteria for sepsis with the raised lactate, and she will require close monitoring over the next hour to assess whether she responds to treatment.

At 19:20, the RN checks that all requirements of the sepsis 6 bundle have been completed. The house officer informs the consultant responsible for the patient that Maja has sepsis, and it is documented in the notes. The plan from the medical team is to give another fluid bolus of 500mL crystalloid and monitor response of urine output and lactate levels.

At 19:45h, reassessment of Maja's status shows RR 22, SpO_2 99% on 4L O_2, (oxygen reduced to 3L to keep within target), HR 100 and BP 117/65; she is alert and orientated, and her temperature 38.0°C. Urine output has been 40mL in the last hour, which is within 0.5mL–1mL/kg/hour.

NEWS (B [2 + 0 + 2], C [0 + 1], D [0], E [0]) **Total = 5**

Blood results reveal:

- Creatinine: 79mcmol/L.
- WWC: raised at 18 x10^9/L.
- CRP: 59mg/L.
- Repeat venous lactate: 2.3mmol/L.

Renal function tests are within normal range; therefore, no AKI is detected. WCC and CRP are both raised, consistent with infection. The repeat lactate has fallen from the initial level of 2.8mmol/L, which is evidence of a positive response to initial therapy. No other abnormalities are detected in the blood results.

The chest X-ray reveals a right lower lobe consolidation, consistent with pneumonia.

Following review by the house officer. The NEWS score is now 5. It is clear that Maja is responding to treatment; this needs to continue with further fluid therapy to reduce her serum lactate and NEWS.

21:00: a further 1L of Plasma-Lyte has been given within the 3 hours required by the sepsis care bundle.

Assessment reveals RR 18 on 3L O_2, SpO_2 95%, HR 98 and BP 117/65; urine output has been 100mL in the last hour, she is alert and orientated, and her temperature 37.5°C.

NEWS (B [0 + 1 + 2 = 3]) (C [0 + 0]) (D [0]) (E [0]) = **3**

A repeat serum lactate is 1.8mm/L.

Maja has responded well to timely interventions. No additional intervention is required at this stage. Close monitoring will ensure early detection, should clinical deterioration occur. This is an example of early recognition and appropriate management of the patient with sepsis.

Septic shock

Patients developing septic shock require immediate transfer to the intensive care unit, where they will receive ongoing support for organ dysfunction/failure. For most patients, this will entail mechanical ventilation, additional inotropic support for cardiac function, haemofiltration for renal impairment and further haematological support for coagulopathy. They will also be nursed in an upright position (of at least 30°) to help prevent any additional pulmonary infection (Rhodes et al. 2017). The Surviving Sepsis Campaign highlights the evidence-based interventions required for patients with septic shock (Rhodes et al. 2017). These include:

- The administration of low-dose steroids to support adrenal function, if fluid therapy and vasopressor agents have proved unsuccessful in treating hypotension.
- Use of a 'lung protective' strategy for mechanically ventilated patients to regulate inspiratory plateau pressures <30cmH_20 and deliver tidal volumes at no greater than 6mL/kg for sepsis-induced ARDS.
- Early establishment of enteral nutrition is vital.
- Communicating with the patient, even when sedated, and communicating with the family is of vital importance. The patient's prognosis and goals of care need to be discussed with the family.

On discharge from ICU, follow-up should ideally be provided by the critical care outreach team, with regular reviews on discharge to ensure no further problems develop and with a view to preventing re-admission. Literature on sepsis and its after-effects should be provided to the patient and family to provide safety netting advice, but also to inform and prepare them of the possible side effects that may occur over the next few months (Smith and Meyfroid 2017). Post-sepsis syndrome (PSS) is a term used to describe a group of problems that commonly occur following sepsis, both physical and psychological. The aetiology is not fully understood of PSS, however, the pro-inflammatory cytokines may play a role (Daniels and Nutbeam 2017).

Conclusion

A fully functioning immune system is vital for the maintenance of good health. An overview of applied physiology of this system has been given, and the clinical problems that may lead to a medical emergency of anaphylaxis and sepsis have been explored. Lack of recognition and appropriate intervention of these problems may lead swiftly to multiple organ dysfunction, cardiac arrest and/or death. Infections, health care-associated infections and the spectrum of sepsis increase mortality, but there is consensus in the literature that early recognition of the deteriorating, septic patient and timely instigation of therapeutic management is key to mortality reduction. Sepsis is a life-threatening condition; by understanding the key principles, healthcare professionals can identify, recognise and escalate care in an appropriate and timely manner. Nurses have a *major role* in the recognition of sepsis, and by working collaboratively with other members of the multidisciplinary team, they can ensure patients receive evidence-based care and ultimately improve patient outcomes.

Glossary

Abscess A collection of pus accumulation in a cavity.

Aetiology The causes or origin of a disease.

Anaerobic metabolism A process of breaking down glucose for energy without the presence of oxygen. This occurs when oxygen cannot enter the mitochondria quickly enough, or when there is tissue hypoxia.

Anaphylaxis An acute, multi-system, severe, type I hypersensitivity allergic reaction.

Angioedema Swelling of the deeper layers of the skin; this is often severe and is caused by a build-up of fluid.

Asepsis The absence of pathogenic organisms.

Basal metabolic rate The base rate at which the body consumes calories for basic metabolic functions, such as maintaining internal temperature and repairing cells.

Care bundle A group of interventions that, when performed altogether, improve patient outcomes.

Commensal Living on or within another organism and deriving benefit without harming or benefiting the host.

Complement Part of the immune system made up of a number of proteins that enhances (or complements) the ability of the immune system to clear microbes and damaged cells and to attack pathogen membranes.

C-reactive protein (CRP) A protein produced by the liver in response to inflammation, injury and infection.

Croup A respiratory condition that is usually triggered by an acute viral infection of the upper airway.

Cytokines Chemical messengers that coordinate an immune response.

Disseminated intravascular coagulation (DIC) A condition that may occur in the critically ill, whereby small blood clots form and block some smaller blood vessels. The excessive clotting can lead to organ damage, and when clotting factors have been consumed, bleeding.

Dysregulated host response to infection This is an abnormal, uncontrolled response to infection that causes organs damage. This is a feature of sepsis.

Enterotoxin A protein toxin released by a microorganism in the intestine.

Enzyme Proteins that catalyse chemical reactions.

Fibrin A fibrous protein involved in the clotting of blood.

Haemolysis The breaking down of erythrocytes.

Heparin An injectable anticoagulant.

Histamine A chemical that is released in the body as part of an allergic reaction.

Hyper-inflammatory phase An excessive response of inflammation causing cytokines, seen in sepsis and septic shock.

Hypo-inflammatory A response to dampen inflammation. The anti-inflammatory response in sepsis mediates and balances the hyper-inflammatory response. In some, this response may actually make the patient more vulnerable to new infection.

Immunoglobulin Also known as an antibody.

Infection Presence of a microorganism in the tissues that causes a host response and classic signs and symptoms, including, redness, heat, swelling and temperature.

Innate Existing since birth.

Lactate Serum lactate reflects the amount of lactic acid in the blood. Lactate is produced when there is not enough available oxygen to metabolise glucose in the mitochondria (anaerobic metabolism) and is used as a marker of organ hypoperfusion/dysfunction.

Meticillin resistant *staphylococcus aureus* A group of Gram-positive bacteria that are distinct from other strains in that they are resistant to many common antibiotics.

Microbes Tiny organisms that cannot be seen by the naked eye.

Microthrombi Small thrombus located in a capillary or other small blood vessel.

Morphology The study of the form and structure of organisms.

Oedema An accumulation of fluid in the interstitial space. This can be caused by heart failure, low protein levels or leaky capillary endothelium (as in sepsis).

Pathogen An infectious agent (a germ).

Pyrexia Refers to a fever or temperature above the normal range.

qSOFA A quick, sequential, sepsis, organ-related failure assessment. A score of >2 is associated with higher mortality.

Refractory Refers to a disease or state that does not respond to treatment.

Relative hypovolaemia A poor distribution of fluids between intravascular and extravascular compartments. Whilst the total fluid in the body may be the same, the proportion in the vascular compartment is lower than normal.

Sepsis A life-threatening organ dysfunction caused by a dysregulated host response to infection.

Sepsis 6 Six steps to take on recognition of sepsis to improve health outcomes.

Septic shock Sepsis with a serum lactate above 2mmol/L despite fluid resuscitation.

Stridor A high-pitched wheezing sound resulting from turbulent air flow in the upper airway.

Toxin A poisonous substance produced within living cells or organisms. Vascular endothelium.

TEST YOURSELF

1. Name the 2 types of immune defence systems in the body.
2. List the 5 major white blood cell groups.
3. Identify the 3 main functions of the complement system.
4. What is the primary function of fever?
5. Define the following terms:
   a. antigen
   b. antibody
6. Name the 4 main classes of microorganisms affecting humans.
7. List 6 key signs and symptoms of anaphylaxis.
8. Name the high-risk criteria for sepsis, as given by NICE (2016), in order to identify sepsis.
9. What is the significance of a raised serum lactate level?
10. Name the 6 initial actions to be taken on the recognition of sepsis.

Answers

1. Innate or natural immunity and adaptive or acquired immunity, specific to each individual.
2. Neutrophils, lymphocytes, monocytes, eosinophils and basophils.
3. Opsonisation, chemotaxis and inflammation
4. To increase metabolic rate and therefore inhibit bacterial growth.
5. a. An antigen is a foreign substance that the host's lymphoid cells and tissues mount a direct response to.
   b. An antibody is a soluble protein that holds the memory of a previous pathogen and binds to the surface of an antigen.
6. Bacteria, viruses, fungi and protozoa.
7. Airway swelling, stridor, wheezing, hypotension, tachycardia and erythema.
8. Objective evidence of new altered mental state.
   HR >130bpm.
   RR $\geq$ 25 or new need to $\geq$40% O_2 to maintain saturation
   >92% (>88% in known COPD).
   Systolic blood pressure <90mmHg or >40mmHg below normal.
   Anuric in the last 18 hours, or, if catheterised, patient's urine output <0.5mL/kg/hr.
   Non-blanching rash of skin.
   Mottled or ashen skin.
   Cyanosis of skin, lips or tongue.
9. There are several reasons why lactate may be raised, usually this is due to organ dysfunction in the form of tissue hypoxia.
10. Antibiotics, fluids, oxygen, cultures (blood), urine output measurement and serum lactate level.

References

Arwyn-Jones, J. and Brent, A. J. (2019). Sepsis. *Surgery (Oxford)*, 37(1), 1–8. doi:10.1016/j.mpsur.2018.11.007. Available from https://www.surgeryjournal.co.uk/article/S0263-9319(18)30257-6/pdf.

Australasian Society of Clinical Immunology and Allergy. (2016). *Anaphylaxis Resources*. Australasian Society of Clinical Immunology and Allergy (ASCIA). Available from https://www.allergy.org.au/hp/anaphylaxis. Accessed 10 August 2019.

Bader, S. (2016). Introduction to forensic genetics. In Jamieson, A. and Bader, S. (eds.), *A Guide to Forensic DNA Profiling*. GB: Wiley.

Blay, A. (2011). Introduction to routine blood tests, normal values and relevance to clinical practice. In Phillips, S., Collins, M. and Dougherty, L. (eds.), *Venepuncture and Cannulation (Essential Clinical Nurses)*. Chichester: Wiley-Blackwell.

Brent, A. (2017). Sepsis. *Medicine*, 45(10), 649–653. doi:10.1016/j.mpmed.2017.07.010.

Churpek, M., Snyder, A., Han, X., Sokol, S., Pettit, N., Howell, M. and Edelson, D. (2017). Quick sepsis-related organ failure assessment, systemic inflammatory response syndrome, and early warning scores for detecting clinical deterioration in infected patients outside the intensive care unit. *American Journal of Respiratory and Critical Care Medicine*, 195(7), 906–911. doi:10.1164/rccm.201604-0854OC. Accessed August 2018.

Colbert, B., Ankney, J., Lee, K., Steggall, M. and Dingle, M. (2012). *Anatomy and Physiology for Nursing and Healthcare Professionals*. Harlow: Pearson Education Limited.

Daniels, R., Nutbeam, T., McNamara, G. and Galvin, C. (2011). The sepsis six and the severe sepsis resuscitation bundle: a prospective observational cohort study. *Emergency Medicine Journal*, 28(6), 507–512.

Daniels, R. and Nutbeam, T. (eds.) (2017). *The Sepsis Manual: Responsible Management of Sepsis, Severe Infection and Antimicrobial Stewardship*, 4th Edition. Birmingham: The UK Sepsis Trust.

Department of Health. (2017). *High Impact Intervention: Central Venous Catheter Care Bundle*. London: DH, pp. 2–3. Available from http://hcai.dh.gov.uk/files/2011/03/2011-03-14-HII.

Drewry, A. M., Fuller, B. M., Skrupky, L. P. and Hotchkiss, R. S. (2015). The presence of hypothermia within 24 hours of sepsis diagnosis predicts persistent lymphopenia. *Critical Care Medicine*, 43(6), 1165.

Dutton, H. and Finch, J. (2018). *Acute and Critical Care Nursing at a Glance*. Oxford: Wiley Blackwell.

Flenady, T., Dwyer, T. and Applegarth, J. (2016). Rationalising transgression: a grounded theory explaining how emergency department registered nurses rationalise erroneous behavior. *Grounded Theory Review*, 15(2), 41–58.

Goering, R., Dockrell, H., Zuckerman, M., Wakelin, D., Roitt, I., Mims, C. and Chiodini, P. (2013). *Mims' Medical Microbiology*, 5th Edition. London: Elsevier Limited.

Gould, D. J., Moralejo, D., Drey, N., Chudleigh, J. H. and Taljaard, M. (2017). Interventions to improve hand hygiene compliance in patient care. *Cochrane Database of Systematic Reviews*, 9(9), CD005186.

Humphreys, H. (2012). Staphylococcus skin infections; osteomyelitis; food poisoning; foreign body infections; MRSA. In Greenwood, D., Barer, M., Slack, R. and Irving, W. (eds.), *Medical Microbiology: A Guide to Microbial Infections: Pathogenesis, Immunity, Laboratory Diagnosis and Control*, 18th Edition. London: Churchill Livingstone Elsevier, pp. 176–182.

Johnson, K. and Henry, K. (2013). Shock, systemic inflammatory response syndrome and multiple organ dysfunction syndrome. In Morton, P. and Fontaine, D. (eds.), *Critical Care Nursing a Holistic Approach*, 10th Edition. London: Wolters Kluwer/Lippincott, Williams & Wilkins.

Kushimoto, S., Gando, S., Saitoh, D., et al. (2013). The impact of body temperature abnormalities on the disease severity and outcome in patients with severe sepsis: an analysis from a multicentre, prospective survey of severe sepsis. *Critical Care*, 17, R271.

Levy, M. M., Evans, L. E. and Rhodes, A. (2018). The surviving sepsis campaign bundle: 2018 update. *Critical Care Medicine*, 46(6). doi:10.1097/ccm.0000000000003119.

Ljunggren, M., Castren, M., Nordberg, M. and Kurland, L. (2016). The association between vital signs and mortality in a retrospective cohort study of an unselected emergency department population.

Scandinavian Journal of Trauma, Resuscitation and Emergency Medicine, 24(1), 21. doi:10.1186/s13049-016-0213-8.

Loveday, H. P., Wilson, J. A., Pratt, R. J., Golsorkh, M., Tingle, A., Bak, A. and Browne, J. (2014). epic3: national evidence-based guidelines for preventing healthcare-associated infections in NHS hospitals in England. *Journal of Hospital Infection*, 86(Supplement 1), S1–S70.

Marieb, E. and Hoehn, K. (2016). *Human Anatomy and Physiology*, Global Edition. San Francisco, CA: Benjamin Cummings Education.

Michaud, D., Houseman, E., Marsit, C., Nelson, H., Wiencke, J. and Kelsey, K. (2015). Understanding the role of the immune system in the development of cancer: new opportunities for population-based research. *Cancer Epidemiology, Biomarkers & Prevention*, 24(12), 1811–1819. doi:10.1158/1055-9965.EPI-15-0681.

Nagalingam, K. (2018). Understanding sepsis. *British Journal of Nursing*, 27(20), 1168–1170. doi:10.12968/bjon.2018.27.20.1168. Available from https://www.magonlinelibrary.com/doi/pdf/10.12968/bjon.2018.27.20.1168.

National Confidential Inquiry into Patient Outcomes and Death (NCEPOD). (2015). *Just Say Sepsis! A Review of the Process of Care Received by Patients with Sepsis*. Available from https://www.ncepod.org.uk/2015 sepsis.html. Last accessed September 2019.

National Institute for Health and Care Excellence. (2011). *Anaphylaxis: Assessment Referral after Emergency Treatment*, cg 134. Available from https://www.nice.org.uk/guidance/cg134/resources/anaphylaxis-assessment-and-referral-after-emergency-treatment-pdf-35109510368965.

National Institute for Health and Care Excellence. (2012). *Neutropenic Sepsis: prevention and management in people with cancer*, cg 151. Available from https://www.nice.org.uk/guidance/cg151/resources/neutropenic-sepsis-prevention-and-management-in-people-with-cancer-pdf-35109626262469.

National Institute for Health and Care Excellence. (2016). *Sepsis: Recognition, Diagnosis and Early Management*. Available from https://www.nice.org.uk/guidance/ng51.

NHS England. (2017). *Sepsis Guidance Implementation Advice for Adults*. Available from https://www.england.nhs.uk/wp-content/uploads/2017/09/sepsis-guidance-implementation-advice-for-adults.pdf. Accessed October 2019.

NHS Improvement and IPS. (2017). *High Impact Interventions. Care Processes to Prevent Infection 4th Edition of Saving Lives: High Impact Interventions*. Available from https://www.ips.uk.net/files/6115/0944/9537/High_Impact_Interventions.pdf.

Nursing and Midwifery Council. (2018). *Standards Framework for Nursing and Midwifery Education*. Available from https://www.nmc.org.uk/globalassets/sitedocuments/education-standards/education-framework.pdf.

O'Driscoll, R., Howard, L., Earis, J., Mak, V., Bajwah, S., Beasley, R., Curtis, K., Davison, A., Dorward, A., Dyer, C., Evans, A., Falconer, L., Fitzpatrick, C., Gibbs, S., Hinshaw, K., Howard, R., Kane, B., Keep, J., Kelly, C., Khachi, H., Asad, M., Khan, I., Kishen, R., Mansfield, L., Martin, B., Moore, F., Powrie, D., Restrick, L., Roffe, C., Singer, M., Soar, J., Small, I., Ward, L., Whitmore, D., Wedzicha, W., Wijesinghe, M. and BTS Emergency Oxygen Guideline Development Group On behalf of the British Thoracic Society. (2017). BTS guideline for oxygen use in adults in healthcare an emergency settings. *Thorax*, 72(S1), i1–i20.

Public Health England. (2018). *Staphylococcus aureus (MRSA and MSSA) Bacteraemia: Mandatory Surveillance 2017/18 Summary of the Mandatory Surveillance Annual Epidemiological Commentary 2017/18*. Available from https://assets.publishing.service.gov.uk/government/uploads/system/uploads/attachment_data/file/724361/S_aureus_summary_2018.pdf.

Public Health England/NHS Improvement. (2017). *Preventing Healthcare Associated Gram-Negative Bloodstream Infections: An Improvement Resource*.

RCUK (Resuscitation Council UK). (2008). *Emergency Treatment of Anaphylactic Reactions. Guidelines for Healthcare Providers*. Available from http://www.resus.org.uk/pages/reaction.pdf. Last accessed August 2019.

Rhodes, A., Evans, L. E., Alhazzani, W., Levy, M. M., Antonelli, M., Ferrer, R., Kumar, A., Sevransky, J. E., Sprung, C. L., Nunnally, M. E., Rochwerg, B., Rubenfeld, G. D., Angus, D. C., Annane, D.,

Beale, R. J., Bellinghan, G. J., Bernard, G. R., Chiche, J. D., Coopersmith, C., De Backer, D. P., French, C. J., Fujishima, S., Gerlach, H., Hidalgo, J. L., Hollenberg, S. M., Jones, A. E., Karnad, D. R., Kleinpell, R. M., Koh, Y., Lisboa, T. C., Machado, F. R., Marini, J. J., Marshall, J. C., Mazuski, J. E., McIntyre, L. A., McLean, A. S., Mehta, S., Moreno, R. P., Myburgh, J., Navalesi, P., Nishida, O., Osborn, T. M., Perner, A., Plunkett, C. M., Ranieri, M., Schorr, C. A., Seckel, M. A., Seymour, C. W., Shieh, L., Shukri, K. A., Simpson, S. Q., Singer, M., Thompson, B., Townsend, S. R., Van der Poll, T., Vincent, J. L., Wiersinga, W. J., Zimmerman, K. L. and Dellinger, R. P. (2017). Surviving sepsis campaign: international guidelines for management of sepsis and septic shock: 2016. *Intensive Care Medicine*, 43, 304–377. doi:10.1007/s00134-017-4683-6.

Royal College of Physicians. (2017). *National Early Warning Score (NEWS) 2 Standardising the Assessment of Acute-Illness Severity in the NHS*. Available from http://www.rcplondon.ac.uk/resources/national-early-warning-score-news. Accessed on 14 January 2019.

Singer, M., Deutschman, C. S., Seymour, C. W., et al. (2016). The third international consensus definitions for sepsis and septic shock (sepsis-3). *JAMA*, 315(8), 801–810.

Smith, M. and Meyfroid, G. (2017). Critical Illness: the brain is always in the line of fire. *Intensive Care Medicine*, 43(6), 870–873.

Stewart, J. (2012). Innate and acquired immunity. In Greenwood, D., Barer, M., Slack, R. and Irving, W. (eds.), *Medical Microbiology A Guide to Microbial Infections: Pathogenesis, Immunity, Laboratory Diagnosis and Control*, 18th Edition. London: Churchill Livingstone Elsevier, pp. 109–135.

Treacy, M. and Stayt, C. L. (2019). To identify the factors that influence the recognizing and responding to adult patient deterioration in acute hospitals. *Journal of Advanced Nursing*, 75, 1–14. doi:10.1111/jan.14138.

Wentowski, C., Mewada, N. and Nielson, N. D. (2019). Sepsis in 2018: a review. *Anaesthesia & Intensive Care Medicine*, 20(1), 6–13. doi:10.1016/j.mpaic.2018.11.009.

Weston, D. (2013). *Fundamentals of Infection Prevention and Control: Theory and Practice for Healthcare Professional*. Chichester: Wiley-Blackwell.

Wiewel, M. A., Harmon, M. B., van Vught, L. A., Scicluna, B. P., Hoogendijk, A. J., Horn, J., Zwinderman, A. H., Cremer, O. L., Bonten, M. J., Schultz, M. J. and van der Poll, T. (2016). Risk factors, host response and outcome of hypothermic sepsis. *Critical Care*, 20(1), 328.

World Health Organisation (WHO). (2009). *WHO Guidelines on Hand Hygiene in Health Care, First Global Patient Safety Challenge Clean Care is Safer Care*. ©World Health Organization. Available from http://whqlibdoc.who.int/publications/2009/9789241597906_eng.pdf. Last accessed August 2011.

World Health Organisation (WHO). (2017). *Improving the Prevention, Diagnosis and Clinical Management of Sepsis*. Available from http://apps.who.int/gb/ebwha/pdf_files/WHA70/A70_R7-en.pdf?ua=1&ua=1.

World Health Organisation (WHO). (2018). *Sepsis, Key Facts*. Available from https://www.who.int/news-room/fact-sheets/detail/sepsis.

Further reading

Wilson, J. (2017). *Infection Control in Clinical Practice Updated Edition*, 3rd Edition. Elsevier.

Zhou, Y., Lei, J., Xie, Q., Wu, L., Jin, S., Guo, B., Wang, X., Yan, G., Zhang, Q., Zhao, H., Zhang, J., Zhang, X., Wang, J., Gu, J., Liu, X., Ye, D., Miao, H., Serhan, C. N., & Li, Y. (2019). Fibrinogen-like protein 2 controls sepsis catabasis by interacting with resolvin Dp5. *Science Advances*, *5*(11), eaax0629. https://doi.org/10.1126/sciadv.aax0629'.

13 The safe transfer of acutely ill patients

Luke Cox

AIM

The aim of this chapter is to increase your knowledge with regard to the safe transfer of acutely ill patients.

OBJECTIVES

After reading this chapter, you will be able to:

- Differentiate between intra- and inter-hospital transfers.
- Identify reasons for transferring acutely ill patients.
- Debate the ethico-legal issues that arise in practice when transferring patients.
- Using the ABCDE format, describe the safe and effective preparation of the patient and the equipment prior to transfer.
- Highlight the physiological and psychological complications that the patient could sustain during the transfer process and how to manage them.
- Critically review the role of the nurse during transfer.

Introduction

In a medical emergency, a patient will require transfer between clinical environments at some point. There are many circumstances in which this would occur. It could involve admission from the community to the **Emergency Department (ED)** and subsequent **intra-hospital transfers** to a ward, a High-Dependency Unit (HDU) or an Intensive Care Unit (ICU). Patients may deteriorate within the hospital setting and be transferred to a higher level of dependency. Patients are also subject to intra-hospital transfers for investigations, imaging, surgery and other interventions.

Transfers *between* hospitals are a routine occurrence. Often, these provide **definitive care** or specialist treatment not offered at the source hospital (for instance, within the structure of an **operational delivery network**). In many circumstances, these inter-hospital transfers will be time critical. There may also be considerations depending on the manner of transport, be this by road, boat or air.

A further (although unusual) consideration is that clinical environments have procedures in place for the transfer of patients in emergency scenarios (e.g., fire), ranging from **'horizontal evacuation'** to the evacuation of whole buildings.

Each transfer instance represents risks to patient safety. These risks will be present regardless of the distance or the method of transport involved. Haemodynamic changes on movement and positioning, leaving behind an area with readily accessible help and resources, and consideration of **human factors** in co-ordinating the transfer process, all contribute to this risk. Practitioners must therefore possess the relevant knowledge, skills and training to safely and effectively transfer patients in their care. Nurses will also need to be aware of the significance of ethical and legal issues arising from the transfer process.

This chapter will explore preparation for transfer and the process itself, considering physiological complications, organisational problems and human factor errors that may occur, as well as strategies through which these risks may be mitigated.

How many patient transfers take place?

The scale of transfers between and within hospitals in the UK is not fully known. Audit of transfer activity tends to take place on a local scale and comparing figures from individual networks is problematic. **The Intensive Care Society (ICS)** (2019) suggests approximately 9500 *critical care* transfers occur between hospitals each year in the UK. In 2018, the Scottish Ambulance Service recorded 56,621 inter-hospital transfers for the area they cover (NHS Scotland 2018). If extrapolated to the whole UK, this would suggest more than 500,000 inter-hospital transfers each year.

Intra-hospital transfers are much more frequent. By way of illustration, available figures show that, in England in the year 2016/7, there were more than 1 million intra-hospital patient journeys between emergency and radiology departments *for* ***computerised tomography (CT)*** *scans alone* (NHS England 2017), and nearly 300,000 admissions to critical care units in the same period (NHS Digital 2017). It is safe to say that *millions of patient transfers take place each year.*

Reasons for transfer

Most movement of patients between areas or settings are intra-hospital transfers. This involves physical movement between wards, departments, or between buildings on the same hospital site. Here, an important distinction is made between transfers and ***transfers of care***, in which another provider or team is taking over the care of a patient. Intra-hospital transfers may well have a transfer of care as their aim (for instance, in transferring a patient from ED to ICU) but also include all aspects of patient movement which the same team oversees, such as moving a patient from a ward environment to the **radiology department** for a CT scan. Some types of transfer may have established protocols, while others may be *ad hoc.* There may be competing priorities in the decisions made around transfers, particularly where a patient is being moved to receive treatment (for instance, surgery) in an emergency.

Inter-hospital transfers also occur for a variety of reasons. Many transfers will be for *clinical* reasons, with a focus on providing patients with definitive treatment. This may occur within an arranged structure in which the specialities of hospitals are shared. In England, **Organisational Delivery Networks (ODNs)** exist to manage complex conditions such as major trauma, critical care and burns, with centres designated to receive patients as severity or dependency dictates. **Critical Care Networks** are an example of this structure. Some hospitals are designated centres at which certain interventions can take place. Transfer to a hospital which can provide **primary percutaneous coronary intervention (PPCI)** will usually be preferable to local medical management of an **ST-elevation myocardial infarction (STEMI)** (National Institute for Health and Care Excellence (NICE) 2013). Similarly, in the care of stroke, transfer to an **acute stroke unit** is recommended (Rudd et al. 2017). In both these examples, evidence-based targets exist for transfer and treatment, and delays in obtaining definitive care can be harmful.

Patients may also be transferred between hospitals for *non-clinical* reasons, for instance to meet socio-geographic demand, such as returning the patient to a place nearer their home. In the case of a hospital receiving patients as part of an ODN or other care network, a likely pathway for patients is that they are returned to their referring hospital once their clinical condition improves or an intervention has been completed. It may also be the case that patients are transferred for *capacity* reasons, which, for critically ill patients, should be the case only as a last resort (Intensive Care Society 2019).

Ethico-legal issues

A decision to transfer a patient will be debated by the multidisciplinary team, ideally as part of a process of **shared decision making** with the patient or their legally designated representative. The overall responsibility for a decision to transfer rests with the consultant overseeing the patient's care (and jointly with the consultant receiving the patient, if applicable). From an ethical perspective, patient transfer should be an act of beneficence, taken in the patient's best interests, especially as the process may cause their clinical condition to deteriorate further.

As key members of the multidisciplinary team, nurses have a professional responsibility to work within ethical and legal frameworks. These responsibilities are outlined in their code of professional conduct. Their foremost concerns are with the prioritisation of the patients in their care and acting in their best interests. This may be at odds with transfers for non-clinical reasons (NMC 2018).

Ideally, no patient should be transferred purely on the grounds of capacity, but a pragmatic approach must be taken when dealing with the realities of clinical practice. Workload constraints mean that transfers for non-clinical reasons, such as bed shortages, do occur. All members of the multidisciplinary team must ensure that this is a safe, well-implemented and well-documented procedure. In all patient transfers, the mode, timing and process of the move should be carefully planned, taking clinical parameters, such as the patient's condition, and environmental factors, such as travel arrangements, into consideration (Intensive Care Society 2019).

Nursing preparation for transfer

The role of the nurse in the transfer of an acutely ill patient is a challenging one, as it requires the practitioner to apply a range of knowledge and clinical skills under unfamiliar circumstances. The patient requires the delivery of a high standard of care throughout the transfer process, much of which may occur outside of the normal clinical environment. Managing a deteriorating patient in a familiar working context is easier than trying to cope in a series of places in which the nurse is not accustomed to working, such as corridors, lifts and ambulances. Problems may occur and, without preparation of the accompanying staff member, the patient and the equipment being used, the results may be disastrous.

During preparation for transfer, there are four key areas to consider:

- Staff training.
- Patient preparedness.
- Equipment
- Communication and documentation.

Staff training

Specialist training in the transfer of patients is recommended for all staff.

Training is a key factor in the successful transfer of patients. Until recently, there has been little formal training of nursing and medical staff in this area. In the past, an assumption was made that, if staff members possess a level of clinical expertise within their own working environment, they will be able to apply their knowledge and skills anywhere. This is not always the case. Many practitioners may be poorly prepared for transferring patients and a lack of specialist training exacerbates this. Often, junior staff are sent to accompany patients on inter- or intra-hospital transfers because senior staff cannot leave the clinical area. Cook and Allan (2008) found that transfer training of medical staff was haphazard and dependent on local initiatives, with no systematic approach to transfer education in place. This is an issue of concern for nursing staff, who may look to their medical colleagues for guidance and support during the transfer process. In many cases, depending on the severity of the patient's condition, the nurse may be the only health care professional present during the transfer process.

All staff should seek to receive some specialist training in this area of clinical practice. The Intensive Care Society (2019) recommends that staff should not undertake unsupervised transfers of critically ill patients without specific training and competencies, and specific training for the unusual features of **aeromedical** transfers is vital (Johnson and Luscombe 2011). In the UK, training for critical care transfers tends to be delivered locally by Critical Care Networks. Training is a pre-requisite for nurses working in acute areas, such as ICU, and for anyone undertaking inter-hospital transfers, but will be equally useful for ward nurses. Ideally, transfer training will cover technical skills related to transfer (such as patient preparation and stabilisation, familiarity with specific equipment and calculating oxygen requirements) alongside **non-technical skills (NTS)**, which include aspects of individual and team performance, such as situational awareness, decision making, communication, leadership and team work. An awareness and understanding of NTS is vital. An Australian study described how, of 191 critical incidents in intra-hospital transfers, 39% were attributed to equipment failures, and 61% to avoidable resource management, with communication between and within teams a predominant theme (Beckmann et al. 2004). Training programmes may include **clinical simulation** as a teaching method, as this can be effective at addressing human factor issues, and this is now a recommendation of the Intensive Care Society (2019).

Patient preparation

Acutely ill patients have an increased risk of deterioration during transfer (Dunn et al. 2007), so the nurse should adopt a systematic approach when planning to move a patient. In previous chapters, we have seen how the use of the ABCDE format for assessment, goal planning, intervention and evaluation enables clinicians to effectively manage patients in their care. Collecting both subjective and objective data during the assessment process can assist with the generation of an early warning score. Track and trigger systems, such as NEWS, provide valuable information on the severity of a patient's condition, and therefore assist the nurse to identify whether or not the patient is ready to be moved or requires additional clinical optimisation.

Before transfer, patients should be assessed systematically, using the ABCDE format. Remember to:

- Look.
- Feel.
- Listen.

Airway

Continuous monitoring of the patient's ability to maintain an airway is required. If there is any doubt, either due to impaired consciousness (see Disability) or sounds of obstruction being heard, such as **stridor**, then the airway should be secured by artificial means. Tracheal **intubation** prior to transfer may be indicated if there are any concerns of this nature. For further information on airway management, please refer to Chapter 7.

Breathing

If patient assessment reveals inadequate breathing, such as changes in the respiratory rate, the use of accessory muscles, evidence of poor gas exchange or the presence of **adventitious breath sounds**, action should be taken to improve the adequacy of ventilation before transfer – either by the administration of oxygen therapy or by initiating non-invasive or invasive mechanical means. Problems with oxygenation are more likely to occur during transfer, because, when a patient is moved, they are exposed to ***g*-forces** associated with acceleration and deceleration. Physiological compensatory mechanisms enable individuals to cope with this force, provided it is not severe or prolonged. In acute illness, the patient's ability to compensate is likely to be insufficient. Changes in the distribution of blood flow in the lungs can quickly result in a mismatch between alveolar ventilation and perfusion, and to a significant drop in a patient's oxygen saturations. Constant monitoring of all respiratory parameters is therefore required.

The identification of specific respiratory problems, such as the presence of a pneumothorax, must be addressed immediately, with chest drain insertion occurring prior to departure.

Every action must be taken to avoid deterioration of the patient's condition during transfer. If physiological problems are evident from the outset, these must be addressed as a priority.

Circulation

A thorough assessment of the patient's cardiovascular status is essential before departure. As noted in previous chapters, information needs to be gathered regarding general appearance; perfusion and capillary refill; skin temperature; skin sensation to touch; and the degree of hydration. The transferring team should proceed only when confident that the patient's condition and their vital signs have been rendered as stable as possible. If there are concerns, the patient should not be moved until the problems have been resolved (Intensive Care Society 2019). Knowledge of the patient's haematological status prior to departure is crucial, with problems, such **anaemia** or a **coagulopathy,** being addressed as a matter of urgency.

Of particular concern is **hypovolaemia**, which can occur for a number of reasons, including **haemorrhage** secondary to trauma, dehydration and sepsis. Volume-depleted patients do not tolerate transportation well. The *g*-forces alter blood flow distribution, and this can be exacerbated if a patient is fluid depleted. Movement towards the head (such as a trolley being pushed forwards), will result in blood moving suddenly towards the feet and pooling there. In contrast, during acceleration towards the feet, blood rushes towards the head. The net effect of these forces is to render the patient hypotensive, with poor cardiac output, because, the more volume depleted they are, the greater the scope there is for volume movement within the body (see Figure 13.1).

In Figure 13.1, we can see how a vessel that is only partially full allows room for movement of the fluid within it during movement. When the vessel is full, the fluid cannot be rapidly shifted from one end to another, because there is no empty space for it to move

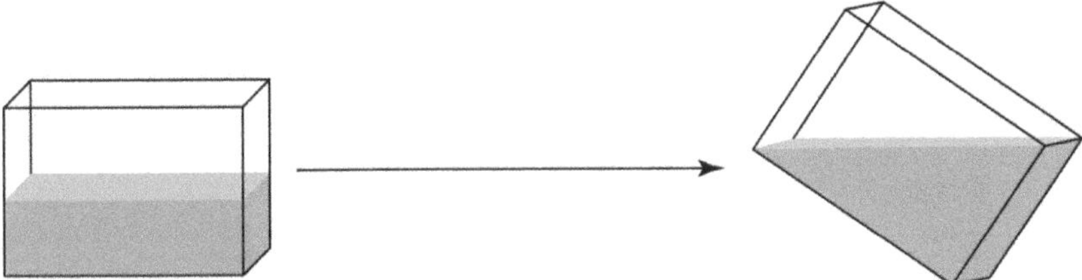

Transport in hypovolaemia: there is rapid movement of fluid in an underfilled patient

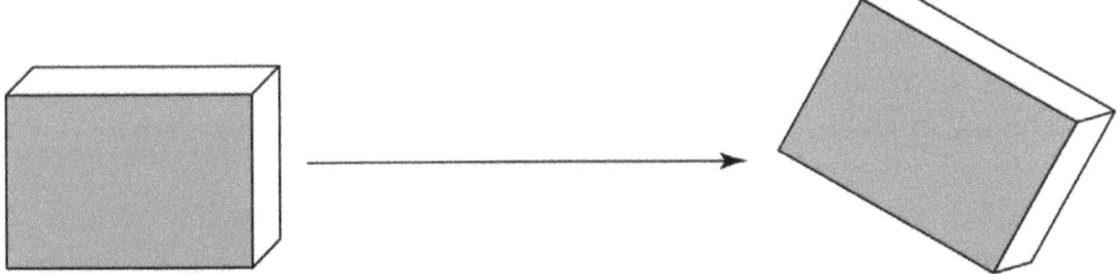

Transport in normovolaemia: less movement of fluid occurs

Figure 13.1 Treating hypovolaemia reduces the physiological effect of movement on blood flow. *Source*: Reproduced with kind permission from Dr J. Handy, NWL Critical Care Network.

into. The same principle applies to patients: if they are normovolaemic, with a good circulating volume, they are less likely to suffer from the effects of acceleration on blood flow. As a general rule, 'full patients travel better' (Handy and van Zwanenberg 2007), although there are specific instances (such as aortic dissection) where fluid resuscitation should be kept to a minimum.

During transfer, acutely ill patients must have at least

- Cardiac monitoring.
- SpO_2 monitoring.
- Non-invasive blood pressure monitoring;
- Intravenous access

It is vital to ensure that patients are haemodynamically stable and that fluid deficits have been addressed before moving them. Acutely ill patients should have in place cardiac monitoring, non-invasive blood pressure monitoring, functioning *in-situ* intravenous access and SpO_2 monitoring. If hypovolaemia has been confirmed, intravenous fluid replacement should be administered promptly, although caution must be taken not to 'overfill', as this may lead to further problems in the form of **pulmonary oedema**. Patients may also have been receiving fluid volume *via* enteral sources; these should be stopped, and tubes left on free drainage during transfer. Free drainage is important because the gut will be exposed to the same forces as other organs and will not function well, leading to poor absorption and an increased risk of aspiration.

Another key factor is urinary output, monitored by hourly measurements if the patient is catheterised. When a patient is already well-filled with fluid, therapy, in the form of **inotropes** or other **vasoactive medication** for additional cardiovascular support, may be started. Anti-arrhythmic agents, such as amiodarone, might also be prescribed if patients are not in sinus rhythm, or are experiencing ectopic beats. Blood chemistry such as urea, electrolyte and blood glucose levels should all be checked prior to moving a patient, so that complications in transit arising from abnormal values can be avoided, wherever possible.

Disability

Neurological assessment is a crucial aspect of patient preparation. For patients with a reduced level of consciousness, constant monitoring, using the **Glasgow Coma Scale (GCS)**, together with pupillary assessment, is essential (see Chapter 9). The nurse must observe the patient's ability to maintain an airway and self-ventilate, the degree to which they have normal verbal and motor function, and changes in pupil size and reaction. Vital signs may be affected if the intracranial pressure is rising. Hypotension can exacerbate this, owing to a reduction in cerebral perfusion pressure, and can contribute to secondary brain injury (Carney et al. 2017). Should deterioration be noted, prompt action will be required to stabilise the patient before transfer. For some patients, the transfer may be indicated by the need for specialist intervention at another hospital, such as in the case of an intracranial haemorrhage. In such cases, the airway should be secured first. Any patient with a GCS of eight or below will require immediate intubation and mechanical ventilation, and this should also be considered if a patient's GCS has dropped two points or more below their baseline (Association of Anaesthetists of Great Britain and Ireland 2006).

For all patients, changes in blood flow related to acceleration can compromise neurological status, especially if blood rushes to the patient's head during a manoeuvre. A patient with raised intracranial pressure would not be able to tolerate this haemodynamic instability and changes to intracranial blood flow could precipitate cerebral oedema, risking further neuronal injury. To reduce the chance of this occurring, patients should be positioned in a 20° 'head-up' position, which will limit the effect of positive and negative acceleratory forces (Handy and van Zwanenberg 2007). **Cervical fracture** (a particular risk for trauma patients) must be excluded before moving the patient from a supine position. A protective **rigid cervical collar** should be worn at all times, until radiological investigation confirms that neck immobilisation is no longer necessary. A **spinal cord injury** may be sustained if the patient's neck is moved prematurely (Walters et al. 2013).

If a patient requires intubation and mechanical ventilation, they will be sedated and might have intravenous analgesia in progress. These measures are necessary to facilitate therapeutic intervention and promote patient comfort. Many patients are transferred while fully conscious and self-ventilating, and the nurse should be aware that these individuals are likely to experience pain and discomfort when being prepared for transfer and during the transfer itself. **Ischaemia,** surgical wound sites, fractures or tissue damage may be present and often the patient will be immobilised. They may also be distressed by other sensory disturbances, such as bright lighting or unfamiliar noises. Pain and discomfort should be assessed by the nurse, and this will include behavioural observation alongside verbal feedback There is an increasing role for objective behavioural observation tools in this process, with the Critical Care Pain Observation Tool (CPOT) being a useful example (Stiles 2013). Should it be required, analgesia should be prescribed and administered before moving the patient, and consideration given to continuous pain management during the transfer process.

Patients should be kept fully informed regarding the transfer and, if conscious, given the opportunity to ask questions and participate in the decision-making process. Informing a conscious patient that they are to be moved may provoke anxiety and even anger. The nurse therefore has a responsibility to work in partnership with patients and their families, using effective communication and interpersonal skills to deliver compassionate, person-centred care (Nursing and Midwifery Council (NMC) 2018). Keeping people informed can allay their fears and concerns, whilst simultaneously reducing their sense of powerlessness when faced with the stressful circumstances accompanying critical illness. Gustard et al. (2008) found, in their study of 249 patients who were being transferred, that, when nursing staff gave repeated information at regular intervals about proceedings, it lessened the patients' anxiety.

Exposure

Corridors and vehicles can be cold places and a patient will lose body heat if exposed to a low temperature. Hypothermia, when the core temperature drops below 35°C, can lead to repetitive muscle contraction in the form of shivering, and the release of hormones from the adrenal and thyroid glands can also occur. The net effect of these physiological responses is for the metabolic rate and oxygen consumption to increase, which can lead to cardiovascular instability (Paal et al. 2018).

Pyrexia is an alternative complication, which may be a feature of the patient's clinical condition. This will also increase metabolic rate and oxygen consumption (Jain and Saxena 2015). Wounds may be present; apart from being a source of pain for the patient, these are access points for infection and so should be well protected and securely dressed.

The location and function of indwelling and invasive devices should be carefully noted, with care taken to stabilise them. It is easy to tug or displace cannula or catheters, particularly during lateral transfers between beds and trolleys. Patency must be checked before departure, as replacing an invasive device is achieved less easily when on the move. For intravenous cannula, ensuring that a second patent cannula is *in situ* is a reasonable consideration, particularly for patients receiving sedation or inotropic support, where the sudden cessation of an infusion can be disastrous.

Equipment preparation

It is not safe practice for the nurse to be gathering together items for transfer when the patient's move is imminent, and this would not be practical in an emergency. All clinical areas should therefore have a stocked and checked **transfer bag**. Assembling and maintaining a transfer bag requires a checklist and a staff commitment to ensuring that the bag is restocked after use and its contents sealed and checked daily. The example checklist in Table 13.1 shows equipment and consumables arranged in an ABCDE format. Staff accompanying a patient should be familiar with the layout of the transfer bag and the functions of its contents.

Not all the equipment necessary for a transfer will fit into the transfer bag, and not all larger items of equipment will be necessary for every transfer. Transfer equipment must be checked, well maintained, ready to use and accessible. A key consideration here is that battery-powered equipment (for instance, a portable suction device or a portable monitor) will work when not on charge and have sufficient power for the duration of the planned transfer. As observed by Beckmann et al. (2004), power supply problems are a frequent and avoidable cause of critical incidents. Just as a secondary cannula is a worthwhile consideration, it may be necessary to take a spare infusion pump or syringe driver for infusions that must not be stopped. Conversely, if infusions can be safely stopped during transfer, this will cut down on the amount of equipment to transport.

To calculate oxygen required

Delivery rate (L/minute) x journey time (minutes) × 1.5= litres of oxygen required

The amount of medication to take on a transfer is also an important consideration. This will depend on the length of the journey and the rate at which infusions are being delivered. Taking 150% of the calculated amount of medicine needed provides leeway in the event of an emergency or delay. This may mean preparing additional infusions before departure. This principle also applies to calculating the amount of oxygen required for a transfer. For a patient who is not mechanically ventilated, this involves calculating the volume of oxygen likely to be used in the journey as follows, allowing for a return journey if appropriate, and then ensuring that that amount is available. In practice, this means selecting a cylinder of appropriate volume and ensuring that it is full. Table 13.2, developed by Colchester Hospital University NHS Trust, shows common tank sizes used in the NHS, their content in litres, when full, and running times when used with different flow rates (National Patient Agency 2009) (Figure 13.2).

Table 13.1 Transfer equipment checklist

Item	*Checked*	*Item*	*Checked*
Airway:		Circulation:	
A selection of face masks		Venous access: 14- to 22-gauge cannula	
Guedel airways sizes 2, 3 and 4		A variety of needles and syringes	
Nasopharyngeal airways, sizes 6 and 7		Scalpel	
Bag valve mask with reservoir		Two silk sutures, sizes 0 or greater	
Two laryngoscopes with size 3 and 4 blades with functioning bulbs (plus spare bulbs)		Sterile scissors	
Endotracheal tubes (ET) sizes 6–9mm		Forceps	
Tracheostomy tubes sizes 6–9mm with obturators		20mL lignocaine 2% with adrenaline	
Tracheostomy dilator		Selection of giving sets and burettes	
Two laryngeal masks sizes 3 and 4		2–4 litres of colloid	
Bougie		2–4 litres of Hartmann's solution	
Lubricant		2 × 50mL 50% glucose	
Magill's forceps		200mL 8.4% bicarbonate	
10mL syringe to inflate endotracheal cuff		250mL 20% mannitol	
Endotracheal tape to secure tube		Portable intravenous infusion stand	
Catheter mount		Glucometer	
Cricothyroidotomy kit		Emergency drugs:	
Portable suction equipment		• Atropine 1mg/10mL	
Yankeur sucker		• Atropine 3mg/10mL	
Suction catheters of different sizes		• Epinephrine 1:10,000/10mL	
		• Amiodarone 300mg/10mL	
Breathing:			
Oxygen cylinder: with sufficient amount of oxygen for a return journey, plus a 50% or one-hour reserve		Mains- and battery-powered monitor with ECG and non-invasive blood pressure capability. Battery to be fully charged and a spare to be available	
SpO_2 monitoring		Syringe drivers for all infusions, with at least one spare	
Chest drain equipment: **Heimlich valves**		Direct current defibrillator (depending on the severity of the patient's condition)	
Aminophylline 25mg/mL (10mL)		**Disability**:	
		Working pen torch and spare battery	
		Diazemul 5mg/mL (2mL)	
		Exposure:	
		Core and peripheral temperature monitoring	
		Warming blankets	
		Wound dressings	
Name and signature:		**Date and time:**	

Flow = ltrs/min

Size → / Flow ↓	D (340 ltrs)	PD (300 ltrs)	CD/DD (460 ltrs)	E (680 ltrs)	F/AF (1360 ltrs)	HX (2300 ltrs)	ZX (3040 ltrs)	G (3400 ltrs)	J (6800 ltrs)
0.25	22.6	20.0	30.6	45.3	90.6	153.6	202.6	226.6	453.3
0.5	11.3	10.0	15.3	22.6	45.3	76.6	101.3	113.3	226.6
0.75	7.5	6.6	10.2	15.1	30.2	51.1	67.5	75.5	151.1
1	5.6	5.0	7.6	11.3	22.6	38.3	50.6	56.6	113.3
2	2.8	2.5	3.8	5.6	11.3	19.1	25.3	28.3	56.6
3	1.9	1.6	2.5	3.7	7.5	12.7	16.8	18.8	37.7
4	1.4	1.2	1.9	2.8	5.6	9.5	12.6	14.1	28.3
5	1.1	1.0	1.5	2.2	4.5	7.6	10.1	11.3	22.6
6	0.9	0.8	1.2	1.8	3.7	6.3	8.4	9.4	18.8
7	0.8	0.7	1.0	1.6	3.2	5.4	7.2	8.0	16.1
8	0.7	0.6	0.9	1.4	2.8	4.7	6.3	7.0	14.1
9	0.6	0.5	0.8	1.2	2.5	4.2	5.6	6.2	12.5
10	0.5	0.5	0.7	1.1	2.2	3.8	5.0	5.6	11.3
12	0.5	0.4	0.6	0.9	1.8	3.1	4.2	4.7	9.4
15	0.4	0.3	0.5	0.7	1.5	2.5	3.3	3.7	7.5

S.CONNEW. EBME. 03/03/05

Time = Hours

Figure 13.2 Content (in litres) of oxygen tanks.

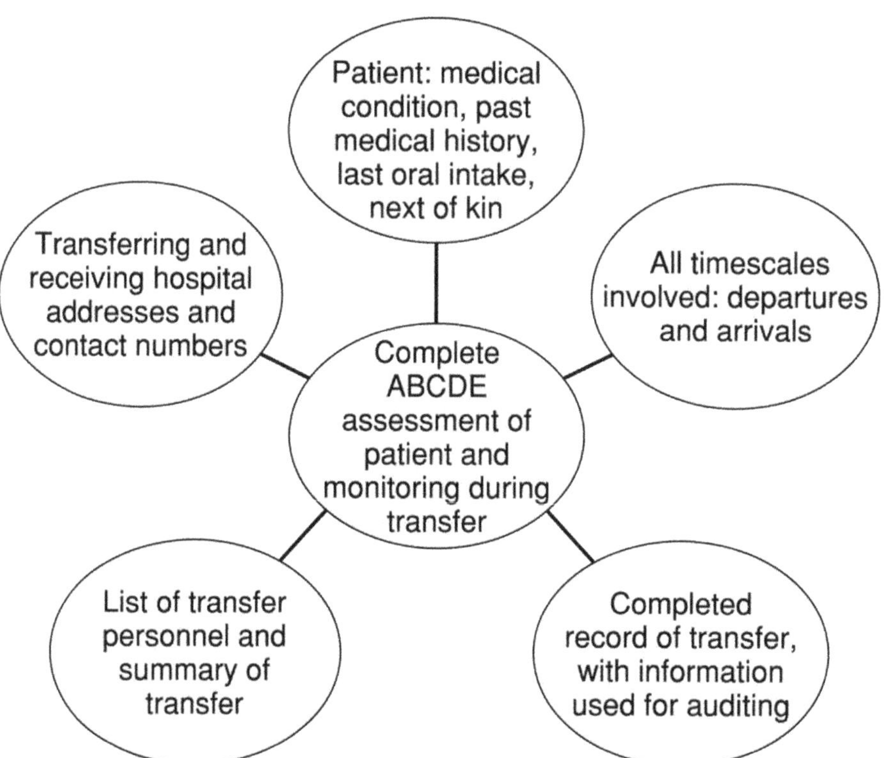

Figure 13.3 Information to be included in a transfer form.

Table 13.2 Nursing responsibilities during the transfer process

Action	*Rationale*
Effectively communicating the decision to transfer to all concerned parties	All staff members at the transferring and receiving ends need to be fully informed that the patient is being moved and why the move is necessary. The patient's family also needs to be informed
Informing all staff involved of the timescales to be observed	All staff members need to know the time of departure and the anticipated time of arrival, so that the process runs smoothly without delays. If ambulance personnel are involved, they must be contacted in advance and everything put in place for their arrival time
Preparing the patient, staff and equipment for the move	The patient should be fully assessed and prepared for transfer: • transfer bag, plus any additional equipment required, should be ready for use • The staff accompanying the patient should be suitably prepared to go in terms of personal readiness, for example, possessing a mobile phone, being appropriately dressed and having money to hand. All are necessary as there may be delays, or, in an intra-hospital transfer they may have to find their own way back to their workplace. Remember ambulances are not taxis - they may be called away to another clinical incident
Executing the move safely and efficiently	All accompanying medical and nursing personnel must constantly monitor the patient in transit and record any problems encountered
Giving a detailed handover to receiving nursing staff	Whereas medical staff will liaise with each other, regarding the patient's condition, a thorough nursing handover must be given to nursing colleagues, and this should include the following information about the patient: • present medical and nursing problems, including the reason for transfer • past medical history • any known allergies • current medication • any known source of infection (for example, methicillin-resistant *Staphylococcus aureus* MRSA) • therapy delivered during transit and any problems encountered • social circumstances (next of kin) and all relevant contact numbers It is recommended that the SBAR tool (situation, background, assessment and recommendation) be used in order to deliver a systematic report (as discussed in Chapter 1)
Producing documentation to support the verbal handover	For legal and professional reasons, there must be clear, legible and accurate nursing documentation accompanying the handover discussion. Good record keeping is essential (NMC 2018). Nursing staff must also ensure that all other relevant clinical information pertaining to the patient is transferred with them, for example, medical notes and chest X-rays
Liaising with the doctor to complete a transfer form	Both the transferring and receiving clinical teams must keep copies of this multidisciplinary documentation
Auditing of the transfer process	Auditing of all transfer events is important so that problems, that may have occurred anywhere in the procedure, can be identified and acted upon quickly in order to prevent a repetition. Auditing can also contribute to the collection of national data

Communication and documentation

Problems occurring during the transfer of a patient from one area to another are often attributed to 'systems failure', where organisational issues have compromised patient safety. Ineffectual communication with other clinical teams, poor preparation of staff, inadequate stabilisation of the patient and insufficient checking of equipment have all contributed to unsafe practice. Access to and completion of a designated **transfer form,** outlining the key areas to be addressed when transporting patients, is one of the ways in which these problems can be minimised. It is recommended that transfer forms are completed, so that there is a detailed record of all transfer events taking place, and that forms are standardised (Intensive Care Society 2019). Whereas many different formats of transfer forms exist, certain requisite information should be included, as illustrated in Figure 13.3.

The NMC (2018) stresses the importance of nurses using a full range of communication methods, demonstrating verbal, non-verbal and written skills. They must also be able to work effectively as part of the multidisciplinary team, providing leadership and coordinating inter-professional care.

All clinicians are professionally accountable for their own actions or omissions, but it is imperative that one person takes overall responsibility for communication and documentation in a transfer. The nurse is often the best-placed team member to do this (Handy and van Zwanenberg 2007), as they have close proximity to the patient and can effectively liaise with other team members, who may be based in different departments or different hospitals.

The preparation process to which the nurse should adhere when transferring a patient is illustrated by the following case study, and the responsibilities of the nurse during transfer are outlined in Table 13.2

CASE STUDY 13.1 AN INTRA-HOSPITAL TRANSFER 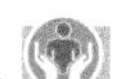

Samira Khan, a teacher, is 56 years old. Overnight, she has been admitted to the acute medical unit (AMU) with a diagnosis of acute pancreatitis. The consultant has requested an urgent CT scan of her abdomen, because pseudocyst formation (a common feature of the disease) is suspected. It is now 08:00 and the nurses on the day shift have just come on duty. During the handover, they are informed that the scan is booked for 11:00 in the radiology department.The porter has been contacted and asked to arrive at 10:30 to transport the patient to the radiology department on the ground floor from the AMU, which is on the 5th floor in the same building.

The nurse allocated to care for Mrs Khan conducts an initial assessment of her condition in order to effectively plan the transfer.

Airway: Mrs Khan is conscious and is able to maintain her own airway.

Breathing: Mrs Khan is sitting in an upright position at a 30° angle. She complains of feeling breathless. Her respiratory rate is assessed for a full minute and is found to be 22 breaths per minute. No use of accessory muscles is observed. She is receiving 2L/minute of oxygen *via* nasal cannula and her SpO_2 reading is currently 92%. Her target saturations are noted to be 94–98%.

On chest auscultation, no adventitious breath sounds are heard. She has a productive cough, and the nurse noted that a sputum sample has already been sent to microbiology for culture and sensitivity.

An arterial blood gas (ABG) sample taken at 04:30 revealed the following results:

pH: 7.32
PaO_2: 8.0kPa
$PaCO_2$: 4.5kPa
HCO_3: 18mmol/L
BE: -6mmol/L

The nurse interprets this as hypoxaemia with evidence of a metabolic acidosis and attributes this finding to anaerobic metabolism, possibly occurring secondarily to sepsis and hypovolaemia.

Breathing NEWS (2+2+2) =6

Circulation: Mrs Khan appears well-perfused, with no indication of peripheral or central cyanosis. Her skin is warm and dry to the touch and her capillary refill time is prolonged, at 4 seconds. Her observations have been recorded hourly and, at 09:00, are as follows:

Arterial blood pressure: 110/72mmHg
Heart rate: 110bpm, sinus tachycardia.

She is receiving intravenous crystalloid fluid (0.9% sodium chloride) at 125mL/hour and has a urinary output of 38mL per hour. Her recorded weight is 82kg. Since admission seven hours ago, she has a recorded positive fluid balance of 580mL.

The nurse concludes that, despite fluid replacement, Mrs Khan remains volume depleted as a result of sepsis and hypovolaemia. She is currently nil by mouth (NBM) and has a nasogastric tube *in situ* on free drainage. A total of 200mL of bile-stained fluid is present in the drainage bag.

Blood tests, taken on admission, reveal an elevated white cell count (WCC), serum amylase, serum lipase and blood glucose. Currently, she is receiving an intravenous sliding-scale insulin infusion.

Circulation NEWS: (2+1) =3

Disability: Mrs Khan is alert, oriented, and, although anxious, is able to hold a coherent conversation with the nurse. The nurse assesses her as 'alert' in the ACVPU section of the NEWS 2 chart. At 03:00, a pain score of 9/10 was recorded, and a patient-controlled analgesia (PCA) pump was initiated. Now, Mrs Khan reports that she feels comfortable.

Disability NEWS =0

Exposure: Mrs Khan's body temperature is 38.5°C. Blood cultures were taken at 02:00 and IV antibiotics were commenced. On examination, no wounds, broken skin or pressure area damage are noted. The nurse notes the position and condition of two intravenous cannula (in the cephalic vein of the left forearm and right antecubital fossa), an arterial cannula (left radial artery), a central venous catheter (right internal jugular vein) and a urinary catheter. The cannula sites are well secured, and the surrounding skin does not appear inflamed.

Exposure NEWS =1

The nurse concludes, from her preliminary assessment, that Mrs Khan is acutely unwell with a risk of deterioration. Her immediate problems are increasing hypoxaemia and hypovolaemia, which, the nurse believes, are associated with sepsis.

The nurse calculates Mrs Khan's early warning score using the NEWS 2 scoring system, with the following findings:

Resipiratory rate: 21–24 breaths per minute = 2
SpO_2: 92–93% = 2
Additional oxygen used: = 2
Systolic blood pressure: 101–110 = 1
Pulse: 91–110 = 1
Conscious level: alert = 0
Temperature: 38.1–39.0°C = 1

NEWS 2 = 9

An aggregate score ≥7 indicates an urgent or emergency response. Despite the urgency of the planned investigation, Mrs Khan must be stabilised before transfer or her condition will deteriorate further. Her haemodynamic instability is likely to be exacerbated by movement during the journey. The nurse contacts the specialist registrar and discusses the need for additional oxygen therapy and fluid resuscitation. Oxygen is increased to 8L/minute *via* a face mask, and the rate of the prescribed fluid is commenced at 250mL/hour, with further fluid prescribed. In addition, blood cultures are taken, and antibiotics are prescribed and administered.

Following this, the nurse continues with her preparation for transfer, and uses a transfer checklist to assist with this as follows:

- She fully informs Mrs Khan of the transfer procedure.
- She collects the transfer equipment she will require:
- The ward keeps two stocked transfer bags and she notes the intact seal on the bag.
- She collects a portable suction unit. She checks that the battery is fully charged, and that the unit works when not on charge.
- She ensures that she has an oxygen cylinder which will provide sufficient oxygen for the journey. The bed has a storage slot for a Size F cylinder, which, when full, holds 1360L. This cylinder is half full. Her experience tells her the transfer will take less than 2 hours in total. Using 5L/min would require 600L and half a full-sized F cylinder would contain 680L. This might be sufficient, but she has been advised to carry 150% of the expected use, and so she exchanges the half-full cylinder for a full tank.

- She ensures that the infusion pumps for the crystalloid, insulin infusion and PCA are fully charged and work when not plugged in, and that these can be securely attached to the bed. She checks that the volume in each of these infusions will be sufficient for the transfer.
- She ensures Mrs. Khan's notes are updated and available on the hospital's electronic patient notes (EPR) system, and that she has the documentation to record the transfer process.
- When the porter arrives at 10:30, the nurse calls the radiology department to advise that Mrs Khan is fully prepared and is ready to be transferred.

Evaluation:

Prior to transfer, the team's interventions stabilised Mrs Khan's condition. At 10:30, her SpO_2 was 96%, her heart rate was 87, and her blood pressure was 114/70mmHg. The nurse recalculated her NEWS 2 as 5. The porter arrived at 10:30 and the porter, Mrs Khan and the nurse left HDU at 10:45, arriving in the radiology department at 10:55. There was an unexpected delay in the department because of a technical problem with the CT scanner, and, in total, the transfer time, from leaving the ward to return, was 70 minutes. As the nurse had prepared sufficiently, stabilising Mrs. Khan's condition, collecting the required equipment and communicating effectively with other members of the multi-disciplinary team, she was able to leave the ward on time. Anticipating delays meant she had sufficient oxygen and medication prepared for the entire transfer. On return to the unit, the nurse completed the transfer form and submitted it to the unit manager as part of the Trust's audit process.

Conclusion

This chapter has discussed intra- and inter-hospital transfers of patients. Regardless of the distance involved and mode of transport used, transfers can be hazardous. They require sufficient planning so that physiological and organisational complications can be avoided. The key areas of concern are the stabilisation of the patient and the preparation of staff and equipment. To safely move patients from one clinical area to another without incident, a systematic, coordinated approach is required. With appropriate training in the role, the nurse is well placed to act as a team leader in this situation and ensure that all patient transfers are conducted in a safe and professional manner

Glossary

Acute pancreatitis Sudden inflammation of the pancreas, often associated with gallstones or chronic alcohol use.

Acute stroke unit A specialised area in the hospital for treating, monitoring and rehabilitating stroke patients, staffed by a specialist stroke multidisciplinary team.

Adventitious breath sounds Abnormal sounds that are heard over a patient's lungs and airways, such as crackles, wheezes (sometimes called rhonchi), pleural rubs and stridor

Aeromedical Relating to the use of aircraft for medical purposes, such as transporting patients to hospital

Anaemia The condition of having fewer than the normal number of red blood cells or less than the normal quantity of haemoglobin in the blood, leading to a reduction in the oxygen-carrying capacity of the blood.

Coagulopathy A condition in which the blood's ability to coagulate (form clots) is impaired. This can cause prolonged or excessive bleeding,

Computerised tomography (CT) The use of a computer to co-ordinate X-ray images taken sequentially from multiple angles. This allows a detailed view of the targeted organ or structure.

Clinical simulation Simulation-based education is an educational model that allows students to rehearse behaviours and skills, and learn from clinical scenarios, without placing patients or resources at risk.

Crew Resource Management (CRM) Management of all available resources for the purpose of promoting safety and effectiveness. Resources include equipment, procedures and people.

Cricothyroidotomy Cannula insertion into the cricothyroid membrane to facilitate ventilation.

Critical Care Networks A type of operational delivery network, focusing on the transfer of patients between and to intensive care units.

Definitive care The delivery of a selected treatment for a disease or injury, or the place at which it will be provided. For instance, definitive care for a patient with a STEMI is likely to be PPCI, requiring transfer to a Coronary Care Unit.

Emergency Department (ED) A treatment facility specialising in the acute care of patients who present without prior appointment. This may also be referred to as an accident and emergency department (A&E), emergency room (ER) or casualty department.

Glasgow Coma Scale (GCS) An observational tool, developed as a way to communicate the level of consciousness of patients with an acute brain injury.

Gravitational force equivalent (*g* force) A measurement of the type of force per unit mass – typically acceleration – that causes a perception of weight.

Haemorrhage An escape of blood from a ruptured blood vessel.

Heimlich valve A type of one-way flutter valve which supports chest drainage by preventing drained gases or fluids from returning to the body.

Horizontal evacuation Where a building's construction means that immediate evacuation is not required, and people can be moved gradually away from an area of danger, typically involving evacuation to other areas on the same level, behind fire-resistant structures. May be phased or progressive horizontal evacuation.

Human factors The application of psychological and physiological principles to the design of processes and systems with the aim of reducing human error and enhancing safety.

Hypovolaemia A state of decreased intravascular volume, either through a loss of water and salt, or through a decrease in blood volume.

Inotrope An agent that alters the force of muscular contractions. Typically, in a critical care context, positive inotropes will be used to increase cardiac muscle contractility and support blood pressure

Ischaemia A restriction in blood supply to tissues, leading to a shortage of the oxygen needed for cellular metabolism

The Intensive Care Society (ICS) The representative body in the UK for intensive care professionals and patients. It performs many functions for the intensive care community in the United Kingdom, including the production of guidelines and standards.

Inter-hospital transfer Moving a patient from one hospital to another.

Intra-hospital transfer Moving a patient from one area to another within the same hospital.

Intubation The insertion of an artificial ventilation tube into the trachea.

Non-Technical Skills (NTS) Cognitive, social and personal resource skills that complement technical skills, contributing to safe and effective practice.

Organisational Delivery Networks A system for coordinating patient pathways between different health care providers, enabling access to specialist resources and expertise.

Pancreatic pseudocyst An abdominal collection of fluid and tissue, formed as a complication of pancreatitis, and accounting for 75% of pancreatic masses associated with pancreatitis.

Pneumothorax A collapse of the lung caused by air or gas in the cavity between the lining of the lungs and the chest wall.

Primary percutaneous coronary intervention (PPCI) A procedure carried out under local anaesthetic in which a narrowing (stenosis) of coronary arteries is dilated with a balloon catheter and treated with a stent (a tubular metal alloy device), which is implanted into the artery as a scaffold to maintain its patency. Also referred to as coronary angioplasty.

Pulmonary oedema Fluid accumulation in the tissue and air spaces of the lungs, leading to impaired gas exchange and possibly respiratory failure.

Radiology department The facility in a hospital where radiological examinations of patients are carried out, using a range of equipment. Often referred to as an X-ray department or imaging department.

Rigid cervical collar May be referred to as a neck brace. A medical device used to support a person's neck. In trauma care, its use can help prevent movement of the neck and protect the patient from spinal cord injury in the case of a cervical fracture.

Shared decision making (SDM) A process whereby both the patient and health care professional contribute to the decision-making process. Treatments and alternatives are explained to patients to help them choose the option that best aligns with their preferences and beliefs.

Spinal cord injury Damage to the spinal cord that causing temporary or permanent changes in its function, often associated with loss of muscle function, sensation or autonomic function in the parts of the body served by the spinal cord below the level of the injury

ST-Elevation Myocardial Infarction (STEMI) A type of myocardial infarction (heart attack) in which a coronary artery is occluded by a blood clot. Distinctive changes to the ST segment of an ECG assist in making this diagnosis.

Stridor A high-pitched, wheezing sound caused by disrupted airflow.

Transfer bag A large rucksack containing essential transfer equipment.

Transfer of care The process whereby one clinician, providing management for some or all of a patient's care, relinquishes this responsibility to another clinician, who explicitly agrees to accept this responsibility

Vasoactive medication A drug with the effect of either increasing or decreasing blood pressure and/or heart rate through its effect on blood vessels.

TEST YOURSELF

1 Name two types of transfer that take place.
2 Identify two reasons for transferring a patient.
3 Name two physiological problems that may occur as a result of the *g* forces experienced during transfer.
4 If a patient is prescribed oxygen therapy, how much should be taken on a transfer?
5 At what point on the Glasgow Coma Scale does a patient require endotracheal intubation?
6 Why should enteral feeding be stopped before transfer?
7 What is the minimum level of monitoring for the transfer of an acutely ill patient?
8 List eight responsibilities of the nurse prior to and during transfer.
9 The decision to transfer the patient is the responsibility of whom?

Answers

1 Intra-hospital
Inter-hospital
2 Two from: transfer to a specialist centre for treatment (e.g., to definitive care within an organisational delivery network); transfer to radiology department or other diagnostic investigations; escalation or de-escalation of care; repatriation; transfer to hospital of origin; emergency transfers (e.g., horizontal evacuation in the event of a fire or other emergency).
3 The most likely complications are hypoxemia and hypotension. Other physiological problems include: hypothermia; secondary damage to tissues where fractures are present; and secondary spinal cord injuries where cervical fractures are present. In the case of head injury, g forces can contribute to raised intra-cranial pressure (ICP).
4 150% (or 1.5 times) the expected use of oxygen during the journey, calculated as delivery rate (L/min) × expected journey time (in mins) × 1.5.
5 A GCS of 8 or below, and endotracheal intubation should be considered if there is a drop of two points below the patient's baseline.
6 The feed will be poorly absorbed because of reduced blood flow to the gut and there will be a risk of aspiration.
7 The patient must have at least: cardiac monitoring, non-invasive blood pressure monitoring, and intravenous access.
8
- Effective communication with the multi-disciplinary team
- Informing all parties of the timescale involved
- Preparing the patient, staff and equipment
- Safely executing the move with colleagues
- Giving a detailed nursing handover
- Producing accurate documentation
- Completion of a transfer form if one is available
- Auditing of the transfer process

9 The overall responsibility rests with the consultant responsible for the patient's care, but the decision to transfer must be a joint decision including the consultant receiving the patient. Ideally a shared decision-making process is applied involving the multi-disciplinary team, the family of the patient, and the patient themselves where this is possible.

References

Association of Anaesthetists of Great Britain and Ireland. (2006). *Recommendations for the Safe Transfer of Patients with Brain Injury*. Available from http://www.nasgbi.org.uk/resources/1/ Documents/braininjury.pdf.

Beckmann, U., Gillies, D. M., Berenholtz, S. M., Wu, A. W., Pronovost, P. (2004). Incidents relating to the intra-hospital transfer of critically ill patients. An analysis of the reports submitted to the Australian incident monitoring study in intensive care. *Intensive Care Medicine*, 30(8): 1579–1585. doi:10.1007/s00134-004-2177-9.

Carney, N., Totten, A. M., O'Reill, C., Ullman, J. S., Hawryluk, G. W., Bell, M. J., Bratton, S. L., Chesnut, R., Harris, O. A., Kissoon, N., Rubiano, A. M., Shutter, L., Tasker, R. C., Vavilala, M. S., Wilberger, J., Wright, D. W., Ghaiar, J. (2017). Guidelines for the management of severe traumatic brain injury, fourth edition. *Neurosurgery*, 80(1): 6–15.

Cook, C., Allan, C. (2008). Are trainees equipped to transfer critically ill patients? *Journal of the Intensive Care Society*, 9(2): 145–147.

Dunn, M., Gwinnuitt, C., Gray, A. (2007). Critical care in the emergency department: patient transfer. *Emergency Medicine Journal*, 24: 40–44.

Gustard, T., Chabover, W., Wallis, M. (2008). *Intensive Care Patients Transfer Anxiety: A Prospective Cohort Study*. Available from http:www.ncbi.n/m.nih.gov/pubmed/18805700.

Handy, J., van Zwanenberg, G. (2007). Secondary transfer of the critically ill patient. *Current Anaesthesia and Critical Care*, 18: 303–310.

Intensive Care Society. (2019). *Guidance On: The Transport of the Critically Ill Adult*, 3rd Edition.

Jain, R., Saxena, D. (2015). Pyrexia: an update on importance in clinical practice. *Indian Journal of Anaesthesiology*, 59(4): 207–211. doi:10.4103/0019-5049.154996.

Johnson, D., Luscombe, M. (2011). Aeromedical transfer of the critically ill patient. *Journal of the Intensive Care Society*, 12(4): 307–312.

National Institute for Health and Care Excellence. (2013). *Mycocardial Infarction with ST-Segment Elevation: Acute Management (*NICE Guideline CG167). Available from https://www.nice.org.uk/guidance/cg167.

National Patient Safety Agency. (2009). *Implementing the Rapid Response Report 'Osygen Safety in Hospitals'*. Available from https://www.sps.nhs.uk/wp-content/uploads/2011/07/Implementing_the_RRR_Oxygen_safety_in_hospitals_FAQs_2009_12_16_v1.pdf.

NHS Digital. (2017). *Hospital Adult Critical Care Activity 2015–16*. Available from https://files.digital.nhs.uk/publicationimport/pub23xxx/pub23426/adul-crit-care-data-eng-apr-15-mar-16-rep.pdf.

NHS England. (2017). *Diagnostic Imaging Dataset Annual Statistical Release 2016/17*. Available from https://www.england.nhs.uk/statistics/wp-content/uploads/sites/2/2017/11/Annual-Statistical-Release-2016-17-DID-PDF-1.5MB.pdf.

NHS Scotland. (2018). Scottish Ambulance Service – *Annual Report and Accounts for Year Ended* 31 March 2018. Available from https://www.parliament.scot/S5_HealthandSportCommittee/Inquiries/Scottish_Ambulance_Service_-_Annual_Report_and_Accounts(1).pdf.

North West London Critical Care Network. (2002). *Adult Critical Care Record of Transfer*. Available from www.nwlcritcarenetwork.nhs.uk.

Nursing and Midwifery Council. (2018). *The Code: Standards of Conduct, Performance and Ethics for Nurses and Midwives*. Available from www.nmc.org/.

Paal, P., Brugger, H., Stappazzon, G. (2018). Accidental hypothermia. *Handbook of Clinical Neurology*, 157: 547–563. doi:10.1016/B978-0-444-64074-1.00033-1.

Rudd, A. G., Bowen, A., Young, G., James, M. A. (2017). National clinical guideline for stroke: 5th edition 2016. *Clinical Medicine*, 17(2): 154–155. doi:10.7861/clinmedicine.17-2-154.

Stiles, M. (2013). Observational pain scales in critically ill adults. *Critical Care Nurse*, 33(3): 66–78. doi:10.4037/ccn2013804.

Walters, B. C., Hadley, M. N., Hurlbert, J., Aarabi, B., Dhall, S. S., Gelb, D. E., Harrigan, M. R., Rozelle, C. J., Ryken, T. C., Theodore, N. (2013). Guidelines for the management of acute cervical spine and spinal cord injuries: 2013 update. *Neurosurgery*, 60(CN Supplement 1): 82–91. doi:10.1227/01.neu.0000430319.32247.7f.

Index

Note: page references in bold indicate end-of-chapter glossary entries.

Milton Keynes UK
Ingram Content Group UK Ltd.
UKHW052028141024
449569UK00017B/736